ADVANCES IN QUANTITATIVE CORONARY ARTERIOGRAPHY

 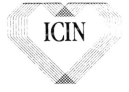 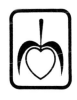

Developments in Cardiovascular Medicine

VOLUME 137

The titles published in this series are listed at the end of this volume.

ADVANCES IN QUANTITATIVE CORONARY ARTERIOGRAPHY

Edited by

JOHAN H.C. REIBER

Laboratory for Clinical and Experimental Image Processing,
Department of Diagnostic Radiology and Nuclear Medicine,
University Hospital Leiden, Leiden,
The Netherlands

and

PATRICK W. SERRUYS

Catheterization Laboratory, Thorax Center,
Erasmus University, Rotterdam,
The Netherlands

KLUWER ACADEMIC PUBLISHERS
Dordrecht/Boston/London

Library of Congress Cataloging-in-Publication Data

Advances in quantitative coronary arteriography / edited by Johan H.C.
Reiber and Patrick W. Serruys.
        p.   cm. -- (Developments in cardiovasculer medicine ; v. 137)
    Includes bibliographical references and index.
    ISBN 0-7923-1863-3 (hb : alk. paper)
    1. Angiocardiography.   2. Coronary heart diseases--Diagnosis.
I. Reiber, J. H. C. (Johan H. C.)   II. Serruys, P. W.   III. Series.
    [DNLM: 1. Angiography--methods.   2. Coronary Vessels--radionuclide
imaging.   3. Vascular Surgery--methods.   W1 DE997VME v.137 / WG 300
A2448]
RC683.5.A5A38   1992
616.1'207572--dc20
DNLM/DLC
for Library of Congress   92-20819

ISBN 0-7923-1863-3

Published by Kluwer Academic Publishers,
P.O. Box 17, 3300 AA Dordrecht, The Netherlands.

Kluwer Academic Publishers incorporates
the publishing programmes of
D. Reidel, Martinus Nijhoff, Dr W. Junk and MTP Press.

Sold and distributed in the U.S.A. and Canada
by Kluwer Academic Publishers,
101 Philip Drive, Norwell, MA 02061, U.S.A.

In all other countries, sold and distributed
by Kluwer Academic Publishers Group,
P.O. Box 322, 3300 AH Dordrecht, The Netherlands.

Printed on acid-free paper

Printed in the Netherlands

Table of Contents

Preface

In this fourth book in the series on quantitative coronary arteriography (QCA) with the earlier three volumes published in 1986, 1988 and 1991, the latest developments in this exciting field are covered. Both the methodological and clinical application aspects of these advances are presented in a comprehensive manner in a total of 37 chapters by world renowned experts. The book is subdivided into a total of eight parts, beginning with the more methodological issues, such as QCA and other modalities (3 chapters), cine-film versus digital arteriography (3 chapters), quality control in QCA (4 chapters), and coronary blood flow and flow reserve (3 chapters). Since QCA has been well established as *the* technique for the assessment of regression and progression in atherosclerotic disease, and of restenosis after recanalization procedures, major clinical trials in both groups are described extensively by their principal investigators in a total of 11 chapters. In addition, the QCA results after the application of various recanalization techniques are presented in another eight chapters. In the last part the experiences with various intracoronary prostheses with the emphasis on QCA are discussed in five chapters.

This large increase in application oriented chapters means that QCA is well alive and gaining momentum. Although the accuracy and precision of the analytical methods steadily improve with the increasing complexity of the algorithms, there is still always the human factor involved in these processes in terms of frame selection, segment definition, etc., which result in variations. To minimize these variations as much as possible, the users should have a complete understanding of all the possibilities and limitations of current QCA acquisition and analysis techniques.

It is our belief that this book provides both the necessary global as well as the in depth information to the interested clinician and physicist.

Johan H.C. Reiber
Patrick W. Serruys

List of Contributors

Andreas Baumbach, Eberhard-Karls-Universität Tübingen, Medizinische Klinik und Poliklinik, Abt. Innere Medizin III, 7400 Tübingen, Germany.
Co-authors: Karl K. Haase and Karl R. Karsch

Michel E. Bertrand, Service de Cardiologie B et Hémodynamique, Hôpital Cardiologique, 59037 Lille Cedex, France.
Co-authors: Fabrice Leroy, Jean M. Lablanche, Eugene McFadden, Christophe Bauters and Gaetan J. Karillon

Glenn J. Beauman, Division of Cardiology, University of Maryland Hospital, 22 5-Green St., Baltimore, Maryland, 21201, U.S.A.
Co-authors: Johan H.C. Reiber, Gerhard Koning and Robert A. Vogel

B. Greg Brown, Department of Cardiology RG-22 University of Washington, Seattle, Washington 98195, U.S.A.
Co-authors: Lynn A. Hillger, Xue-Qiao Zhao, Dianne Sacco, Brad Bisson and Lloyd Fisher

Adam D. Cannon, Interventional Cardiology, Division of Cardiovascular Diseases, The University of Alabama, 701 South 19th St., Suite 310, UAB Station, Birmingham, Alabama 35294, U.S.A.
Co-author: Gary S. Roubin

Jack T. Cusma, Department of Medicine, Duke University Medical Center, Cardiac Catheterization Laboratories, Box 3012, Durham, North Carolina 27710, U.S.A.
Co-authors: Kenneth G. Morris and Thomas M. Bashore

Michael J. Davies, Department of Histopathology Pathology, St. Georges Hospital Medical School, Cranmer Terrace, SW17 0RE London, United Kingdom.

David P. Faxon, Boston University, School of Medicine, 80 East Concord street, Boston, MA 02118, U.S.A.
Co-author: Raphael Balcon

Pim J. de Feyter, Thorax Center Bd 432, Erasmus University and University Hospital Rotterdam-Dijkzigt, Bd 432, P.O. Box 1738, 3000 DR Rotterdam, The Netherlands.
Co-authors: Jeroen Vos, Johan H.C. Reiber and Patrick W. Serruys

David L. Fischman, Thomas Jefferson University Hospital, Cardiac Catheterization Laboratory, 1025 Walnut Street, Suite 403 College, Philadelphia, Pennsylvania 19107, U.S.A.
Co-authors: Michael P. Savage, Stephen Ellis, Donald S. Baim, Richard A. Schatz, Martin B. Leon and Sheldon Goldberg

Donald F. Fortin, Department of Medicine, Division of Cardiology, Box 3111, Duke University Medical Center, Durham NC 27710, U.S.A.
Co-authors: Michael H. Sketch, Jr., Harry R. Phillips III and Richard S. Stock

Walter R.M. Hermans, Thorax Center, Erasmus University and University Hospital Rotterdam-Dijkzigt, P.O. Box 1738, 3000 DR Rotterdam, The Netherlands.
Co-authors: Benno J. Rensing, Jaap Pameyer and Patrick W. Serruys

David M. Herrington, Department of Cardiology, The Bowman Gray School of Medicine, Wake Forest University, Winston-Salem, NC 27157, U.S.A.
Co-author: Gary D. Walford

Guy R. Heyndrickx, Department of Cardiology, OLV-hospital, Moorselbaan 164, 9300 Aalst, Belgium.

David R. Holmes Jr., Cardiac Catheterization Laboratory, Department of Cardiology, Mayo Foundation 200, 1st St SW, Rochester, MN 55905, U.S.A.
Co-authors: Kirk N. Garratt, Stephen G. Ellis and Jeffrey J. Popma

Peter P. de Jaegere, Thorax Center Bd 432, Erasmus University and University Hospital Rotterdam-Dijkzigt, P.O. Box 1738, 3000 DR Rotterdam, The Netherlands.
Co-authors: Pim J. de Feyter and Patrick W. Serruys

Kenneth M. Kent, Washington Cardiology Center, 110 Irving street, NW RM 4B14, Washington, DC 20010–2931 U.S.A.
Co-authors: Marie L. Foegh, Mun Hong and Peter W. Ramwell

Paul R. Lichtlen, Medizinische Hochschule, Department für Innere Medizin, Abteilung für Kardiologie, Postfach 610108, 3000 Hannover 61, Germany.
Co-authors: Wolfgang Rafflenbeul, Stefan Jost, Peter Nikutta, Paul Hugenholtz, Jaap Deckers, Birgitt Wiese and the INTACT study group

G.B. John Mancini, Department of Medicine, The University of British Columbia, University Hospital-UBC Site, 2211 Wesbrook Mall, Vancouver B.C., Canada.
Co-authors: Paula R. Williamson, Scott F. DeBoe, Bertram Pitt, Jacques Lespérance and Martial G. Bourassa

Steven E. Nissen, Division of Cardiology, Department of Medicine, University of Kentucky, College of Medicine MN 670, 800 Rose Street, Lexington, KY 40536–0084, U.S.A.
Co-author: John C. Gurley

Kirk L. Peterson, Department of Medicine H-811–A, UCSD Medical Center, 255 W. Dickinson Street, San Diego, California 92067, U.S.A.
Co-authors: Isabel Rivera, Martin McDaniel, John Long, Allan Bond and Valmik Bhargava

Nico H.J. Pijls, Department of Cardiology, Catharina Hospital, P.O. Box 1350, 5602 ZA, Eindhoven, The Netherlands.
Co-authors: Joost den Arend, Karel van Leeuwen, Truus Pijnenburg, Evert Lamfers, Jacques D. Barth, Gerard J.H. Uijen and Tjeerd van der Werf

Thijs H.W. Plokker, Department of Cardiology, St. Antonius Hospital, P.O. Box 2500, 3430 EM Nieuwegein, The Netherlands.
Co-authors: Richard J. Spears, Gijs E. Mast, Sjef M.P.G. Ernst, Egbert T. Bal and Melvyn Tjon Joe Gin

Johan H.C. Reiber, Laboratory for Clinical and Experimental Image Processing, Department of Diagnostic Radiology and Nuclear Medicine, University Hospital Leiden, Building 1, C2–S, P.O. Box 9600, 2300 RC Leiden, The Netherlands.
Co-authors: Pieter M.J. van der Zwet, Graig D. von Land, Gerhard Koning, Bert van Meurs, Beert Buis and Ad E. van Voorthuisen

Jean Renkin, Coronary Care Unit, St-Luc University Hospital, Avenue Hippocrate 10, B-1200 Brussel, Belgium.
Co-authors: Emmanuel Haine, Victor Umans, Pim J. de Feyter, William Wijns and Patrick W. Serruys

Wolfgang Rutsch, Department of Cardiology, University Rudolf-Virchow, Spandauer Damm 130, D-1000 Berling 19, Germany.
Co-authors: Patrick W. Serruys, Guy R. Heyndrickx, Nicolas Danchin, E. Gijs Mast, Willem Wijns, Jeroen Vos and J. Stibbe

Robert H. Selzer, Jet Propulsion Laboratory, California Institute of Technology, 4800 Oak Grove Drive, Pasadena, CA 91109, U.S.A.
Co-authors: David H. Blankenhorn, Anne M. Shircore, Paul L. Lee, Janice M. Pagoda, Wendy J. Mack and Stanley P. Azen

Patrick W. Serruys, Thorax Center, Erasmus University and University Hospital Rotterdam-Dijkzigt, P.O. Box 1738, 3000 DR Rotterdam, The Netherlands.
Co-authors Chapter 19: Walter R.M. Hermans, Benno J. Rensing and Pim J. de Feyter
Co-author Chapter 35: Bradley H. Strauss

Rüdiger Simon, 1st Medical Clinic, Klinikum der Christian-Albrechts-University zu Kiel, D-2300 Kiel, Germany.

Richard S. Stack, Catheterization Laboratory, Duke University Medical Center, Box 3111, Duke North, Durham, North Carolina 27710, U.S.A.
Co-authors: Donald F. Fortin, Michael H. Sketch Jr. and Harry R. Phillips III

Bradley H. Strauss, Thorax Center, Erasmus University and University Hospital Rotterdam-Dijkzigt, P.O. Box 1738, 3000 DR Rotterdam, The Netherlands. Current address: St. Michael's Hospital, 30 Bond St., Toronto, Ontario MSB 1WB, Canada.
Co-authors: Marie-Angele M. Morel, Eline J. Montauban van Swijndregt, Walter R.M. Hermans, Victor A.W. Umans, Benno J.W.M. Rensing, Peter P. de Jaegere, Pim J. de Feyter, Johan H.C. Reiber and Patrick W. Serruys

Willem J. van der Giessen, Thorax Center, Erasmus University and University Hospital Rotterdam-Dijkzigt, P.O. Box 1738, 3000 DR Rotterdam, The Netherlands.
Co-authors: Heleen M.M. van Beusekom, Cornelis J. Slager, Johan C.H. Schuurbiers and Pieter D. Verdouw
Robert A. Vogel, Internal Medicine, Division of Cardiology, University of Maryland Hospital, 22 South Green st., Baltimore, MD 21201, U.S.A.
Co-authors: Glenn J. Beauman, Johan H.C. Reiber and Gerhard Koning
David Waters, Institute de Cardiologie de Montréal, 5000 Est, rue Bélanger, Montréal, Quebec H1T 1C8, Canada.
Co-author: Jacques Lespérance
Christopher J. White, Cardiac Catheterization Laboratory, Alton Ochsner Medical Institutions, 1516 Jefferson Highway, New Orleans, Louisiana 70121, U.S.A.
Co-authors: Stephen R. Ramee and Tyrone J. Collins
James T. Willerson, Department of Internal Medicine, Health Science Center, University of Texas, P.O. Box 20708, Houston, Texas 77225, U.S.A.
Co-authors: Sheng-Kun Yao, Janice McNatt, Claude R. Benedict, H. Vernon Anderson, Paolo Golino, Sidney S. Murphree and L. Maximilian Buja
Adam Workman, The University of Leeds, Department of Medical Physics, The Wellcome Wing, The General Infirmary, Leeds LS1 3EX, UK.
Co-authors: Arnold R. Cowen and Stuart Vaudin

PART ONE

Quantitative coronary arteriography (QCA) versus other modalities

1. A Pathologist's view of quantitative coronary arteriography

MICHAEL J. DAVIES

Summary

The arteriographic lumen outline has major drawbacks in assessing wall disease. Atherosclerotic vessels dilate in a remodelling response to preserve lumen dimensions; only when the capacity of this response is overcome does stenosis occur. In diffuse atherosclerosis the media remodels to allow an overall increase in the external diameter of the vessel often with an increase in lumen diameter above normal at that site. Localised plaques are associated with atrophy of the subjacent media and rupture of the internal elastic lamina allowing the plaque to bulge outward into the adventitia. Vessels which appear angiographically normal or slightly irregular may therefore contain large plaques. Arteries which have been distended during fixation show that normal segments have a round lumen; at sites of eccentric stenosis the residual segment of normal vessel wall has a round profile while the more rigid plaque is straighter giving a D shape to the lumen.

The implications of these facts for methods of quantification which compare the lumen diameter at a point of stenosis with an adjacent normal reference segment are:
1. The lumen shape at eccentric stenosis is not round and will alter both in shape, and size, with variation of tone within the normal residual wall segment.
2. The reference segment, taken as normal, may either be narrowed or dilated.

The progression of coronary atherosclerosis is dependent, in part, on episodes of thrombosis the majority of which are clinically silent. Unless major intraluminal thrombosis has occurred, angiography may be relatively insensitive at detecting these unstable plaques The repair response in these plaques involves smooth muscle proliferation to smooth the lumen outline. Angiographic changes due to these repair responses may considerably alter both the test and reference segment in the time interval between two angiograms and may be erroneously regarded as regression of the basic atherosclerotic process.

J.H.C. Reiber and P.W. Serruys (eds), Advances in Quantitative Coronary Arteriography, 3–14.
© 1993 *Kluwer Academic Publishers. Printed in the Netherlands.*

Introduction

Coronary arteriography in life is currently used for two quite separate purposes. First the investigation is used as a means of demonstrating segmental stenosis in order to confirm a clinical diagnosis of angina due to coronary atherosclerosis. The extent, severity and distribution of stenotic lesions is a guide to the need for intervention either by surgery or angioplasty, and a guide to long term prognosis. Inherent in these aims for angiography is an attempt to predict the physiological significance of segments of stenosis in terms of flow limitation when myocardial oxygen demand rises [1]. The method involves comparison of the diameter of the narrowed segment with that of an adjacent apparently normal segment in the same artery. Analogy with the flow in tubes in vitro suggests that 50% diameter (75% cross sectional) reduction is needed before flow is significantly altered at the viscosity and pressures which pertain within the coronary arteries in vivo [2]. The methods used to measure stenosis range from simple subjective observations to sophisticated edge detection algorithms and computer measurement, but the concept of a 50% diameter reduction has stood the test of being clinically relevant and useful.

The second major purpose of coronary angiography has now become the assessment of the progression, or regression, in the disease within the arterial wall itself i.e. atherosclerosis. For this purpose the measurement and detection of lesions causing less than 50% diameter stenosis, and in particular the recognition of new minor lesions is necessary [3]. Comparison of sequential angiograms has become a major tool in assessing the effect of antiatherogenic drugs [4].

It has to be declared at once that angiography either as a means of determining the physiological significance of stenoses [1], or measuring the amount of atherosclerotic disease which is present has inherent limitations. The angiogram is no more, nor less, than a cast of the lumen dimensions from which the desired parameters concerning the vessel wall are inferred. Knowledge of the factors limiting this derivation is essential to allow the figures obtained to be seen in their true clinical context. This review considers the structural factors which prevent accurate measurement of both the physiological significance of stenoses and the volume of atherosclerotic plaque tissue present.

Definition and nature of atherosclerosis

Atherosclerosis is an intimal disease which, at focal points within medium or large arteries, causes connective tissue proliferation and lipid accumulation to occur. The focal nature of the disease leads to use of the term plaque and these are traditionally displayed "en face" by pathologists as elevated humps on the internal surface of arteries opened longtitudinally in the autopsy room. Unphysiological as this means of demonstrating plaques is, it allows assessment of the proportion of the intimal surface covered by plaques and is a valuable quantification method in comparative population studies of humans or in experimental animals. It is however a method that can only be used at post mortem. Such studies in man have shown that on a population basis the number of plaques is related directly to the risk of ischaemic heart disease in that population [5], and that elevated plasma lipid levels, smoking [6], and hypertension [7] are all associated with more atherosclerotic plaques being present than found in controls. In animals with atherosclerosis induced by high fat diets reduction of the intimal area occupied by plaques occurs following any lowering of plasma lipids [8]. Thus to know the extent of atherosclerosis in the vessel wall in a living human subject would be a powerful research and prognostic tool.

Plaques may be of sufficient size to cause reduction of the lumen in medium sized arteries such as those in the coronary bed. The volume of the plaque is made up of the connective tissue matrix proteins (collagen, proteoglycans, elastin) produced by proliferating smooth muscle cells and lipid, either contained within macrophage/monocyte derived foam cells or occurring as extracellular deposits. Calcification is common in advanced atherosclerosis being deposited both within the lipid and connective tissue component of the plaque. Calcium thus may make a major contribution to the mass of some plaques but does not in itself increase plaque volume. There is a very considerable plaque to plaque variation in the relative proportion of plaque volume contributed by connective tissue as compared to lipid, even within one coronary artery. The evolutionary relation, if any between lipid rich "soft" plaques and collagen rich "hard" plaques is not known in man.

If plaque growth in man were entirely dependent on the accumulation of lipid and connective tissue proliferation it might be anticipated that the progression of atherosclerosis in man would approximately be linear with time. Numerous sequential coronary angiographic studies in man demonstrate that progression is in fact unpredictable and episodic. New high grade stenoses may appear within segments of artery which were normal at a previous angiogram and conversely moderate stenoses may remain static for many years [9, 10]. The sites at which thrombosis causing acute myocardial infarction will develop cannot be predicted from earlier angiograms [11], mildly diseased segments of artery often progress more rapidly than more severely diseased segments [12] and there is little relation between the rate of progression of stenoses at different sites in one individual.

The inflammatory nature of atherosclerosis is now being recognised [13] with the plaque being regarded as the site of interactions between monocytes, macrophages, T lymphocytes and smooth muscle cells. One factor initiating this inflammatory lesions is oxidation of plasma LDL within the intima to form products which are chemoattractants, chemoactivators and cytotoxic for monocytes. The process is however not equally active in all the plaques present in an individual, at any one point in time. There are quiescent relatively acellular plaques and cellular "hot" plaques which are probably entering an accelerated growth phase.

The unpredictable progression of atherosclerosis can also in part be explained by the contribution that episodic thrombosis over a plaque plays in disease progression [14]. It has been now accepted that acute ischaemic syndromes such as acute myocardial infarction, unstable angina of the crescendo type and a proportion of cases of sudden ischaemic death are due to thrombosis over an unstable "culprit" plaque [15]. It is less commonly realised that the majority of episodes of plaque thrombosis are clinically silent in terms of myocardial ischaemia but do lead to an episode of plaque growth and progression [14, 16].

Plaques undergo thrombosis because of two quite distinct processes [14]. In the first the endothelium over a plaque becomes denuded thus exposing the immediate subendothelial connective tissue and leading to local platelet adhesion. The majority of thrombi related to this superficial injury to the plaque are small and below the limits of angiographic recognition. Despite the fact that antegrade blood flow is not reduced these thrombi will invoke smooth muscle proliferation as a repair response and thus growth of the plaque. In some cases superficial endothelial loss is sufficiently extensive to invoke larger mural, or even occlusive, coronary thrombi. Precipitating factors for the development of larger thrombi, in relation to superficial plaque injury, are preexisting high grade stenosis at the site.

In contrast deep intimal injury involves the lipid rich plaque tearing open to expose its lipid rich core to the blood within the lumen. This core contains collagen, lamellar lipid on the surfaces of which coagulation is enhanced, and tissue factor produced by macrophages within the plaque. The interior of a lipid rich plaque is therefore extremely thrombogenic. When a plaque tears, fissures or cracks, blood enters the depths of the plaque from the lumen and a mass of thrombus forms within the plaque itself [14]. Plaque volume is thus suddenly increased and plaque configuration is radically altered. Thrombosis may, or may not, form subsequently in the arterial lumen. Initially this thrombus may be mural i.e. project into the lumen but not prevent antegrade flow, but in a proportion of cases progresses to become occlusive. The formation of intralumural thrombi is often associated with evidence of acute myocardial ischaemia and the angiographic features of type II stenosis with a ragged edge and an intraluminal filling defect which are now known on one hand to be due to plaque fissuring with overlying thrombus [17, 18] and on the other to be associated clinically with unstable angina and acute myocardial infarction [19, 20]. What is equally important is that a similar process, which stops short of the formation of intraluminal thrombus, is responsible for plaque growth without clinical evidence of myocardial ischaemia. Subjects with hypertension and or diabetes have a greater risk of undergoing these sub-clinical episodes of plaque instability fissuring and intraplaque thrombosis [21].

Plaque fissuring and thrombosis, whether this be confined to within the plaque itself or also extending into the lumen is followed by rapid repair response within the vessel wall. This repair response has three components, first the lysis of thrombus and second smooth muscle proliferation. Lysis of thrombosis will restore lumen patency and also reduce plaque volume, if there has been intraplaque thrombosis, while smooth muscle proliferation covers the areas of torn intima and restabilies the plaque. Endothelial regeneration can be considered as the third and final stage in this repair process. During the repair phase, therefore, there may be both considerable reduction in plaque volume and a smoothing of the outline of the lumen. The end result may range from total chronic occlusion, where thrombus has not been lysed and therefore been replaced by connective tissue, to virtually complete restoration of a good lumen. This latter end of the spectrum indicates lysis of both intraplaque and intraluminal thrombus with just sufficient smooth muscle proliferation to reseal the plaque without encroaching on the arterial lumen.

Estimation of plaque size by angiography – errors introduced by medial remodelling

It is unfortunately true that however good the angiogram may be at measuring the dimensions of the lumen it is very poor at indicating plaque volume. An apparently normal or mildly irregular vessel can harbour large plaques. The reason for this discrepancy is the very considerable remodelling of the media that occurs in atherosclerotic arteries; in effect this allows the plaque to bulge outward toward the adventitia rather than inward toward the lumen.

Atherosclerotic plaques within the coronary arteries very commonly involve only an arc of the arterial wall thus leaving a segment of normal vessel wall on the opposite side of the artery (Figure 1A) [22, 23]. The arc of the circumference of the artery occupied by the plaque varies widely but those occupying 50% or less of the vessel wall are clearly eccentric and do have some normal vessel wall while those occupying more than 75% of the circumference are regarded as concentric and have no residual segment of normal wall. Plaques between these extremes may have the lumen displaced from the centre point of the vessel but often do not have a segment of normal vessel wall, i.e. one in which the intima is sufficiently thin to allow medial muscle contraction to influence the lumen size.

The media behind eccentric atherosclerotic plaques undergoes atrophy and thinning with a reduction in the number of smooth muscle cells [24, 25]. The plaque shifts outward toward the adventitia and can be seen as a bulge from outside the artery. This outward shift is associated with fracture of the internal elastic lamina (Figure 1B) and in some instances the plaque is virtually extruded from the artery leaving the lumen unaffected. Such plaques may however still be liable to undergo fissuring and can invoke occlusive thrombosis in what was apparently an angiographically normal artery. The

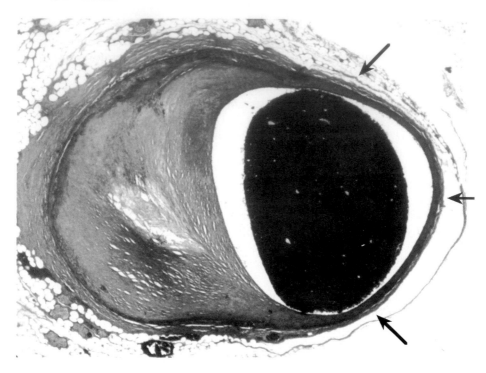

Figure 1A Histological cross section of a plaque within a segment of coronary artery which was only slightly irregular in outline. The lumen contains a barium/gelatine suspension for postmortem angiography; in tissue processing this retracts from the vessel wall. There is an eccentric fibrous plaque (P) which leaves a large segment of normal vessel wall (arrows). The plaque actually occupies approximately 45% of the cross-sectional area of the vessel but has bulged outward rather than inward allowing the lumen to remain of normal dimensions. (Elastin H-E Stain × 30.)

mechanisms of this localised atrophy of the media in relation to plaques is a matter of some controversy. It has been regarded as a form of pressure atrophy or as a hypoxic phenomenon developing due to intimal thickening increasing the perfusion distance between the arterial lumen and the smooth muscle cells in the media. Neovascularisation of the media from the adventitia develops behind plaques which will allow the ingress of inflammatory cells into the vessel wall. Atherosclerosis is now regarded as a local inflammatory process and the accumulation of activated macrophages capable of producing proteolytic enzymes may account for the medial destruction. The outward shift toward the adventitia of eccentric plaques means that such lesions may initially not affect the outline of the lumen and go undetected. In the context of angiography therefore "new" is not a term relevent to the age of the plaque; the threshold of detection is not reached until the plaque occupies over 40% of the original cross sectional area of the vessel. Angio-

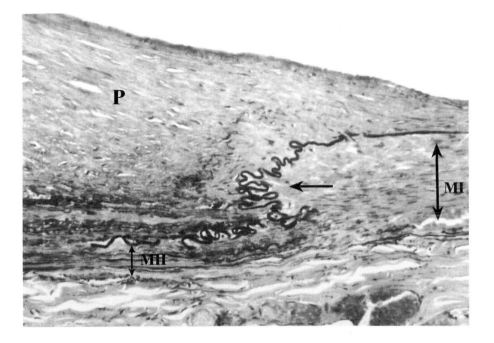

Figure 1B Coronary artery wall at the junction of a plaque with more normal vessel wall. The media (MI)in the normal segment is far thicker than that (MII) behind the plaque (P). The internal elastic lamina has fractured and the broken end coiled back at the edge of the plaque (arrow). (Elastin H-E Stain × 250.)

graphically new lesions are those which have had a rapid growth phase, and are not those which have recently been initiated "de novo".

Even apart from the very localised medial atrophy that occurs behind eccentric plaques, Glagov and others [26, 27] have emphasised that a general remodelling of the artery wall occurs in order to accommodate the development of atherosclerosis within the intima and to preserve the lumen dimensions. In general this remodelling is sufficiently pronounced that the intima has to be increased by more than 40% of the original cross sectional area of the artery before a reduction in lumen size occurs. The phenomenon of medial loss is associated with diffuse atherosclerosis, but an increase rather than a reduction in lumen size reaches its zenith in what is usually called ectasia, and can occur in segments of artery alternating with other segments which have become narrowed. It is unclear why in some patients there is generalised dilation, or in other patients segments within individual arteries in which this dilatation overrides the stenotic potential of intimal proliferation. The morphological hallmark of ectasia is extreme medial muscle loss and very diffuse intimal involvement by atherosclerosis often rich in foam cells but these features describe what ectasis is rather than providing an understanding of the mechanism.

Errors introduced by reference segment comparison

The conventional method of measuring stenosis compares the diameter of a test stenotic segment with that of an adjacent control reference segment. The two values are expressed as a relative percentage diameter. Such a method is extremely dependent on the reference segment being normal. In reality, the reference segment although smooth in outline may have a lumen which is narrowed due to diffuse concentric disease thus leading to an overestimation of the degree of stenosis, or dilated due to some ectasia leading to an underestimation of the degree of stenosis.

Pathologists often regard their measurements as the "gold standard" albeit one carried out after the death of the patient. In reality measurement of stenosis from histological cross sections also has considerable errors. If the artery has not had the lumen distended during preparation estimation of lumen area can only be made by measuring the lumen circumference and calculating the area as if the lumen were circular. This introduces an error based on the lumen shape variation (see below).

The lumen of arteries which have been fixed after postmortem injection with gelatine/barium mixtures, or have been fixed by perfusion at physiological pressures of around 100 mg within the lumen, will approximate to the shape which occurs in life, and the area can be measured accurately by planimetry. It is usually assumed that the cross-sectional area of the vessel inside the media at the internal elastic lamina is the "normal reference" value. The ratio of the lumen area to the area inside the elastic lamina is used to calculate% stenosis. In reality, this reference area is unreliable because of the overall dilatation of the vessel with an increase in its external dimensions has almost inevitably occurred to compensate for atherosclerosis. In consequence, comparisons of postmortem and antemortem stenosis are rarely exact [28–31]; the degree of concordance however rises with increasing severity of the narrowing and in general if high grade stenosis is found in life it can be identified at post mortem.

Errors introduced by lumen shape

The normal vessel has a lumen which is round and, unless totally collapsed and empty of blood, this shape is independent of the filling pressure. Abnormal vessels, particularly those in which the atherosclerotic plaques are eccentrically situated, may however not have a round lumen even when filled. When examined at autopsy in the totally collapsed state the lumen over plaques is often crescentic or slit-like in shape [31]. This extreme appearance

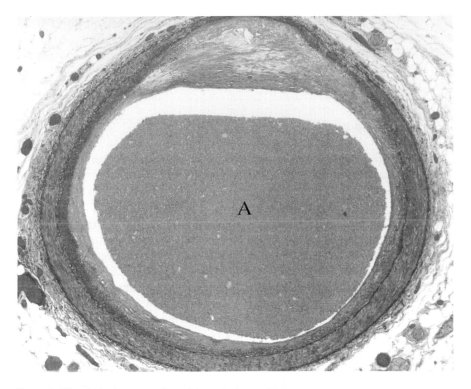

Figure 2. Histological cross section of a small plaque (P) in a human coronary artery which has been perfused at systemic pressure during fixation. The outline of the lumen over the plaque is straight while that of the large residual segment of normal vessel wall is circular. The lumen contains angiographic media (A) which as in Figure 1A has retracted from the vessel wall to leave a clear space. (Elastic H-E Stain × 50.)

is however an artefact of an absence of pressure in the lumen; when arteries are examined post mortem after perfusion fixation at physiological pressures the lumen shape approximates more closely to being round. In some instances however the lumen is not entirely round but D-shaped or oval [32]. The former is seen in association with eccentric hard plaques which occupy between 20 and 50% of the circumference of the vessel wall. The lumen edge over the plaque remains straight (Figure 2), while that of the normal segment of vessel wall is circular [27, 32]. Elevation of the fixation pressure to levels above that of systolic blood pressure does not lead to such plaques adopting a curved configuration, and suggests that plaque rigidity precludes flexion of the lesion itself. It is therefore likely that such D-shaped arterial lumens exist in life. Two plaques on opposite sides of the vessel wall in the same segment will produce an oval lumen. The shape of the lumen and, in particular the difference between the longest and shortest transverse axis of the lumen over plaques which are eccentric in situation and having a normal segment of vessel wall will probably alter with variations in smooth muscle tone in the media. The lumen shape deviating from circular implies that errors are introduced by uniplane views and that in comparing successive angiograms both the plane and degree of medial muscle tone need to be identical.

Errors introduced by intimal remodelling and repair

It is now well established that eccentric ragged stenoses with overhanging edges and an intraluminal filling defect indicate an unstable plaque with thrombosis. Such type II angiographic lesions are the hallmark of unstable angina [33–35]; yet there are a significant minority of cases in which an intraluminal filling defect cannot be detected. It seems likely that the current angiographic methods and criteria in life are relatively insensitive as regards detecting plaque instability. The importance of this fact is that a subsequent angiogram may indicate a stenosis which has undergone marked improvement. This may spuriously be regarded as regression of the basic atherosclerotic process, whereas it is really lysis of intraplaque thrombosis. In the extreme case a plaque may undergo major tearing amounting to ulceration in which the intraplaque lipid is washed out leaving a crater outlined in the angiogram. Once again, the lumen will have enlarged between two successive angiograms but this is hardly regression of the basic disease. This process of plaque ulceration is more common in the carotid than coronary arteries. With time smooth muscle proliferation fills in the ragged outline of the lumen and an apparently normal segment of vessel is restored.

Remodelling of the intima also occurs both distal and proximal to high grade stenoses and takes the form of concentric intimal thickening occurring possibly as a response to turbulent flow. Sequential angiographic studies in human coronary artery disease using absolute lumen diameters have demonstrated this apparent progression of disease in the normal reference segment adjacent to high grade stenoses, thus causing the use of% diameter stenosis to be a misleading measure of disease progression in the original lesion [12] and of the physiological significance of the stenosis [36].

References

1. Marcus ML, Skorton DJ, Johnson MR, Collins SM, Harrison DG, Kerber RE. Visual estimates of percent diameter coronary stenosis: "a battered gold standard". J Am Coll Cardiol 1988; 11: 882–5.
2. Gould KL, Kelley KO, Bolson EL. Experimental validation of quantitative coronary arteriography for determining pressure-flow characteristics of coronary stenosis. Circulation 1982; 66: 930–7.
3. Lichtlen PR, Hugenholtz PG, Rafflenbeul W, Hecker H, Jost S, Deckers JW. Retardation of angiographic progression of coronary artery disease by nifedipine. Results of the Interna-

tional Nifedipine Trial on Antiatherosclerosis Therapy (INTACT). INTACT Group Investigators. Lancet 1990; **335**: 1109–13.

4. Brown G, Albers JJ, Fisher LD, et al. Regression of coronary artery disease as a result of intensive lipid-lowering therapy in men with high levels of apolipoprotein B. N Engl J Med 1990; **323**: 1289–98. Comment in: N Engl J Med 1990; **323**: 1337–9.

5. Strong JP, Solberg LA, Restrepo C. Atherosclerosis in persons with coronary heart disease. Lab Invest 1968; **18**: 527–37.

6. Relationship of atherosclerosis in young men to serum lipoprotein cholesterol concentrations and smoking. A preliminary report from the Pathological Determinants of Atherosclerosis in Youth. (PDAY) Research Group JAMA 1990; **264**: 3018–24. Comment in: JAMA 1990; **264**: 3060–1.

7. Robertson WB, Strong JP. Atherosclerosis in persons with hypertension and diabetes mellitus. Lab Invest 1968; **18**: 538–51.

8. Blankenhorn DH, Kramsch DM. Reversal of atherosis and sclerosis. The two components of atherosclerosis. Circulation 1989; **79**: 1–7.

9. Rafflenbeul W, Nellessen U, Galvao P, Kreft M, Peters S, Lichtlen P. Progression und Regression der Koronarsklerose im angiographischen Bild. Z Kardiol 1984; **73** (Suppl 2): 33–40.

10. Bruschke AV, Wijers TS, Kolsters W, Landmann J. The anatomic evaluation of coronary artery disease demonstrated by coronary angiography in 256 nonoperated patients. Circulation 1981; **63**: 527–36.

11. Ambrose JA, Tannenbaum MA, Alexopoulos D, et al. Angiographic progression of coronary artery disease and the development of myocardial infarction. J Am Coll Cardiol 1988; **12**: 56–62.

12. Gibson M, Stone P, Pasternak R, Sandor T, Rosner B, Sacks F. The natural history of coronary atherosclerosis using quantitative angiography: implications for regression trials. J Am Coll Cardiol 1991; **17** (Suppl A). 231A (Abstract).

13. Libby P, Hansson GK. Involvement of the immune system in human atherogenesis: current knowledge and unanswered questions. Lab Invest 1991; **64**: 5–15.

14. Davies MJ. A macro and micro view of coronary vascular insult in inschaemic heart disease. Circulation 1990; **82** (Suppl 3): II 38–46.

15. Fuster V, Badimon L, Cohen M, Ambrose JA, Badimon JJ, Chesebro J. Insights into the pathogenesis of acute ischemic syndromes. Circulation 1988; **77**: 1213–20.

16. Waters D, Hudon G, Lemarbre L, Francetich M, Lesperance J. Regression of coronary atherosclerosis: a prospective, quantitative angiographic study. J Am Coll Cardiol 1991; **17** (Suppl A): 231A (Abstract).

17. Levin DC, Fallon JT. Significance of the angiographic morphology of localized coronary stenoses: histopathologic correlations. Circulation 1982; **66**: 316–20.

18. Davies MJ, Thomas AC. Plaque fissuring – the cause of acute myocardial infarction, sudden ischaemic death and crescendo angina. Br Heart J 1985; **53**: 363–73.

19. Ambrose JA, Winters SL, Arora RR, et al. Angiographic evolution of coronary artery morphology in unstable angina. J Am Coll Cardiol 1986; **7**: 472–8.

20. JA, Hjemdahl-Monsen CE, Borrico S, Gorlin R, Fuster V. Angiographic demonstration of a common link between unstable angina pectoris and non Q-wave acute myocardial infarction. Am J Cardiol 1988; **61**: 244–7.

21. Davies MJ, Bland JM, Hangartner JR, Angelini A, Thomas AC. Factors influencing the presence or absence of acute coronary artery thrombi in sudden ischaemic death. Eur Heart J 1989; **10**: 203–8.

22. Waller BF. Coronary luminal shape and the arc of disease free wall: morphologic observations and clinical relevance. J Am Coll Cardiol 1985; **6**: 1100–1.

23. Hangartner JR, Charleston AJ, Davies MJ, Thomas AC. Morphological charactertistics of clinically significant coronary artery stenosis in stable angina. Br Heart J 1986; **56**: 501–8.

24. Crawford T, Levene CI. Medial thinning in atheroma. J Pathol Bacteriol 1953; **66**: 19–23.

25. Isner JM, Donaldson RF, Fortin AH, Tischler A, Clarke RH. Attenuation of the media of coronary arteries in advanced atherosclerosis. Am J Cardiol 1986; **58**: 937–9.
26. Glagov S, Weisenberg E, Zarins CK, Stankunavicius R, Kolettis GJ. Compensatory enlargement of human atherosclerotic coronary arteries. N Engl J Med 1987; **316**: 1371–5.
27. Stiel GM, Stiel LS, Schofer J, Donath K, Mathey DG. Impact of compensatory enlargement of atherosclerotic coronary arteries on angiographic assessment of coronary artery disease. Circulation 1989; **80**: 1603–9.
28. Marcus ML, Armstrong ML, Heistad DD, Eastham CL, Mark AL. Comparison of three methods of evaluating coronary obstructive lesions: postmortem arteriography, pathologic examination and measurement of regional myocardial perfusion during maximal vasodilation. Am J Cardiol 1982; **49**: 1699–706.
29. Schwartz JN, Kong Y, Hackel DB, Bartel AG. Comparison of angiographic and postmortem finds in patients with coronary artery disease. Am J Cardiol 1975; **36**: 174–8.
30. Hutchins GM, Bulkley BH, Ridolfi RL, Griffith LS, Lohr FT, Piasio MA. Correlation of coronary arteriograms and left ventriculograms with postmortem studies. Circulation 1977; **56**: 32–7.
31. Vlodaver Z, Frech R, van Tassel RA, Edwards JE. Correlation of the antemortem coronary arteriogram and the postmortem specimen. Circulation 1973; **47**: 162–9.
32. Thomas AC, Davies MJ, Dilly S, Dilly N, Franc F. Potential errors in the estimation of coronary arterial stenosis from clinical arteriography with reference to the shape of the coronary arterial lumen. Br Heart J 1986; **55**: 129–39.
33. Freeman MR, Williams AE, Chisholm RJ, Armstrong PW. Intracoronary thrombus and complex morphology in unstable angina. Relation to timing of angiography and in-hospital cardiac events. Circulation 1989; **80**: 17–23.
34. Gotoh K, Minamino T, Katoh O, et al. The role of intracoronary thrombus in unstable angina: angiographic assessment and thrombolytic therapy during ongoing anginal attacks. Circulation 1988; **77**: 526–34.
35. Rehr R, Disciascio G, Vetrovec G, Cowley M. Angiographic morphology of coronary artery stenoses in prolonged rest angina: evidence of intracoronary thrombosis. J Am Coll Cardiol 1989; **14**: 1429–37. Comment in: J Am Coll Cardiol 1989; **15**: 1438–9.
36. Leung WH, Lee T, Stadius ML, Alderman EL. Quantitative measurements of apparently normal coronary segments in patients with coronary artery disease. J Am Coll Cardiol 1991; **17** (Suppl A): 230A (Abstract).

2. Angioscopy versus angiography for the detection of coronary artery disease surface morphology

CHRISTOPHER J. WHITE, STEPHEN R. RAMEE and
TYRONE J. COLLINS

Summary

We observed the surface morphology of normal and diseased segments of coronary arteries using percutaneous intracoronary angioscopy and coronary angiography. We examined patients undergoing coronary angioplasty for stable angina ($n = 4$), unstable angina ($n = 16$), and patients with restenosis following balloon angioplasty ($n = 5$). In these angioplasty patients, the angioscope was more sensitive for the detection of intracoronary thrombus and intimal dissection than was the angiogram. We also had the opportunity to image coronary allograft arteries in 10 patients following cardiac transplantation. The angioscope was superior to angiography in detecting early evidence of accelerated atherosclerosis in this patient subset. There were no complications related to the performance of intracoronary angioscopy in any patient.

Introduction

Selective coronary angiography is currently and will likely remain the "gold standard" for imaging modalities of the coronary arteries. Inherent limitations of negative contrast imaging have been reported to reduce the sensitivity and specificity of this technique for coronary artery pathology [1–12]. These limitations of angiography include errors caused by viewing a three-dimensional, tortuous, vascular structure in only two dimensions and the inability to assess the absolute severity of atherosclerotic disease with a negative contrast image of the vessel lumen. This negative luminal image provides only the relative severity of the vascular obstruction while making the generally inaccurate assumption that the adjacent non-obstructive region of the coronary artery is, in fact, normal. Other limitations of angiography include the inability to accurately define plaque fracture, arterial dissections, intracoronary thrombi, and the degree of residual stenosis following angioplasty [13–16].

15

J.H.C. Reiber and P.W. Serruys (eds), Advances in Quantitative Coronary Arteriography, 15–27.
© 1993 *Kluwer Academic Publishers. Printed in the Netherlands.*

Early in this century, attempts to image intracardiac structures with cardio-scope were performed intraoperatively [17]. To clear blood from the field of view, transparent balloons were inflated on the ends of these scopes to allow visualization of the cardiac chambers and large vessels [18–20]. As angioscopes became smaller in size, they were initially used in peripheral and coronary arteries intraoperatively [21–23]. The clinical utility of these intraoperative scopes was explored and included attempts to quantify coron-ary stenoses [24], the intraoperative assessment of technical errors in con-structing distal graft anastomoses [25], and the demonstration of the superior sensitivity of the intraoperative coronary angioscopy for detecting thrombus when compared to angiography in patients with unstable angina [26].

The emergence and rapid growth of interventional coronary procedures, including percutaneous transluminal coronary angioplasty (PTCA) and intra-coronary thrombolytic therapy in the early 1980's, created the necessary incentive for catheter engineers to develop smaller and more flexible catheter systems for intracoronary use. These catheter advances coincided with a technological explosion in the fiberoptic industry making available extremely thin, high-quality optical fibers and included the development of miniature lenses. The marriage of fiberoptic technology and catheters designed for intracoronary use led to a new generation of smaller, more flexible angio-scopes.

Methods

The percutaneous angioscope. The design of the percutaneous coronary an-gioscope (Microvision™, Advanced Cardiovascular Systems, Santa Clara, CA) is based on the design of a coronary balloon angioplasty catheter. Key features of this device which facilitate its use in the coronary arteries are its small diameter, flexibility and steerability. The polyethylene catheter is 1.4 mm in diameter (4.3 French), has 11 illumination fibers, and contains a 0.2 mm fiberoptic bundle with 2,000 fibers for imaging. The angioscope has a distal lumen for guidewire passage and distal flushing. In order to reduce the amount of solution that must be infused to clear the viewing field during angioscopy, a low-pressure polyethylene balloon (inflated diameter of 2.5, 3.0, or 3.5 mm) has been incorporated at the distal tip for intermittent occlusion of arterial blood flow. This unique design allows the operator to image in the coronary artery for up to 45 seconds during balloon occlusion while infusing less than 10 ml of crystalloid. A special 0.14–inch angioscopy guidewire containing a series of preformed bends allows the operator to deflect the tip of the angioscope and image the vessel circumferentially by withdrawing and rotating the wire. The video chain includes a video camera, character generator, high-resolution video monitor, and 3/4–inch videotape recorder.

Angiography. Patients were sedated with oral diazepam and diphenhydramine prior to the procedure. After local infiltration with 1% xylocaine, the femoral artery was cannulated percutaneously with an 8 French sheath using the modified Seldinger technique and 10,000 U of heparin was administered. Baseline angiography of the target vessel was performed in orthogonal views after administration of 200 micrograms of intracoronary nitroglycerin using an 8 French coronary angioplasty guiding catheter (Advanced Cardiovascular Systems, Santa Clara, CA).

Angioscopy. Using standard coronary angioplasty technique, the stenotic lesion was crossed with the angioscopy guidewire. The angioscope was then advanced over the guidewire using fluoroscopic guidance so that the distal tip marker on the angioscope was located just proximal to the target lesion. The angioscope balloon was then inflated with low pressure [1–2 atm) to occlude antegrade blood flow. After balloon inflation, warm lactated Ringer's solution (2–10 ml) was infused through the distal port to create a blood-free field during viewing. Angioscopic images were recorded on videotape for immediate review and archiving. Guiding catheter pressure, ST-segment changes, cardiac rhythm, and patient comfort were monitored continuously during angioscopy.

Angioplasty. After angioscopy, the angioscope was exchanged for a coronary angioplasty balloon, and balloon angioplasty was performed by standard technique. After balloon angioplasty, the coronary angioplasty balloon was exchanged for the angioscope and post-coronary angioplasty angioscopy was performed as described previously. A final angiogram was then performed. The patients received standard post-angioplasty care and treatment as dictated by their clinical status.

The imaging chain. The imaging system is made up of components that perform several functions, including illumination fibers, a fiberoptic imaging bundle, a television camera, a video monitor, and a videotape recorder. The illumination source should provide a high-intensity "cold" light so as to avoid causing thermal damage within the vessel being illuminated. The imaging bundle should contain at least 2,000 individual fibers for adequate resolution of the picture. A video display allows live viewing of the procedure, and a video recorder provides archival storage for review of the images. A 35 mm camera may also be used for high-resolution still frames, if desired.

Coronary artery morphology

Atherosclerotic plaque. The coronary angioscope provides a unique opportunity to observe the surface morphology of the coronary arteries during cardiac catheterization. One of the most distinctive features of a diseased

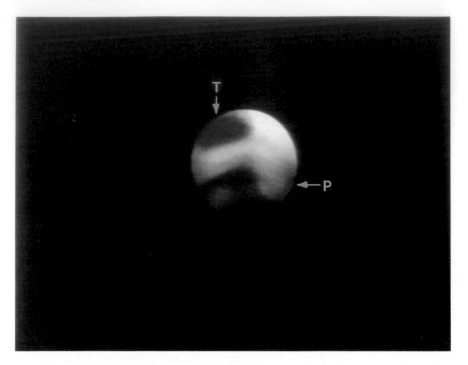

Figure 1. Angioscopic image of a coronary vessel after angioplasty showing a mural thrombus (T), and yellow plaque (P).

coronary artery is the contrast between atherosclerotic plaque and normal arterial endothelium. The normal coronary artery intima appears as a smooth, glistening, white surface. In contrast, atherosclerotic plaque is commonly pigmented ranging from yellow to yellow-brown in color. White plaque, probably representing a fibrotic lesion, is more commonly seen in patients with restenosis following balloon angioplasty.

Surface features of plaque include textures which may appear as roughened corrugations or smooth, raised undulations. Complex plaque morphologies such as ulcerations and dissections have been imaged and are seen more commonly in patients with unstable angina. In saphenous vein bypass grafts, plaque may appear as friable chunks of material loosely attached to the vessel wall.

Intracoronary thrombi. The characteristic finding of thrombus during coronary angioscopy is its red color against the white or yellow background of atherosclerotic plaque (Figures 1 and 2). It is our impression that the relative age of thrombi be assessed with fresher clots having a brighter red color versus the duller, darker red-brown color of older thrombi. Intraluminal thrombi have the appearance of globular masses attached to the vessel wall

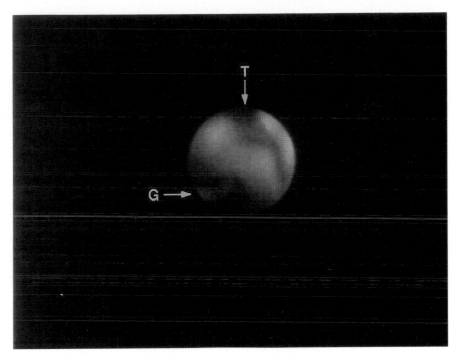

Figure 2. Angioscopic image of a coronary artery after angioplasty showing the guidewire within the lumen (G), and a mural thrombus (T) and plaque fracture.

and protruding into the lumen. Mural thrombi are patches of red color which are smoothly attached and lie flat against the vessel wall. These mural thrombi are commonly associated with ulcerated lesions seen in patients with unstable angina.

Dissection. Disruption of the intimal surface may be seen as white fronds of tissue seeming to dangle into the lumen or deep crevices or cracks in atherosclerotic plaque extending into the media of the arterial wall (Figure 3). These intimal disruptions are more commonly seen in patients with acute ischemic syndromes and are often present following balloon angioplasty in a coronary artery.

Clinical findings

Stable angina pectoris. Intracoronary angioscopy was performed before and after coronary angioplasty in four patients with stable angina. All had atherosclerotic plaque visualized. Intracoronary thrombi were not seen in any patient either by angiography or angioscopy (Table 1). Intimal disruption or

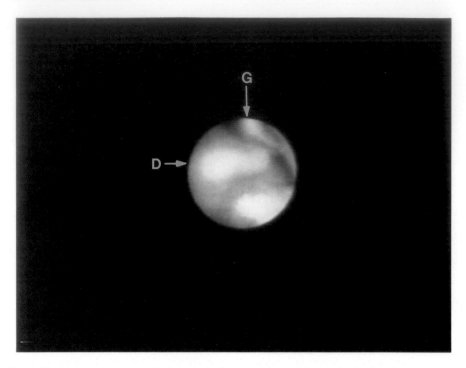

Figure 3. Intracoronary image before angioplasty showing evidence of a healed dissection (D) following angioplasty. The guidewire (G) is visible within the eccentric lumen.

dissection was not detected by angiography or angioscopy in any of these stable angina patients prior to PTCA. Following balloon angioplasty, plaque fracture and dissections which were not detected by angiography were seen in three of four (75%) stable angina patients (Table 1).

Unstable angina pectoris. Pre- and post-PTCA angioscopy has been performed in 16 patients with unstable angina. All of these patients had atherosclerotic plaque associated with their coronary lesions which most commonly were yellow to yellow-brown in color. Before angioplasty, intracoronary thrombi were visualized angioscopically in 8 of 16 (50%) patients of which only 2 were seen angiographically. Following coronary angioplasty, intraco-

Table 1. Angioscopy verus angiography for detecting thrombi and dissection

	Stable angina		Unstable angina	
	Thrombus	Dissection	Thrombus	Dissection
Angioscopy	0/4	3/4	15/16	16/16
Angiography	0/4	0/4	2/16	7/16

Table 2. Restenosis patient data

Patient	Age	Artery	Clinical status	Prior PTCA (weeks)	PTCA No. (n)
1	40	LCX	SA	69	2
2	78	RCA	UA	8	2
3	48	RCA	UA	34	3
4	53	LAD	UA	6	2
5	60	RCA	UA	31	2

PTCA = percutaneous transluminal coronary angioplasty, LAD = left anterior descending artery, LCX = left circumflex artery, RCA = right coronary artery, SA = stable angina, UA = unstable angina.

ronary thrombi were seen in 15 of 16 (94%) patients with angioscopy, of which only 2 were identified with angiography (Table 1). These results confirm the intraoperative angioscopy study by Sherman et al. [26] in which they documented a surprisingly high incidence of intracoronary thrombi in patients with unstable angina and the insensitivity of angiography for detecting these thrombi.

Dissections were either delicate, white fronds of tissue that appeared to be shallow intimal dissections or deep plaque fractures which extended deeply into the arterial wall and appeared to be medial dissections. Prior to angioplasty, no dissections were detected by angiography; but seven patients were seen to have dissections by angioscopy. Following angioplasty, dissections were seen angioscopically in all, 16 of 16 (100%) of the unstable angina patients as opposed to angiographic detection of dissection in 7 of 16 (44%) (Table 1). This superior ability of the angioscope to detect intimal disruptions is due to the high resolution optics that enable the operator to image subtle details of the surface morphology of the artery. The majority of the arterial dissections seen were very small, shallow tears which were not of sufficient magnitude to be detected by angiography.

Restenosis after angioplasty. Angioscopy has been performed in five patients presenting clinical and angiographic evidence of restenosis following coronary balloon angioplasty (Table 2). Atherosclerotic plaque in this group of patients was distinctive in that, in four of the five patients, the lesions were white and had a fibrotic appearance Figure 4). The white fibrotic appearance of the restenosis lesions is consistent with the hypothesis that restenosis is secondary to smooth muscle and fibrointimal proliferation. The single lesion that contained yellow pigmentation was from a patient who had early restenosis six weeks following balloon angioplasty (Figure 3). Angioscopically, there was evidence of a very large dissection that had healed in such a manner as to significantly narrow the lumen of the coronary artery.

Cardiac transplantation and accelerated atherosclerosis. Coronary athero-

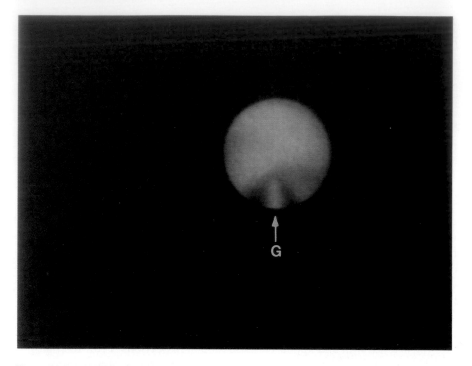

Figure 4. A pre-PTCA image of a restenosis lesion. Note the absence of pigmentation in the plaque (white plaque), consistent with fibrosis. There is an eccentric stenosis at the bottom of the image and the guidewire (G) is visible within the lumen.

sclerosis involving allograft coronary arteries is a significant cause of morbidity and mortality in patients following cardiac transplantation [27]. The pathogenesis is unknown, but it may result from chronic cellular or humoral injury to the coronary vascular endothelium. In addition, it has also been found to be associated with some of the risk factors for native coronary atherosclerosis, particularly hyperlipidemia [28]. It has been reported that angiography is an insensitive method for detecting the presence of early allograft coronary disease due to the frequently diffuse and concentric nature of the plaque in arteries [29].

We have performed coronary angioscopy in ten cardiac transplant patients during routine annual coronary angiography (Table 3). The length of time after heart transplantation ranged from one to four years. Of the ten patients, seven had normal coronary angiography. One of the seven patients with normal coronary angiography, who was one year from his transplantation, had evidence of a non-obstructive yellow plaque visualized in the right coronary artery. Of the three patients with abnormal coronary angiography, tw·
had evidence of non-obstructive luminal irregularities by angiography with yellow pigmented non-obstructive lesions by angioscopy. The third patient,

Table 3. Angioscopy versus angiography in allograft coronary arteries

Patient	Allograft age	Angiographic findings	Angioscope findings
1	1 year	NI	NI
2	1 year	NI	NI
3	1 year	NI	YP
4	1 year	NI	NI
5	2 years	NI	NI
6	2 years	NO	YP
7	2 years	OP	WP
8	3 years	NI	NI
9	4 years	NO	YP
10	4 years	NI	NI

NI = Normal, NO = Non-obstructive luminal irregularities; OP = Obstructive plaque; YP = Yellow plaque; WP = White plaque.

who was two years from transplantation, had diffuse three-vessel obstructive disease by angiography. Angioscopy of this patient's coronary arteries revealed diffuse white plaque which significantly compromised the coronary lumen.

Potential clinical utility

Natural history studies. The correlation of atherosclerotic lesion morphology with clinical outcomes has been the cornerstone of our understanding of this disease and guided our treatment of these patients. The landmark study by DeWood et al. [30] made clear the role of intracoronary thrombosis in the pathogenesis of myocardial infarction and has dramatically changed the standard therapy of this disease from supportive care to interventional therapy with thrombolytic agents. Angiographic morphology studies of coronary arteries in patients with stable and unstable angina has allowed us to stratify patients with high-risk lesions [31–33]. These studies have been limited by the documented insensitivity of angiography for detecting subtle changes in coronary artery surface morphology such as plaque fractures, dissections, intracoronary thrombi, and the assessment of residual stenosis following angioplasty [13–16].

When compared to angiography, angioscopy offers a superior sensitivity and specificity for identifying these subtle changes in atherosclerotic plaque morphology. Like angiography, this is a percutaneous technique which can be used during diagnostic angiography to more closely examine suspicious regions or lesions and, hopefully, provide more precise data concerning the progression of coronary disease. Angioscopy allows the in vivo examination of the surface pathology present in the coronary artery. Our early studies suggest that angioscopy has the potential to improve our understanding of coronary artery lesion morphology in patients with acute ischemic syndromes, restenosis following angioplasty, and atherosclerotic allograft coronary disease.

Guiding interventional therapy. Percutaneous coronary angioscopy may play a role in guiding interventional coronary therapy. The angioscope has a superior ability to detect small amounts of intracoronary thrombus which may be important in determining the clinical outcome of patients with acute ischemic syndromes. Current studies are underway to determine if the angioscopic detection of intracoronary thrombus in patients undergoing balloon angioplasty can identify those at higher risk for complications of the procedure. Perhaps the administration of adjunctive thrombolytic therapy, either before or after balloon dilation, will be guided by angioscopic findings.

Other seemingly useful roles requiring further investigation for angioscopy include reducing the risk of reocclusion of the infarct artery possibly due to incomplete resolution of the intracoronary thrombus following intravenous thrombolytic therapy for acute myocardial infarction. The angioscope may have clinical utility in stratifying the risk of complications after angioplasty in arteries that have "hazy" appearance by angiography. In patients with abrupt occlusion following angioplasty, the angioscope should be able to reliably differentiate thrombotic occlusion from intimal dissection. This distinction would lead to more specific therapy for the occluded artery and possibly increase the success of salvage angioplasty, thereby reducing the need for emergency coronary bypass surgery. As alternative angioplasty techniques such as atherectomy, laser angioplasty, and stent implantation are more commonly used, perhaps the surface morphology of coronary lesions will become an important factor in determining indications for these procedures.

Our early experience in patients with stenotic saphenous vein coronary bypass grafts has demonstrated our ability to differentiate shaggy atheroma from smooth fibrotic-appearing lesions, which has not been possible with angiography alone. This suggests that the risk of atheroembolism in older vein grafts following balloon dilation may be better assessed by angioscopy and that the choice of revascularization procedure in patients with stenotic bypass grafts could be guided by angioscopic findings.

Limitations. At present, percutaneous coronary angioscopy has achieved clinical success in a research environment. The image quality is excellent, and we are able to obtain diagnostic images of selected lesions virtually every time. However, the ability to obtain circumferential images of coronary lesions requires a significant learning curve for the operator. The manipulation of the angioscope guidewire necessary to achieve a coaxial view of the coronary lumen is significantly different than manipulating a conventional coronary angioplasty guidewire and requires patience and experience to achieve optimal results. Currently, we must exchange the diagnostic angioscope for the therapeutic balloon catheter which is cumbersome and somewhat time-consuming. In the future, it is hoped that these two devices will be combined, thereby shortening and simplifying the procedure.

Conclusion

The future of coronary angioscopy as an everyday tool for the interventional cardiologist is uncertain at present. Clearly the angioscope has demonstrated superior sensitivity for intracoronary pathology when compared to angiography. The question is whether or not the information provided by angioscopy has a significant impact on improving the current results of coronary angioplasty.

Angioscopy allows us to examine the surface morphology of coronary arteries during cardiac catheterization. In many ways, the technique is analogous to gastrointestinal or pulmonary endoscopy. With angioscopes, we now have clinical access to information regarding arterial wall pathology that has only been available at autopsy. Whereas angiography provides us with a two-dimensional, black and white image of the coronary vessels, angioscopy complements this with a full-color, three-dimensional perspective of the intracoronary surface morphology.

Coronary angioscopy will not replace diagnostic angiography as the "gold standard" for imaging stenotic lesions in coronary arteries. Angiography provides a rapid and relatively safe means for identifying critical lesions and for mapping the coronary artery tree. However, there may well be a clinical niche for a technology that gives accurate information regarding a specific lesion if the information can be used to improve the acute or chronic outcome of the interventional procedure.

Color discrimination makes it relatively easy to distinguish between thrombus, dissection, and coronary spasm. The presence or absence of complex lesion morphology, thrombosis, and dissection in patients with stable and unstable ischemic syndromes has tremendous implications regarding the therapy of these conditions and may determine prognosis as well. In addition, angioscopy may allow us to better predict the progression of coronary lesions in patients by studying the intracoronary surface morphology.

In today's cost conscious environment, the novelty of directly viewing the coronary arteries will not be sufficient to justify the additional cost of the device. There is no question that there is significant room for improvement in our current angioplasty results, and I am optimistic that, in selected cases, angioscopic information can be translated into better treatment for the patient.

Acknowledgment

Inclusion of the colour illustrations in this chapter has been made possible by support of Advanced Cardiovascular Systems, Inc., Santa Clara, CA, U.S.A.

References

1. Vlodaver Z, Frech R, Van Tassel RA, Edwards JE. Correlation of the antemortem arteriogram and the postmortem specimen. Circulation 1973; **47**: 162–9.
2. Grondin CM, Dyrda I, Pasternac A, Campeau L, Bourassa MG, Lesperance T. Discrepancies between cineangiographic and postmortem findings in patients with coronary artery disease and recent myocardial revascularization. Circulation 1974; **49**: 703–8.
3. Pepine CJ, Nichols WW, Feldman RL, Conti CR. Coronary arteriography: potentially serious sources of error in interpretation. Cardiovasc Med 1977; **2**: 747–52.
4. Arnett EN, Isner JM, Redwood CR, et al. Coronary artery narrowing in coronary heart disease: comparison of cineangiographic and necropsy findings. Ann Intern Med 1979; **91**: 350–6.
5. Isner JM, Kishel J, Kent KM, Ronan JA Jr, Ross AM, Roberts WC. Accuracy of angiographic determination of left main coronary arterial narrowing. Angiographic-histologic correlative analysis in 28 patients. Circulation 1981; **63**: 1056–64.
6. Spears JR, Sandor T, Baim DS, Paulin S. The minimum error in estimating coronary luminal cross-sectional area from cineangiographic diameter measurements. Cathet Cardiovasc Diagn 1983; **9**: 119–28.
7. White CW, Wright CB, Doty DB, et al. Does visual interpretation of the coronary arteriogram predict the physiologic importance of a coronary stenosis? N Engl J Med 1984; **310**: 819–24.
8. Isner JM, Donaldson RF. Coronary angiographic and morphologic correlation. Cardiol Clin 1984; **2**: 571–92.
9. Gould KL. Quantification of coronary artery stenosis in vivo. Circ Res 1985; **57**: 341–53.
10. Zijlstra F, van Ommeren J, Reiber JH, Serruys PW. Does the quantitative assessment of coronary artery dimensions predict the physiologic significance of a coronary stenosis? Circulation 1987; **75**: 1154–61.
11. Marcus ML, Skorton DJ, Johnson MR, Collins SM, Harrison DG, Kerber RE. Visual estimates of percent diameter coronary stenosis: "a battered gold standard." J Am Coll Cardiol 1988; **11**: 882–5.
12. Katritsis D, Webb-Peploe M. Limitations of coronary angiography: an underestimated problem? Clin Cardiol 1991; **14**: 20–4.
13. Block PC, Myler RK, Stertzer S, Fallon JT. Morphology after transluminal angioplasty in human beings. N Engl J Med 1981; **305**: 382–5.
14. Duber C, Jungbluth A, Rumpelt HJ, Erbel R, Meyer J, Thoemes W. Morphology of the coronary arteries after combined thrombolysis and percutaneous transluminal coronary angioplasty for acute myocardial infarction. Am J Cardiol 1986; **58**: 698–703.
15. Essed CE, Van den Brand M, Becker AE. Transluminal coronary angioplasty and early restenosis. Fibrocellular occlusion after wall laceration. Br Heart J 1983; **49**: 393–6.
16. Mizuno K, Kurita A, Imazeki N. Pathological findings after percutaneous transluminal coronary angioplasty. Br Heart J 1984; **52**: 588–90.
17. Rhea L, Walker IC, Cutler EC. The surgical treatment of mitral stenosis: experimental and clinical studies. Arch Surg 1924; **9**: 689–90.
18. Harken DE, Glidden EM: Experiments in intracardiac surgery: intracardiac visualization. J Thorac Surg 1943; **12**: 566–72.

19. Bolton HE, Bailey CP, Costas-Durieux J, Gemeinhardt W. Cardioscopy – simple and practical. J Thorac Surg 1954; **27**: 323–9.
20. Sakakibara S, Iikawa T, Hattori J, Inomata K. Direct visual operation for aortic stenosis: cardioscopic studies. J Int Coll Surg 1958; **29**: 548–62.
21. Litvack F, Grundfest WS, Lee ME, et al. Angioscopic visualization of blood vessel interior in animals and humans. Clin Cardiol 1985; **8**: 65–70.
22. Grundfest WS, Litvack F, Sherman T, et al. Delineation of peripheral and coronary detail by intraoperative angioscopy. Ann Surg 1985; **202**: 394–400.
23. Sanborn TA, Rygaard JA, Westbrook BM, Lazar HL, McCormick JR, Roberts AJ. Intraoperative angioscopy of saphenous vein and coronary arteries. J Thorac Cardiovasc Surg 1986; **91**: 339–43.
24. Lee G, Garcia JM, Corso PJ, et al. Correlation of coronary angioscopic to angiographic findings in coronary artery disease. Am J Cardiol 1986; **58**: 238–41.
25. Grundfest WS, Litvack F, Glick D, et al. Intraoperative decisions based on angioscopy in peripheral vascular surgery. Circulation 1988; **78** (3 part 2): I 13–7.
26. Sherman CT, Litvack F, Grundfest W, et al. Coronary angioscopy in patients with unstable angina pectoris. N Engl J Med 1986; **315**: 913–9.
27. Kosek JC, Bieber C, Lower RR. Heart graft arteriosclerosis. Transplant Proc 1971; **3**: 512–4.
28. Gao SZ, Schroeder JS, Alderman EL, et al. Clinical and laboratory correlates of accelerated artery disease in the cardiac transplant patient. Circulation 1987; **76** (5 part 2): V56–61.
29. Gao SZ, Johnson D, Schroeder JS, et al. Transplant coronary artery disease: histopathologic correlations with angiographic morphology. J Am Coll Cardiol 1988; **11** (Suppl A): 153A (Abstract).
30. DeWood MA, Spores J, Notske R, et al. Prevalence of total coronary occlusion during the early hours of transmural myocardial infarction. N Engl J Med 1980; **303**: 897–902.
31. Ambrose JA, Winters SL, Stern A, et al. Angiographic morphology and the pathogenesis of unstable angina pectoris. J Am Coll Cardiol 1985; **5**: 609–16.
32. Rehr R, Disciascio G, Vetrovec G, Cowley M. Angiographic morphology of coronary artery stenoses in prolonged rest angina: evidence of intracoronary thrombosis. J Am Coll Cardiol 1989; **14**: 1429–37. Comment in: J Am Coll Cardiol 1989; **14**: 1438–9.
33. Levin DC, Fallon JT. Significance of the angiographic morphology of localized coronary stenoses: histopathologic correlations. Circulation 1982; **66**: 316–20.

3. Development and application of coronary intravascular ultrasound: comparison to quantitative angiography

STEVEN E. NISSEN and JOHN C. GURLEY

Summary

Technologic advances have permitted development of miniaturized intravascular ultrasound catheters capable of real-time coronary imaging. For quantitative assessment of coronary artery disease (CAD), the cross-sectional orientation of ultrasound offers many advantages, particularly the ability to visualize the intramural anatomy of the vessel wall. Two alternative approaches to intraluminal ultrasound have emerged, mechanically rotated devices and electronic imaging arrays. In initial animal studies, comparison of vessel diameter by angiography and intravascular ultrasound revealed a close correlation, $r = 0.98$. Coronary intravascular ultrasound has been performed safely in more than 200 patients with CAD. For each of a series of coronary sites, both intravascular ultrasound and contrast cineangiography were performed simultaneously. In approximately two-thirds of CAD patients, a relatively concentric lumen was present and the correlation between ultrasound and angiography was close, $r = 0.93$. In approximately one third of CAD patients, the lumen was eccentric and comparisons between angiography and ultrasound diameter revealed significant differences, $r = 0.78$. In normal subjects, morphologic analysis revealed an echogenic intimal leading-edge with a maximum thickness averaging $0.18 \pm .06$ mm and a sub-intimal sonolucent layer averaging 0.11 ± 0.04 mm. A spectrum of abnormalities in wall morphology were detected in patients with atherosclerotic CAD including thickening of the leading edge and/or sonolucent zone. Abnormalities in coronary morphology were also detected at many sites in which no lesion was present by angiography. Minimum diameter by angiography and intravascular ultrasound immediately following balloon angioplasty correlated poorly, $r = 0.30$. A probe combining both imaging capability and an angioplasty balloon is undergoing human testing.

J.H.C. Reiber and P.W. Serruys (eds), Advances in Quantitative Coronary Arteriography, 29–51.

Introduction

New electronic and acoustic technology has permitted development of miniaturized intravascular ultrasound systems capable of real-time tomographic coronary imaging [1–8]. The development of intravascular ultrasound provides the first practical new technique for evaluating the anatomy of coronary artery disease (CAD) since the introduction of angiography more than 30 years ago. Many observers believe that intraluminal imaging will play an increasingly important role in the quantitative evaluation of CAD. Intravascular ultrasound also holds great promise as a means to evaluate and guide therapeutic coronary interventions such as balloon angioplasty.

Although the precise clinical role of intravascular ultrasound is still rapidly evolving, several inherent properties of intraluminal imaging suggest how this new modality will augment diagnostic capabilities in the cardiac catheterization laboratory. Current research is beginning to define the relationship between intravascular ultrasound and the current "gold standard" for coronary evaluation, quantitative angiography. In this regard, it has become apparent that there are fundamental differences in the orientation and perspective of tomographic coronary imaging techniques such as intraluminal ultrasound and planar methods such as angiography.

Limitations of angiography

Much of impetus for development of intraluminal coronary imaging originates from an understanding of the inherent limitations of conventional angiographic methods [9–16]. For several decades, clinical studies have demonstrated large intra- and interobserver variability in the visual interpretation of coronary angiograms. Investigators have also reported large differences in stenosis severity determined by antemortem angiography in comparison to necropsy findings. Most such studies report that angiography underestimates the extent of atherosclerosis in comparison to postmortem histologic measurements. Clinical studies have also demonstrated a dissociation between the apparent angiographic severity of lesions and physiologic measures of stenosis severity such as hyperemic flow reserve [17].

A variety of phenomena account for the inaccuracies and high observer variability of angiography. Histologic studies demonstrate that coronary obstructions are frequently complex and may be highly eccentric in cross-section. Angiographic methods depict this eccentric arterial anatomy from a projected two-dimensional silhouette of the vessel lumen. Accordingly, any single arbitrary angle of view may significantly misrepresent the extent of luminal narrowing for a complex coronary lesion (Figure 1). Theoretically, two orthogonal angiograms should accurately reflect the severity of many lesions, but orthogonal views may be unobtainable since optimal imaging angles are frequently unavailable due to overlapping sidebranches, disease at bifurcation sites and radiographic foreshortening. Mechanical interven-

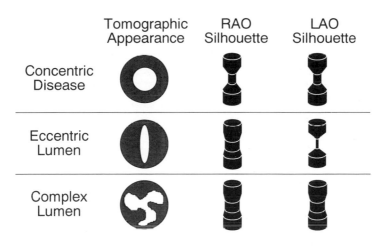

Figure 1. Differences between tomographic and planar coronary imaging techniques. For concentrically diseased vessels, the angiographic silhouette general will accurately depict the severity of narrowing. However, when the coronary is narrowed eccentrically, angiography becomes highly dependent on the angle of view. For complex coronary obstructions, no angle of view may accurately reflect the severity of disease.

tions such as balloon angioplasty distort the lumen and further complicate the problem of vessel eccentricity.

The widespread practice of describing lesion severity based upon percentage reduction in luminal area generates additional limitations. Computation of percent stenosis requires identification and measurement of dimensions for the atherosclerotic lesion and an adjacent "normal" segment. However, necropsy studies demonstrate that coronary disease is frequently diffuse and contains no truly normal segment from which to calculate the percent area reduction [9–14]. Thus, in the presence of diffuse disease, angiography will always systematically underestimate disease severity (Figure 2). Angiography is also insensitive to the phenomenon of "remodeling", a process observed histologically as the outward displacement of the external vessel wall in vascular segments with atherosclerotic luminal encroachment (Figure 3).

Potential advantages of coronary ultrasound

For quantitative assessment of coronary disease, the cross-sectional orientation of intravascular ultrasound offers several potential advantages. Theoretically, the tomographic perspective of ultrasound should enable precise quantitative measurements of cross-sectional area independent of radiographic projection. Measured dimensions obtained from cross-sectional imag-

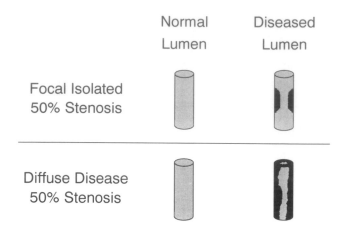

Figure 2. Impact of diffuse disease on stenosis evaluation. The percent stenosis will underestimate disease severity whenever the vessel is diffusely involved by atherosclerosis.

ing will be accurate even when the coronary is eccentrically diseased or the lumen shape distorted by a mechanical revascularization procedure. Intravascular imaging should also permit quantitative assessment of segments difficult to image radiographically, such as bifurcation sites or arteries obscured by the presence of overlapping vessels.

Intravascular ultrasound brings additional quantitative information to the diagnostic armamentarium – the intramural anatomy of the vessel wall. Necropsy studies have demonstrated that atherosclerotic plaque morphology

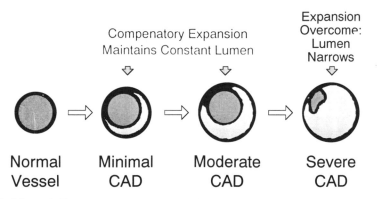

Figure 3. Schematic illustration of coronary remodeling. During initial stages of atherosclerosis, outward expansion of the vessel wall maintains lumen size. A stenosis is evident only when the luminal expansion is overcome by the disease process.

is complex and may include soft lipid atheroma as well as fibrocalcific plaque. The ability to directly visualize these plaques may provide valuable insights into the pathophysiology and natural history of CAD. For example, ultrasound may enable identification of morphologic features that predict a high likelihood of plaque rupture and acute thrombotic occlusion. Similarly, lesion morphology may predict the propensity for restenosis following mechanical revascularization. Imaging of the intramural anatomy of atherosclerotic plaques should enable highly precise studies of atherosclerosis regression or progression.

The theoretic and practical advantages of ultrasound for quantitation of atherosclerosis are routinely utilized in the evaluation of noncoronary vascular disease. During the last decade, duplex Doppler ultrasound has emerged as the dominant noninvasive technique for assessment of peripheral vascular and carotid disease. However, attempts to image the coronaries by transthoracic or transesophageal echocardiography have achieved limited success, primarily because the low ultrasound frequencies required to penetrate the chest wall provide inadequate spatial resolution for coronary diagnosis. Intraluminal ultrasound moves the transducer in close proximity to the vessel wall which provides excellent spatial resolution. Since the intravascular device operates in a fluid environment, attenuation by air or bone is avoided.

Development of intravascular ultrasound

Although initial efforts to develop coronary ultrasound began nearly 20 years ago, only recently have such efforts yielded success [1–8, 18–28]. The small size and tortuous nature of human coronaries have represented a significant technical challenge to development of imaging catheters. For safe application in the coronaries, intravascular ultrasound requires highly miniaturized and mechanically flexible transducer delivery systems. Such devices are inherently difficult and costly to develop and manufacture in large quantities. Coronary ultrasound has also been slowed by safety concerns. Since intracoronary instrumentation is required, some centers have been reluctant to utilize coronary ultrasound until large clinical studies demonstrate the safety of intraluminal examination performed during routine cardiac catheterization.

In addition, difficulty with image interpretation represents a major research problem that has impeded clinical application of coronary ultrasound. Previous experience with angiography cannot be applied readily to evaluation of the tomographic images produced by intraluminal ultrasound devices. Although several published studies have compared histology and ultrasound using necropsy specimens, elastic recoil and other alterations in the acoustic appearance in postmortem arteries represent an important confounding variable. Accordingly, ultrasound studies must be performed in vivo to define normal and abnormal anatomy prior to widespread clinical application of intraluminal imaging in human coronary disease. However, it remains difficult to identify and study a normal cohort, since patients admitted for cardiac catheterization are rarely true normals.

Probe size and flexibility

Practical diagnostic application of intraluminal imaging in coronary disease requires a transducer-tipped catheter small enough to successfully image the major epicardial coronary branches. Normal first order coronaries are usually 2.0 to 5.0 mm in diameter, but second-order vessels and atherosclerotic lumina are generally in the range of 2.0 mm or less. In the past several years, considerable reduction in ultrasound probe sizes has yielded coronary imaging devices ranging from 3.5 to 5.0 F (1.16 to 1.67 mm). Such probes are suitable for evaluation of major epicardial vessels and most lesions post-PTCA, but are too large to cross tight stenoses.

Successful coronary imaging requires not only small transducers, but also catheter delivery system with a high degree of mechanical flexibility. This feature permits optimal safety in cannulating the tortuous vessels frequently encountered in humans. However, miniaturization of ultrasound transducers for intracoronary application limits available acoustic power and thus compromises signal to noise ratio. In comparison to imaging probes developed for peripheral vascular imaging, all coronary ultrasound devices suffer from a noticeable decrement in image quality.

Practical coronary ultrasound imaging has also required engineering solutions to the troublesome problem of transducer ring-down artifact. The ring-down phenomenon is characterized by high amplitude oscillations of the piezoelectric transducer material that obscures imaging of structures located close to the catheter surface. No matter how small the physical dimensions of the ultrasound catheter, it is ultimately the size of the ring-down artifact that determines the practical limits in imaging small or stenotic coronary vessels. Thus, successful coronary ultrasound devices require both a small physical size and minimal "acoustic" size.

Alternative catheter designs

A variety of technical strategies have been employed to construct ultrasound probes capable of intraluminal coronary examination [1, 2, 5, 6] (Figure 4). Two alternative approaches have emerged, mechanically rotated devices and electronic imaging arrays. Each design must overcome different engineering problems to successfully image the coronary arteries. The first practical commercial ultrasound systems have utilized rotating mechanical transducers. To decrease or eliminate ring-down artifacts, recent mechanical designs often employ a rotating acoustic mirror to permit a longer signal path from the transducer to the vessel lumen. This approach confines the ring-down within the catheter and theoretically permits imaging up to the surface of the device.

Mechanical imaging catheters have inherent advantages and disadvan-

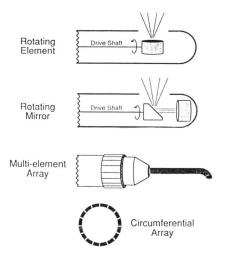

Figure 4. Technical strategies for development of intravascular imaging devices. Initial devices used a rotating transducer, whereas recent designs employ a rotating acoustic mirror. A more complex approach utilizes a multi-element array.

tages. In comparison to multi-element electronic arrays, the comparatively large size of the transducer element used in mechanical coronary ultrasound devices provides greater acoustic power. Improved acoustic power will potentially yield higher image quality, in particular, improved penetration and better gray scale. Practical disadvantages of rotating transducer systems include significant mechanical stiffness which impairs safe passage through tortuous coronaries. In mechanical probes, the presence of a drive shaft obviates a central lumen guidewire, although monorail systems are in common use. However, the monorail strut obscures imaging for part of the vessel circumference.

Any imprecision in the manufacture of a rotating device will result in image flaws capable of influencing quantitative measurements. Rotation speed may increase or decrease because of mechanical drag, particularly when the drive-shaft is bent by a tortuous vessel. The resulting nonuniform rotational velocity produces an unpredictable warping of the image. This distortion can be quite significant and may affect measurements of lumen size or alter the apparent location of structures. Nonuniform rotational distortion has been improved, but not eliminated by recent designs.

Multi-element ultrasound probe

Although most prototype intravascular ultrasound probes employ mechanical transducer rotation, an electronic array is also feasible [5, 6, 8]. In our laboratory, initial animal and human studies were performed using a multi-element 20 MHz intravascular ultrasound device with no mechanical moving parts (Endosonics Corp, Rancho Cordova, CA). This system employs a 32 or 64 element transducer array mounted on a central lumen catheter that accommodates a standard 0.014 inch guidewire to facilitate safe over-the-wire coronary placement (Figure 4). The absence of a mechanical drive shaft enhances catheter flexibility and thereby improves passage through tortuous coronaries. Initial 64 element probes were 5.5 F (1.83 mm) in diameter, while more recent designs have permitted even smaller transducers, 5.0 F (1.66 mm) and 3.5 F (1.16 mm) in diameter.

The image reconstruction algorithm of this unique multi-element device employs an imaging approach described as a "synthetic aperture array." This design differs from the "phased-array" approach commonly employed in transthoracic echocardiography. The imaging catheter individually transmits and receives ultrasound signals from each of the elements of the annular array. These signals are electronically amplified and multiplexed by micro-miniaturized integrated circuits contained within the catheter tip. A complex image reconstruction algorithm analogous to computed tomography is utilized to synthesize the gray scale image. To reconstruct pixels near to the catheter surface, the algorithm utilizes only a few adjacent elements, whereas more distant pixels are generated using data from larger groupings of elements. This results in a variable aperture device ("synthetic aperture") that theoretically maintains constant focus from the surface of the catheter to infinity. To produce a complete image, the computer must generate 1800 radial scan lines at 10 frames per second.

Multi-element designs have inherent advantages and disadvantages. The acoustic power available with multi-element probes is significantly less than for mechanical devices, although the clinical significance of this difference is uncertain. The lack of mechanical moving parts yields a flexible catheter with better handling properties. Since the transducer elements are surface-mounted, the electronic array cannot eliminate ring-down by increasing the signal path length. However, ring-down artifact is reduced by computer image processing using digital subtraction. The subtraction procedure uses a reference image containing the ring-down artifact that is collected during ultrasound in a large vessel such as the aorta. During real-time imaging, the central portion of the reference image is subtracted from all subsequent frames to electronically remove ring-down. This process reduces, but may not always completely eliminate the ring-down signal.

Limitations of all intravascular ultrasound

Several limitations are common to all intraluminal ultrasound devices, regardless of design. Tomographic imaging techniques such as intravascular ultrasound, are vulnerable to distortion produced by oblique imaging planes. Thus, a vessel lumen with a circular cross-sectional profile will appear elliptical whenever the transducer is not orthogonal to the long axis of the vessel. This phenomenon can represent a significant confounding variable in quantitative measurements. Axial positioning is also important in optimizing image quality because current devices employ very low acoustic power to produce images and "drop-out" is often evident when imaging off-axis structures. This problem is most troublesome in normal subjects who often have an intimal leading-edge of minimal acoustic reflectance which may poorly reflect ultrasound.

For all ultrasound systems, fibrotic or calcified intimal plaques can impede transmission of low energy, high-frequency ultrasound signals and may obscure the underlying structure of the arterial wall. These "shadowing" plaques prevent accurate measurement of atheroma area because the full thickness of the vessel wall is not visualized. It must also be emphasized that intravascular ultrasound can characterize structures as echogenic or echolucent, but cannot determine precise histology. Thus, "tissue" composition is inferred from "acoustic" properties, an inherently imprecise approach. More sophisticated tissue evaluation techniques such as texture or backscatter analysis are promising, but still experimental.

Quantitative measurements: experimental validation

Vessel dimensions in an animal model

Initial in vivo studies were designed to compare measurements of vessel dimensions by intravascular ultrasound and angiography to identify any systematic differences between the two techniques. We compared vascular diameter and cross-sectional area by angiography and intravascular ultrasound in an animal model using a prototype 32 element probe [6]. In each animal, cineangiography was performed during simultaneous ultrasound imaging at each of a series of peripheral vascular sites.

Arterial diameter was measured from cineangiograms using a radiographic grid for magnification correction. Videotaped intravascular ultrasound images were digitized using an image processing computer and cross-sectional area and diameter measured directly from the image with an electronic cursor. Comparison of vessel diameter by angiography and intravascular ultrasound revealed a close correlation, $r = 0.98$, with a regression equation approaching the line of identity, $y = 0.86x + 0.78$. Similar results were obtained for comparisons of cross-sectional area by angiography and ultrasound [6]. These data demonstrated the expected concordance between angiographic and ultrasound dimensions for non-atherosclerotic vessels in an idealized experimental setting.

In the animal model, artificial stenoses were formed using a ligature fashioned from a segment of femoral nerve, and the resulting lesions imaged by both intravascular ultrasound and angiography. Subsequent measurement of these lesions revealed a close correlation between intravascular ultrasound and angiography, $r = 0.88$ [6]. Thus, measurements of stenosis severity by intravascular ultrasound was comparable to conventional radiographic methods in this nonatherosclerotic experimental model. No systematic measurement differences between angiography and ultrasound were documented.

At additional sites, balloon dilation was performed in the peripheral vessels to produced ectasia of the artery, sometimes yielding asymmetrical distortion of luminal shape. Following balloon dilation, the correlation between angiography and intravascular ultrasound was less close, $r = .81$ [6]. Thus, when luminal distortion and eccentricity was produced by balloon dilation, dimensions derived from intravascular ultrasound differed significantly from angiography. Intuitively, a cross-sectional imaging technique such as ultrasound should be superior for examining these noncircular vessels.

Although the luminal size measurements obtained from intravascular ultrasound in our initial animal studies were promising, the image quality of the prototype 32–element probe did not permit adequate discrimination of the intramural morphology of the arterial wall. The spatial resolution of the 32–element catheter was limited and the images were relatively lacking in gray scale which prevented detailed analysis of vessel wall structures. An improved, higher resolution device was developed to permit more detailed observations of wall morphology in human coronaries.

Human studies: quantitative measurements

Imaging protocol

Initial human studies of coronary intravascular ultrasound were performed with the improved, 64–element synthetic aperture device [8, 22–27]. This probe has a maximum diameter of 5.5 F (1.83 mm) and incorporates a 0.014 inch central lumen guidewire to facilitate safe subselective coronary placement. Imaging was restricted to vessels with an estimated diameter greater than 2.0 millimeter to avoid reduction in flow or mechanical occlusion of the coronary. The investigational protocol consisted of standard diagnostic arteriography followed by intravascular ultrasound in patients who were clinically stable. In initial studies, full doses of heparin (5,000 to 10,000 units) were administered systemically prior to the procedure.

An 8 F guiding catheter with minimum lumen size of 0.074 inches (1.88 mm) was required to permit unrestricted passage of the 5.5 F intravascular ultrasound device. The coronary was engaged with the guiding catheter and the angioplasty guidewire was advanced into the distal coronary under fluoroscopic guidance. The imaging probe was advanced over the wire to achieve a subselective position in the coronary vessel to be examined. Because an over-the-wire approach was utilized, the ultrasound transducer could be safely advanced and withdrawn to systematically examine a segment of the coronary.

Clinical results: *safety*

We assessed the risk of the intravascular ultrasound in a typical patient cohort undergoing diagnostic coronary arteriography [8]. Other investigators have reported experience with intracoronary ultrasound performed following interventional procedures, typically balloon angioplasty [7]. However, we deliberately examined patients following routine catheterization to determine the safety and utility of intravascular ultrasound in a representative diagnostic setting. Although intraluminal ultrasound was used as an adjunct to diagnostic catheterization, the imaging probe was always placed by an interventional cardiologist with extensive angioplasty experience.

We have performed coronary intravascular ultrasound in more than 200 patients with CAD undergoing routine diagnostic catheterization. This cohort includes more than 50 patients with acute coronary syndromes such as unstable angina or evolving myocardial infarction. The only significant adverse effect in this group was transient coronary spasm occurring in 8 patients. Occasionally, the device produced temporary reduction in coronary flow when advanced into the distal vessel, but only two patients experienced chest pain and in each case withdrawal of the catheter resulted in normal distal flow. The ability of the electronic multi-element probe to accommodate a central lumen guidewire was highly advantageous, because handling and placement was similar to standard angioplasty techniques. These data establish the safety of intravascular ultrasound imaging of coronaries performed following routine coronary angiography.

Quantitative measurement methods

For each of a series of coronary sites, both intravascular ultrasound and contrast cineangiography were performed [8]. For each analyzed site, a cineangiogram was performed with the catheter in situ to document precise probe location. This procedure yielded a series of ultrasound and angiographic images from identical sites for quantitative analysis (Figure 5). For each site examined, the cineangiogram was optically magnified and the diameter of the guiding catheter measured to correct for radiographic magnification. For each coronary site, the radiographic projection yielding minimum diameter was measured at the location of the ultrasound imaging catheter. At stenosis sites, angiographic cross-sectional area reduction was calculated from diameter measurements.

Ultrasound images were stored on S-VHS videotape and quantitative analysis performed using an image processing system (Mipron-D, Kontron Electronics) equipped with 32 megabytes of video RAM to enable digitization of full motion ultrasound imaging sequences. Although all measurements were performed using single stop-frames, the large video memory permitted review of dynamic sequences which was valuable in the identification of moving structures to determine the frame with optimal delineation of vessel

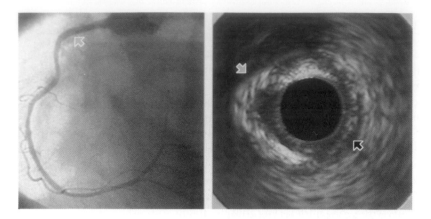

Figure 5. Comparison of angiography and intravascular ultrasound at the same site. In the left panel, the gray arrow indicates the site examined by ultrasound. In the right panel, the gray arrow indicates a densely thickened intimal leading edge that shadows underlying structures. The black arrow identifies a more normal side of the artery.

borders. Ultrasound analysis was also aided by the injection of iodinated contrast media during imaging which produces microbubble luminal opacification and assisted in the identification of the intimal leading-edge (Figure 6).

Because atherosclerotic coronaries in patients are frequently complex and eccentric, we anticipated that a tomographic imaging technique such as intravascular ultrasound might yield measurements that differed significantly from angiography. To evaluate the impact of vessel eccentricity upon quantitative

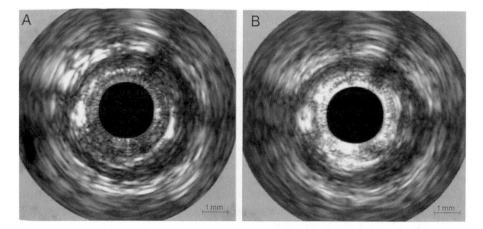

Figure 6. Opacification of the lumen with microbubble contrast. The left panel illustrates the image just prior to contrast administration, while the right panel shows the lumen fully opacified.

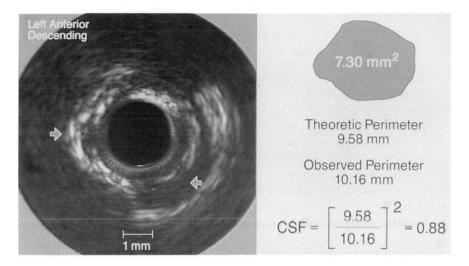

Figure 7. Computation of the circular shape factor (CSF). The cross-sectional area of the lumen is measured and a theoretic perimeter is computed for a perfect circle of the measured cross-sectional area. The actual observed perimeter is compared to the theoretic perimeter to determine the CSF.

measurements, we analyzed ultrasound images using a computer index of eccentricity, the circular shape factor. The planimetered vessel cross-sectional area (CSA) was used to calculate the mean vessel diameter as $d = \sqrt{CSA/\pi}$. The perimeter (P) for a perfect circle of this diameter was determined as $P = \pi d$. This calculated perimeter was compared to the actual measured perimeter (by planimetry) of the vessel lumen. This calculation yielded an index of eccentricity, the circular shape factor (CSF), defined as:

$$CSF = \left(\frac{\text{calculated perimeter}}{\text{observed perimeter}}\right)^2.$$

This computer shape index yields a value of 1.0 for a perfect circular lumen, whereas vessels with increasing eccentricity yield values progressively smaller than 1.0 (Figure 7).

Comparison: angiographic and ultrasound dimensions

Measurements of lumen dimensions by ultrasound and angiography were compared for a variety of patient subsets including normal subjects and patients with atherosclerotic CAD [8, 25]. Comparisons in normals provided a measure of the variability inherent in comparing two different techniques such as angiography and ultrasound. Comparisons in CAD patients were separately analyzed for subgroups of sites with a concentric vs. an eccentric lumen by ultrasound determined by the circular shape factor. These analyses were designed to evaluate the impact of lumen eccentricity upon comparative measurements by ultrasound and angiography.

The lumen was nearly circular in patients with normal coronaries with the circular shape factor averaging 0.96 ± 0.02. This analysis yielded 95% confidence limits of 0.92 to 1.0 for CSF in normals [8]. The correlation between angiographic and ultrasound minimum coronary diameter was close, $r = 0.92$, in these normal subjects. Thus, intravascular ultrasound and angiography yield highly comparable measures of vessel dimension in normal vessels with a circular cross-sectional profile.

In approximately two-thirds of CAD patients, a relatively concentric lumen was present, defined as a CSF within the normal range (> 0.92). In the subset of patients with concentric shaped lumina, the correlation between ultrasound and angiography was also close, $r = 0.93$ [8, 25]. In approximately one third of CAD patients, the lumen was eccentric (CSF < 0.92). In the subgroup of CAD patients with an eccentric lumen, comparisons between angiography and ultrasound diameter revealed significant differences, $r = 0.78$. We believe this reduced correlation is explained by inability of angiography to accurately measure the irregular, noncircular cross-sectional vessels in patients with atherosclerotic CAD. These data demonstrate the potential superiority of a tomographic technique, such as intravascular ultrasound, in measurement of coronary dimension for the complex eccentric vessels commonly encountered in CAD patients.

Assessment of stenoses

Both cineangiography and intravascular ultrasound demonstrated a stenosis of more than 25% at 41 coronary sites. Comparison of mean percent area reduction, was similar by cineangiography, $48.9 \pm 13.8\%$, and intravascular ultrasound, $52.3 \pm 16.3\%$ ($p = 0.10$) [8, 25]. However, the correlation between percent stenosis by cineangiography and ultrasound was only moderate, $r = 0.63$. The regression equation demonstrated considerable divergence from the line of identity, $y = 0.54x + 20.7$. Standard error of the estimate was also moderately large, 10.9%. These data demonstrate major differences between ultrasonic and angiographic assessment of stenosis severity.

Other investigators have reported discrepancies between ultrasound and angiography for assessment of residual stenosis following coronary angioplasty [7]. Because balloon dilation distorts the shape of vessel lumen and wall, the reported differences between angiographic and ultrasonic measurements following angioplasty are not surprising. Our data confirm that stenosis measurements by angiography and ultrasound also frequently disagree for native lesions in vessels not distorted by prior balloon dilation.

Coronary wall morphology

Wall structure: normal cohort

Because of the significant alterations in wall morphology observed following removal and fixation of vessels, we established normal values for ultrasound based upon in vivo imaging. The normal subjects consisted of patients with atypical chest pain in whom angiography demonstrated absence of any coronary luminal irregularity [8, 23, 24]. Other rigorous exclusion criteria for the normal cohort included any history of myocardial infarction, hypertension, diabetes, claudication, cerebral vascular events, valvular or congenital heart disease. Normal subjects were also carefully screened for any physical findings of atherosclerosis in peripheral vascular vessels.

Ultrasound images in these normal subjects were digitized for quantitative analysis of wall morphology. The 95% confidence limits obtained in normal subject were used to classify abnormal coronary anatomy in the patients with CAD. In approximately 60% of normal subjects, the anatomy consisted of two distinct vessel wall layers, an echogenic intimal leading-edge and a sonolucent sub-intimal zone. At the remaining 40% of normal sites, ultrasound failed to reveal distinct laminations of the vessel wall despite continuous imaging and catheter manipulation. When evident, the maximal thickness of these two structures was measured with an electronic cursor and the mean and standard deviation values determined. These values provided a normal range from which to analyze coronary ultrasound images in CAD patients.

At sites suitable for measurement, the maximum thickness of the echogenic intimal leading-edge averaged 0.18 ± 0.06 mm [8]. The maximal thickness of the sub-intimal sonolucent layer averaged 0.11 ± 0.04 mm. Using the mean plus/minus two standard deviations, this analysis yielded upper limits of 0.30 mm for the echogenic intimal leading-edge and 0.20 mm for the subintimal sonolucent zone. These findings demonstrate that the intimal leading edge and subadjacent sonolucent zones are thin and discrete in most normal subjects (Figure 8). However, individual ultrasound frames frequently demonstrated a distinctly laminar wall structure only for a portion of the vessel circumference. In normal subjects, ultrasound images frequently exhibited "drop-out" of endothelial reflections. The low echogenicity of the intimal leading-edge required careful review of the dynamic imaging sequences to obtain optimal measurement of wall structures. In all patients, manipulation of the catheter to achieve a central and coaxial position in the lumen was often effective in reducing drop-out.

Abnormal wall morphology: CAD patients

In CAD patients, a wall layer was classified as abnormal if the thickness of the structure was more than two standard deviations greater than the normal value. Echogenicity of a wall layer was considered abnormal if fibrosis or

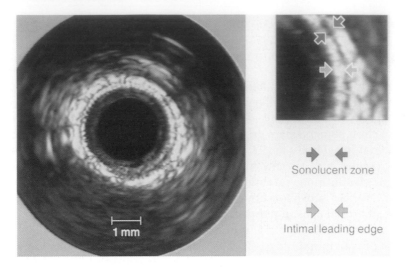

Figure 8. Intravascular ultrasound in a normal subject. The lumen is nearly circular and the intimal leading-edge and sonolucent zones are both thin and discrete. (Reproduced with permission of Circulation and the American Heart Association)

calcification impeded transmission of ultrasound thus obscuring underlying anatomy. Using these criteria, a spectrum of abnormalities in coronary wall morphology were detected in patients with atherosclerotic CAD [8, 24]. The thickness of the intimal leading-edge or sonolucent zone were abnormally increased at more than 50% of all examined sites in CAD patients. In some segments, the vessel exhibited both abnormal thickening and increased echogenicity of the intimal leading-edge, so call "hard plaques" (Figure 9). In the most severe plaques, dense fibrocalcific intimal structures impeded ultrasound transmission thus shadowing underlying anatomic features. For segments with angiographic disease, wall measurements by ultrasound were abnormal at nearly 90% of sites.

A distinct sub-intimal sonolucent zone was evident at approximately 70% of sites in the CAD patients. The maximal thickness of this sonolucent structure was abnormal (30.20 mm) at more than one half of all sites in CAD patients. Some sonolucent plaques were eccentric, appearing as crescent shaped bands located within a portion of the vessel circumference (Figure 10). These sonolucent crescents represent less echogenic, presumably more lipid-laden "soft" atherosclerotic plaque. These sonolucent atheroma were frequently covered by a thickened more echogenic fibrous cap. At some sites, an expanded symmetrical thickened leading-edge and sonolucent zone were present resulting in a distinctive triple-layer appearance (Figure 11). This exaggerated tri-laminar appearance was not evident in any of the normal subjects and represents concentric atherosclerotic disease.

The adventitial surface of the vessel wall appeared as a poorly defined

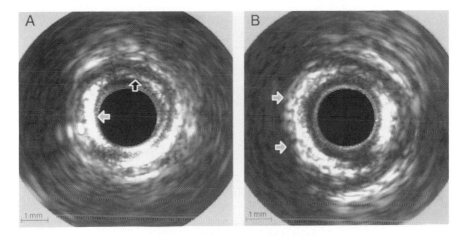

Figure 9. Ultrasound images from two coronary sites. In the left panel, a zone with a thickened intimal leading edge is illustrated by the gray arrow, while the black arrow shows an area with normal intimal thickness. In the right panel, the ultrasound shows greatly thickened intima with shadowing of underlying structure, also known as "hard plaque." See text.

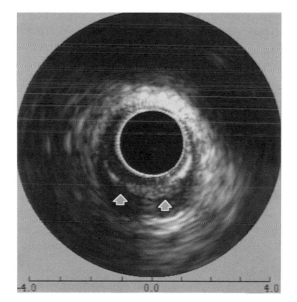

Figure 10. Crescent shaped sonolucent plaque. The gray arrows indicate an eccentric plaque with a reduced acoustic reflectance. The adventitia overlying this plaque is remodeled outward. See text.

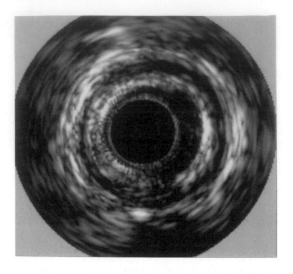

Figure 11. Symmetrical trilayered vessel appcarance. In this case, both the intimal leading-edge and sonolucent zone are abnormally thickened.

third layer of the arterial wall at most coronary sites. The leading-edge of this structure was often evident, but a distinct interface at the trailing edge was not apparent except within bypass grafts. The ambiguity of the trailing edge precluded measurement of total vessel wall thickness. It is apparent from these findings that there are no prominent acoustic features to distinguish the adventitia from other tissues encasing the vessel.

Findings: *angiographically normal sites*

We also sought to evaluate the utility of intravascular ultrasound in the detection of angiographically occult CAD. In patients with any luminal irregularity, abnormalities in coronary wall morphology were detected at most sites in which no lesion was present by angiography. In some cases, it was evident that preservation of angiographic lumen size was a consequence of compensatory remodeling of the vessel wall (Figure 10). In other patients with angiographically occult disease, diffuse atherosclerosis involved the entire vessel. In such cases, the angiogram was negative because there was no superimposed focal luminal encroachment. The extent of disease in angiographically normal vessels confirms the finding, previously reported from necropsy studies, that coronary disease is frequently more diffuse than apparent by angiography.

Intravascular imaging following PTCA

Background

Although PTCA has achieved worldwide clinical acceptance, imaging problems continue to impede optimal application of catheter-based mechanical interventions. Necropsy studies demonstrate that balloon angioplasty frequently produces cracks, splits and dissections in the vessel wall. These complex alterations in wall morphology are often difficult to evaluate by a planar technique such as angiography. In many cases a "hazy" appearance is evident on the post-PTCA angiogram and the observer is uncertain how to measure the vessel dimensions. Restenosis continues to represent a troublesome problem in the management of patients following apparently successful angioplasty. Unfornately, angiography is a poor predictor of which patients will return with a recurrent lesion.

Intravascular ultrasound hold great promise as an independent technique for evaluation of the results of PTCA. Other investigators have demonstrated that residual stenosis measurements by angiography and ultrasound correlate poorly following PTCA [7]. Because of the differences between ultrasound and angiography observed in eccentric coronaries, we hypothesized that distortion of the vessel lumen by balloon dilation would explain these discrepancies. Therefore, we compared luminal dimensions by angiography and intravascular ultrasound in a group of patients examined immediately following angioplasty [27]. We also examined the morphology of the vessel wall following PTCA.

Minimum diameter and residual stenosis

The minimum diameters of residual coronary lesions by angiography and intravascular ultrasound were compared immediately following balloon dilation. This analysis revealed a very poor correlation between minimum diameter by angiography and intravascular ultrasound, $r = 0.30$ [27]. Importantly, measurements of luminal diameter and cross-sectional area following angioplasty were often smaller when assessed by intravascular ultrasound in comparison to angiography ($p \leqslant .01$). It is likely that these difference represents an enhancement of the apparent angiographic diameter produced by extra-luminal contrast within cracks or splits in the intima and/or media of the vessel wall (Figure 12). Thus, angioplasty-related alterations in vessel wall structure dramatically impair the reliability of conventional quantitative angiographic methods.

The differences between angiography and ultrasound in assessment of PTCA results have important clinical implications. We believe that "restenosis" may sometimes represent inadequate dilation and not exclusively a process of cellular proliferation. Further studies will be required to determine if intravascular ultrasound can predict long-term results following angioplasty,

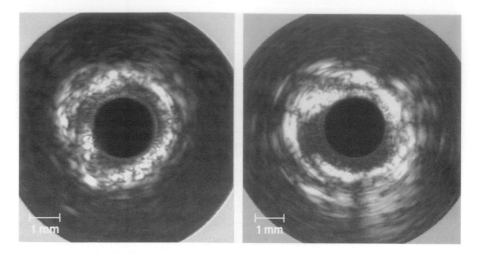

Figure 12. Distortion of the vessel lumen at PTCA sites. In the left panel a kidney-bean shaped lumen is evident, while, in the right panel, multiple cracks or splits in the vessel wall are apparent. In both cases, the angiographic silhouette misrepresented the lumen size.

particularly restenosis. Large scale multi-center trials will likely be required to determine the ability of intravascular imaging to improve assessment of PTCA results. However, is is reasonable to predict that a tomographic technique such as intravascular ultrasound will be more accurate in assessment of the residual cross-sectional area following mechanical interventions that distort the coronary.

In initial studies post-PTCA, we identified some limitations of intravascular ultrasound. Following PTCA, it was often difficult to distinguish therapeutic from pathologic dissection by intravascular ultrasound. In some cases, dissection planes was difficult to differentiate from other sonolucent plaque features such as lipid laden atheromas. We also encountered difficulty in reliably identifying the presence of thrombosis by intravascular ultrasound, primarily because the acoustic properties of intraluminal thrombus are similar to blood.

A catheter exchange following PTCA was required to allow imaging post-procedure, a requisite that impaired optimal utilization of intravascular ultrasound. This procedural requirement diminished the feasibility of performing serial ultrasound imaging after each balloon inflation.

Combination probes

To facilitate the practical application of intravascular ultrasound during PTCA, a combination probe was developed that incorporated both imaging capability and an angioplasty balloon. Thus, imaging could be performed without the necessity for catheter exchange. The initial combination device was based upon the 5.5 F (1.83 mm) imaging array. Although useful, the prototype combination probe incorporated a balloon with a relatively large cross-sectional profile and was therefore suitable only for relatively moderate stenoses in the proximal coronary. Subsequently, an improved low-profile combination device was developed and is currently undergoing initial human testing. This improved device incorporates the 3.5 F, 64 element array and utilizes a balloon with a deflated profile of 0.71 to 0.83 mm for balloon sizes of 2.0 to 3.5 mm. We believe that such devices may well become the "gold standard" for balloon angioplasty in the future.

Coronary ultrasound: current status

Studies published to date demonstrate that coronary intravascular ultrasound is a safe technique for routine evaluation of coronary lumen size and wall morphology in patients admitted for diagnostic or therapeutic catheterization. The tomographic perspective of ultrasound is likely superior to planar methods such as angiography for precise cross-sectional area measurement. Ultrasound measurements of coronary luminal diameter and cross-sectional area may have particular clinical value in eccentrically diseased vessels. Tomographic measurements may also be advantageous when the lumen is distorted by mechanical interventions. However, it must be emphasized that current intravascular ultrasound devices are too large to assess lumina smaller than 1.0 mm.

Detailed images of atherosclerotic coronary plaques are provided by intravascular ultrasound. Intraluminal imaging is a highly sensitive technique for the detection of CAD and frequently demonstrates atherosclerosis at angiographically normal sites. The sensitivity of intraluminal imaging has great potential for research to improve understanding of the relationship between vessel wall anatomy and the pathophysiology of CAD. The morphology of the vessel wall following revascularization may hold important clues to phenomena such as restenosis and abrupt occlusion. Ultrasound assessment of the morphologic characteristics of plaques will also likely prove valuable in the evaluation of atherosclerosis progression or regression, although definitive studies are not yet available.

Intravascular ultrasound technology is still rapidly evolving. Ongoing technical developments will continue to expand the utility of intraluminal imaging. For example, an imaging catheter is under development that incorporates a tip-mounted Doppler flow probe and thereby allows simultaneous cross-sectional area and flow velocity measurements. This device will provide continuous beat-to-beat assessment of coronary blood flow in vivo. Combination imaging and therapy devices have the potential to become the future standard for balloon angioplasty technique. Other technical developments will continue to improve the image quality and utility of intraluminal imaging devices. Accordingly, we believe that intravascular ultrasound will continue to play an expanding role in the diagnosis and therapy of CAD.

References

1. Bom N, Lancee CT, Van Egmond FC. An ultrasonic intracardiac scanner. Ultrasonics 1972; **10**: 72–6.
2. Yock, PG, Johnson EL, Linker DT. Intravascular ultrasound: development and clinical potential. Am J Card Imaging 1988; **2**: 185–93.
3. Pandian NG, Kreis A, Brockway B, et al. Ultrasound angioscopy: real-time, two-dimensional, intraluminal ultrasound imaging of blood vessels. Am J Cardiol 1988; **62**: 493–4.
4. Roelandt JR, Serruys PW, Bom N, Gussenhoven WG, Lancee CT, Ten Hoff H. Intravascular real-time, two-dimensional echocardiography. Int J Card Imaging 1989; **4**: 63–7.
5. Hodgson JM, Graham SP, Savakus AD, et al. Clinical percutaneous imaging of coronary anatomy using an over-the-wire ultrasound catheter system. Int J Card Imaging 1989; **4**: 187–93.
6. Nissen SE, Grines CL, Gurley JC, et al. Application of a new phased-array ultrasound imaging catheter in the assessment of vascular dimensions: in vivo comparison to cineangiography. Circulation 1990; **81**: 660–6.
7. Tobis JM, Mallery J, Mahon D, et al. Intravascular ultrasound imaging of human coronary arteries in vivo. Analysis of tissue characterizations with comparison to in vitro histological specimens. Circulation 1991; **83**: 913–26.
8. Nissen SE, Gurley JC, Grines CL, et al. Intravascular ultrasound assessment of lumen size and wall morphology in normal subjects and coronary artery disease patients. Circulation 84; **3**: 1087–99.
9. Roberts WC, Jones AA. Quantitation of coronary arterial narrowing at necropsy in sudden coronary death. Analysis of 31 patients and comparison with 25 control subjects. Am J Cardiol 1979; **44**: 39–45.
10. Arnett EN, Isner JM, Redwood DR, et al. Coronary artery narrowing in coronary heart disease: comparison of cineangiographic and necropsy findings. Ann Intern Med 1979; **91**: 350–6.
11. Grondin CM, Dydra I, Pasternac A, Campeau L, Bourassa MG, Lesperance J. Discrepancies between cineangiographic and postmortem findings in patients with coronary artery disease and recent myocardial revascularization. Circulation 1974; **49**: 703–8.
12. Blankenhorn DH, Curry PJ. The accuracy of arteriography and ultrasound imaging for atherosclerosis measurement: A review. Arch Pathol Lab Med 1982; **106**: 483–91.
13. Isner JM, Kishel J, Kent KM, Ronan JA jr, Ross AM, Roberts WC. Accuracy of angiographic determination of left main coronary arterial narrowing. Angiographic-histologic correlative analysis in 28 patients. Circulation 1981; **63**: 1056–64.
14. Vlodaver Z, Frech R, van Tassel RA, Edwards JE. Correlation of the antemortem coronary arteriogram and the postmortem specimen. Circulation 1973; **47**: 162–9.
15. Zir LM, Miller SW, Dinsmore RE, Gilbert JP, Hawthorne JW. Interobserver variability in coronary angiography. Circulation 1976; **53**: 627–32.
16. Galbraith JE, Murphy ML, de Soyza N. Coronary angiogram interpretation: Interobserver variability. JAMA 1978; **240**: 2053–6.
17. White CW, Wright CB, Doty DB, et al. Does visual interpretation of the coronary arteriogram predict the physiologic importance of a coronary stenosis? N Engl J Med 1984; **310**: 819–24.
18. Potkin BN, Bartorelli AL, Gessert JM, et al. Coronary artery imaging with intravascular high-frequency ultrasound. Circulation 1990; **81**: 1575–85.

19. Nishimura RA, Edwards WD, Warnes CA, et al. Intravascular ultrasound Imaging: in vitro validation and pathologic correlation. J Am Coll Cardiol 1990; **16**: 145–54.
20. Tobis JM, Mallery JA, Gessert J, et al. Intravascular ultrasound cross-sectional arterial imaging before and after balloon angioplasty in vitro. Circulation 1989; **80**: 873–82.
21. Gussenhoven EJ, Essed CE, Lancee CT, et al. Arterial wall characteristics determined by intravascular ultrasound imaging: an in vitro study. J Am Coll Cardiol 1989; **4**: 947–52.
22. Gurley JC, Nissen SE, Diaz C, Fischer C, O'Conner WN, DeMaria AN. Is the tri-layer arterial appearance an artifact? Differences between in vivo and in vitro intravascular ultrasound. J Am Coll Cardiol 1991; **17** (2 Suppl A): 112A (Abstract).
23. Nissen SE, Gurley JC, Grines CL, Booth DC, Fischer C, DeMaria AN. Coronary atherosclerosis is frequently present at angiographically normal sites: evidence from intravascular ultrasound in man. Circulation 1990; **82** (4 Suppl III): III–459 (Abstract).
24. Nissen SE, Gurley JC, Booth DC, McClure RR, Berk MR, DeMaria AN. Spectrum of intravascular ultrasound findings in atherosclerosis: wall morphology and lumen shape in CAD patients. J Am Coll Cardiol 1991; **17** (2 Suppl A): 93A (Abstract).
25. Nissen SE, Gurley JC, Grines CL, Booth DC, Fischer C, DeMaria AN. Comparison of intravascular ultrasound and angiography in quantitation of coronary dimensions and stenoses in man: impact of lumen eccentricity. Circulation 1990: **82** (4 Suppl III): III–440 (Abstract).
26. Gurley JC, Nissen SE, Booth DC, Grines CL, Grigsby G, DeMaria AN. Evaluation of peripheral vascular diameter and cross-sectional area with a multi-element ultrasonic imaging catheter: correlation with quantitative angiography. J Am Coll Cardiol 1990; **15** (2 Suppl A): 28A (Abstract).
27. Gurley JC, Nissen SE, Grines CL, Booth DC, Fischer C, DeMaria AN. Comparison of intravascular ultrasound and angiography following percutaneous transluminal angioplasty. Circulation 1990; **82** (4 Suppl III): III–72 (Abstract).

PART TWO

QCA: cinefilm versus digital arteriography

4. Quantitative analysis of the cineangiogram: Why bother?

JOHN G. B. MANCINI, PAULA R. WILLIAMSON,
SCOTT F. DEBOE, BERTRAM PITT, JACQUES LESPERANCE
and MARTIAL G. BOURASSA

Summary

Background: Numerous studies have demonstrated that subjective analysis of cineangiograms is highly variable. While this has fostered use of quantitative methods in research projects, clinical utilization is uncommon. Because many clinical decisions in cardiology are based on an evaluation of the cineangiogram, the variability inherent in subjective analyses must also mean that the clinical decisions are subject to inconsistency. Thus, we set out to determine whether quantitative parameters obtainable from the cineangiogram were of prognostic importance. This would provide a more clinically relevant impetus for greater utilization of quantitative methods in practice in addition to the already demonstrated value in providing more reproducible results.

Methods: Baseline cineangiograms of 283 patients with at least 10 years of clinical follow-up were randomly selected from the 3,566 patients in the Coronary Artery Surgery Study Registry and subjected to quantitation of ejection fraction, regional wall motion, regional shape analysis and quantitative coronary arteriography. These parameters were considered in isolation ("quantitative coronary arteriography" and "regional wall function" predictive models), in combination ("quantitative cineangiographic" predictive model) and in combination with subjective angiographic analysis and clinical information such as age and history of prior infarction ("clinical" predictive model). Prognostic indicators of death, infarction, unstable angina and other cardiac syndromes were determined by multiple logistic regression. Event free survival curves based on the various quantitative parameters were also constructed using log-rank testing.

Results: The most important quantitative parameters were the ejection fraction and the percent diameter narrowing of left anterior descending coronary territory stenoses. Regional wall motion provided additional prognostic power beyond that of the ejection fraction in the prediction of lethal myocardial infarction. Regional shape contributed additional power in the prediction of any cardiac event and the need for bypass surgery. Surprisingly, percent diameter stenosis measurements, predominantly of the left anterior

J.H.C. Reiber and P.W. Serruys (eds), Advances in Quantitative Coronary Arteriography, 55–73.

descending were even more frequently of prognostic significance. When quantitative parameters were analyzed in the "clinical" model, the factors of overriding prognostic importance were the ejection fraction and the subjective determination of the number of vessels involved with "significant" stenoses. However, even under these circumstances, quantitative coronary arteriography retained independent prognostic value. This was not the case for any of the regional wall motion or shape parameters. There were no quantitative parameters that predicted the syndrome of unstable angina.

Conclusions: Quantification of the cineangiogram, particularly with respect to the ejection fraction and severity of coronary lesions, provides objective, verifiable and reproducible parameters that are also of prognostic importance. Wider spread use of such methodologies could have the impact of promoting greater consistency in the delivery of cardiac care. Quantitative methodologies provide a clinically important mechanism for establishing greater quality control and accountability of the ever increasing number of catheterization laboratories that have been fostered by the current era of interventional cardiology.

Introduction

The need for quantitative and reproducible measurements of global and regional ventricular function and coronary lesion severity is unquestioned in research arenas because visual estimates of these parameters, especially parameters of lesion severity, are highly variable [1, 2]. While the implications for research are obvious, what is not as readily appreciated is that this same problem must also impart a tremendous degree of variability to major, clinical decisions commonly based on the cineangiogram. Although various quality assurance standards exist for the performance of cardiac catheterization and cineangiography, none exist for the accuracy of the actual clinical data extracted from the cineangiograms. Given the pivotal importance of cineangiography in cardiac clinical decision making, emerging issues of third party reimbursement for self-referred interventional therapy and exploding costs of cardiac care, the issue of verifiable quantitation of the cineangiogram is not merely a pedantic or esoteric one but one that has major implications for the consistent and appropriate delivery of care to cardiac patients. Based on the well documented variability of subjective analyses, one can conclude that decisions based on cineangiographic data are almost capricious. While subjective cineangiographic analysis is often justified on the basis of practicality, this argument pales in the era of digital imaging and the ubiquitous presence of desktop computers. Nevertheless, it is unclear whether quantitative analyses performed on a routine basis would add merely the element of reproducibility to angiographically-based clinical decisions or whether the quantitative parameters are also truly important in predicting the clinical course of patients. This study was undertaken to determine the latter in a group of patients with a decade of clinical follow-up after an initial cineangiogram. The primary purpose was to determine the prognostic importance of quantitative measures of regional wall motion, wall shape and quantitative percent diameter stenosis measurements in a clinically relevant framework.

Methods

296 cineangiograms were randomly selected by investigators at the Montreal Heart Institute from studies of 3,566 patients in the Coronary Artery Surgery Study (CASS) Registry who had at least ten years of clinical follow-up after the initial angiogram [3]. Some patients had follow-up data up to 11.2 years. Clinical information was collated about patient characteristics (sex, age, prior myocardial infarction, bypass surgery or angioplasty, number of diseased vessels, location of stenoses). The number of diseased vessels was determined by the original CASS investigators who considered disease to be present when a visually apparent stenosis estimated to be ≥50% was detected.

Cineangiograms were delivered to the Ann Arbor Veterans Administration Medical Center for quantitative analysis using previously developed and validated methodologies. Cineangiograms were displayed on a Vanguard XR15 Projector interfaced via a video chain to an ADAC 4100C Digital Image Processing Computer (Milpitas, CA). Poorly opacified left ventriculograms or studies lacking a non-post-ectopic beat were excluded from ventricular analysis (13 cases). The largest (end-diastolic) and smallest (end-systolic) ventricular images in the right anterior oblique projection were traced and digitized in a 256×256 matrix and stored. Global ejection fraction was measured using the area-length method [4]. Volumes were not measured due to absence of routinely available calibration grids. Regional wall motion was calculated using the centerline method developed at the University of Washington and previously described in detail [5, 6]. Similarly, regional ventricular shape was measured using a previously described and validated methodology developed at the University of Michigan [7–10]. The optimal threshold values for optimizing sensitivity and specificity of these two regional analysis programs have been previously determined at the University of Michigan [9]. Therefore, all wall motion and shape results were normalized by these previously determined values so that the numerical results could be more easily compared. The wall motion and wall shape parameters are, therefore, reported in "critical value" units. One critical value unit for detection of abnormal wall motion corresponds to -1.1 standard deviations/chord and for detection of shape abnormalities it corresponds to -0.4 standard deviations/point [9].

The most severe focal lesion in each involved vascular territory designated by the CASS investigators was subjected to quantitative analysis using a previously described and validated method developed at the University of

Michigan [11]. The projection showing the lesion in its most severe perspective and without overlapping side branches was digitized, stored and analyzed. Normal and occluded vessels were designated as having 0% and 100% diameter stenoses respectively. Absolute measures of lumen size were not recorded due to lack of information about angiographic catheter size.

Over the term of follow-up, the following complications were recorded: unstable angina, myocardial infarction, congestive heart failure, arrhythmias, syncope, cardiogenic shock, peripheral emboli, stroke and death as well as the cause of death, and need for bypass surgery or angioplasty.

Multiple logistic regression analysis was used to determine independent predictors of adverse events [12]. Four specific models were tested. The first, termed the "clinical model" incorporated both qualitative and quantitative data as well as clinical information such as sex, age, and prior infarction. The second, termed the "quantitative angiography model" incorporated only quantitative parameters of ejection fraction, wall motion, wall shape and stenosis severity. The third, termed the "regional wall function model" incorporated only quantitative parameters of wall motion and shape. The final, termed the "quantitative coronary arteriography model" incorporated only quantitative percent diameter stenosis data. Each of these four models was tested for the prediction of death, cardiac events, any initial cardiac event that proved lethal, sudden death, myocardial infarction, lethal myocardial infarction, congestive heart failure, unstable angina, and bypass surgery. Event-free survival curves were calculated for groups with ejection fractions below 55% and ≥55%, anterior and inferior shape or wall motion indexes ≤−2 and >−2 critical values, and percent diameter stenosis of <70% and ≥70% of the left anterior descending, circumflex and right coronary vascular distributions [12]. Bonferroni adjusted log-rank tests were used to determine the time at which differences in event-free survival curves occurred [13].

Results

Clinical Characteristics: Of the original 296 studies, complete angiographic data was obtained in 283. Table 1 summarizes characteristics of the study group. At entry, ages ranged from 30 to 68 years and ejection fractions ranged between 6 and 80%. When visually identified and quantitated, the least severe left main, left anterior descending, circumflex and right coronary lesions were 50, 41, 41 and 43%, respectively. The most severe left main stenosis was 75% whereas in the other territories total occlusions occurred. Despite a normal mean ejection fraction on the whole, mean regional wall motion and shape indexes were abnormal in this group reflecting the high proportion of patients with prior infarctions (184 of 283). In 6 cases, the exact timing of the first significant cardiac event was unknown. Therefore, all subsequent statistical analyses were based on 277 cases. Quantitative

Table 1. Baseline characteristics of the study group (*n* = 283)

Male	243	
Female	40	
Age (years)	51 ± 8	
Previous MI	184	
# vesel disease:	0	4
	1	85
	2	98
	3	96
Location of stenoses:	IM	4
	LAD	216
	CX	162
	RCA	189
Ejection fraction (%)		52 ± 15
Wall motion (critical values):		
anterior		−1.73 ± 0.99
inferior		−1.87 ± 1.01
Wall shape (critical values):		
anterior		−3.20 ± 2.73
inferior		−1.46 ± 2.63

CX = circumflex bed, LAD = left anterior bed, IM = left main, MI = myocardial infarction, RCA = right coronary artery bed, continuous data presented as mean ± standard deviation.

cineangiographic findings in these patients are further summarized in Table 2.

Table 3 summarizes the clinical events that occurred during follow-up. For purposes of this study, stroke and periperal emboli were considered non-

Table 2. Number of patients with designated quantitative index (*n* = 277)

	Visually	Quantitative diameter stenosis	
	insignificant	<70%	≥70%
IM	273	3	1
LAD	65	68	144
CX	116	50	111
RCA	92	45	140
	>−2 Critical values	≤−2 Critical values	
ANT motion	174	103	
INF motion	148	129	
ANT shape	86	191	
INF shape	140	137	
	≥55%	31–54%	≤30%
EF	143	111	23

Abbreviations as in Table 1.

Table 3. Number of clinical events occurring during follow-up period in 277 patients

Cardiac		Noncardiac	
Unstable angina	85	Stroke	14
Bypass surgery	77	Peripheral embolism	3
Myocardial infarction	66		
Congestive heart failure	37		
Sudden death	25		
Arrhythmias	14		
Ventricular tachycardia	5		
Cardiogenic shock	7		
Coronary angioplasty	1		

cardiac events. 102 patients had an event-free follow-up. In the remaining, the commonest event was the onset of unstable angina in 63 patients (85 occurrences) followed by bypass surgery in 74 patients (77 occurrences) and myocardial infarction in 53 (66 occurrences). The single percutaneous coronary angioplasty reflects the emergence of the technique after the time of patient enrollment and during the course of follow-up.

Tables 4, 5, 6 and 7 summarize the important factors within each model that were predictive of cardiac events and specific cardiac syndromes. The coefficients and *p* values are provided in these tables. Table 8 summarizes all the models and important parameters. Quantitative coronary angiography of all four vascular sites were independently predictive of death (Table 4). In the regional wall function model (Table 5), only the wall motion indexes were predictive, the anterior wall motion moreso than inferior wall motion. However, in the quantitative cineangiography model (Table 6), the ejection fraction was of overriding importance, eliminating all wall function indexes but none of the quantitative percent diameter stenosis variables. The latter were eliminated in the clinical model wherein the predictors in order of importance, were the quantitated ejection fraction, the number of diseased vessels assessed qualitatively and the patient age at entry (Table 7).

Predictors of cardiac events (i.e. of a complicated clinical course) were determined. Quantitative percent diameter stenosis of the left anterior coronary bed, followed by quantitative percent diameter stenosis of the right coronary artery bed were the most important factors in the quantitative coronary arteriography model (Table 4). When regional wall function was considered, the shape of the anterior wall, followed by the shape of the inferior wall were most predictive (Table 5). Regional wall motion was not predictive at all. Moreover, when all quantitative parameters, including ejection fraction, were included in the quantitative cineangiography model, quantitative percent diameter stenosis of the left anterior descending bed and the shape of the inferior wall retained predictive powers that were greater than the ejection fraction (Table 6). Percent diameter stenosis of the right coronary also retained predictive, but less important, power in this

Table 4. Summary of factors predicting clinical outcomes, ranked in order of importance, for the Quantitative Coronary Arteriography Model

	Parameter	Coefficient	p value
Death	%DS CX	1.50	.009
	%DS LAD	1.77	.001
	%DS RCA	1.59	.003
	%DS LM	3.99	.04
Cardiac event	%DS LAD	1.61	.00001
	%DS RCA	1.36	.0005
Lethal cardiac event	%DS LAD	2.56	.00001
	%DS RCA	1.96	.0005
Sudden death	%DS RCA	2.89	.0004
	%DS LAD	3.25	.0004
Myocardial infarction	%DS LM	4.11	.04
	%DS LAD	1.48	.04
Lethal myocardial infarction	%DS LM	13.09	.002
	%DS CX	3.06	.003
	%DS LAD	2.16	.04
Congestive heart failure	%DS RCA	2.41	.003
Unstable angina	–	–	–
Bypass	–	–	–

%DS = percent diameter stenosis, CX = circumflex bed, LAD = left anterior descending bed, LM = left main, RCA = right coronary artery.

analysis. In the clinical model, all wall motion and shape indexes were eliminated leaving the qualitative assessment of the number of vessels involved, the quantitative ejection fraction and the quantitative percent diameter stenosis of the left anterior descending bed (Table 7).

The latter analysis gives an indication of the predictors of a complicated clinical course of a patient. The analysis of lethal cardiac events looks at predictors of a first, major event that proves fatal. That is, the clinical course is uncomplicated but is terminated by a single, lethal cardiac event. In this analysis, when only quantitative arteriography is considered, percent diameter stenosis of the left anterior descending bed, followed by the right coronary artery bed are predictive (Table 4). Indexes of both anterior and inferior wall motion were predictive in the regional wall function model (Table 5). However, when ejection fraction was included in the model, all indexes of regional function were eliminated. The ejection fraction was the most important predictor even though quantitative percent diameter stenosis of each coronary bed also retained independent, predictive power (Table 6). In the clinical model, the overriding factors of importance were the quantitative ejection fraction, the number of diseased vessels as assessed qualitatively

Table 5. Summary of factors predicting clinical outcomes, ranked in order of importance, for the Regional Wall Function Model

	Parameter	Coefficient	*p* value
Death	INF motion	3.04	.00001
	ANT motion	2.83	.0001
Cardiac event	ANT shape	1.90	.0003
	INF shape	1.73	.0006
Lethal cardiac event	ANT motion	3.68	.0001
	INF motion	3.19	.0009
Sudden death	ANT motion	3.29	.02
	INF motion	7.56	.0002
	ANT shape	8.43	.008
Myocardial infarction	–	–	–
Lethal myocardial infarction	ANT motion	3.57	.02
Congestive heart failure	–	–	–
Unstable angina	–	–	–
Bypass	INF shape	2.21	.01

ANT = anterior wall, INF = inferior wall.

and quantitative percent diameter stenosis of the left anterior descending bed (Table 7).

In the prediction of sudden death, it was surprising to note that the presence of a right coronary lesion and its severity were of greater predictive value than quantitation of left anterior descending bed stenoses (Table 4). These, however, were not as important as the ejection fraction (Tables 6 and 7). The regional wall function model in this instance is also interesting (Table 5) because the shape of the anterior wall had residual, independent predictive value.

Myocardial infarction, lethal or not, was not predicted by the ejection fraction under any circumstance (Table 8). Only lethal infarctions were predicted by the severity of anterior wall motion, presumably reflecting a prior anterior infarction. This was not as important as the quantitative severity of arterial lesions, especially the left main. But even quantitative arteriographic measurements of the left main were not as important in the clinical model as were the presence of a left anterior descending stenosis assessed qualitatively (predictive of myocardial infarction) or simply the number of vessels diseased (predictive of a lethal myocardial infarction). Although it was not surprising that development of congestive heart failure was best predicted by the ejection fraction, we did not expect a lack of predictive value of any parameter of regional wall motion or wall shape. Furthermore, the presence of a right coronary artery stenosis in the clinical predictive

Table 6. Summary of factors predicting clinical outcomes, ranked in order of importance, for the Quantitative Angiography Model

	Parameter	Coefficient	*p* value
Death	EF	2.82	.0001
	%DS CX	1.51	.005
	%DS LM	4.06	.03
	%DS LAD	1.52	.02
	%DS RCA	1.42	.02
Cardiac event	%DS LAD	1.59	.00001
	INF shape	1.44	.04
	EF	1.35	.01
	%DS RCA	1.22	.05
Lethal cardiac event	EF	2.56	.00001
	%DS LAD	2.16	.0001
	%DS RCA	1.58	.02
	%DS CX	1.58	.03
	%DS LM	3.81	.04
Sudden death	EF	4.00	.00001
	%DS RCA	2.40	.004
	%DS LAD	2.84	.004
Myocadial infarction	%DS LM	4.11	.04
	%DS LAD	1.48	.04
Lethal myocardial infarction	%DS LM	14.16	.0009
	%DS CX	3.02	.003
	ANT motion	3.67	.02
Congestive heart failure	EF	3.04	.0007
	%DS RCA	2.12	.01
Unstable angina	–	–	
Bypass	INF shape	2.91	.001
	%DS LAD	1.64	.01

EF = ejection fraction, other abbreviations as in Tables 4 and 5.

model and its quantitative severity in both the quantitative cineangiography and coronary arteriography models were unexpected (Table 8).

Unstable angina was the most frequent cardiac event in this study population. Only the clinical model revealed a predictor of this important syndrome (Table 7). The visually detected presence of a significant left anterior descending stenosis, but not its quantitative severity, was the only important variable associated with unstable angina.

Bypass surgery was also a frequent event but few predictors were noted. The number of diseased vessels (clinical model, Table 7) and the shape of the inferior wall (regional wall function and quantitative cineangiography models, Tables 5 and 6, respectively) were predictive. Quantitative arteriography by itself was not contributory (Table 4) but when considered in con-

Table 7. Summary of factors predicting clinical outcomes, ranked in order of importance, for the Clinical Model

	Parameter	Coefficient	p value
Death	EF	3.08	.00001
	# VD	2.03	.0001
	Age	1.05	.009
Cardiac event	# VD	1.53	.00001
	EF	1.48	.001
	%DS LAD	1.28	.02
Lethal cardiac event	EF	2.78	.00001
	# VD	2.16	.0006
	%DS LAD	1.69	.05
Sudden death	EF	4.31	.00001
	ST RCA	6.80	.002
	%DS LAD	2.79	.004
Myocardial infarction	ST LAD	3.88	.002
	%DS LM	3.79	.05
Lethal myocardial infarction	# VD	3.16	.003
	%DS LM	4.86	.02
Congestive heart failure	EF	3.24	.0003
	ST RCA	4.84	.01
Unstable angina	ST LAD	2.24	.02
Bypass	# VD	1.60	.01

ST = presence of stenosis by visual (qualitative) assessment, # VD = number of vessels diseased (i.e. no, single, double or triple vessel disease), all other abbreviations as in Tables 4, 5 and 6.

junction with ejection fraction and regional wall function indexes, the percent diameter stenosis of the left anterior descending was of independent value (Table 6).

Event-free survival curves were constructed for the quantitative indexes and are demonstrated in Figures 1 and 2. The event-free survival curves were significantly different with respect to each of the quantitative parameters except when based on inferior wall motion, or percent diameter stenosis of the right coronary artery. Significant overall differences in the event-free survival curves ($p < .02$) between patients with and without a normal ejection fraction $\geqslant 55\%$ were found but these curves were not significantly different at any specific time point during the follow-up period. The curves based on anterior wall motion were also significantly different ($p < .003$) and, in contrast to the ejection fraction curves, diverged significantly from the fourth year to the end of the follow-up period. Anterior shape abnormalities $\leqslant -2$ critical values were also associated with a worse event-free survival ($p < .004$) and the curves were significantly divergent from the third year on. Inferior wall shape abnormalities also imparted a worse event-free survival ($p < .007$)

Table 8. Summary of factors predicting clinical outcomes, ranked in order of importance, for each model ($n = 277$)

	Model			
	Clinical	Quantitative cineangiography	Regional wall function	Quantitative coronary arteriography
Death	EF # VD Age	EF %DS CX %DS LM %DS LAD %DS RCA	INF motion ANT motion	%DS CX %DS LAD £DS RCA %DS LM
Cardiac event	# VD EF %DS LAD	%DS LAD INF shape EF %DS RCA	ANT shape INF shape	%DS LAD %DS RCA
Lethal cardiac event	EF # VD %DS LAD	EF %DS LAD %DS RCA %DS CX %DS LM	ANT motion INF motion	%DS LAD %DS RCA
Sudden death	EF ST RCA %DS LAD	EF %DS RCA %DS LAD	ANT motion INF motion ANT shape	%DS RCA %DS LAD
Myocardial infarction	ST LAD %DS LM	%DS LM %DS LAD		%DS LM %DS LAD
Lethal myocardial infarction	# VD %DS LM	%DS LM %DS CX ANT motion	ANT motion	%DS LM %DS CX %DS LAD
Congestive heart failure	EF ST RCA	EF %DS RCA		%DS RCA
Unstable angina	ST LAD			
Bypass	# VD	INF shape %DS LAD	INF shape	

Abbreviations as in Tables 4 to 7.

but the curves did not diverge significantly except at the end of the follow-up period. Patients with left anterior descending territory stenoses that were <70% had a better event-free survival than those with more severe stenoses ($p < .002$). These curves diverged significantly from the fourth year on except in year 6 where the curves did not quite reach statistically significant differences. Patients with stenoses of the circumflex that were < 70% also had a better event-free survival ($p < .03$) but these curves were not statistically divergent at any specific time point.

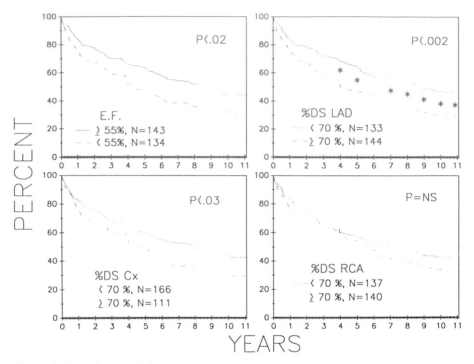

Figure 1. Event-free survival curves were constructed for groups of patients having normal or abnormal quantitative indexes of ejection fraction and percent diameter stenosis of the left anterior descending, circumflex and right coronary arterial beds. N refers to the number of patients with the quantitative index value determined from the baseline angiogram. The y-axis designates the percent of the original number with event-free survival. The x-axis is given in years. Significant overall differences are designated by the *p*-values which are based on log-rank tests. Symbols between curves designate specific time points when the curves are statistically different based on Bonferronni adjustments of the log-rank test. EF = ejection fraction, LAD = left anterior descending, CX = circumflex, RCA = right coronary artery, * = $p < .05$, + = $p < .01$.

Discussion

This study was motivated by a desire to put into perspective several of the currently available quantification methods that are applied to cineangiographic images. While variability of subjective cineangiographic analysis is readily acknowledged, the detrimental effects of this variability on the consistent and appropriate delivery of care is not often considered. Accordingly, we assessed the importance of quantitative cineangiography in a population with at least a decade of well-defined clinical follow-up to determine whether more rigorous measurements are of prognostic power and therefore of value in the clinical arena as well as in research projects. Our a priori expectation was that parameters of ventricular function and shape would be of overriding

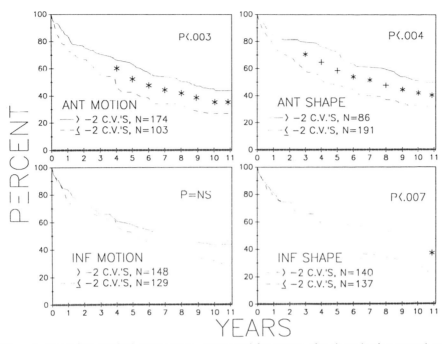

Figure 2. Event-free survival curves were constructed for groups of patients having normal or abnormal quantitative indexes of regional wall motion or regional shape on their baseline ventriculogram. The format is the same as in Figure 1. ANT = anterior, INF = inferior, CV = critical values.

clinical importance and that quantitative coronary arteriography would provide little, if any, prognostic power. But the results of this investigation were not as anticipated. In general, the ejection fraction was the prime determinant of most cardiac syndromes and regional wall motion and shape were of only minor prognostic value in most instances. In contrast, quantitative coronary arteriography was often of independent prognostic value even in the "clinical" and "quantitative cineangiographic" models which incorporated ejection fraction measurements.

The overwhelming importance of ejection fraction measurements is not a new finding [14]. However, it should be recognized that even this easily quantified parameter is not often measured in practice from the cineangiogram. The results of the current investigation provide support for more meticulous measurement of this important parameter during routine studies and suggest that quality assurance testing of the accuracy and reproducibility of the measurement are advisable. It is important to emphasize that the angiographic ejection fraction as measured from a single plane ventriculogram has numerous well recognized limitations especially in the presence of wall motion abnormalities. Such limitations, however, did not override or eliminate the practical and powerful importance of this parameter in this study which included many patients with prior infarctions and wall motion abnormalities.

Despite the importance of the ejection fraction, other factors were also of independent, prognostic importance. Surprisingly, these were generally not related to more detailed or sophisticated measures of regional function or shape. Instead, these were often the quantitative measures of percent diameter stenosis, especially of the left anterior descending coronary bed or the left main coronary artery. This was particularly the case when considering lethal or non-lethal cardiac events, sudden death, and lethal or non-lethal myocardial infarction. In fact, in the latter case, the ejection fraction was of no prognostic value.

Several specific clinical syndromes deserve special comment. The syndrome of sudden death was most closely related to ejection fraction as well as the presence of significant coronary disease. The "wall function" model, which excluded clinical characteristics, qualitative parameters and quantitative coronary arteriographic parameters, demonstrated that, the shape of the anterior wall was of independent prognostic value. Given the large number of patients in this cohort with prior infarctions, this finding probably reflects the presence of anterior aneurysm formation which may be the site of genesis of ventricular arrhythmia, a putative cause of this syndrome [15]. The quantitative regional curvature analysis method used in this study may be useful in defining a very high risk group of patients with depressed ejection fraction and coronary disease who also have a quantifiable ventricular aneurysm of the anterior wall. Such a group might be most suitable for determining in the most cost effect way the efficacy of new drugs or interventions that may be useful in preventing this syndrome.

The syndrome of unstable angina is the current subject of many investigations to determine pathogenetic mechanisms and effective therapies [16, 17]. It is extremely interesting to note that few predictors of this syndrome were found in our analysis. Specifically, this study confirms prior reports noting the lack of utility of quantitative measures of relative or absolute stenosis severity in predicting this syndrome. The important observations of Ambrose and coworkers [18, 19] suggest that lesion complexity may be of overriding importance in this syndrome and that such complexity provides a substrate for, or is a consequence of, thrombotic mechanisms associated with spontaneous plaque rupture and fissuring. Algorithms for more rigorously and mathematically quantitating lesion roughness are being undertaken in our laboratory and appear to provide quantitative parameters that are associated with unstable angina [20]. This methodology was not available during the course of the current study nor could it be applied due to lack of catheter images used to correct for intrinsic image noise. However, the lack of simple prognostic indicators of the occurrence of unstable angina, as corroborated in this study, mandate further exploration of these methods and a determination of their value relative to qualitative measures of lesion morphology.

Bypass surgery was a common event in this group of patients with chronic stable angina at the outset of the observation period. It is not surprising that this therapy was predicted by both the number of diseased vessels and the percent diameter stenosis of left anterior descending lesions. We did not expect, however, that the shape of the inferior wall would be of predictive value and do not have an explanation for this finding. Whether this anatomical configuration is a precursor of worsening symptoms and medically refractory angina or is merely a relection of the extent and severity of both the underlying coronary disease and depressed ventricular function cannot be determined with certainty.

A recent study has made the provocative observation that severe lesions are often not the sites of subsequent occlusion and causation of myocardial infarctions [21]. Others have shown an association between lesion severity and infarction [22]. The current study suggests that over a long follow-up period, the quantitative severity of coronary lesions, especially of the left main or left anterior descending, is indeed predictive of infarction. Whether these severe lesions are actually the sites of occlusion leading to infarction in the current study group cannot be established with certainty because follow-up angiograms were not available. One can only conclude that the presence of severe lesions was a marker of a higher risk of subsequent infarction. The observations underscore the need for additional, detailed studies of which types of stenoses are at highest risk of progressing or occluding.

We chose to study four prognostic models to take into account different degrees of integration of information and to assess the most important parameters within the context of each of the quantitative software programs. The quantitative angiographic model is relevant to the way in which many studies of new devices are undertaken. That is, the focus is only on the arteries themselves. In these analyses, the percent diameter stenosis of the left anterior descending, while not always the most important in predicting the clinical course, was commonly invoked. The regional function model mimics many studies of thrombolysis which focus on segmental effects and minimize attention to either arteriographic findings or overall ejection fraction measurements. In these analyses, the most consistently found factor was the quantitative anterior wall motion analysis. It is noteworthy, however, that shape parameters, especially of the anterior wall, are of overriding or of complementary value in prediction of cardiac events, sudden death and bypass surgery. In addition, since these parameters were often eliminated in the "clinical" and "quantitative cineagiographic" models, one might question the use of isolated measures of wall function as surrogate end points in many clinical trials. Our results suggest that these parameters should not be evaluated separate from the quantitative coronary arteriographic findings and support the use of overall ejection fraction results in such studies [23]. Importantly, it has been demonstrated in studies of thrombolysis that patency of an infarct-related artery confers a better outcome [24]. Our study is supportive of this concept in that the quantitative severity of coronary lesions is of definite prognostic importance.

The "clinical" model was chosen because it approximates most closely the cognitive aspects of clinical decision making that take into account many factors influencing the interpretation of test results [25]. Thus, this model included patient age, sex, the presence of prior infarction and subjective assessments of the number of vessels with "significant" stenoses, their number and location. These are not the only factors and perhaps not even the main factors that a practicing cardiologist would use to make an overall clinical assessment of risk and a clinical decision regarding therapy. For example, results of exercise testing and especially functional radionuclide studies commonly sway clinical decisions and such results were not incorporated into this study. Our best effort was made to mimic the "clinical" setting by using all the information that was readily available to us. It is also worth emphasizing that all of these patients had chronic, stable angina at the time of the initial cineangiogram. In this context, it is still impressive and even reassuring that the ejection fraction and the number of diseased vessels are the most consistent and important determinants of adverse clinical outcomes. Even so, quantitative coronary arteriography, in contrast to regional wall motion or shape, provided additional, independent prognostic power in numerous clinical syndromes.

The "quantitative cineangiography" model is the one that is most generalizable to cardiac practice because such measurements could be performed by virtually any laboratory. This analysis showed that although the ejection fraction was of overriding importance in the prediction of 4 of the 9 clinical syndromes, quantitative arteriography was also commonly of independent prognostic importance. Indeed, quantitative arteriography was of even greater importance in predicting cardiac events, and lethal or non-lethal myocardial infarction than was the ejection fraction. Even regional motion, predictive of lethal myocardial infarction, and regional shape parameters, predictive of cardiac events and bypass surgery, contributed independent prognostic value. The only exception to these general findings was in the case of unstable angina which, as discussed earlier, could not be predicted from these simple quantitative efforts.

The event-free survival curves serve to underscore these findings. All long-term follow-up of groups dichotomized with respect to these quantitative parameters showed significant differences in event-free survival over the decade of follow-up except in the case of percent diameter stenosis of the right coronary artery and inferior wall motion quantitation. The most highly divergent curves were associated with anterior shape analysis, anterior wall motion analysis and percent diameter stenosis of the left anterior descending coronary artery territory. Prognosis was statistically but less dramatically dependent on inferior shape as well.

The percent diameter stenosis parameter, even measured meticulously, has been roundly criticized in recent years based on recognition of the diffuse nature of atherosclerosis and the resultant difficulty in selecting normal reference diameters [26], the fact that such measurements do not take into account other important morphological features such as length or entrance and exit angles [27], the realization that many stenoses are eccentric and cannot be accurately represented by a single plane measurement [28], the new knowledge that remodelling and dilatation of vessels occurs in response to atherosclerosis [29, 30] and the imprecise relation between the measurement and other directly measured indexes of functional stenosis severity [31, 32]. While all of these arguments are cogent, this study suggests that percent diameter stenosis, much like the ejection fraction with its well recognized limitations, is still of tremendous prognostic importance when measured quantitatively and is an appropriate parameter upon which to base routine clinical judgments [25]. Much greater experience and long-term follow-up analyses, such as the one presented in this study, will need to be undertaken with the alternative proposed indexes of stenosis severity before replacing the simple quantification of percent diameter stenosis.

The final and most important implication of this study is that the quantification of the cineangiogram and the improvement in reproducibility afforded by quantitative methods are not merely subjects of pedantic or esoteric value restricted to research projects. The parameters are truly of critical prognostic importance. This study, therefore, provides perhaps the most compelling and most clinically relevant reason to promote the use of quantitative and verifiable methods in cardiac catheterization laboratories. The results suggest that quality assurance efforts to ensure accuracy and reproducibility of cineangiographic results should be undertaken. It is anticipated that such efforts would help make more uniform the angiographically based clinical decisions that are currently being made on an almost capricious basis using subjective analysis. Self imposition by the cardiology community of higher diagnostic standards are to be encouraged and should be preferred over involvement of governmental, licensing or insurance agencies who might impose such standards in an overly onerous and counterproductive fashion.

Acknowledgements

This chapter is adapted from a paper originally published in the American Journal of Cardiology, April 15, 1992. This study was supported by the National Institutes of Health, Bethesda, Maryland, RO1HL36813

References

1. Detre KM, Wright E, Murphy ML, Takaro T. Observer agreement in evaluating coronary angiograms. Circulation 1975; **52**: 979–86.

2. Zir LM, Miller SW, Dinsmore RE, Gilbert JP, Harthorne JW. Interobserver variability in coronary arteriography. Circulation 1976; **53**: 627–32.
3. Principal Investigators of CASS and their associates. The National Heart, Lung and Blood Institute Coronary Artery Surgery Study. A multicenter comparison of the effects of randomized and surgical treatment of mildly symptomatic patients with coronary artery disease, and a registry of consecutive patients undergoing coronary angiography. Circulation 1981; **63**: I1–81.
4. Sandler H, Dodge HT. The use of single plane angiocardiograms for the calculation of left ventricular volume in man. Am Heart J 1968; **75**: 325–34.
5. Bolson EL, Kliman S, Sheehan FH, Dodge HT. Left ventricular segmental wall motion: a new method using local direction information. Comput Cardiol 1980; 245–8.
6. Mancini GBJ, Hodgson JM, Legrand V, et al. Quantitative assessment of global and regional left ventricular function with low-contrast dose digital subtraction ventriculography. Chest 1985; **87**: 598–602.
7. Mancini GBJ, LeFree MT, Vogel RA. Curvature analysis of normal ventriculograms: Fundamental framework for the assessment of shape changes in man. Comput Cardiol 1985; 141–4.
8. Mancini GBJ, DeBoe SF, Anselmo E, Simon SB, LeFree MT, Vogel RA. Quantitative regional curvature analysis: an application of shape determination for the assessment of segmental function in man. Am Heart J 1987; **113**: 326–34.
9. Mancini GBJ, DeBoe SF, Anselmo E, LeFree MT. A comparison of traditional wall motion assessment and quantitative shape analysis: a new method for characterizing ventricular function in man. Am Heart J 1987; **114**: 1183–91.
10. Mancini GBJ, DeBoe SF, McGillem MJ, Bates ER. Quantitative regional curvature analysis: a prospective evaluation of ventricular shape and wall motion measurements. Am Heart J 1988; **116**: 1616–21.
11. Mancini GBJ, Simon SB, McGillem MJ, LeFree MT, Friedman HZ, Vogel RA. Automated quantitative coronary arteriography: In-vivo morphologic and physiologic validation of a rapid digital angiographic method. Circulation 1987; **75**: 452–60. [Published erratum appears in Circulation 1987; **75**: 1199].
12. Mathews DE, Farewell VT. Using and understanding medical statistics. 2nd rev. ed. Basel: Karger 1988: 156–66.
13. Neter J, Wasserman W. Applied linear statistical models: regression, analysis of variance, and experimental designs. Homewood, Ill: R.D. Irwin, 1974: 730–4.
14. Multicenter Post-infarction Research Group. Risk stratification and survival after myocardial infarction. N Engl J Med 1983; **309**: 321–36.
15. Weaver WD, Lorch GS, Alvarez HA, Cobb LA. Angiographic findings and prognostic indicators in patients resuscitated from sudden cardiac death. Circulation 1976; **54**: 895–900.
16. Fuster V, Badimon L, Cohen M, Ambrose JA, Badimon JJ, Chesebro J. Insights into the pathogenesis of acute ischemic syndromes. Circulation 1988; **77**: 1213–20.
17. Theroux P, Ouimet H, McCans J, et al. Aspirin, heparin, or both to treat acute unstable angina. N Engl J Med 1988; 319: 1105–11. Comment in: N Eng J Med 1989; **320**: 1014–5.
18. Ambrose JA, Winters SL, Stern A, et al. Angiographic morphology and the pathogenesis of unstable angina pectoris. J Am Coll Cardiol 1985; **5**: 609–16.
19. Ambrose JA, Hjemdahl-Mosen CE, Borrico S, Gorlin R, Fuster V. Angiographic demonstration of a common link between unstable angina pectoris and non-Q wave acute myocardial infarction. Am J Cardiol 1988; **61**: 244–7.
20. Kalbfleisch SJ, McGillem MJ, Simon SB, DeBoe SF, Pinto IMF, Mancini GBJ. Automated quantitation of indexes of coronary lesion complexity. Comparison between patients with stable and unstable angina. Circulation 1990; **82**: 439–47.
21. Little WC, Constantinescu M, Applegate RJ, et al. Can coronary angiography predict the site of a subsequent myocardial infarction in patients with mild-to-moderate coronary artery disease? Circulation 1988; **78**: 1157–66.

22. Ellis S, Alderman EL, Cain K, Wright A, Bourassa M, Fisher L. Morphology of left anterior descending coronary territory lesions as a predictor of anterior myocardial infarction: a CASS Registry Study. J Am Coll Cardiol 1989; **13**: 1481–91.
23. White HD. Relation of thrombolysis during acute myocardial infarction to left ventricular function and mortality. Am J Cardiol 1990; **66**: 92–5.
24. Ritchie JL, Cerqueira M, Maynard C, Davis K, Kennedy JW. Ventricular function and infarct size: the Western Washington Intravenous Streptokinase in Myocardial Infarction Trial. J Am Coll Cardiol 1988; **11**: 689–97.
25. Klocke FJ. Cognition in the era of technology: "Seeking the shades of gray." J Am Coll Cardiol 1990; **16**: 763–9.
26. Vlodaver Z, Frech R, Van Tassel RA, Edwards JE. Correlation of antemortem coronary arteriogram and the postmortem specimen. Circulation 1973; **47**: 162–9.
27. Kirkeeide RL, Gould KL, Parsel L. Assessment of coronary stenoses by myocardial perfusion imaging during pharmacologic coronary vasodilation. VII. Validation of coronary flow reserve as a single integrated functional measure of stenosis severity reflecting all its geometric dimensions. J Am Coll Cardiol 1986; **7**: 103–13.
28. Arnett EN, Isner JM, Redwood DR, et al. Coronary artery narrowing in coronary heart disease: comparison of cineangiographic and necropsy findings. Ann Intern Med 1979; **91**: 350–6.
29. Glagov S, Weisenberg E, Zarins CK, Stankunavicius R, Kolettis GJ. Compensatory enlargement of human atherosclerotic coronary arteries. N Engl J Med 1987; **316**: 1371–5.
30. Stiel GM, Stiel LSG, Schofer J, Donath K, Mathey DG. Impact of compensatory enlargement of atherosclerotic coronary arteries on angiographic assessment of coronary artery disease. Circulation 1989; **80**: 1603–9.
31. Legrand V, Mancini GBJ, Bates ER, Hodgson JM, Gross MD, Vogel RA. Comparative study of coronary flow reserve, coronary anatomy and results of radionuclide exercise tests in patients with coronary artery disease. J Am Coll Cardiol 1986; **8**: 1022–32.
32. White CW, Wright CB, Doty DB, et al. Does visual interpretation of the coronary arteriogram predict the physiologic importance of a coronary stenosis? N Engl J Med 1984; **310**: 819–24.

5. Quantitative coronary arteriography: equipment and technical requirements

JOHAN H.C. REIBER, PIETER M.J. VAN DER ZWET, CRAIG D. VON LAND, GERHARD KONING, BERT VAN MEURS, BEERT BUIS and AD E. VAN VOORTHUISEN

Summary

In the first part of this chapter the requirements for modern X-ray systems suitable for coronary arteriography are defined. It may be concluded that all modern X-ray systems from the different vendors satisfy the basic requirements for adequate coronary arteriography, although for some applications or institutions small but relevant differences do exist. Secondly, an overview of the currently most widely used digital cardiac imaging systems is presented. On the basis of the data presented, the following conclusions can be drawn: 1) all reviewed systems allow image acquisition at 25 or 30 frames/s at the 512^2 matrix size or even 1024^2 size; 2) sufficient real-time disk space can nowadays be made available to store all the pictorial information acquired in a catheterization laboratory during a single day; and 3) a universal long-term storage medium (archival of the data) with the same degree of transportability, durability and cost of cinefilm is not yet available. In the third part of this chapter the state-of-the-art analytical software packages for quantitative digital (Philips, DCI/ACA-package) and cine (MEDIS, CMS software) coronary arteriography are described and preliminary validation results presented. It has been shown for both approaches that by virtue of modifications in the edge detection software to correct for the limited resolution of the X-ray imaging chain, vessel sizes down to 0.66 mm can be measured accurately and precisely. Also, inter- and intra-observer variability of absolute obstruction dimensions with the ACA-package were found to be equal to 0.11 mm and 0.10 mm, respectively. This means that analytical techniques are now available to the angiographer for the objective assessment of the optimal choice of recanalization devices and for the instantaneous assessment of the effects of such recanalization procedures during the cardiac catheterization based an on-line acquired digital data. Finally, for the off-line assessment of the morphology of coronary vessels for multi-center, longitudinal coronary research studies on the basis of cinefilm, a robust quantitative coronary arteriographic software package is available as well.

J.H.C. Reiber and P.W. Serruys (eds), Advances in Quantitative Coronary Arteriography, 75–111.

Introduction

Since the first papers on quantitative coronary arteriography (QCA) were published in 1977 and 1978, this field has grown substantially and will continue to do so in the coming years [1, 2]. Two major clinical developments have stimulated this growth. First of all, the exponential rise in interventional catheterization procedures following the first coronary balloon dilatation (PTCA) by Andreas Grüntzig in 1979 [3]. Since that time, PTCA has been established as a routine revascularization procedure with a known restenosis rate of approximately 33%. Many other new approaches have been invented since then, including thrombolysis in the acute myocardial situation with various pharmacological agents [4, 5], and the use of various recanalization devices, such as stents [6–9], mechanical atherectomy devices [10–12], lasers [13–16], spark erosion techniques [17], etc. To study the efficacy, restenosis rates and other limitations of these approaches, carefully acquired coronary arteriographic data pre- and immediate post-intervention as well as at follow-up need to be interpreted in great detail [18]. In this book various chapters have been devoted to descriptions of the basic principles of many of these devices, to the currently obtained results and to discussions about the expected areas of application by experts in the field. Secondly, there has been an enormous growth in the development and use of pharmacological drugs directed at the regression or no-growth of existing coronary artery disease or the delay in the formation of new lesions [19–21]. These approaches require the precise comparison of the arterial dimensions in a control group versus those in a treated group studied over a long period of time (typically 2–3 years). Also for this particularly exciting field, the basic principles and results from several of the most well-known QCA intervention studies have been described in this book by their principal investigators.

It has been well accepted that the conventional visual interpretation of coronary arteriograms is no longer acceptable to study the efficacy and limitations of all these different intervention procedures [22]. The results should be evaluated in an objective and reproducible manner on the basis of absolute parameters describing accurately the baseline and subsequent changes in coronary morphology.

The sample size of the number of patients that need to be investigated to demonstrate a certain effect by a proposed drug regimen is proportional to the variability of the measurement technique divided by the number of years between the arteriograms squared [23]. From a view-point of the population size, duration and cost-effectiveness of a study, it is therefore of great importance to minimize the variability of the arteriographic data acquisition and computer analysis procedures.

In parallel to and partly triggered by these clinical developments, there has been a significant progress in X-ray imaging technology. Image quality is continually improving due to the availability of higher quality X-ray sources, image intensifiers, TV chains, the use of pulsed fluoroscopy, and real-time image enhancement. It is now also possible to store the dynamic pictorial information on-line in digital format at relatively high spatial and temporal resolution [24, 25]. The application of gap filling techniques allows a reduction in the acquisition frame rates with a concommitant reduction in X-ray radiation dose. Quantitative data on coronary arterial dimensions can now be made available at the time of the catheterization procedure (on-line) measured directly from digitally acquired arteriograms [26–28].

Cinefilm-based analysis systems have also followed the rapid changes in computer technology. There has been a definite shift from the more traditional PDP and Vax computers to workstations and very powerful personal computers (PC's), characterized by decreased cost and highly increased performance [29]. In addition, major advances have taken place in the development of quantitative coronary arteriographic software packages. Progress has been made towards more routinely applicable user-interfaces, more robustness of the software itself coupled with a higher degree of automation (less user interaction) and reproducibility in the derivation of the clinically relevant parameters [30].

In this chapter an overview will be given on the currently available X-ray technology and the latest digital systems for cardiac angiography; in addition, the state of the art in digital and cinefilm-based quantitative analysis approaches will be presented.

Requirements X-ray systems

It is fair to say that all modern X-ray systems from the different vendors satisfy the basic requirements for adequate coronary arteriography, although for some applications or institutions relevant differences do exist [31]. Any system should allow recordings in standard right and left anterior oblique positions, as well as cranial and caudal angulations, which are of particular relevance for the modern intervention procedures. This should be achieved by independent rotation and angulation of the stand on which the X-ray source and image intensifier are mounted. On older X-ray systems, the rotation was achieved by actual rotation of the patient table; however, this is a much more cumbersome and therefore less practical procedure.

For the majority of the applications, single-plane X-ray systems suffice. On the other hand, there are a number of advantages in using biplane systems, among others: 1) it reduces the amount of contrast material necessary for a particular investigation, since two projections are obtained simultaneously. This is particularly important in patients in unstable hemodynamic situation and in patients with impaired renal function; 2) shorter procedure times in the hands of angiographers who are experienced in the use of biplane systems; and 3) in catheter interventions simultaneous biplane acquisition may facilitate the positioning of the intervention devices. Disadvantages of biplane systems include the significantly higher price, and the fact that the angiographer has less access to the patient. It requires considerable training and a mental capability to combine the images of a biplane system into a three-dimensional representation to make optimal use of the biplane configuration. If these requirements are not fulfilled, use of a biplane system may actually lead to deterioration of the overall diagnostic information.

There is no doubt that biplane imaging systems are preferred for clinical research studies; in these cases the simultaneously acquired information from two views can be combined into a pseudo three-dimensional calculation of the derived parameters, such as left ventricular volume, the severity of coronary stenoses, etc. This means that for institutions with two or more catheterization laboratories and with an interest in research studies, one laboratory should be a biplane laboratory and the others could be single plane. In pediatric cardiology, biplane systems are used exclusively because of the contrast dye aspect.

Nowadays, multi-mode image intensifiers are widely available. For left ventriculography the 7″ (17.8 cm) or 9″ (22.9 cm) mode is to be preferred, while for diagnostic coronary arteriography a good choice is the 7″ image mode. A small field such as 6″ (15 cm) requires more panning to visualize the entire coronary tree. However, panning should be discouraged during the first three to four cardiac cycles after the contrast administration, as frames suitable for QCA are usually selected in this time period. When the distal portion of the coronary tree needs to be viewed, panning is allowed during the subsequent cardiac cycles. For intervention studies, a 5″ (12.5 cm) image mode is a valuable asset, allowing a magnified presentation of the coronary segment studied. Consequently, a triple mode 5″/7″/9″-image intensifier should be a good compromise if interventional and diagnostic procedures need to be carried out on one system.

Larger multiple mode input screens are also currently available. If, for logistic reasons, the equipment for coronary arteriography should also be used for other vascular studies, this may be an acceptable choice; however, these X-ray systems are cumbersome to use because of their dimensions. Thus far, clinical experience with modern large size systems for coronary arteriography is very limited.

Older image intensifiers show significant geometric distortion at the edges of the images, particularly in the largest image-mode – the so-called pincushion distortion [29]. Over the last several years, improvements in the quality of the image intensifiers have resulted in a much lower degree of image distortion. The geometric distortion can be assessed by acquiring a cm-grid held against the input screen of the image intensifier; this needs to be done only once as long as no major service procedures on the X-ray system have been carried out [32]. Onnasch et al. and Solzbach et al. have demonstrated that the distortion is rotation dependent due to the earth magnetic field [33, 34]. If the additional errors are small, one does not need to worry about this rotational dependency; otherwise, the correction vector data have to be established for individual angiographic views which would make it rather cumbersome. More research is necessary at this point in time to come up with a definite solution for this particular problem. Therefore, for intervention studies in which the arterial dimensions are to be compared in identical views, it seems acceptable not to correct for pincushion distortion, until this rotation dependency has been studied in more detail. Otherwise, if one would apply the correction data as acquired in the standard AP-view to another arteriographic view, one may introduce more artefacts than correct for any distortion present.

The growing importance of intervention studies, demanding uncompromisingly good image quality, requires a high performance of the X-ray tubes particularly with respect to the heat management [24]. Even with fluoroscopy the requirement for high image quality during the catheterization procedure using the high tube current technique, results in a significant thermal loading. When cineruns have to be made with a tube that is already hot, many X-ray tubes with barely adequate specifications are brought close to the limits of their loadability, particularly when several runs are made in rapid succession. This may lead to inconveniently long waiting times for the tube to cool down. An X-ray source for a busy interventional laboratory should offer the following facilities: 1) high continuous load; 2) virtually unlimited series length; 3) a steep cooling curve; 4) short waiting times; and 5) grid switch (for pulsed fluoroscopy). In addition, the X-ray tube should also be virtually noiseless. Modern X-ray tubes satisfy such requirements by virtue of large anode discs with extremely efficient heat radiation and a high heat storage capacity. In addition, new types of bearings with liquid metal lubrication permit direct cooling of the rotation anode. Such tubes are available with small and medium focal spot sizes, for example 0.5/0.8 mm.

Radiation exposure to the laboratory personnel is an important factor, particularly with recanalization procedures which require a higher average X-ray time than do conventional diagnostic procedures. Lowering the frame speed has a direct, although nonlinear relation with the total radiation exposure; the nonlinearity comes from the fact that the radiation contribution due to fluoroscopy is not influenced by the frame rate. Frame speeds as low as 12.5/15 frames/s, in conjunction with gap filling techniques have shown promising results and merit further evaluation. Using a system with optimal image quality in itself also limits the radiation dose, in the sense that only a limited number of views are required for clinical decision making. Among others this effect has played a role with the introduction of pulsed fluoroscopy.

Minimizing radiation dose is of course a matter of extreme importance; however, the X-ray flux should not be decreased to the extent that the image quality and thus the ability to obtain reliable quantitative measurements and to take the appropriate clinical decisions are compromized.

Digital cardiac imaging

Digital imaging has considerably improved the quality of the fluoroscopic and radiographic video images, which facilitates the interpretation of arteriographic findings during catheterization; in addition, options like "road mapping", image subtraction, etc. are available. At present, digital recordings cannot replace film recordings, mostly because of the lack of a practical and universally available long-term storage medium with the same degree of transportability, durability and cost of cinefilm, but we envisage that this will change in the next five to ten years [35]. A personal, philosophical look on and some predictions for catheterization laboratories in the 1990's was recently given by C.J. Pepine [36]. In general terms, expectations are towards high-definition systems, recording directly to solid-state memory using fluoroscopic techniques, increased resolution at reduced noise and enhanced contrast, larger sizes of the image intensifiers and of course, filmless laboratories. At this point in time a few laboratories have indeed done away with cinefilm, a trend that will increase in the coming years. However, this will limit the opportunities of such laboratories at the present time to participate in longitudinal, multi-center intervention studies for the reasons mentioned above. It is unacceptable to provide super-VHS analog video recordings for quantitative coronary analysis for the following reasons: 1) a video recorder provides in still frame mode only one of the two interlaced video fields, thereby reducing the vertical resolution by a factor of two; 2) the limited signal/noise ratio of these recorders; and 3) the images recorded from a digital imaging system represent processed (image enhanced) data, not the original information. One solution to this problem could be to store the angiographic runs on a digital streamer tape and to interface such tape streamer to the quantitative angiographic workstation. However, since the manufacturers of the digital cardiac systems have not yet standardized on the tape streamers, this would require developing tape streamer interfaces for the individual digital systems. Another limitation of the current generations of tape streamers is the low transfer rate on the order of 6 frames/s.

Recent developments in digital cardiac imaging have been directed towards the development and implementation of analytical software packages which allow quantitative measurements on-line during the catheterization procedure from the video digitized images [28, 37]. By this approach, the system will function as a tool providing the cardiologist with quantitative data useful for the selection of the appropriate sizes of recanalization devices (e.g. intracoronary balloons, stents, atherectomy catheters, lasers, spark erosion catheters, etc.). In addition, the effect of an intervention (e.g. PTCA) can be assessed directly during the procedure; the angiographer can continue with the procedure until a quantitatively assessed acceptable result in terms of morphology and/or function has been obtained. Therefore, this approach is particularly useful for diagnostic and/or therapeutic decision making during the catheterization procedure. The digital systems are characterized by a high density resolution (256 levels – 8 bits, or 4096 levels – 12 bits) and in principle a linear transfer function of the imaging chain from the output of the image intensifier to the brightness levels in the digitized images. In most systems the linear transfer function has been modified into a well-defined nonlinear function (socalled white compression) to achieve a better image display quality, and to obtain an almost linear relation between the contrast concentrations in the body and the brightness levels in the digital images, which makes this approach theoretically more suitable for densitometric analysis than the conventional cinefilm approach. Matrix size of the digital images is usually 512^2 pixels; further details will be given in the following section.

As the terms on-line, off-line, etc. in general have been used rather loosely, it is appropriate here to define these more accurately. The ultimate requirements of the hardware and software are met in the *on-line* situation, where quantitative results must become available immediately after the acquisition of a coronary arteriogram in a particular angiographic view with the patient still on the table. *Postprocessing* refers to the situation that analysis of the image data takes place after the complete cardiac catheterization has been finished, usually after the patient has left the catheterization laboratory; however, at that time the image data are still available on the real-time harddisk of the system. Of course, processing times are not so critical anymore in this situation. We would define *reviewing* as the processing of a previously performed patient study which is not available anymore on the real-time disk of the system, and therefore has to be recovered from long-term mass storage into the imaging system. Finally, *off-line* is applicable in situations where the image data are processed on another workstation, which has no direct link to the digital imaging system or which has been interfaced to the digital imaging system via a computer network (e.g. Ethernet) allowing the transmission of selected images. Such off-line systems are typically based on either microcomputers or workstations. The relevant single or sequences of images can be transferred to the analysis system via digital tapes or the computer network, or selected cineframes can be acquired via a cine-projection system and analog-to-digital conversion.

Overview of digital cardiac imaging systems

In Table 1 an overview is given of the most relevant characteristics of the most widely used modern integrated or add-on digital imaging systems as of June 1991. These data were obtained from five manufacturers (ADAC, General Electric CGR (GE CGR), Philips, Siemens and Toshiba), by having a corresponding questionnaire filled in by representatives from these companies. The names of the various digital systems are given under item 1 of Table 1. Philips has now two versions, the DCI-S which is based on a 80286–processor and the new DCI-SX using a 80486–processor. In the following paragraphs all the details will be discussed.

To quantitate the coronary morphology, the minimal requirement for image acquisition must be 512^2 matrices at a rate of 25 frames/s (Europe) or 30 frames/s (USA) with a density resolution of minimally 8 bits. In addition, pulsed X-ray radiation should be used to minimize motion blur in

Table 1. Image acquisition/digitization on-line digital cardiac systems

	ADAC	General Electric CGR
1. Name of Digital Cardiac System	DPS 4100 Plus	DXC-Hiline
2. Limitations in matrix acquisition – Matrix size (pixels)	256^2 512^2 1024^2	512^2
– Max. frame rate in frames/s (f/s) (X-ray pulse width)	60/50 f/s 256^2 (1–20 ms) 30/25 f/s 512^2 (1–20 ms) 7.5/6.25 f/s 1024^2 (1–20 ms)	30/25 f/s (<10 ms)
– Density resolution	8 bits	8 bits
3. Type video camera	DTV 4114	Advantx-VIC
Size video tube (inch)	1 inch	1 inch
Interlaced or progressive (noninterlaced) scanning mode	interlaced 625/1249 lines; progressive scan mode 625/1249; Multiscan	progressive
4. *Image storage* How many images can be stored on the real-time disk(s) of the system and at what matrix size?	2700/1024^2 10800/512^2 43200/256^2 with 4 real-time disks each of 889 Mbyte; uncompressed data	basic: 12000 (512^2) option: 24000 (512^2); data compressed by an average factor of 3 (range 2–4.6)
How many images can be stored in the semi-conductor memory of the system, and at what matrix size?	8 images (512^2) in ref memory	12 MB semi-conductor memory (4MB for CPU, 8MB for image processor); data stored directly to disk.
5. *Long-term storage* Which medium and system do you propose for long-term storage of the data	1) digital optical disk; transfer rate; 2 f/s; 2) VLDS-tape (5.2 GByte); frame rates: 8 f/s plus verification; 16 f/s without verification; no data compression 3) analog optical disk.	8 mm DAT tape; up to 50000 images per tape, $512^2 \times 8$ bits; transfer rate: 5 f/s compressed data; tape price <$30.

Table 1. Continued

Philips	Siemens	Toshiba
DCI-S (80286-based) DCI-SX (80486-based)	HICOR	DFP-60A
512^2	1024^2	256×512 (v × h) 512^2 1024^2
60/50 f/s 512^2 (3–8 ms); 2 × 30/25 f/s biplane	30/25 f/s (max. 8 ms)	60/50f/s 512×256 (0.3–8 ms) 30/25 f/s 512^2 (0.3–8 ms) 7.5/6.25 f/s 1024^2 (0.3–8 ms)
8 bits	8 bits	12 bits
Plumbicon	Diode Gun	Diode Gun Saticon
1 and 2 inch	1 inch	1 inch
progressive	progressive	progressive and interlaced
DCI-S 12000 (512^2) with 4 real-time disks each of 850 Mbyte (un- compressed data); with 2 : 1 compression max. 24000 images (512^2). *DCI-SX* 48000 (512^2) with 4 : 1 data compression.	*Monoplane* basic: 4000 images (512^2) data compressed by a factor of 2 (USA) or 1.8 (Europe) on real-time digital disks; option: 11000 images *Biplane:* basic: 8000 images option: 22000 images	3360 (1024^2) 12000 (512^2) 22400 (512×256) with 4 (8″) real-time disks, each of 889 Mbyte (raw data stored; no data compression)
no semiconductor memory; all data stored directly to disk; max. 100 photo- file images plus 16 refer- ence images stored on disk.	200 images (512^2); 300 images in photofile on disk.	32–80 MB temporary memory depending on the harddisk capacity; real-time storage in parallel to semiconductor memory, disks and DVR-10.
1) VLDS streamer tape; one pt per tape; transfer rate approx. 7 f/s; price $100 k; 2) Analog optical disk (12″): ±50 patient studies (for USA only). Price: $50k. Incl. Super-VHS recorder and PC for database, price $200k; optical disk $150; transfer rate: real time.	digital tape; standard: 2000 images; usage: 1 pt/tape; transfer rate: 2–4 f/s, fast tape: 12.5 f/s; Archiving takes place in background (during the procedure without user interference)	Real-time digital video- cassette recorder DVR-10; max. 160000 frames $512^2 \times 12$ bits; price $75 k; tapes: 22 GB ($50) and 69 GB ($100); 22 GB tape can contain 30 patient studies

Table 1. Continued

	ADAC	General Electric CGR
6. At what matrix size (pixels) are images displayed to the user?	512^2	1024^2
Interpolation technique used?	256^2; bilinear interpol.; 512^2; none; 1024^2: downscale to 512^2; option: high resolution to 1024^2 with (repeated) bilinear interpol.	bilinear interpolation
7. Is digital zoom available for coronary quantitation? If YES, provide zoom factor.	YES 2, 4, 8×	YES 2× on ROI around coronary segment automatically selected;
Interpolation technique used?	bilinear interpolation	bilinear interpolation
8. Horizontal pixel size in 512^2 image (without zoom) as measured at the input screen of the II.	290 µm/6″ FOV 440 µm/9″ FOV	287 µm/6″ FOV 430 µm/9″ FOV
9. 35 mm Cinefilm acquisition possible simultaneously with digital acquisition? If YES, are there any limitations?	YES; 25 fr/s 512^2 50 fr/s 256^2	YES; no limitations

the images. From Table 1, item 2 it becomes clear that four out of five manufacturers offer a 512^2 image acquisition mode with 8 bits or 12 bits (Toshiba). Both ADAC and Toshiba also provide lower resolution acquisitions at 256^2 and 256×512 pixels, respectively; both companies also have a 1024^2 matrix acquisition mode. The Siemens HICOR has a single 1024^2 matrix mode, although the images are stored at a matrix size of 512^2 pixels on the real-time disk. All four earlier mentioned systems allow 25 or 30 frames/s (f/s) frame rate at the 512^2 imaging mode and Siemens for the 1024^2 mode. In monoplane mode the Philips DCI even allows 50 or 60 f/s. If the 1024^2 matrix size is selected on the ADAC or Toshiba equipment, the maximum frame rate is limited to 6 1/4 and 7 1/2 frames/s, respectively, which is, however, not practical for cardiac applications. Again all companies have short X-ray pulse width selections available; most likely a value of 4–5 ms is used most frequently in routine practice.

Nowadays all manufacturers use 1 inch video tubes of various types (Table 1, item 3) in the progressive scan mode. For more detailed information on these different readout techniques, the reader is referred to ref. [38].

Table 1. Continued

Philips	Siemens	Toshiba
512^2	1024^2	1024^2 512^2 512×256 conform acquisition
none option: scan converter to 1024^2 by replication	linear interpolation	none
YES	YES	YES
2×	2×	any zoom factor up to 1500 acceptable;
bilinear interpolation	linear interpolation	cubic interpolation
247 μm/6″ FOV	231 μm/6″ FOV 270 μm/7″ FOV	292 μm/6″ FOV in normal mode; 238 μm/6″ FOV in cine-mode (overframing)
YES; no limitations	YES; no limitations	YES; no limitations

Over the years, disk technology has steadily improved to the extent that digital images can be stored in real-time; in most digital systems this is achieved by using parallel disk technology. Of great concern in the practical application of these systems is the size of the real-time disks on which the cardiac images are stored during the actual catheterization procedures. If this size would be too small, previous runs could be overwritten, or frequent transfers of the data to medium or long-term storage media would be required. As is apparent from Table 1, item 4, the maximal number of 512^2 images that can be stored on standard configurations on the real-time disks vary from 4,000 (Siemens; data compression of factor 2; optional 11,000 images), to 10,800 (ADAC; no data compression), to 12,000 (both Toshiba (no data compression), and GE CGR (average data compression factor 3; range 2–4.6; optional 24,000 images)), to 24,000 (Philips DCI-S; data compression factor 2), and 48,000 (Philips DCI-SX; data compression factor 4). To get an idea about how much this really means in clinical practice, let us make the following calculation. We assume a heart rhythm of the patient of 80 beats/min. with the angiographic data typically acquired over 6 cardiac cycles per angiographic view at a frame speed of 25 frames/s. In an average catheterization procedure the number of runs will not exceed 10, including left ventriculography. Therefore, for one particular patient study $10 \times 6 \times 60/80 \times 25 = 1,125$ frames will be acquired with a monoplane system, and thus double this number is 2,250 frames for a biplane system. This means that 10 biplane patient studies representing at the average one to two days of work for one catheterization laboratory can be stored on the real-time disks having a capacity of 24,000 images, as provided by GE CGR and Philips (DCI-S). For smaller capacities (ADAC, Siemens and Toshiba) a proportionally smaller number of studies can be saved on the disks. These maximum numbers are usually achieved with 4 real-time disks in parallel; these represent the top of the line products as far as storage capacity is concerned. For a busy catheterization laboratory where one wishes to keep a number of studies on the system for later reference, the basic system with one real-time disk is too small.

Only three companies (ADAC, Siemens, Toshiba) provide an additional semiconductor memory for the storage and quick retrieval of selected images. On the ADAC system, 8 images of size 512^2 pixels can be stored in such a reference memory, while Siemens has a capacity for 200 images at 512^2 resolution. Toshiba provides a semiconductor image memory with a size ranging from 32 to 80 MB depending on the harddisk capacity; on the Toshiba DFP-60A the image data are stored in parallel to this semiconductor memory, the real-time disks and to the real-time archiving system DVR-10. On the Philips DCI 100 photofile images plus 16 reference images can be stored on the real-time disks for reference purposes only. Since these images have been processed (edge enhancement, window width and level, etc.), these are not suitable anymore for quantitative analysis.

At this point in time, a universal long-term storage medium that has been accepted by all companies is not available. As mentioned earlier, there is a great need for such a universal long-term storage medium with the same or better performance than cinefilm in terms of price, transportability, durability and transfer rate. A good overview of the present and most likely future approaches can be found in [35]. At this point in time various techniques are proposed by the manufacturers. ADAC proposes a digital optical disk with low transfer rate of 2 frames/s, as well as an analog optical disk with real-time transfer rates. This last approach has resulted in the creation of a low cost ($ 12k–15k) viewing station, which is now being extended with a jukebox for the optical disks. Preferred is a 5.2 GByte VLDS-tape with a frame rate of 8 frames/s including verification of the data, or 16 frames/s if verification is not included. GE CGR uses an 8 mm DAT streamer tape which can contain maximally 50,000 images of $512^2 \times 8$ bits; however, the transfer rate is limited to 5 frames/s. Philips uses a high-speed VLDS streamer tape for digital backup of the DCI images. One tape contains data for only one patient. The transfer rate at 7 frames/s requires approximately 8 minutes to store a complete patient-study. The price of the streamer drive is approximately $100,000.-.

Furthermore, as a replacement for cinefilm, Philips proposes the 12″ analog magneto-optical laser disk (Sony for PAL and NTSC, Panasonic for NTSC only). One disk can contain 40 minutes of video, which corresponds to approximately 50 patient studies. Transfer to disk is done in real time during acquisition, or during reviewing for processed images. The price for a recorder is approximately $50,000.- ($25,000.- for a player only). At present the laser optical disk is integrated in one rack with a S-VHS recorder and a patient database management system on a PC. This entire system is now sold in the USA only for approximately $200,000.-.

Siemens uses a digital tape that can contain 2,000 images. In routine practice, most likely one tape per patient as with the cinefilm will be used. The transfer rate is rather low at 2–4 frames/s, although a fast tape with 12.5 frames/s is also available. It should be mentioned that the archiving process takes place in the background during the regular procedures without user interference.

Finally, Toshiba uses for archival purposes a real-time digital videocassette recorder (DVR-10) with a maximal storage capacity of 160,000 images $512^2 \times 12$ bits on the D2–tape. As mentioned earlier the image data are stored on the DVR-10 in parallel with the real-time disks, i.e. there is no additional time loss or effort from the user necessary to transfer the data from the disks to the archival medium. The price for this DVR-10 is $75,000.- and the price per tape $50.- for 22 GB and $100.- for a 69 GB tape. The 22 GB tape has a capacity for approximately 30 patient studies. Toshiba also sells a stand-alone viewing station (socalled digital Tagarno) for this D2–tape. This means that this archival approach is an excellent candidate for the long-sought universal solution.

Table 1, item 6 was concerned with the matrix size at which images are displayed to the user, and in case the display matrix size is larger than the original one, the kind of interpolation technique used.

ADAC and Philips use standard 512^2 displays. On the ADAC system the 256^2 images are bilinearly interpolated, and the 1024^2 images downscaled to 512^2 pixels. Both companies have an option for a scan converter to upscan the images to 1024^2 pixels by (repeated) bilinear interpolation and by image replication, respectively. Philips is the only company at present providing synchronized biplane viewing; Siemens expects to have this feature available by the end of 1991. GE CGR and Siemens both use only 1024^2 matrix displays with bilinear and linear interpolation, respectively. Toshiba displays the images in the same format as these were acquired (512×256, 512^2 or 1024^2).

The question was also posed whether regions of interest (ROI's) in the image can be magnified for subsequent coronary quantitation, and if so, to what degree and by which interpolation technique (Table 1, item 7). It turns out that all five manufacturers have a facility for digital zoom on their image data with zoom factors ranging from 2–8 times; Toshiba allows any zoom factor up to the theoretical value of 1,500. Most common is a two-fold digital magnification with either linear interpolation (Siemens), bilinear interpolation (ADAC, GE CGR, Philips) or cubic interpolation (Toshiba).

Item 8 was concerned with the horizontal pixel size for a 512^2 matrix (no zoom) as measured at the input screen of the image intensifier (II). If we normalize all the values provided on the questionnaire to a 6″ field-of-view (FOV), it becomes apparent that the Siemens system has the smallest pixel size (231 μm) and ADAC the largest value (290 μm); other values include 238 μm for Toshiba in the cine-mode (292 μm in normal mode), 247 μm for Philips, and 287 μm for GE CGR. Basically two categories can be distinguished: Philips, Siemens and Toshiba with sizes below 247 μm; and the other two companies with values around 290 μm. These different pixel sizes are related to the definition of the 512^2 digitizing matrix with respect to the size of the image intensifier output screen. In some systems the entire circular shape of the II output screen is included in the digitizing matrix (socalled exact framing), which means that a certain portion of the 512^2 pixels does not contain useful information. In the other extreme, the digitizing matrix fits within the circular shape of the II output screen (total overframing), which means that significant portions of the area of the II output screen are lost. Finally, in other systems (e.g. Philips DCI) an attempt was made to optimize the superimposition of the matrix on the II output screen (subtotal overframing), resulting in a small pixel size. In this situation a compromise is reached between the number of pixels at the corners not containing useful information and the areas of the II output screen not been digitized. It is of course true, that the smaller the pixel size, the more pixels are available for contour detection. In general, however, one cannot state that a smaller pixel size results in a more accurate edge detection performance; the accuracy is to a large degree dependent on the actual edge detection algorithm implemented. It should be noted that ADAC and Toshiba allow acquisitions at a matrix size of 1024^2 with resulting decrease in the pixel size by 50%. However, the number of frames per second on these systems at this size is low (max. 7.5 frames/s), making this mode not useful for cardiac applications. On the other hand, Siemens allows image acquisition at 25 frames/s at a matrix size of 1024^2 pixels.

Finally, it was investigated whether 35 mm cinefilm can be acquired simultaneously with the digital acquisition. Basically all manufacturers provide this feature, without any limitation mentioned (Table 1, item 9). However, it should be realized that at a frame speed less than 12.5 frames/s, which is not practical for coronary arteriography anyway, cinefilm acquisition is not possible. This is the case for all manufacturers. Secondly, to allow simultaneous digital and cine acquisition a 50/50 or 30/70 splitting mirror is introduced in the image formation chain resulting in a decreased film quality; ADAC uses a 10/90 mirror which does not seem to compromise the film image quality.

Extensive validation studies need to be carried out to determine the accuracy and precision of these digital approaches as compared to the established cinefilm techniques with optical zooming [39]. Thus far, a limited number of studies have been carried out and most of these failed to demonstrate superiority of either method in this respect [40–42]. On the basis of phantom and catheter measurements we have recently been able to demonstrate a 10–15% improvement in the precision of cinefilm analysis with $2.3 \times$ optical zoom as compared to 512^2 digital images [30]. Meticulous studies using a matrix size of 1024^2 have so far not demonstrated a substantial improvement in quantitative accuracy over a matrix size of 512^2 when used in currently available X-ray systems [43, 44].

Quantitative coronary (cine)arteriography

An extensive overview of developments carried out by various investigators in the field of quantitative coronary *cine*arteriography has been published elsewhere [29, 45]. From these overviews the following conclusions were drawn: 1) modern workstations and very powerful personal computers were increasingly being used; 2) analytical software packages were mostly written in Pascal and C; 3) in the majority of the cases the edge definition for the arterial structures was based on a combination of 1st-and 2nd-derivative functions; 4) correction for the limited bandwidth of the X-ray system was still insufficiently used; 5) in the majority of the cases image calibration was based on the measurement of the size of the coronary contrast catheter; 6) there had been no signal of new developments in the definition of clinically relevant parameters except for the stenotic flow reserve and more recently roughness calculations of the arterial boundaries [46]; 7) densitometry remained a problematic technique; and 8) the use of more extensive and particularly standardized validation procedures should be encouraged.

Instead of updating this overview, which would only result in a limited number or changes, I have chosen to describe in some more detail a state of the art analytical software package which has been developed for both digital and cinefilm applications on the Philips DCI and the MEDIS Cardiovascular Measurement System (CMS), respectively. Where appropriate, differences in the underlying algorithms will be indicated.

Image acquisition

The architecture of the Philips DCI has been described in the overview of the digital systems in this chapter. Matrix size of the entire image is $512 \times 512 \times 8$ bits.

The Cardiovascular Measurement System (CMS) uses a high quality CAP-35E telecine converter allowing a selected cineframe to be projected onto the target of a CCD camera via a zoom lens (range $1–6 \times$); in practice, an optical magnification of $2.3–2.9 \times$ is used. This means that a region of interest (ROI) in a cineframe encompassing the catheter or coronary segment can be selected by x,y-positioning of the CCD-camera to center the CCD-target on this ROI. The video signal (either PAL or NTSC) is subsequently digitized at a matrix size of $512 \times 512 \times 8$ bits by means of a frame grabber/image memory (Imaging Technologies VFG) installed in the host processor being a Compaq 80386/80486 at 33 MHz. The digitized image is then available for subsequent analysis.

Basic principles analytical software

For a quantitative coronary analysis package to be applicable in a routine environment, a number of requirements must be met:

1. minimal user-interaction should be required in the selection and processing of a coronary segment to be analyzed;
2. a high success-score; preferably in at least 90% of the cases the user should agree with the first obtained automatically determined results and not feel the necessity to manually edit the intermediary results, such as the detected contours of the arterial segments particularly at the lesion;
3. a sufficient number of both absolute and relative clinically relevant parameters should be presented;
4. a short processing time in the order of 15 seconds or less;
5. high accuracy and precision in the assessment of the morphologic data to be determined from extensive phantom and routinely acquired clinical studies.

Based on these requirements we have set out to develop the ACA-package for the Philips DCI [28, 37] and a similar package for the MEDIS CMS [30]. In the processing of a coronary segment, the following steps can be distinguished: 1) calibration of the image data; 2) definition of coronary segment to be analyzed; 3) automated detection of the arterial contours; 4) derivation of the clinically relevant parameters; and finally, 5) presentation of the results. These different steps will be briefly clarified in the following sections; calibration is based on the same basic principles as arterial analysis and therefore will be described third.

Definition of coronary segment to be analyzed. From the standpoint of minimal user-interaction and primary suitability for on-line and high throughput off-line use, we have been convinced that simply defining the start and end point of the segment to be analyzed is the most preferable procedure. The mouse of these analysis systems is used to define these points inside the arterial segment. In the next step, an arterial path through the segment of interest will be computed automatically.

In our implementation, the arterial path functions as a rough model for the subsequent contour detection, so it does not have to follow the actual centerline of the vessel. For this reason, we shall refer to the line connecting the start and end points as the *pathline*. The automated pathline technique is based upon two algorithms: the socalled *tracer* algorithm and the *box* algorithm, which have been described in detail elsewhere [47]. Figure 1 shows the results of this technique on the CMS for a proximal segment of a left anterior descending (LAD) artery. This pathline is defined as acceptable when it remains within the arterial boundaries along the entire length of the selected segment. On the rare occasion, when the detected pathline does not follow the path the user had in mind, (s)he can provide, in an iterative manner, one additional point in the missing part of the arterial segment. The program then searches for a new path from the start point, via the correction point, to the end point. On the DCI the pathline is detected in the original nonmagnified image, while on the CMS it is determined in the optically magnified region-of-interest encompassing the arterial segment to be analyzed.

Automated detection of arterial contours. The contour detection procedure is carried out in 2 iterations: the first one relative to the detected pathline, and the second one relative to the individual contours detected in the first iteration. The contour detection technique itself is based on resampling the image perpendicular to a model (in the 1st iteration the pathline; in the 2nd iteration the contours detected in the 1st iteration) and applying the *minimal cost* contour detection technique to the resampled matrix [28, 29, 37]. This technique has been shown to be very robust and computationally fast. To correct for the limited bandwidth of the X-ray imaging system, the minimal cost contour detection technique is modified in the second iteration based on an analysis of the point spread function of the imaging chain, which is of particular importance for the accurate measurement of small vessels. The detected contours are subsequently transformed back to the magnified image (Figure 2). In the actual implementations, differences exist between the digital DCI/ACA-package and the cinefilm-based CMS package. In the ACA-implementation, the initial contour detection in the first iteration is carried out in the original nonmagnified (512^2 pixels) image. In the second iteration, a region of interest (ROI) centered around the defined arterial segment is digitally magnified by a factor of two with bilinear interpolation. If the length of the selected arterial segment was chosen such that the digitally magnified segment would not fit within the 512^2 matrix size, digital magnification is not carried out and the second iteration is performed in the orgininal matrix size. In the CMS-implementation, both iterations are carried out in the optically zoomed (magnification factor 2.3–2.9×) image without subsequent digital magnification.

If the user does not agree with one or more parts of the detected contours, manual corrections can be applied after the second iteration. Two possibilities have been implemented. If the erroneous part can be approximated by a straight line, the user erases this part using the mouse. Next, the two remaining contour parts are connected by a straight line and the contour detection technique is again applied in a restricted area around this part (3rd iteration), so that in the end all contour points are based upon the actual grey level distribution in the image. If this straight line approximation is not applicable, the user erases the erroneous part and manually redraws the correct contour

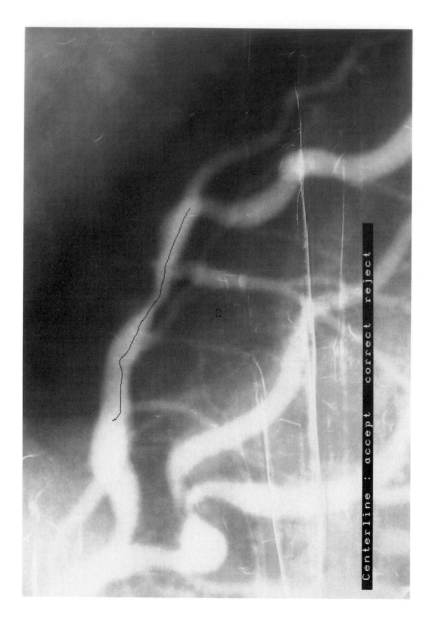

Figure 1. Arterial pathline detected automatically between manually defined start and end points of the arterial segment.

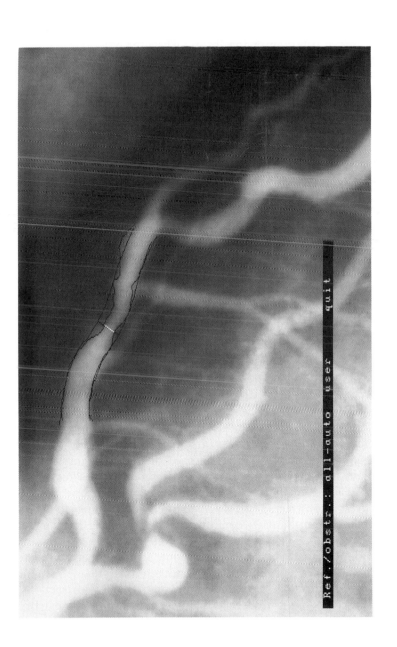

Figure 2. Result of the contour detection algorithm. The arterial contours are found by the minimum cost algorithm, the reference contours by the iterative linear regression technique.

as accurately as possible. However, if this corrected part deviates significantly from the initial, erroneous contour part, the contour detection process is also repeated in a restricted area around this redrawn part. This means that in the majority of the cases, the finally accepted contour will be based on the actual grey level distribution in the image. The user only identified the unacceptable contour parts. All these manual interactions have been made as user-friendly as possible.

Calibration. To be able to provide absolute morphological data (vessel and obstruction sizes in mm) a calibration procedure needs to be carried out prior to the coronary analysis. For this purpose, a nontapering part of the contrast catheter is used. Basically, the same procedure is followed for the automated edge detection of this segment of the contrast catheter as for an arterial segment, as described above (Figure 3). However, in this case, additional information is used in the 2nd iteration of the edge detection process, knowing that the nontapering part of the catheter is characterized by parallel, although not necessarily straight, boundaries. The calibration factor (mm/pixel) can then be computed on the basis of the average diameter of the catheter segment in pixels, and the known French size of the catheter, or the true size of the catheter in mm as measured with a micrometer.

Derivation of clinically relevant parameters. From the two sets of contour positions of the arterial segment a new accurate centerline is computed. Next, a diameter function is determined by measuring for every second position along this centerline the distances between the two contours. From these data the following parameters are automatically calculated: the site of maximal percent diameter stenosis, the corresponding lesion diameter (does not need to be at the point of absolutely minimal vessel diameter, as the lesion was selected by the *maximal percent* diameter stenosis), the extent of the obstruction and the corresponding reference diameter (Figures 2 and 4A). To be able to automatically determine the reference diameter value, an estimation of the size of the vessel prior to the occurrence of a focal obstruction has to be reconstructed (the socalled reference diameter function, shown as a straight line in the diameter function). The reference diameter value is taken at the site of the obstruction, so that neither overestimation nor underestimation occurs. This automated approach has been found to be very reproducible. From the obstruction and reference diameters, the percentages diameter and area stenoses (assuming circular cross sections) are derived. On the basis of this reference diameter function, and the actual arterial contours, the reference contours (outer contours in Figures 2 and 4A) can be reconstructed. Situations may occur in which the user does not agree with the automatically determined reference position, or a second obstruction needs to be measured within the same segment. The user interfaces of both the Philips DCI and the MEDIS CMS allow the user to

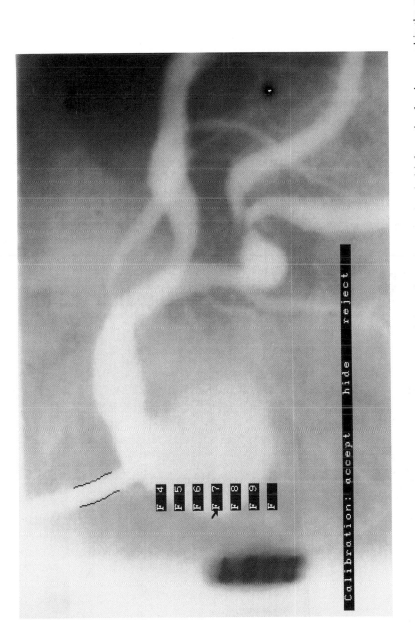
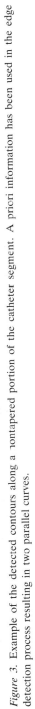

Figure 3. Example of the detected contours along a nontapered portion of the catheter segment. A priori information has been used in the edge detection process resulting in two parallel curves.

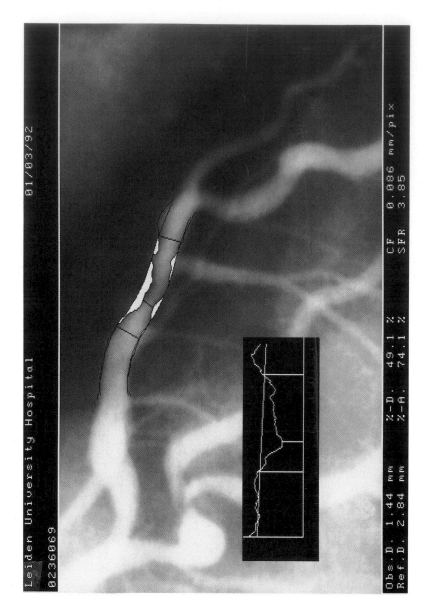

Figure 4A.

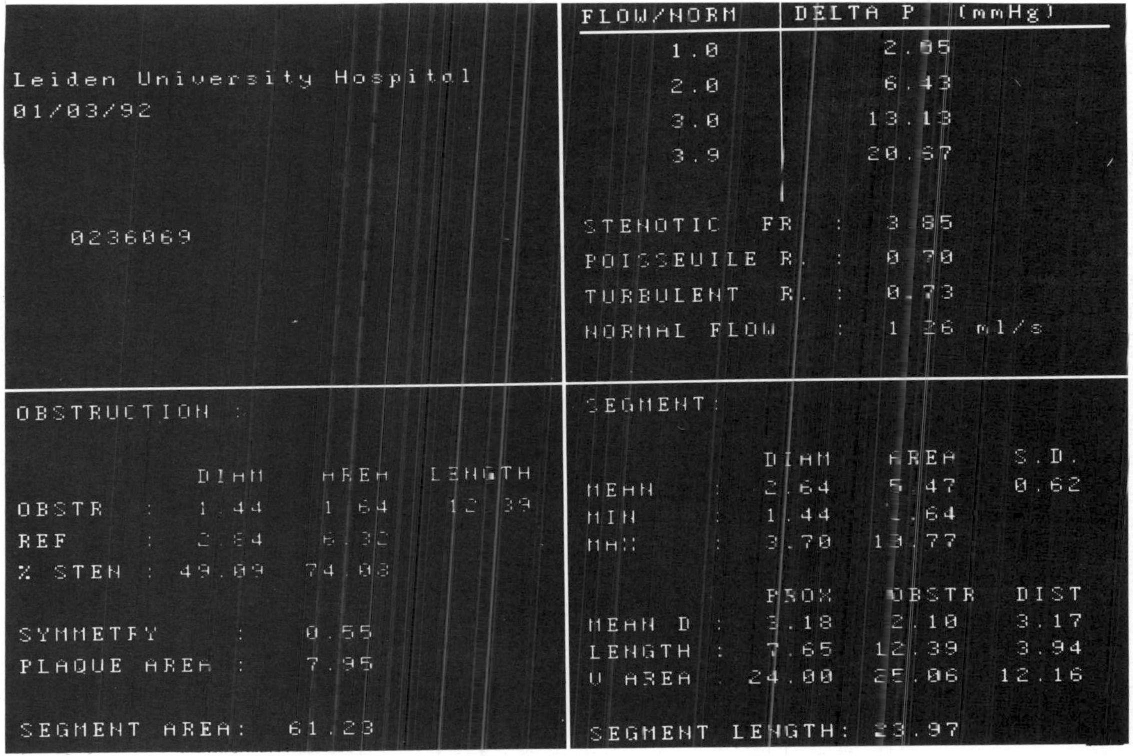

Leiden University Hospital
01/03/92

0236069

OBSTRUCTION :

	DIAM	AREA	LENGTH
OBSTR	1.44	1.64	10.34
REF	2.84	6.36	
% STEN	49.09	74.03	

SYMMETRY   : 0.55
PLAQUE AREA : 7.95

SEGMENT AREA: 61.23

FLOW/NORM	DELTA P (mmHg)
1.0	2.65
2.0	6.43
3.0	13.13
3.9	20.57

STENOTIC FR. : 3.85
POISSEUILE R. : 0.70
TURBULENT R. : 0.73
NORMAL FLOW : 1.26 ml/s

SEGMENT:

	DIAM	AREA	S.D.
MEAN	2.64	5.47	0.62
MIN	1.44	1.64	
MAX	3.70	13.77	

	PROX	OBSTR	DIST
MEAN D	3.18	2.10	3.17
LENGTH	7.65	12.39	3.94
U AREA	24.00	25.06	12.16

SEGMENT LENGTH: 23.97

Figure 4B.

Figure 4. Final result pages of the analysis of the coronary segment of Figure 1. Shown are the automatically detected luminal contours, the computer-defined reference contours, and the diameter function (lower left quadrant), plus the most relevant quantitative measurements. (Figure 4A). In Figure 4B the second result page is displayed with all the detailed derived quantitative data (see text).

simply change the obstruction and/or reference positions and carry out the corresponding quantitative analyses.

Presentation of the results. The first result pages of the ACA and CMS packages show the same kind of data, being the actual angiographic image with the boundaries superimposed, the diameter function with the straight line being the interpolated reference diameter function, demographic data in a top panel in the image, and the most important derived parameters in a bottom panel.

The second result page provides a complete overview of all parameters derived (Figure 4B). The layout for the second result pages on the ACA and CMS packages differ slightly; since the CMS package provides the most extensive description of the arterial morphology, this will be used as an example. Those parameters that are not presently available with the ACA-package will be identified with an asterix. The upper left quadrant of the CMS output shows the patient administration data, the upper right quadrant functional information about the selected obstruction, the lower left quadrant provides detailed obstruction information, while in the lower right quadrant overall segment and subsegment related data are given.

The left upper quadrant of the ACA output shows the standard diagram for the calculation of the stenotic flow reserve (SFR) as described by Kirkee-ide and Gould [48]. For space limitations this plot is not shown anymore on the CMS; the actual SFR-value is, however, listed in the right upper panel. All these quantitative data will be described in more detail in the following paragraphs.

The lower left quadrant provides in addition to the parameters already mentioned for the first result page:

OBST AREA	Obstruction cross-sectional area (assuming circular cross section). Unit: mm^2.
REF AREA	Reference cross-sectional area (assuming circular cross section). Unit: mm^2.
%-D STEN	Percentage diameter stenosis. Unit:%.
%-A STEN	Percentage area stenosis. Unit:%.
SYMM	Obstruction symmetry measured from the relative amounts of plaque area on either side of the vessel. Range: 0.0 (asymmetric) to 1.0 (symmetric).
PLAQUE	Plaque area measured between the luminal contours and the reference contours within the given obstruction limits. Unit: mm^2.
SEGM AREA	Projected vessel area of the entire segment. Unit: mm^2.

The lower right quadrant shows a summary of segment related data, and contains the following parameters:

*MEAN DIAM	Mean diameter over the entire arterial segment. Unit: mm.
*MEAN AREA	Mean cross-sectional area (assuming circular cross sections) over the entire segment. Unit: mm^2
*MEAN S.D.	Standard deviation of diameter measurements. Unit: mm.
*MIN DIAM	Minimum segment diameter. Unit: mm.
*MIN AREA	Minimum cross-sectional area assuming a circular cross section at the point of minimum segment diameter. Unit: mm^2.
*MAX DIAM	Maximum segment diameter. Unit: mm.
*MAX AREA	Maximum cross-sectional area assuming a circular cross section at the point of maximum segment diameter. Unit: mm^2.

Following this is a subsegmental analysis, where the arterial segment is divided into three sections: proximal, obstruction and distal as defined by the obstruction. Subsegment projected vessel areas are defined in the same manner as the total vessel area enclosed by the vessel contours in the given angiographic projection, however now for the corresponding subsegments.

*MEAN D PROX	Mean diameter in the proximal subsegment. Unit: mm.
*MEAN D OBSTR	Mean diameter within the obstruction limits. Unit: mm.
*MEAN D DIST	Mean diameter in the distal subsegment. Unit: mm.
*LENGTH PROX	Length of the proximal subsegment Unit: mm.
LENGTH OBSTR	Length of the obstruction. Unit: mm.
*LENGTH DIST	Length of the distal subsegment. Unit: mm.
*V AREA PROX	Vessel area measured proximal to the obstruction. Unit: mm^2.
*V AREA OBSTR	Vessel area of the obstruction. Unit: mm^2.
*V AREA DIST	Vessel area measured distal to the obstruction. Unit: mm^2.
*SEGMENT LENGTH	Length of the entire arterial segment measured along the centerline of the vessel. Unit: mm.

In the upper right quadrant functional information is given, such as the normal flow (ml/s) based on the assumption of a constant flow velocity of 20 cm/s and taking into account the computed reference area, the Poiseuille and turbulent resistances, as well as the radiographic Stenotic Flow Reserve

(SFR-)value computed according to the techniques described by Kirkeeide and Gould [48]. Finally, pressure gradients (mmHg) are given for various normalized flow situations.

Validation results

With the introduction of improved quantitative techniques which provide on-line support to the angiographer during the angiographic examination as well as a detailed description of the morphology for clinical research studies, it has become absolutely essential to carry out thorough validation studies to demonstrate the strengths and weaknesses of the analytical programs. First of all, the reliability of the edge detection technique should be demonstrated on realistic phantom studies [29]. Secondly, the reproducibility of the image analysis procedure should be clarified with a sufficient number of routinely acquired digital and cine-arteriograms. It has been suggested to describe the results from validation studies in terms of the mean signed differences (accuracy) and the standard deviation (precision) of these signed differences (measurement 1– measurement 2; not absolute differences) between the true and measured values or between the values from repeated measurements [29, 49]. Finally, we have tested the suitability of the socalled Softouch catheter for QCA. Some preliminary evaluation results for the ACA and CMS-packages on several of these topics will be described in the following paragraphs.

Accuracy and precision of the edge detection algorithm. To determine the accuracy and precision of the edge detection algorithm, a plexiglass phantom with eleven tubular "vessel" sizes ranging from 0.660 to 5.055 mm, filled with different contrast concentrations (100% and 50%), acquired at different kV-levels (70 and 90 kV), and at the 5″ and 7″ image intensifier modes was analyzed (Figure 5). Each segment was analyzed over a length of approximately 2 cm, providing a mean value and a standard deviation per segment; this standard deviation is a measure for the irregularity of the detected contours. Per segment the mean difference between the calculated mean diameter and its true diameter was calculated. To obtain an overall measure for the phantom acquired under a certain imaging condition, the mean difference values were averaged over all eleven segments providing an accuracy value, and the pooled standard deviation was calculated being a measure for the precision of the measurements. The overall results for all the different imaging modes for both the CMS and the ACA analytical packages are given in Table 2. The results in Table 2 demonstrate that all accuracy values are very close to zero, with ACA consistently showing a slight underestimation (negative accuracy values), while CMS shows both slight under- and overestimations. The precision values for CMS range from 0.081–0.115 mm and for ACA 0.082–0.136 mm. Under all circumstances, except for the 7″ image

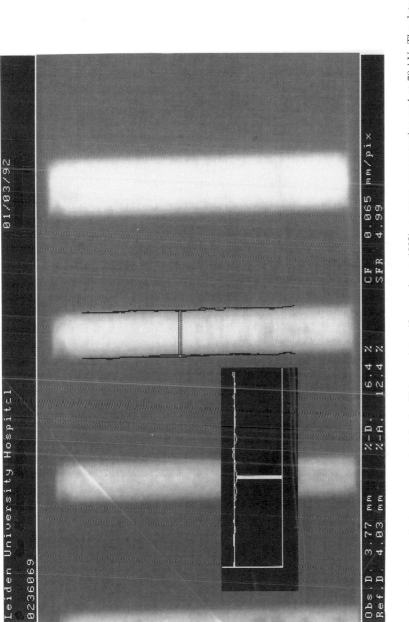

Figure 5. Example of the vessel phantom acquired in the 7″ image intensifier mode, at 100% contrast concentration and at 70 kV. The detected contours for the tube with a true size of 4.34 mm are superimposed on the images. In this case a mean diameter of 3.99 mm and a standard deviation of 0.08 mm were found.

Table 2. Accuracy and precision of edge detection technique as assessed from plexiglass phantom (sizes 0.66–5.055 mm) with the CMS and ACA analytical software packages

II mode	Contrast concentration (%)	Load (kV)	Overall mean difference = accuracy (mm)		Pooled standard deviation = precision (mm)	
			CMS	ACA	CMS	ACA
7"	100	70	0.027	−0.001	0.100	0.096
7"	100	90	0.016	−0.013	0.090	0.110
7"	50	70	−0.014	−0.024	0.112	0.130
7"	50	90	−0.025	−0.015	0.115	0.136
5"	100	70	−0.012	−0.021	0.090	0.095
5"	100	90	0.001	−0.005	0.081	0.082
5"	50	70	−0.041	−0.041	0.093	0.104
5"	50	90	−0.069	−0.025	0.105	0.118

intensifier (II-)mode, 100% contrast and 70 kV, the precision values for CMS are smaller than for ACA.

To provide some further insights in the individual measurements, the results for the phantoms acquired in the 7" image intensifier mode at 70 kV both for 100% and 50% contrast concentrations are given in Figures 6A and 6B for the CMS and ACA analytical packages, respectively. The true diameters of the "vessels" are plotted along the x-axis and the mean differences with respect to the true values along the y-axis. The two horizontal lines represent the pooled standard deviation values with respect to the overall mean difference computed from all the individual standard deviation values for the 100% and 50% contrast concentration measurements. Figures 6A and 6B make clear that the usual roll-off at the smaller sizes does not occur anymore (except for one overestimated measurement at 0.66 for the CMS at 50% contrast concentration) due to the correction technique for image blur applied in the contour detection procedure; this means that obstruction values down to 0.66 mm can be measured with high accuracy and precision.

Reproducibility on routine coronary arteriograms. To assess the inter- and intra-observer variabilities of the ACA-package, 16 routinely acquired digital coronary arteriograms were processed with a total of 39 obstructions. Images were selected in the diastasis period. One or more coronary obstructions were analyzed in a standardized manner, i.e. from one major bifurcation to the following one according to the recommendations by the AHA, by two observers (GK, HR) independently of each other. This same image set was reanalyzed at average 6 weeks later by one of the two observers (GK) without using knowledge from the first analysis session. For each study, a calibration factor was obtained on the basis of the contrast catheter. The

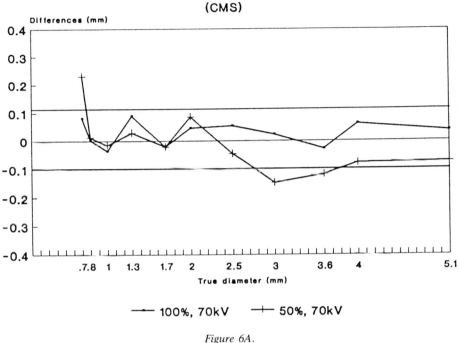

Figure 6A.

image selected for calibration was not necessarily the same as the image in which the obstruction was measured. Criteria for the calibration frame selection included: 1) nontapering segment of the catheter visible; and 2) catheter not obscured by contrast flowing back into the aorta. As a result, the catheter image was usually selected in the early phase of the cardiac study. From these inter- and intra-observer data the mean signed differences (accuracy) between the repeated measurements, and the standard deviation of these differences (precision) were calculated. The inter- and intra-observer variabilities as assessed from the total of 39 coronary obstructions are presented in Table 3. The range data in Table 3 shows that the obstructions represented a wide range from 0.63–2.85 mm in obstruction diameter and 21.4–79.9% in percentage diameter stenosis. It can be observed that all accuracy values are close to zero. This indicates that neither significant systematic over- nor under-estimations occur. Furthermore, the precision in the obstruction measurements for the inter- and intra-observer studies is only 0.11 and 0.10 mm, respectively, and in the automatically determined reference diameters 0.13 and 0.13 mm, respectively. The inter- and intra-observer precision for the percentage diameter stenosis is 5.64 and 3.18%, respectively.

The inter- and intra-observer variabilities in the obstruction length are

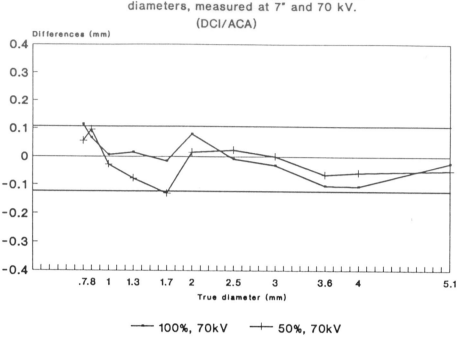

Figure 6B.

Figure 6. Individual measurements for the plexiglass phantom acquired at the 7″ image intensifier mode at 70kV for 100% and 50% contrast fillings for the CMS (Figure 6A) and the ACA (Figure 6B) analytical packages. The true diameters of the vessels from 0.66 mm to 5.055 mm are plotted along the abscissa and the mean differences with respect to the true values along the ordinate. The two horizontal lines represent the pooled standard deviation values with respect to the overall mean difference. A negative difference represents underestimation, a positive difference overestimation.

Table 3. Accuracy and precision, repeated analysis of digital coronary analysis

	Range	Inter-observer (N = 39)		Intra-observer (N = 39)	
		Acc.	Prec.	Acc.	Prec.
Calibration factor (mm/pixel)	0.160–0.240	−0.001	0.003	0.000	0.005
Obstruction diam. (mm)	0.63–2.85	−0.016	0.107	0.027	0.098
Reference diam. (mm)	1.56–4.08	−0.013	0.125	0.026	0.130
Percentage diam. sten (%)	21.45–79.90	0.253	5.641	−0.189	3.184
Percentage area sten (%)	38.29–95.95	−0.225	6.595	−0.027	3.393
Obstruction length (mm)	3.71–35.90	−0.240	1.458	0.357	1.222
Area of plaque (mm²)	1.24–35.13	−0.033	1.289	0.222	1.288
Stenotic flow reserve	0.68–4.87	−0.052	0.360	0.056	0.213

small at 1.46 mm and 1.22 mm, respectively. The values for the area of the atherosclerotic plaque are similar at 1.29 and 1.29 mm^2, respectively. Finally, the variabilities in the derived stenotic flow reserve were 0.36 and 0.21, respectively.

Further studies are underway to determine the inter- and intra-observer variabilities for the CMS-package, and the short-, medium-, and long-term variabilities for repeated angiographies with and without repositioning of the X-ray system for both digital and cinecoronary arteriograms.

Suitability of 6F and 7F Mallinckrodt Softouch^R coronary contrast catheters for QCA from digital and cine arteriograms. In the quantitative assessment of coronary arterial dimensions from cine and digital coronary arteriographic images, the contrast catheters are almost exclusively used as a calibration device. So far only 7F and 8F catheters have been recommended, provided they satisfy certain image quality criteria [50]. From this study in Ref. [50], for example, it became clear that nylon catheters are not suitable for QCA, because of the very low X-ray opacity of these catheters. With the increased use in routine clinical practice of 5F and 6F catheters, questions have frequently been raised whether these smaller catheters may also be used for QCA. Sofar responses to these questions had to be negative if previous generations of QCA equipment were used. Two new developments have spurred interest in restudying catheter performance.

First of all, Mallinckrodt[1] recently developed new Softouch^R tip nylon catheters with improved image quality specifications. Secondly, the new ACA and CMS packages are now available.

In our study we analyzed nontapering parts of the Softouch tips and of the nylon shafts of 6F and 7F catheters with three different fillings: 1) only saline; 2) 175 mg I/cc (50% concentration); and 3) 350 mg I/cc (100% concentration). Each situation was filmed at three different kilovoltages of the X-ray tube: approximately 60 kV, 75 kV and 90 kV, and at two image intensifier modes: 5″ and 7″ input screen sizes. Since all the details have been described elsewhere [51], we will only summarize here the most important results (Table 4).

The average signed differences between the angiographically measured dimensions at 100% contrast fillings and acquired at 3 different kV-levels (60, 75 and 90kV) were − 3.3% and 0.6% for the 6F and 7F catheter tips, respectively as measured with the ACA-package on digital images, and − 0.4% and 2.1%, respectively, as measured with the CMS-system on cinefilm images. The pooled standard deviations were 0.102 mm and 0.107 mm for the 6F and 7F catheter tips, respectively, as measured with the ACA-package, and 0.080 mm and 0.083 mm, as measured with the CMS-system. The deviations for the nylon shafts were much larger. It became also clear that the filling of the catheters, nor the kV-level used, had any appreciable effect on the measurement accuracy for the Softouch tips, which facilitates the frame selection in QCA-studies. From these data it can be concluded

Table 4. Mean values and pooled standard deviations of the catheter Softouch^R tip dimensions for two images intensifier modes, as measured from **digital** and **cinefilm** images*. The numbers in parentheses denote the average percent under- or overestimation of the catheter tip measurements

Catheters	5″ II-mode	7″ II-mode	Both II-modes
	Digital ACA		
6F tip	1.895 ± 0.084 (−4.1%)	1.926 ± 0.118 (−2.5%)	1.910 ± 0.102 (−3.3%)
7F tip	2.270 ± 0.108 (0.5%)	2.274 ± 0.106 (0.7%)	2.272 ± 0.107 (0.6%)
	Cinefilm CMS		
6F tip	1.975 ± 0.079 (0.0%)	1.958 ± 0.081 (−0.9%)	1.967 ± 0.080 (−0.4%)
7F tip	2.310 ± 0.079 (2.3%)	2.303 ± 0.086 (1.9%)	2.307 ± 0.083 (2.1%)

* Note: Measurements averaged over 100% contrast medium concentration and saline.

that the nontapering parts of the 6F and 7F Mallinckrodt Softouch tips are very well suitable for QCA calibration purposes.

Pathline tracer. Validation studies on the pathline tracer have shown that in 89.3% of a total of 110 short and long coronary segments an acceptable pathline was found in only one iteration; in 99% the pathline was acceptable in two iterations [47]. This makes clear that this technique is suitable for on-line routine applications.

Computation time. The entire analysis procedure, including calibration when carried out on the same frame selected for the coronary segment, takes only approximately 10–12 seconds on the CMS (80386 processor) and 15 seconds on the Philips DCI-SX. When separate frames need to be selected for calibration and vessel analysis, additional time is needed to select the appropriate frames. However, these data make clear that the execution times of these packages are now so short, that the other user manipulations such as selection of the appropriate frames and administration of the derived results, have now become the limiting factors in the quantitative analysis of coronary arteriograms.

Short-ACA package. Based on these favorable results and the fact that in practice hardly any or even no contour corrections are necessary in the majority of cases, a second version of the ACA-package has been made available. This so-called Short ACA-package skips the correction possibilities in the pathline and contour detection procedures, as well as the positioning of the obstruction and reference sites. After having defined the start and end point of the vessel, the contour detection and analysis procedure run fully automatically. This is clearly the furthest step that one can go at this point in time with the automated quantitative analysis of a coronary arterial segment. In those situations where the user may expect some manual editing, the standard ACA-package should be used. Extensive experiences with these two versions in the many clinical sites, should make clear in which percentages of the cases the different packages will be used.

Conclusions

In this chapter the requirements for modern X-ray systems suitable for coronary arteriography have been defined. It was concluded that all modern X-ray systems from the different vendors satisfy the basic requirements for adequate coronary arteriography, although for some applications or institutions small but relevant differences do exist. In the second section an overview of the most widely used digital cardiac imaging systems was presented. From this overview it could be concluded that:

1. all systems allow image acquisition at 25 or 30 frames/s at the 512^2 matrix size or even 1024^2 size (Siemens);
2. sufficient disk space can be made available to store all the image information acquired in a catheterization laboratory during a single day;
3. a universal long-term storage medium (archival of the data) with the same degree of transportability, durability and cost of cinefilm is not yet available; and
4. although not described in this overview, it is well known that significant differences exist in the availability and performance of coronary analytical software packages.

In the third part of this chapter a state-of-the-art analytical software package for quantitative digital and cinecoronary arteriography has been described and preliminary validation results have been presented.

The Automated Coronary Analysis (ACA) package has been developed for the Philips DCI-system to allow the objective assessment of coronary vessel dimensions during and after the catheterization procedure from digital angiograms (matrix size $512^2 \times 8$ bits). A second version has been implemented for quantitative coronary cinearteriography on the MEDIS CMS-system which features optical zooming (magnification factor 2.3–2.9 $\times$ of regions of interest).

Results from plexiglass phantom studies indicate that the precision of the CMS is approximately 10–15% better than for digital coronary arteriography making it extremely suitable for multi-center, longitudinal research studies in which cinefilm is still the universal medium of image transport. With the use of modern small field-of-view image intensifiers (4" and 5" FOV), the present resolution of $512^2 \times 8$ bits at 30 frames per second may even be sufficient to assess on-line the long-term efficacy of intervention studies if highly accurate edge detection algorithms, such as the Philips ACA-package, are applied. Appropriate linear or cubic interpolations may compensate largely for the limited matrix size in the digital images, although, this topic requires further research. If this turns out to be true, it would mean that with the rapid improvements in hardware and clinical application software for digital systems, it is to be expected that on-line approaches will play an increasingly important role in clinical and therapeutic decision making, and possibly, in the near future, in the assessment of the efficacy of intervention studies.

Validation studies have made clear that the original development goals have been fully met. These QCA-packages require a minimal amount of user-interaction and provides highly objective and reproducible data.

The features of the ACA and CMS QCA-packages can be summarized as follows:

- in most cases the amount of user-interaction is limited to the manual definition of only the start and end points of the vessel segment to be analyzed;
- the reference diameter of an obstructed segment is determined fully automatically;
- many clinically relevant morphologic and functional parameters are derived;
- phantom studies have proven the high accuracy and precision of the edge detection technique down to "vessel" sizes of 0.66 mm;
- the inter- and intraobserver variability of absolute obstruction dimensions with the ACA-package is equal to 0.11 mm and 0.10 mm, respectively, and for the automatically determined reference diameter 0.13 and 0.13 mm, respectively.

Further developments in this field from our laboratory will be directed towards a biplane or dual plane coronary analysis package, revisiting the densitometric approaches and an automated calibration procedure (not based on the current edge detection approach on the contrast catheter).

In conclusion, a new analytical technique has been made available to the angiographer for the objective assessment of the optimal choice of recanalization devices and for the instantaneous assessment of the effects of such recanalization procedures during the catheterization procedure. For the off-line assessment of the morphology of coronary vessels for multicenter, longitudinal coronary research studies on the basis of cinefilm, a robust software package is available. The strength of these developments are the high quality of the clinical application software in conjunction with extensive, well conducted clinical validation studies.

Acknowledgements

The authors wish to thank mrs. B. Smit-van der Deure for her secretarial assistance in the many versions of this chapter.

Note

1. Mallinckrodt Medical GmbH, Hennef, Germany.

References

1. Brown BG, Bolson E, Frimer M, Dodge HT. Quantitative coronary arteriography: estimation of dimensions, hemodynamic resistance, and atheroma mass of coronary artery lesions using the arteriogram and digital computation. Circulation 1977; **55**: 329–37.
2. Reiber JHC, Booman F, Tan HS, Slager CJ, Schuurbiers JCH, Gerbrands JJ, Meester GT. A cardiac image analysis system. Objective quantitative processing of angiocardiograms. Comput Cardiol 1978: 239–42.
3. Gruentzig AR, Senning A, Siegenthaler WE. Nonoperative dilatation of coronary-artery stenosis: percutaneous transluminal coronary angioplasty. N Engl J Med 1979; **301**: 61–8.
4. Verstraete M, Bernard R, Bory M, et al. Randomized trial of intravenous recombinant tissue-type plasminogen activator versus intravenous streptokinase in acute myocardial infarction. Report from the European Cooperative Study Group for Recombinant Tissue-type Plasminogen Activator. Lancet 1985; **1**: 842–7.
5. Simoons ML, Arnold AE, Betriu A, et al. Thrombolysis with tissue plasminogen activator in acute myocardial infarction: no additional benefit from immediate percutaneous coronary angioplasty. Lancet 1988; **1**: 197–203.
6. Puel J, Joffre F, Rousseau H, et al. Percutaneously implantable endo-coronary prosthesis. In: Reiber JHC, Serruys PW (Eds.), New developments in quantitative coronary arteriography. Dordrecht: Kluwer Accademic Publishers 1988: 271–7.
7. Sigwart U, Puel J, Mirkovitch V, Joffre F, Kappenberger L. Intravascular stents to prevent occlusion and restenosis after transluminal angioplasty. N Engl J Med 1987; **316**: 701–6.
8. Sigwart U, Golf S, Kaufmann U, Kappenberger L. A coronary endoprosthesis to prevent restenosis and acute occlusion after percutaneous angioplasty: one and a half year of clinical experience. In: Reiber JHC, Serruys PW (Eds.), New developments in quantitative coronary arteriography. Dordrecht: Kluwer Academic Publishers 1988: 278–84.
9. Serruys PW, Beatt KJ, van der Giessen WJ. Stenting of coronary arteries: are we the sorcerer's apprentice? In: Reiber JHC, Serruys PW (Eds.), Quantitative coronary arteriography. Dordrecht: Kluwer Academic Publishers 1991: 297–311.
10. Ritchie JL, Hansen DD, Vracko R, Auth D. In vivo rotational thrombectomy. Evaluation by angioscopy. Circulation 1986; **74** (4 Suppl II): II-457 (Abstract).
11. Simpson JB, Zimmerman JJ, Selmon MR, et al. Transluminal atherectomy: initial clinical results in 27 patients. Circulation 1986; **74** (4 Suppl II): II-203 (Abstract).
12. Bertrand ME, LaBlanche JM, Bauters C. Mechanical recanalization of coronary arteries. In: Reiber JHC, Serruys PW (Eds.), Quantitative coronary arteriography. Dordrecht: Kluwer Academic Publishers 1991: 341–50.
13. Isner JM, Clarke RH. Laser angioplasty: unraveling the Gordian knot. J Am Coll Cardiol 1986; **7**: 705–8.
14. Lee G, Garcia JM, Chan MC, et al. Clinically successful long-term laser coronary recanalization. Am Heart J 1986; **112**: 1323–5.
15. Spears JR, Reyes VP, Wynne J, et al. Percutaneous coronary laser balloon angioplasty: initial results of a multicenter experience. J Am Coll Cardiol 1990; **16**: 293–303.
16. Spears JR. Laser balloon angioplasty (LBA). In: Reiber JHC, Serruys PW (Eds.), Quantitative coronary arteriography. Dordrecht: Kluwer Academic Publishers 1991: 329–39.
17. Slager CJ, Essed CA, Schuurbiers JCH, Bom N, Serruys PW, Meester GT. Vaporization of atherosclerotic plaques by spark erosion. J Am Coll Cardiol 1985; **5**: 1382–6.
18. Serruys PW, Luijten HE, Beatt KJ, et al. Incidence of restenosis after successful coronary

angioplasty: a time-related phenomenon. A quantitative angiographic study in 342 consecutive patients at 1, 2, 3, and 4 months. Circulation 1988; **77**: 361–71.

19. Arntzenius AC, Kromhout D, Barth JD, et al. Diet, lipoproteins, and the progression of coronary atherosclerosis. The Leiden Intervention Trial. N Engl J Med 1985; **312**: 805–11.

20. Lichtlen PR, Hugenholtz PG, Rafflenbeul W, Hecker H, Jost S, Deckers JW. Retardation of angiographic progression of coronary artery disease by nifedipine. Results of the International Nifedipine Trial on Antiatherosclerotic Therapy (INTACT). Lancet 1990; **335**: 1109–13.

21. Barth JD. Progression and regression of atherosclerosis. In: Marcus ML, Skorton DJ, Schelbert HR, Wolf GL (Eds.), Cardiac Imaging. Philadelphia: Saunders 1991: 267–70.

22. Marcus ML, Skorton DJ, Johnson MR, Collins SM, Harrison DG, Kerber RE. Visual estimates of percent diameter coronary stenosis: "a battered gold standard". J Am Coll Cardiol 1988; **11**: 882–5.

23. Blankenhorn DH, Brooks SH. Angiographic trials of lipid-lowering therapy. Arteriosclerosis 1981; **1**: 242–9.

24. A special issue on X-ray tubes. Medicamundi 1990; **35**: 1–70.

25. Verhoeven LAJ. Digital cardiac imaging. Medicamundi 1987; **32**: 111–6.

26. Fleck E, Oswald H. Digital cardiac imaging: an effective aid in complex coronary angioplasties. Medicamundi 1988; **33**: 69–73.

27. Mancini GBJ. Digital coronary angiography: advantages and limitations. In: Reiber JHC, Serruys PW (Eds.), Quantitative coronary arteriography. Dordrecht: Kluwer Academic Publishers 1991: 23–42.

28. Reiber JHC, van der Zwet PMJ, von Land CD, et al. On-line quantification of coronary arteriograms with the DCI system. Medicamundi 1989; **34**: 89–98.

29. Reiber JHC. An overview of coronary quantitation techniques as of 1989. In: Reiber JHC, Serruys PW (Eds.), Quantitative coronary arteriography. Dordrecht: Kluwer Academic Publishers 1991: 55–132.

30. Reiber JHC, van der Zwet PMJ, Koning G, et al. Quantitative coronary measurements from cine and digital arteriography; methodology and validation results. Abstract book 4th International Symposium on Coronary Arteriography, Rotterdam, June 23–25, 1991: 36.

31. Bruschke AVG, Reiber JHC, Relik-van Wely L, van Wesemael JWJ. Guidelines. Coronary arteriography. Neth J Cardiol 1991; **5**: 210–21.

32. Meijer DJH, van der Zwet PMJ, Reiber JHC. Fully automated PC-based assessment of pincushion distortion. Abstract book 4th International Symposium on Coronary Arteriography, Rotterdam, June 23–25, 1991: 180.

33. Buschmeyer L, Onnasch DGW, Heintzen PH. Korrektur magnetfeldbedingter Bildverzeichnungen in bewegten Röntgen-Bildverstärker-Fernseh-Systemen. Biomed Tech 1989; **34**: 209–10.

34. Solzbach U, Wollschläger H, Zeiher A, Just H. Optical distortion due to geomagnetism in quantitative angiography. Comput Cardiol 1989: 355–7.

35. Simon R. The filmless catheterization laboratory: when will it be reality? In: Reiber JHC, Serruys PW (Eds.), Advances in Quantitative Coronary Arteriography. Dordrecht: Kluwer Academic Publishers 1992.

36. Pepine CJ. The cardiac catheterization laboratory – 1990. Am J Cardiol 1990; **66**: 37F–40F.

37. Van der Zwet PMJ, von Land CD, Loois G, Gerbrands JJ, Reiber JHC. An on-line system for the quantitative analysis of coronary arterial segments. Comput Cardiol 1990: 157–60.

38. Kruger RA, Riederer SJ. Basic concepts of digital subtraction angiography. Boston: GK Hall Medical Publishers 1984.

39. Mancini GBJ, Simon SB, McGillem MJ, LeFree MT, Friedman HZ, Vogel RA. Automated quantitative coronary arteriography: morphologic and physiologic validation in vivo of a rapid digital angiographic method. Circulation 1987; 75: 452–60 (published erratum appears in Circulation 1987; **75**: 1199).

40. LeFree MT, Simon SB, Mancini GBJ, Bates ER, Vogel RA. A comparison of 35 mm

cine film and digital radiographic image recording: implications for quantitative coronary arteriography. Film vs. digital coronary quantification. Invest Radiol 1988; **23**: 176–83.

41. Ratib OM, Mankovich NJ. Quantitative coronary arteriography: design and validation. Radiology 1988; **167**: 743–7.
42. Bruschke AVG, Padmos I, Buis B, Van Benthem A. Arteriographic evaluation of small coronary arteries. J Am Coll Cardiol 1990; **15**: 784–9.
43. Ovitt TW, Newell JD 2nd. Digital subtraction angiography: technology, equipment, and techniques. Radiol Clin North Am 1985; **23**: 177–84.
44. Mistretta CA, Peppler WW. Digital cardiac X-ray imaging: fundamental principles. Am J Card Imaging 1988; **2**: 26–39.
45. Reiber JHC, Serruys PW. Quantitative coronary arteriography. In: Marcus ML, Skorton DJ, Schelbert HR, Wolf GL (Eds.), Cardiac Imaging. Philadelphia: Saunders 1991: 211–80.
46. Mancini GBJ, DeBoe SF, Anselmo E, Simon SB, LeFree MT, Vogel RA. Quantitative regional curvature analysis: an application of shape determination for the assessment of segmental left ventricular function in man. Am Heart J 1987; **113**: 326–34.
47. Van der Zwet PMJ, Pinto IMF, Serruys PW, Reiber JHC. A new approach for the automated definition of path lines in digitized coronary angiograms. Int J Card Imaging 1990; **5**: 75–83.
48. Kirkeeide RL. Coronary obstructions, morphology and physiologic significance. In: Reiber JHC, Serruys PW (Eds.), Quantitative coronary arteriography. Dordrecht: Kluwer Academic Publishers 1991: 229–44.
49. Herrington DM, Walford GA, Pearson TA. Issues of validation in quantitative coronary angiography. In: Reiber JHC, Serruys PW (Eds.), New developments in quantitative coronary arteriography. Dordrecht: Kluwer Academic Publishers 1988: 153–66.
50. Reiber JHC, Kooijman CJ, Den Boer A, Serruys PW. Assessment of dimensions and image quality of coronary contrast catheters from cineangiograms. Cathet Cardiovasc Diagn 1985; **11**: 521–31.
51. Koning G, van der Zwet PMJ, von Land CD, Reiber JHC. Angiographic assessment of dimensions of 6F and 7F Mallinckrodt Softouch[R] coronary contrast catheters from digital and cine arteriograms. Int J Card Imaging 1992; **8**: 153–61.

6. The filmless catheterization laboratory: when will it be reality?

RÜDIGER SIMON

Summary

Film techniques have been for a long time the standard in vascular and cardiac imaging. Whereas large spot films have been replaced by digital subtraction angiography in peripheral vascular radiology within the last decade, cinefilm has remained the standard in cardiac angiography until recently. With the advent of new hardware technology and fast algorithms for image acquisition and display, digital techniques have now matched the cinefilm in spatial as well as temporal resolution. Thus, cinefilm is no longer needed in the digital catheterization laboratory for proper diagnosis and decision making. The problem of long-term storage of digital images, however, has so far not been solved. There is no digital archival medium or system available that provides sufficient durability, data quality, that is cost effective and allows easy handling of the medium. Thus, the cinefilm is assumed to remain in function as a back-up and exchange medium for some time, and the totally filmless catheterization laboratory will probably not be a widespread reality within the very next future.

When heart catheterization was introduced to clinical cardiology in the 1940's, imaging techniques were rather restricted. Fluoroscopy meant that the investigator had to concentrate on barely discernible pictures displayed on a dimly lightened screen in a totally dark room. Angiograms at that time were taken as large spot films at a rate of only a few exposures per second.

In the sixties, the development of image intensifiers, television or "video" imaging systems and cineangiography fostered a major change in heart catheterization techniques. Fluoroscopy was now possible under daylight conditions and with much better image quality at considerably lower X-ray exposure, and 35 mm cinefilm acquisition during angiography allowed frame rates up to 100 frames/sec. As a result, a much better description of cardiac anatomy as well as a subtle analysis of coronary anatomy became possible. The widespread application of these techniques was a major step forward in cardiac diagnosis, that was followed by new treatment modalities such as

113

J.H.C. Reiber and P.W. Serruys (eds), Advances in Quantitative Coronary Arteriography, 113–122.
© 1993 *Kluwer Academic Publishers. Printed in the Netherlands.*

coronary bypass surgery [1, 2] and interventional catheter techniques such as PTCA [3].

Since then cineangiography has been the standard in cardiology for more than 20 years. There are a number of advantages that have made this technique superior to large spot filming in the sixties. Cinefilming allow high frame rates resulting in a high temporal resolution. In combination with modern image intensifiers, spatial resolution is quite high (4 linepairs/mm). This high quality information is stored reliably for long times (> than 10 years) and can easily be retrieved and displayed using optical filmprojectors. Since 35 mm cine-film is an industrial standard and worldwide available, cineangiograms can be reviewed with standard equipment in any place, which makes the film a preferred medium for storage and exchange. There are, however, disadvantages with cinefilm. The original negative film has to be developed in a rather expensive machinery. The development takes time, requires personel, and may sometimes go wrong. Due to this time consuming development process, decision making in most catheterization laboratory is postponed until the developed film is available. Furthermore, the extraction of quantitative data, that has become more and more an integral part of diagnostic catheterization, requires additional equipment and is doomed to be an off-line procedure outside the catheterization laboratory and after the procedure. It seems logical, therefore, to look for novel imaging techniques that do not have these disadvantages.

Video imaging could provide a solution for some of these drawbacks of the cinefilm. For once, a dynamic review is immediately available. There is no need for a development process, and quantitative data extraction can be done in the catheterization laboratory during replay. Although video tape recorders or disks are available and in use in almost all catheterization laboratories, however, video techniques have never replaced the film because of relatively low image quality. So called "high resolution" video systems using more than 1,000 scanlines per video frame, have improved image quality, but not to an extent to make it really comparable to the cinefilm images.

In the seventies and eighties, another technical break-through has started to revolutionize angiographic techniques. Originating from laboratories in Rochester, Minnesota, Kiel, Germany, and Madison, Wisconsin [see 4, 5], hardware and software techniques have been designed for fast digitization and subtraction of angiographic images. This method of digital subtraction angiography has become "state-of-the-art" for vascular radiology.

The advent of digital imaging in the cardiovascular laboratories, however, has not occurred at the same pace. Due to basic problems such as the constant movement of the heart and underling structures during each heart cycle, simple mask-mode subtraction techniques as used in vascular angiography were not applicable. More sophisticated acquisition systems and computer programs for image processing had to be made available, before conventional cineangiography could be matched in quality by digital techniques.

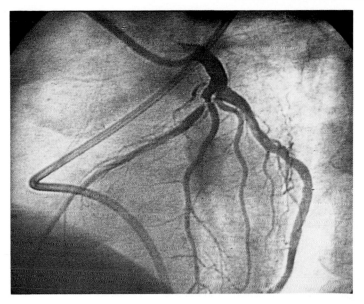

Fig. 1a.

For a considerable amount of time, cinefilm remained superior due to its better spatial and temporal resolution when compared to digital images. The recent development of very fast algorithms for image presentation, contrast enhancement and correction of image distortion or artifacts by sophisticated filtering routines in conjunction with the advent of high-resolution video systems has changed the situation. Optimized coupling of the image intensifier output and the videocamera target, as well as fast acquisition and display algorithms in conjunction with large storage facilities have provided a quality of real-time electronic imaging that is at least comparable in quality with cinefilm. Although pixel matrices of 1024×1024 elements and a high grey level resolution are possible today, a matrix size of 512×512 pixels at a grey level resolution of 8 bits seems sufficient to provide an acceptable image quality [6, 7]. This is of considerable importance since a restriction to this standard matrix would cut down the necessary storage capacity and speed of image processing significantly when compared to extended size matrices or grey scale resolution. With these standard matrices, frame rates up to 60 frames/s are possible with imaging systems that are today offered by the industry; these systems will be acceptable for diagnostic and interventional procedures in adult patients and for most procedures in children.

Integral digital systems can provide further advantages not available with cinefilm. Complex filtering and zooming techniques as well as "windowing" and "leveling" allow the individual adjustment of image quality over a wide range (Figure 1A–C). Additional processing facilities such as dynamic subtraction can reduce the amount of contrast for certain routines considerably,

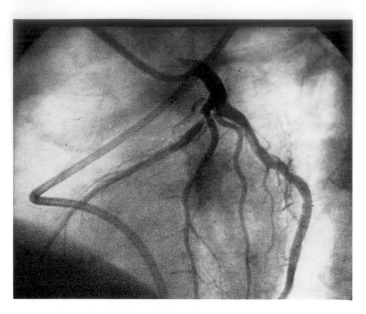

Fig. 1b.

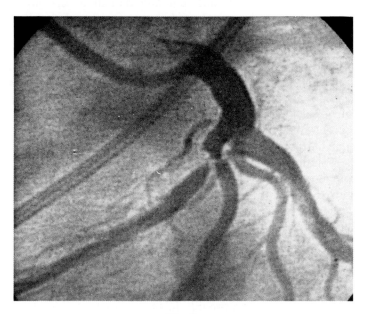

Fig. 1c.

Figures 1A, B & C. Digital coronarography – filtering and zooming. 1A: Original image. 1B: effect of complex filtering (including high-pass filter and edge-enhancement). 1C: additional zooming (including two-directional linear interpolation).

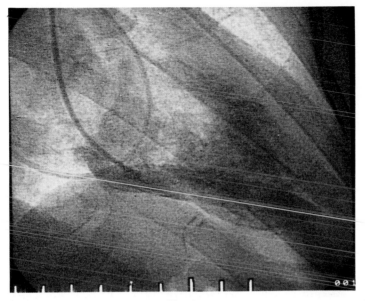

Fig. 2a.

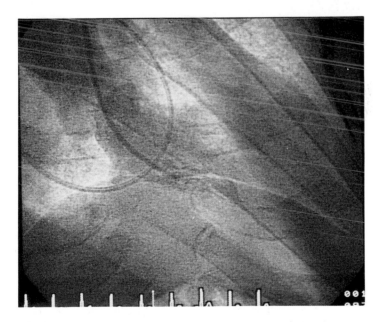

Fig. 2b

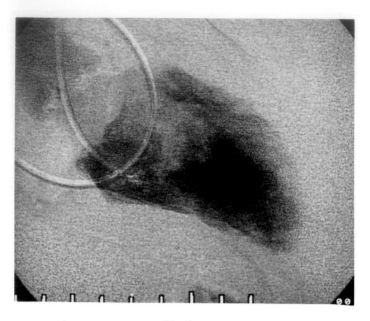

Fig. 2c

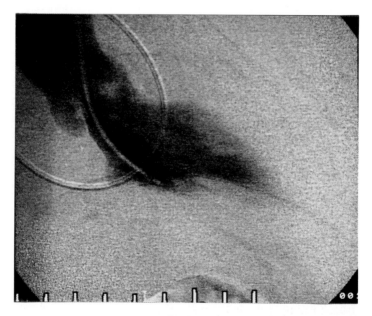

Fig. 2d

Figures 2A–D. Contrast enhancement by phase-matched digital subtraction. 2A, 2B: original images in end-diastole and end-systole after injection of 8 cc of nonionic contrast medium. 2C, 2D: the same images after phase-matched background subtraction and contrast enhancement.

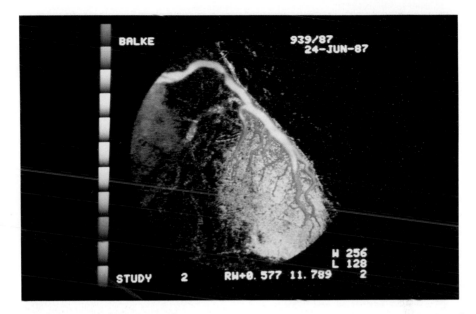

Figure 3. An example of parametric imaging during coronary angiography with an injection of contrast material into aorto-coronary bypass graft to the left anterior descending artery. The arrival of contrast medium is color-coded for each heart beat (color bars on left side correspond to heart beat after start of injection, i.e. purple corresponds to beat No. 1 and the arrival of contrast in the bypass, blue corresponds to beat No. 12 and arrival of contrast in the coronary sinus). The image is a comprehensive representation of contrast flow velocities through the coronary arteries and the myocardium. (Inclusion of this colour illustration has been made possible by support of CIBA GEIGY Foundation.)

which may be of particular relevance in severely ill patients (Figure 2A–D).Furthermore, feature extraction and functional imaging can be done immediately adding valuable information during the procedure (Figures 3 and 4) and allowing immediate decision making.

Finally, new technologies developed only recently such as gap filling in combination with low frequency generator pulsing can reduce the X-ray dosage for fluoroscopy as well as contrast angiography significantly, which is of particular interest in interventional procedures. Accordingly, digital cardiovascular imaging systems have become an increasingly appreciated modality in the interventional catheterization laboratory.

If modern fast digital imaging can provide all these advantageous modalities, why then has it so far not replaced the cinefilm, which is still in use in many cathlabs today?

The main reason, why the filmless catheterization laboratory has not become a widespread reality, has to do with data storage and data exchange. Although real time harddisks are available today that can provide short-term storage capacities for 30,000–50,000 images in a particular laboratory, and

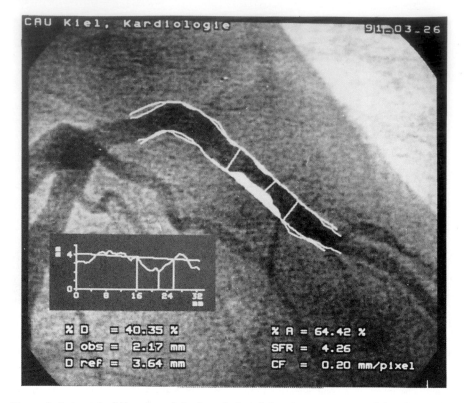

Figure 4. Automatic delineation of the boundaries of the coronary artery and description of a coronary stenosis by a computerized edge-detection method, applied to a digitally stored coronary angiogram. Diameter stenosis was about 40%, area stenosis about 64%, the minimal size of the vessel in the obstructed region 2.17 mm and the reference diameter 3.64 mm. SFR: stenosis flow reserve. CF: calibration factor.

thus handle easily the workload of an entire day, the problem of long-term storage has not been solved in a convincing manner. The requirements for a storage medium that could replace cinefilm in the future are outlined in Table 1. A system for long-term storage of images should provide a high image quality at retrieval, a sufficiently high speed for real-time acquisition and retrieval, and long-term durability, i.e. data security for at least 10 years. The storage medium (e.g. disks or tapes) should be smaller than cinefilm to reduce the space needed for archiving. One "unit" should provide enough capacity to store the entire set of images of one patient (one per one principle). The system hardware and the storage medium should preferably be a worldwide industry standard, it should provide off-line viewing in a simple fashion for the user, and it should be affordable. Finally, a uniform data format should be used by all companies to enable a simple image data exchange between institutions and different types of equipment.

Table 1. Requirements for storage media that could replace the cinefilm

1. Quality	Image quality at least as good as with cinefilm
2. Capacity	Should be sufficient to store all images of *one* patient's investigation
3. Speed	Real-time acquisition and retrieval (30 frames/s or faster)
4. Size	Smaller than a 35 mm cinefilm container
5. Security	Storage should be reliable for at least 10 years
6. Medium	The storage medium should be an industry standard
7. System specifications	Off-line viewing required Handling should be simple; A uniform protocol for all available equipment should be used; The hardware must be affordable

Table 2. Digital archiving systems currently available or under development

	Optical disk 12″	IBM 3480	IBM 3490	8 mm exa-byte	3400 laser tape	DD2
Capacity (GB)	6	0.2	1.6	5	50	25/75/165
Media cost ($)	350	5	5	10	250	40/75/95
Cost/mb (¢)	5.8	2.5	0.003	7	0.5	.001
Transfer rate (mb/sec)	0.6	3	7	0.5	5	15
Access time (sec)	0.4	15	15	45	15	50/94/206
Drive cost (1,000$)	12	8	15	6	20	110
Single unit cost ($)	N/A	N/A	5	10	N/A	40
Media life	>20 yrs	2 yrs	2 yrs	2 yrs	>20 yrs	<5 yrs

(According to Kidd, pers. comm.). N/A: not available.

Today, there is no system or medium available that can fulfill all these criteria. Analog video storage is either poor in image quality or expensive, and not handy (large disks or cassettes). It is also a dead end, since all advantages of image digitization would be lost. Digital storage systems, on the other hand, are so far either slow, expensive, or nonreliable (see Table 2). To make things worse, no uniform protocol for data storage is at hand or even in sight that would be accepted by all companies. On the basis of currently available information, one could estimate that it will take perhaps another five years until a standard protocol as well as a storage medium has emerged, that will allow a reliable storage and a simple data exchange between different types of equipment [8]. It is therefore very likely that the cinefilm will remain in use for some time as a medium for back-up, long-term storage and exchange. In the mean time, we should encourage industry to combine all efforts to reach this very desirable task as soon as possible: the filmless catheterization laboratory.

References

1. Goetz RH, Rohman M, Haller JD, Dee R, Rosenak SS. Internal mammary-coronary artery anastomosis. A nonsuture method employing tantalum rings. J Thorac Cardiovasc Surg 1961; **41**: 378–86.
2. Favaloro RG, Effler, DB, Groves LK, Sheldon WC, Sones FM Jr. Direct myocardial revascularisation by saphenous vein graft. Present operative technique and indications. Ann Thorac Surg 1970; **10**: 97–111.
3. Grüntzig A. Transluminal dilatation of coronary artery stenosis (letter). Lancet 1978; **1**: 263.
4. Heintzen PH, Bürsch JH, Eds. Röntgen-video-technique for dynamic studies of structure and function of the heart and circulation. Stuttgart: Thieme, 1978.
5. Heintzen PH, Brennecke R, Eds. Digital imaging in cardiovascular radiology. Stuttgart: Thieme, 1983.
6. Vogel RA, LeFree MT, Mancini GBJ. Comparison of 35 mm cine film and digital radiographic imaging for quantitative coronary arteriography. In: Heintzen PH, Bürsch JH, (Eds.), Progress in digital angiocardiography. Dordrecht: Kluwer Academic Publishers 1988: 159–72.
7. Mancini GBJ. Digital coronary angiography: advantages and limitations. In: Reiber JHC, Serruys PW, (Eds.), Quantitative coronary arteriography. Dordrecht: Kluwer Academic Publishers 1991: 23–42.

PART THREE

Quality control in QCA

7. Optimal frame selection for QCA

DAVID M. HERRINGTON and GARY D. WALFORD

Summary

Proper frame selection is essential to obtain optimal results from QCA. Understanding the potential sources of frame-to-frame variations in the radiographic appearance of vessels provides a rationale for a frame selection strategy. Data are presented concerning the optimal choice of projection, use of single vs. orthogonal views, timing within the cardiac cycle, and variations between adjacent frames. In addition, results of a study concerning interoperator variability in frame selection and the impact of this variability on the ultimate QCA results will be discussed.

Introduction

Frame selection is a critical element in the successful application of QCA methodology to evaluate coronary physiology and disease. Not only are there frame- to-frame differences in factors that change the radiographic appearance of vessels [1–3]; but also there are physiologic [4–7] and pharmacologic [8, 9] factors which may alter the actual size of the vessel over the course of several frames. Randomly selected frames could potentially lead to dramatically different QCA results from the same cineangiogram of the same coronary artery segment. Optimal frame selection, therefore, should be defined as a practical strategy for selecting frames from a coronary angiogram which will consistently yield the same QCA results for a given segment of the coronary tree. Currently there is no consensus on the optimal approach for selecting frames, although several approaches have been suggested [1, 6, 7, 10–14]. This chapter will review the potential sources of variability that may be influenced by frame selection, identify the key issues that need to be addressed when defining a frame selection strategy, and make specific recommendations about frame selection based on currently available data.

J.H.C. Reiber and P.W. Serruys (eds), Advances in Quantitative Coronary Arteriography, 125–135.
© 1993 Kluwer Academic Publishers. Printed in the Netherlands.

Sources of variability in QCA

There are a number of potential sources of variability in QCA (Figure 1). These sources can be divided into two groups, factors that affect the radiographic appearance of vessels and factors that affect frame analysis. Factors that affect the radiographic appearance include factors related to the physics of X-ray generation, attenuation and detection, patient factors including cardiac and noncardiac parameters, factors related to the angiographic procedure, and factors related to the processing of film. Frame selection serves as a filter through which films with these inherent sources of variability must pass prior to moving on to the actual analysis of selected frames. The following four sections will discuss each of the categories of variability related to the radiographic appearance of vessels as they pertain to frame selection (Table 1). The other major source of QCA variability is related to the process of analyzing a selected frame (Figure 1). As these factors are not affected by frame selection, they will not be discussed.

X-ray physics

There are a number of relevant X-ray imaging phenomena including quantum mottle, scatter and veiling glare, beam hardening, pincushion and magnification distortion, and blurring of the image related to the focal spot size, object motion and characteristics of the image intensifier [15]. The effects of some of these factors, such as quantum mottle, scatter, veiling glare, and beam hardening are relatively subtle to the human observer and are likely only to play a small role in QCA variability. In fact, quantum mottle is a statistically random phenomenon and thus is somewhat unavoidable. Nonetheless, care should be taken to avoid frames where there is a significant mottled appearance in the region of edges of interest. The focal spot size and characteristics of the image intensifier are fixed determinants of the line spread function of the imaging chain which results in blurring of the image. Their effects are relatively constant from frame-to-frame. On the other hand,

Sources of Variability in QCA

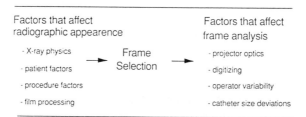

Figure 1. Sources of variability in QCA.

Table 1. Source of variability in QCA–factors affecting radiographic appearance of vessels

X-ray physics
- quantum mottle, scatter, veiling glare, beam hardening
- pincushion and magnification distortion
- focal spot size, input phosphor thickness, motion artifacts

Patient factors
- vasomotor tone, perfusion pressure
- patient, respiratory, and cardiac motion
- cardiac cycle dependent changes in luminal dimensions
- asymmetry in the lumen
- overlapping structures

Equipment and procedure factors
- camera positions (height, skew, relationship to the geomagnetic field)
- collimation and magnification mode
- mixing of contrast in the vessel

Film processing
- temperature
- under, or over replenishment of the developer solution
- variations in fixing, washing, and drying of the film

motion artifacts, the third major component of the line spread function, can change from frame-to-frame. Therefore, frames in which the vessel segment of interest is stationary are desirable.

Pincushion distortion is enhanced in the peripheral zones of the image field and, therefore, selection of frames where the region of interest is as close to the center of the field of view as possible will help diminish the impact of this distortion. If a section of the angiographic catheter is being used to establish scale, then it is important to choose frames in which the distal tip of the catheter, which is usually closest to the vessel segment of interest, is well visualized. This will avoid variability related to magnification (or out-of-plane) distortion.

Patient factors

Important patient factors that may influence frame selection include changes in vasomotor tone, patient position, respiratory effort, cardiac motion, cardiac cycle dependent changes in luminal dimensions, asymmetry in the lumen, and significant overlapping structures. Obviously, frames with as few overlapping structures as possible should be sought. A few minutes coaching the patient in breath holding can greatly reduce extraneous movement and simplify the task of choosing frames with minimal motion artifact. In addition, knowledge about the timing of administration of vasoactive drugs such as nitroglycerin can help the operator select frames less likely to produce results confounded by excessive differences in vasomotor tone. The issues

Table 2. General guidelines for frame selection

Frames should be selected that have the following properties:
– maximal, homogeneous opacification
– no structures overlapping the vessel segment of interest
– vessel segment in the center of the field of view
– projection perpendicular to the long axis of the vessel
– appropriate collimation

of lumen asymmetry and cardiac cycle dependent changes in luminal filling and size will be addressed in subsequent sections.

Angiographic procedure

The angiographic procedure itself also introduces potential sources of variability that can be avoided with proper frame selection. Low contrast concentration has a significant adverse effect on accuracy of QCA results [16]. Therefore, frames should be selected in which there is vigorous injection and full opacification of the vessel segment of interest, preferably with regurgitation of excess contrast into the aorta. Magnified image intensifier modes improve spacial resolution and frames from such sequences are desirable. Occasionally, there are differences from one injection sequence to the next in the degree of columnation. Frames in which appropriate columnation is used helps reduce the effects of scatter. Also, frames from projections close to perpendicular to the long axis of the vessel segment of interest are desirable to avoid errors related to foreshortening of the lesion.

Film processing

Finally, the film processing is an often overlooked potential source of variability. Fluctuations in temperature or variations in the replenishment of the developer solution or fixing, washing, and drying of the film result in differences in the subsequent images of the vessels in question [17]. These problems are unlikely to be readily apparent over the span of a few frames or even several hundred frames during a portion of an angiographic study. Nonetheless, care should be taken to avoid frames where there are obvious problems in the film development process.

Thus, from an understanding of the sources of variability in the radiographic appearance of vessels, some general guidelines about frame selection can be derived (Table 2). These general guidelines can be summarized by the "common sense" statement: Optimal frames for QCA analysis are those in which the vessel segment of interest is most clearly seen. However, after agreeing on the general approach to frame selection, there remain a number of important issues that need to be addressed when defining a frame selection strategy for QCA. These include questions about the optimal projection to select frames from, the optimal portion of the cardiac cycle during which frames should be selected, and which frame (or frames) during a defined portion of the cardiac cycle should be used. Furthermore, even with specific recommendations concerning projection, timing within cardiac cycle, and frame selection, there remains the issue of whether or not there still will be significant inter-subject variability in the actual frames selected and what the impact of that variability on the ultimate QCA results will be. Each of these issues will now be examined in turn.

Most severe projection?

Some investigators [18] choose frames for subsequent QCA analysis in which the lesion of interest appears to be most severe. Although this strategy has some intuitive appeal, it is subject to certain logical flaws and may prove to be detrimental if it's use results in a compromise in the clarity of the images selected. If a lesion appears more severe in one view than another, the vessel lumen must be asymmetric (assuming equivalent filling, perpendicular views, etc.). However, when this is true, the view in which the lesion appears to be most severe will underestimate the cross-sectional area of the vessel (assuming a circular shape), just as selecting a view in which the lesion appears less severe will likely result in an overestimate. Thus, a single projection showing the lesion as most severe has no particular advantage over a projection in which the lesion appears less severe, unless there is a desire to systematically err towards more severe estimates. Furthermore, if the QCA measurements are to be used in the context of a progression/regression study, there is no guarantee that change in luminal dimensions due to regression or progression of disease will occur in the portion of the vessel most easily seen from the projection that the lesion appeared most severe (Figure 2). Therefore, the most severe projection offers no particular advantage for detecting changes due to progression or regression of disease.

   Finally, as a practical matter, the number of lesions in which there is true, significant asymmetry is relatively small. Downes et al. [19] demonstrated that the major to minor axis ratio of diseased vessel segments measured by intravascular ultrasound has an average ratio of 1.08. Teleologically, this observation is not surprising since round lumen remain the most hemodynamically efficient conduit for blood. Even following an acute catastrophic disruption of lumen shape, such as with ulceration of a plaque, the body attempts to restore the round lumen over time through the reparative and healing process which, in fact, is part of the atherosclerotic process as well. Thus, there are no major advantages to selection of frames in which the lesion of interest appears most severe and such frames should not be selected over frames from other views in which the lesion of interest is more clearly seen.

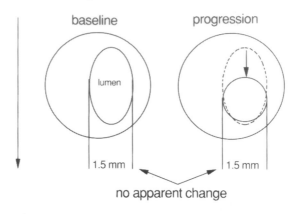

Figure 2. Choosing a projection in which the lesion appears most severe will not necessarily be the best projection to detect changes in luminal dimensions due to progression or regression of disease.

Orthogonal views?

Some authors have suggested that the orthogonal views are helpful to reduce the variability in QCA measures of luminal dimensions. However, selection of orthogonal views is not uniformly possible with all coronary vessel segments. Fifteen to fifty percent of vessel segments are not analyzable in paired orthogonal views from routine diagnostic coronary angiograms [12, 13, 20]. Furthermore, Lesperance et al. [13] demonstrated very small differences between results obtained from single views and results obtained from orthogonal views for vessel segments pre- and post-PTCA as well as from repeat angiograms six months following the balloon dilatation (Figure 3). This suggests that orthogonal views add little or no additional information over a well selected single view. Clearly, averaging multiple measures of the same vessel segment will reduce variability; however, it is not clear that averaging orthogonal views would be significantly better than averaging results from two or more frames from the same or similar projections. Therefore, it may not be worth the additional effort required to identify and analyze paired orthogonal views.

Which part of the cardiac cycle?

Once a projection has been selected from the angiogram, another decision needs to be made concerning when during the cardiac cycle a frame should be selected. Selzer et al. [6, 7] systematically examined this question by comparing the differences between adjacent frames from end diastole, mid-

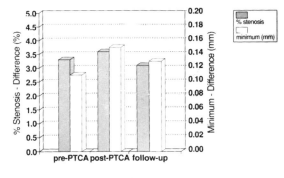

adapted from Lesperance et.al. Am J Cardiol 1989

Figure 3. Mean differences between results obtained from a single view and average of orthogonal views for % diameter stenosis and minimum diameter.

diastole and beginning systole as well as randomly selected frames from anywhere in diastole, anywhere in systole and anywhere in the cardiac cycle (Figure 4). The coefficients of variation generated from these comparisons provide an estimate of the relative variability associated with frame selection from various parts of the cardiac cycle. Adjacent frames selected from end diastole had the lowest coefficient variation. This suggests that end diastole is the portion of the cardiac cycle least likely to introduce frame-to-frame variations in the results obtained from subsequent QCA analysis. This is probably related to the fact that end diastole is associated with relatively little cardiac motion and, therefore, may be less subject to frame to-frame variations in motion artifacts, or changes in intraluminal mixing of contrast.

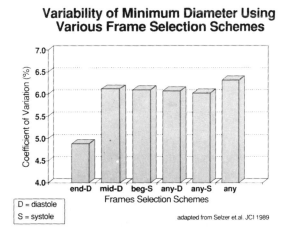

Figure 4. Coefficient of variation for adjacent frames in various parts of the cardiac cycle.

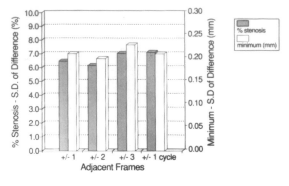

Adapted from Reiber et al. Cathet Cardiovasc Diagn 1985

Figure 5. Standard deviation of the differences between QCA results from frames separated by ±1, ±2, ±3 frames and ±1 cardiac cycle.

Selzer et al. [4, 5] also demonstrated that the actual dimensions of the artery are more stable at the end diastole than at other times during the cardiac cycle.

Once the portion of the cardiac cycle has been selected, the only remaining question is which frame should be used. Reiber et al. [10, 11] examined the variability of differences between frames that were ± 1, ±2 or ±3 frames apart within the same portion of the cardiac cycle (Figure 5). In addition, the variability between frames ± 1 cardiac cycle apart were examined. This study demonstrated a very small increase in variability between frames separated by ± 3 frames compared to those separated by one or two frames. This suggests that within a given portion of a cardiac cycle, there may be a small degree of latitude one way or the other with respect to the actual frame to be selected without imposing too harsh a penalty in terms of significant additional variability in results. Furthermore, Reiber demonstrated that frames from the same portion of one cardiac cycle are likely to yield very similar results to frames from exactly the same time in a subsequent or preceding cardiac cycle.

Observer variability?

Even with a specific and well defined strategy for frame selection, the question still remains whether or not there is significant interobserver variability in the actual frames that would be selected using these criteria, and whether or not these differences in frame selection result in meaningful differences in the actual QCA results. To examine whether or not there is significant interobserver variability in frame selection, angiograms from 30 coronary lesions were examined (author's unpublished data). Investigator 1 selected

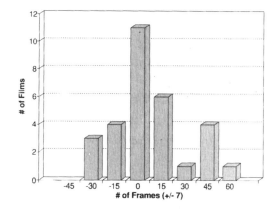

Figure 6. Distribution of the number of frames separating the optimal frame selected by operator #1 vs. operator #2 for 30 lesions.

the optimal frame for QCA analysis based on a predefined set of frame selection criteria. These criteria included the selection of frames in which the vessel segment of interest was well seen, with maximum opacification, no significant overlapping structures, and occurring as close to end diastole as possible. A second investigator, using the same selection criteria, also selected the optimal frame for QCA analysis from the same angiographic injection sequence. The frames selected by the two investigators were subsequently analyzed in a standardized fashion by a trained QCA operator. For each lesion, the frame number selected by the first and second observer were recorded and compared. Figure 6 shows the frequency distribution of number of frames separating the two selections. The average absolute number of frames between the first and second observer selection was 19.4, range 0–52. Only once did the two observers select the exact same frame. Fifty percent of the time, the two observers selected frames within the same cardiac cycle. Thirty-five percent of the time, the two selections were in adjacent cardiac cycles, and 15% of the selection pairs were separated by two cardiac cycles. There were no selection pairs greater than two cardiac cycles apart.

The coefficient variation for minimum diameter from frames selected by the two different observers was 4.4%. This compares favorably with the results generated by Selzer et al. [6, 7] which were generated from frames analyzed in a highly controlled and sequential fashion as opposed to the frames in this study which were selected by different observers and analyzed independently and at completely separate times. These data demonstrate that, although QCA operators using the same selection criteria may select different frames for analysis, the final results are likely to be very similar.

Conclusions

In conclusion, certain recommendations can be made based on an understanding of the process of X-ray imaging and QCA analysis and data from the literature concerning optimal frame selection strategy. In general, a high priority should be placed on the clarity of the image to be analyzed including selection of frames with maximal homogeneous opacification of the vessel of interest, no significant overlapping structures or adjacent vessels, in which the vessel segment of interest is in the center of the field of view, with its long axis perpendicular to the projection angle. Appropriate radiographic technique including columnation and magnification mode are also important. Although there is an intuitive appeal for selecting frames in which the lesion may appear most severe, there is little evidence to suggest that there is a distinct advantage for adopting this approach. As a practical matter, the number of times that there is significant asymmetry is probably small and unlikely to be a major source of additional variability. Similarly, while orthogonal views have some intellectual appeal for providing a more complete evaluation of the vessel segment, in reality, a true pair of orthogonal views is often difficult to obtain and may not be worth the additional effort for the relatively small increase in precision on the estimate of luminal dimensions. Clearly, end diastole is the optimal time for selection of frames for subsequent QCA analysis. Within end diastole, there may be relatively little meaningful difference from one frame to the next in terms of the final results. Similarly, frames from end diastole from one cardiac cycle are likely to yield similar results to frames from end diastole in adjacent cardiac cycles. Finally, with a well defined set of selection criteria, it is possible for two observers to independently select frames which, although may not coincide perfectly in the angiogram itself, will be likely to yield equivalent results from subsequent QCA analysis. Thus, use of appropriate criteria for frame selection can avoid many potential sources of variability resulting in more accurate and precise measurements using QCA.

References

1. Reiber JH, Serruys PW, Kooijman CJ, Slager CJ, Schuurbiers JH, Boer A. Approaches towards standardization in acquisition and quantitation of arterial dimensions from cineangiograms. In: Reiber JH, Serruys PW, (Eds.), State of the art in quantitative coronary arteriography. Dordrecht: Nijhoff 1986: 145–72.
2. Reiber JHC, Serruys PW, Kooijman CJ, et al. Assessment of short-, medium-, and long-term variations in arterial dimensions from computer-assisted quantitation of coronary cineangiograms. Circulation 1985; **71**: 280–8.
3. Brown BG, Bolson EL, Dodge HT. Arteriographic assessment of coronary atherosclerosis. Review of current methods, their limitations, and clinical applications. Arteriosclerosis 1982; **2**: 2–15.
4. Sandor T, Spears JR, Paulin S. Densitometric determination of changes in the dimensions of coronary arteries. Proc SPIE 1981; **314**: 263–72.

5. Hori M, Inoue M, Shimazu T, et al. Clinical assessment of coronary arterial elastic properties by the image processing of coronary arteriograms. Comput Cardiol 1983: 393–5.
6. Selzer RH, Siebes M, Hagerty C, et al. Effects of cardiac phase on diameter measurements from coronary cineangiograms. Comput Cardiol 1988: 363–6.
7. Selzer RH, Hagerty C, Azen SP, et al. Precision and reproducibility of quantitative coronary angiography with applications to controlled clinical trials. A sampling study. J Clin Invest 1989; **83**: 520–6.
8. Brown BG. Response of normal and diseased epicardial coronary arteries to vasoactive drugs: quantitative arteriographic studies. Am J Cardiol 1985; **56**: 23E–29E.
9. Badger RS, Brown BG, Gallery CA, Bolson EL, Dodge HT. Coronary artery dilation and hemodynamic responses after isosorbide dinitrate therapy in patients with coronary artery disease. Am J Cardiol 1985; **56**: 390–5.
10. Reiber JH, van Eldik-Helleman P, Kooijman CJ, Tijssen JG, Serruys PW. How critical is frame selection in quantitative coronary angiographic studies? Eur Heart J 1989; **10** (Suppl F): 54–9.
11. Reiber JH, van Eldik-Helleman P, Visser-Akkerman N, Kooijman CJ, Serruys PW. Variabilities in measurement of coronary arterial dimensions resulting from variations in cinefframe selection. Cathet Cardiovasc Diagn 1988; **14**: 221–8.
12. Brown BG, Bolson E, Frimer M, Dodge HT. Quantitative coronary arteriography: estimation of dimensions, hemodynamic resistance, and atheroma mass of coronary artery lesions using the arteriogram and digital computation. Circulation 1977, **55**. 329–37.
13. Lesperance J, Hudon G, White CW, Laurier J, Waters D. Comparison by quantitative angiographic assessment of coronary stenoses of one view showing the severest narrowing to two orthogonal views. Am J Cardiol 1989; **64**: 462–5.
14. Alderman EL, Berte LE, Harrison DC, Sanders W. Quantitation of coronary artery dimensions using digital image processing. Proc SPIE 1981; **314**: 273–8.
15. Sprawls P Jr. Image blur and resolution. In: Sprawls P Jr. The physical principles of diagnostic radiology. Baltimore: University Park Press 1977: 193–217.
16. Spears JR, Sandor T, Als AV, et al. Computerized image analysis for quantitative measurement of vessel diameter from cineangiograms. Circulation 1983; **68**: 453–61.
17. Curry TS 3d, Dowdey JE, Murry RC Jr. Physical characteristics of x-ray film and film processing. In: Curry TS 3d, Dowdey JE, Murry RC Jr. Christensen's introduction to the physics of diagnostic radiology. Philadelphia: Lea & Febiger, 3rd ed. 1984: 124–33.
18. Waters D, Lespérance J, Francetich M, et al. A controlled clinical trial to assess the effect of a calcium channel blocker on the progression of coronary atherosclerosis. Circulation 1990; 82: 1940–53. Comment in: Circulation 1990; **82**: 2251–3.
19. Downes TR, Braden GA, Herrington DM, Applegate RJ, Kutcher MA, Little WC: Mechanism of PTCA dilatation in coronary vessels: intravascular ultrasound assessment. Cardiol 1990; 17(2 Suppl. A): 126A (Abstract).
20. Popma JJ, Eichhorn EJ, Dehmer GJ. In vivo assessment of a digital angiographic method to measure absolute coronary artery diameters. Am J Cardiol 1989; **64**: 131–8.

8. Variability of QCA-core laboratory assessments of coronary anatomy

GLENN J. BEAUMAN, JOHAN H.C. REIBER,
GERHARD KONING and ROBERT A. VOGEL

Summary

Quantitative coronary arteriography (QCA) has become an essential part of centralized core laboratory evaluations for clinical investigations. Most evaluations of variability of quantitative arteriography have been internally controlled studies with little relevancy to factors associated with core laboratory analyses of large populations. We therefore investigated the variability of repetitive quantitative analyses performed on randomly chosen films from ongoing clinical trials, comparing the relative and absolute parameters determined from internally and externally controlled evaluations. In addition, as quantitative methods and systems are known to vary among core facilities, we evaluated the variability of differing frame selection methods and assessed inter-laboratory variability on differing automated quantitative systems.

Assessments of variability between externally and internally controlled evaluations were found to be dissimilar. The variability (standard deviation) of relative assessment parameters (percent diameter stenosis) in the externally controlled evaluations was 56% greater than the variability of the internally controlled evaluations and absolute parameter variability was found to be 70% greater. Averaged minimal lumen diameter (MLD) from orthogonal projections was found to be the least variable parameter.

Frame selection methodology was not found to be of consequence to the variability of quantitative assessments. No significant differences were found between analyses performed on frames chosen by differing methods, or between frames of each method and frames selected from end-diastole, end-systole, or end-diastasis.

Inter-laboratory variability was determined from automated computer analysis of the randomly chosen frames performed by independent laboratories. Subjectively defined reference diameter values correlated poorly with automated computer reference values ($r = 0.66$). Consequently, percent diameter stenosis comparisons were found to reflect this variability. In addition, differences in MLD values between laboratories (0.23 ± 0.37 mm) were

J.H.C. Reiber and P.W. Serruys (eds), Advances in Quantitative Coronary Arteriography, 137–159.

found to be significantly different ($p < 0.05$), despite similar assessment techniques.

These studies of core laboratory variability emphasize the need for independent and externally controlled evaluations of core laboratory performance, and standardization of QCA calibration and validation techniques.

Introduction

Automated Quantitative Coronary Arteriographic (QCA) methods have been developed over the past decade to increase the reproducibility and accuracy of evaluating coronary artery anatomy over standard visual analysis methods [1–6]. Although aids to visual analysis, such as electronic calipers, have been used to address the limitations of visually based methods, the inherent problems associated with such assessments persist [7–8]. Conversely, QCA techniques, which were initially cumbersome and time consuming, have been vastly improved.

Throughout the decade of development, QCA techniques have been validated in studies using plexiglass phantoms, intraluminally positioned plastic stenoses, human arteries obtained at autopsy, and various angiographic balloons, catheters, and guidewires [9–14]. The accuracy and variability of automated quantitative methods have convincingly been shown to be superior to that of visual assessments [15–16]. However, assessments of accuracy and variability are most frequently assessed from internally controlled experiments. In addition, quantitative systems and methods are known to differ among core facilities, and little is known of inter-laboratory variability or intra- and inter-observer variability of quantitative analyses in large populations of cinefilm. This chapter describes our findings of intra- and inter-laboratory variability of quantitative coronary arteriography.

Variability in core laboratory QCA analysis of cinearteriograms

The assessment of QCA variability is subject to a wide variety of factors. In addition to describing variability by a variety of evaluation parameters (i.e. correlation coefficient, mean difference ± standard deviations, and coefficient of variation), QCA variability can be described from studies involving a variety of image analysis options. For example, variability has been described from: 1) side by side analyses, where projection and cardiac cycle orientation of targeted segments are closely matched between differing arteriograms; 2) unblinded analysis of arteriograms repeated at varying intervals; and 3) repeated analyses of the same image. Variability assessed by each method is unique and therefore cannot be used as a broad descriptor of

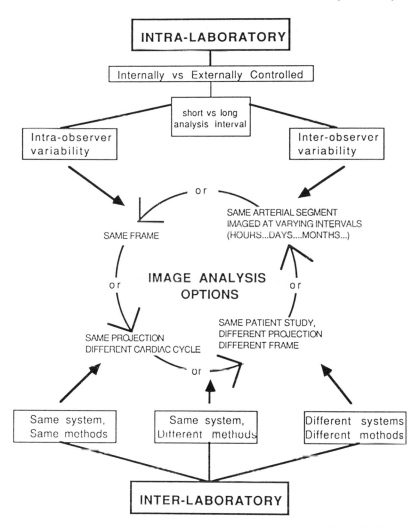

Figure 1. Methods and analysis options associated with the assessment of quantitative coronary arteriographic variability.

QCA variability. The complexity of associated factors and the multiplicity of assessment permutations is described in Figure 1.

Initial reports of variability compared side by side analyses of sequentially acquired arteriographic images [18] or unblinded analysis of arteriograms repeated at varying intervals controlled for magnification and projection [19]. These early evaluations helped to establish confidence limits for assessing change in coronary anatomy using QCA techniques and are frequently referenced as descriptors of "QCA variability". Most descriptions of intra- and inter-observer variability show excellent correlation coefficients, low variability (mean difference and standard deviation), and low coefficients of variance. However, upon closer evaluation, it is apparent that the excellent results commonly reported are often the result of internally controlled studies, where repeated analysis of an identical image, optimized for QCA techniques, has been performed with limited operator blindedness to initially determined values.

The variability assessed from a side by side comparisons of arteriograms is not equivalent to the variability determined from a completely blinded re-analysis of routinely acquired arteriograms. To date, most evaluations of analysis variability have little relevance to factors that describe analysis variability of core laboratory function. We have therefore evaluated: 1) the differences between internally and externally controlled analysis variability; 2) the variability of analyses as a result of operator or methodologic variations; and 3) the inter-laboratory variability of automated computer analyses of coronary anatomy.

Quantitative methods and equipment

Quantitative methodology requires an operator/computer interface which may be the greatest source of variability in quantitative assessments. A brief description of the quantitative methods and equipment used to assess core laboratory variability follows.

Analyses performed at the University of Maryland Core Quantitative Facility followed pre-established guidelines for projection/frame selection and for describing reference, stenotic, and percent diameter stenosis parameters. These standardized operational guidelines are applied to all analyses performed in our laboratory. In brief, suitable projection selection is based on orthogonality and greatest visualization of target segment (i.e. optimally opacified arterial segments, optimal signal to noise differentiation, minimal neighboring vessel or anatomical structure overlap). Individual frame selection from designated projections follows a sharpest focus/narrowest visualization method, where the stenotic portion of the targeted segment is viewed at maximal narrowing and the image of the arterial silhouette is in sharpest focus. In our laboratory, selection of an individual frame from orthogonal projections (or near orthogonal projections) is not based on a specific cardiac cycle timing.

Analyses were performed using commercially available quantitative software (Artrek, version 10) and a digital angiographic computer system (ADAC 4100C Plus, ADAC Laboratories., Milpitas, CA). This quantitative system has been extensively validated and described in detail elsewhere [9, 10, 16, 17]. Briefly, the analysis process follows a sequential progression of frame digitization, operator identification of targeted segment, and report generation. Individual cineframes are positioned on a standard cinefilm projector (Vanguard XR-35) optically coupled to a high resolution video camera.

Assessments of densitometric profiles through the projected field allows for appropriate exposure adjustments, prior to direct digitization of the optically magnified image (2:1) into a 512×512 pixel matrix with 8 bits of density levels.

The analysis process is initiated by operator identification of the targeted segment. This results in an electronic magnification ($2\times$) of the area of interest and a linear expansion of the dynamic range, facilitating full use of the 8 bit range. The operator then identifies the approximate center of the arterial segment undergoing analysis and adjusts the diameter of a circular area of interest to define the limits of the segment analysis. No further operator intervention is required. The centerline of the defined segment is labeled first from consecutive circumferential density profiles of progressively decreasing radii. The arterial borders are then determined in a 2 stage process. First, linear density profiles are drawn perpendicular to the centerline at approximately 0.3 mm intervals. Pixels with density values equal to 75% of the difference between the first and second derivative functions (1st derivative weighted) are labeled for each arterial border. On a second pass, following a screening for spatial continuity, points found to lie outside a specified range are replaced with more appropriate points whose values are determined from gray scale values of acceptable neighboring pixels. As a result of this local thresholding technique, smooth, continuous edges are determined for each vessel border. Magnification calibration, for determining absolute dimensions, is accomplished by applying the same algorithm to a portion of an angiographic catheter of uniform diameter. The validity of computer determined arterial borders is verified visually. Although generally successful, overlapping anatomical or angiographic structures can result in erroneously defined edges, therefore an operator controlled edge point editor is available for minor corrections.

Computer output of the analysis reports absolute arterial dimensions and relative percent diameter stenosis measurements; the latter based on an operator determined "normal" reference segment and the smallest luminal diameter found in the stenotic area of interest. Whenever possible, a standardized formula for describing the reference segment was used. As such, the reference segment represented a portion of the arterial segment minimally 1 mm in length ($\geqslant 5$ diameter points), proximal to the stenotic area of interest, and distal to intervening side branches of significant caliber. A single, computer determined, minimal lumen diameter was used to describe the stenotic segment. Minor operator controlled editing was permitted on a limited basis for obviously errant arterial border detection. Manual repositioning of edge points or simple linear interpolation was limited to 5 or fewer contiguous edge points in areas identified as reference or stenotic portions of the target segment. If more points in these key regions required correction, the analysis for that projection was reported to have "failed" and excluded from the evaluation.

At the University of Leiden QCA core laboratory the following projection and frame selection criteria are followed. Projections should be chosen such that foreshortening of the segments of interest is minimal, i.e. the coronary segment should be visualized at its longest length. Segments with significant foreshortening are excluded from analysis. Each coronary segment is preferably analyzed from two orthogonal or nearly orthogonal views (differences in rotational angles at least 60°C). For frame selection purposes the following guidelines are pertinent:

1. select a frame in the 2nd or 3rd cardiac cycle following contrast injection;
2. make sure that the segment of interest is fully opacified; if not go to another cardiac cycle;
3. select the frame at end-diastole or in the diastasis period so that the effect of motion blur is minimal;
4. if the angiographic view shows the segment minimally foreshortened, the frame with largest luminal size is chosen;
5. on the other hand, if foreshortening occurs at the obstruction, the frame with maximal narrowing (smallest luminal size) is chosen;
6. if no appropriate frame can be found at end diastole or in the diastasis period for example due to vessel or catheter overlap, go to another part in the cardiac cycle, e.g. end systole.

Analyses in Leiden were performed with the Cardiovascular Measurement System (CMS) (Medis Medical Imaging Systems, Nuenen, the Netherlands). The CMS uses a high quality CAP-35E telecine converter allowing a selected cineframe to be projected onto the target of a CCD camera via a zoom lens (range 1–6×); in practice, an optical magnification of 2.3–2.9× is used. The video signal from the CCD camera is subsequently digitized at a matrix size of $512 \times 512 \times 8$ bits by means of a frame grabber/image memory (Imaging Technologies VFG) installed in the host processor being a Compaq 80386/80486 at 33 MHz. The digitized image is then available for subsequent analysis.

To define the coronary segment to be analyzed, the user selects with the mouse of the system a start point and an end point inside the arterial segment. Next, an arterial pathline through the segment of interest is computed automatically. The automated pathline technique is based upon two algorithms: the socalled tracer algorithm and the box algorithm, which have been described in detail elsewhere [20].

The contour detection procedure is carried out in 2 iterations: the first one relative to the detected pathline, and the second one relative to the individual contours detected in the first iteration. The contour detection technique itself is based on resampling the image perpendicular to a model (in the 1st iteration the pathline; in the 2nd iteration the contours detected in the 1st iteration) and applying the minimal cost contour detection technique to the resampled matrix [21, 22]. This technique has been shown to be very robust and computationally fast. To correct for the limited bandwith of the entire X-ray imaging system, the minimal cost contour detection technique is modified in the second iteration based on an analysis of the point spread function of the imaging chain, which is of particular importance for the accurate measurement of small vessels.

For calibration purposes, a nontapering part of the contrast catheter is used. Basically, the same procedure is followed for the automated edge detection of this segment of the contrast catheter as for an arterial segment, as described above. However, in this case additional information is used in the 2nd iteration of the edge detection process, knowing that the nontapering part of the catheter is characterized by parallel, although not necessarily straight, boundaries.

From the two sets of contour points of the arterial segment a new accurate centerline is computed. Next, a diameter function is determined by measuring for every second position along this centerline the distances between the two contours. From these data the following parameters are automatically calculated: the site of maximal percent diameter stenosis, the corresponding lesion diameter (does not need to be at the point of absolutely minimal vessel diameter, as the lesion was selected by the *maximal percent* diameter stenosis), the extent of the obstruction and the corresponding reference diameter. To be able to automatically determine the reference diameter value, an estimation of the size of the vessel prior to the occurrence of a focal obstruction has to be reconstructed (the socalled reference diameter function). The reference diameter value is taken at the site of the obstruction, so that neither overestimation nor underestimation occurs.

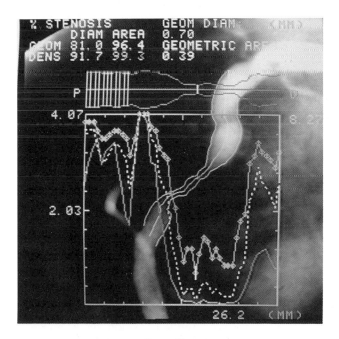

Figure 2a.

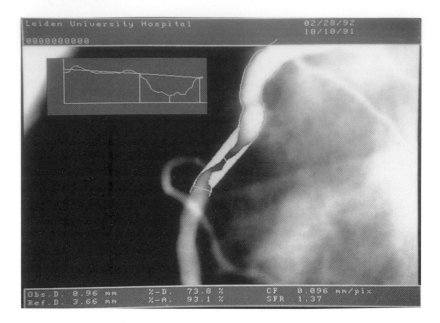

Figure 2b.

Figures 2a, b Typical examples of the output of both quantitative software packages for a proximal RCA coronary segment.Figure 2A shows the results from the ADAC system, Figure 2B from the CMS.

Figure 2 illustrates the output of both quantitative software packages on a typical example from our patient population; in this case a proximal RCA coronary segment. Figure 2A shows the results from the ADAC system, Figure 2B those from the CMS. In this example the following data were obtained:

	ADAC	CMS
Obstruction diameter	0.70 mm	0.96 mm
%-D stenosis	81.0%	74.3%

Study film populations

Core laboratory variability was evaluated using three populations (I, II and III) of cinefilm. Initial internally controlled investigations were made on thirteen films (Population I) randomly selected from the archives of the University of Maryland catheterization laboratory. Angiograms in this population were reviewed twice in blinded fashion by a single observer. The operator was blinded to frame selections, reference and stenotic segments identified in the initial reading, but was unblinded to previously selected projections from which individual frames were identified.

The second film population (II) consisted of 11 patient cine-arteriograms randomly selected from a prospective multicenter clinical trial (V.A. Cooperative Study #267, comparing medical therapy to PTCA). From this population, intra- and inter-observer variability was assessed from the analysis of frames identified as most appropriate for analysis by 2 observers following selection schema specific to their independent quantitative core laboratories. The independently identified cineframes were digitized and analyzed at the QCA core laboratories of the University of Maryland and University Hospital Leiden to assess inter-laboratory variability. In addition, a series of contrast filled plexiglass arterial phantom images were analyzed to determine inter-system variability. The phantoms were imaged over patient chest anatomy at an outside laboratory so as to simulate clinically relevant radiographic parameters. Both core laboratories were blinded to the actual dimensions of the phantom. The external dimensions of a diagnostic angiographic catheter (present in the field) and a centimeter grid were provided for calibration purposes.

Evaluation of core laboratory variability was also assessed by an externally controlled process. As part of the quantitative analysis of films included in the 1985–86 NHLBI PTCA Registry, a pre-designed proportion of the total population was resubmitted to the University of Maryland to assess core laboratory variability. Over a period of 24 months, 640 patient films were submitted to our laboratory for analysis. From this population, 123 paired (pre- and post-angioplasty) arterial segments (Population III) were randomly resubmitted at varying intervals. The operator was completely blinded to previously chosen projections, individual cineframes, and reference and stenotic segments. Unlike the multicenter cinefilm population that made up the V.A. trial, these films were analyzed in retrospective fashion. Cineacquisitions in this population were widely variable with regards to radiographic quality and angiographic technique. Variability as described in this population should be considered to represent the worst case scenario.

Internal vs. external evaluations

To more realistically assess core laboratory function with regards to quantitative analysis in clinical investigations, we compared the variability (mean difference, standard deviations, and correlation coefficients) of repeated quantitative analyses that were performed on the first and third study film populations. The film group from the University of Maryland archives (the first study film population) represents an internally controlled evaluation. Although the films were randomly chosen and analyzed in a blinded fashion, all cinearteriograms were generated using the same radiographic catheterization laboratory equipment, by a small group of experienced angiographers whose techniques were similar. The images used were exposed and processed in a uniform fashion and quantitatively analyzed as a group by in-house personnel, with a short interval between repeated analyses (60 days). Variability in this study group was compared with the multi-variable NHLBI Registry film population (third study film group). Management of the assessment process in this population was completely external to the core quantitative facility. Films were encoded to facilitate a blinded evaluation and the frequency and interval between repeated analyses was variable, ranging from 2–24 months. The multicenter, retrospective nature of the study effectively contrasted all radiographic/angiographic variables of the first study group in that the population was acquired via widely varying radiographic systems and angiographic techniques and was completely uncontrolled for factors known to affect QCA methods. In addition, nontechnical factors such as, transcription errors, errant coronary segment identification and operator variability, that are an inherent part of large clinical investigations, were purposely not excluded to provide the most realistic assessment of core laboratory variability in such quantitative applications.

Dimensional differences were determined between quantitative analyses for the following: Right Anterior Oblique projections, Left Anterior Oblique projections, averaged value for two projections, the maximal value (i.e. largest diameter) of two projections, and the minimal value (i.e. smallest diameter) of two projections. Table 1 describes the mean difference, standard deviation of the differences, and correlation coefficients for minimal lumen diameter and percent diameter stenosis measurements for the preceding parameters in each film population. Differences in analysis reproducibility between the two study groups was large. Whereas the small, internally controlled population of films maintained a good correlation ($r \geqslant 0.88$) between repeated analyses, reproducibility in the larger, externally controlled population was poorer ($r = 0.68$–0.85). These differences clearly reflect the ideal nature of the internally controlled analysis process, where, in a limited population, even when read and analyzed in blinded fashion, observers are more likely to choose the same projection, cardiac cycle, individual frame, and reference segment at subsequent readings, thereby enhancing reproducibility and minimizing variability. In the evaluation of the externally controlled film population, the analyses that resulted in a minimal lumen diameter difference greater than 0.2 mm between readings were found to result from: different cine-angiographic acquisitions in 27% of studies, different cardiac cycles in 41% of instances where the same projections were selected, and when both the same projection and cardiac cycle was identified, 93% of analyses were performed on different frames. These data underscore the effect of totally randomized, blinded evaluations and emphasizes the need for external and independent control of core quantitative laboratory performance evaluations. Despite differences in the population number, overall image quality and the control exerted over the analysis process, no significant difference ($p < 0.05$) was found in the mean differences of repeated analyses for the parameters assessed.

Table 1. Mean differences ± standard deviations and linear regression correlation coefficients of absolute and relative dimension parameters for internally and externally controlled evaluations of core laboratory variability. (MLD = minimal lumen diameter, % DS = percent diameter stenosis, RAO = right anterior oblique, LAO = left anterior oblique, Minimum = minimal of RAO/LAO value, Maximum = maximal of RAO/LAO value, Average = mean of RAO/LAO value)

		RAO	LAO	Minimum	Maximum	Average
Internal (U of Maryland)	MLD	0.02 ± 0.23 mm (r = 0.91)	-0.04 ± 0.28 mm (r = 0.91)	-0.04 ± 0.25 mm (r = 0.89)	0.02 ± 0.17 mm (r = 0.97)	0.01 ± 0.18 mm (r = 0.96)
	% DS	-1.00 ± 9.1% (r = 0.88)	-1.31 ± 9.0% (r = 0.90)	-1.08 ± 7.7% (r = 0.90)	-1.23 ± 8.4% (r = 0.90)	-1.15 ± 6.6% (r = 0.93)
External (NHLBI Pregistry)	MLD	0.07 ± 0.42 mm (r = 0.75)	0.02 ± 0.43 mm (r = 0.75)	0.0002 ± 0.33 mm (r = 0.80)	0.04 ± 0.37 mm (r = 0.81)	0.02 ± 0.29 mm (r = 0.85)
	% DS	-0.28 ± 15.6% (r = 0.68)	-0.02 ± 13.1% (r = 0.76)	-1.11 ± 13.0% (r = 0.77)	1.33 ± 11.3% (r = 0.77)	0.11 ± 10.4% (r = 0.82)

From the analyses of these two study film populations, we further sought to determine the least variable parameter of coronary anatomy. For both relative (percent stenosis) and absolute (minimal lumen diameter) dimensional measurements, parameters derived from orthogonal pairs of projections provided more reproducible data. We found the most reproducible and least variable parameter to be the mean minimal lumen diameter for both the in-house study and the larger, externally controlled population from the NHLBI Registry (Table 1).

Although a biplane analysis is widely viewed as the optimal means of decreasing QCA variability, adequate visualization is frequently not possible in orthogonal planes. We found that paired orthogonal (or near orthogonal) projection analysis was not possible in approximately 35% of the NHLBI film population used as the third study group (biplane analysis was possible in 100% of the in-house population) and other investigators have reported that obtaining adequate visualization in orthogonal planes may not be possible in 40–50% of cases [23, 24].

Initially, videodensitometric techniques held promise as an analysis method independent of projection. The theoretical single projection advantage of this approach, supported in early investigations [25] was not found in later studies [26, 27] where ideal projections were not acquired. Such techniques are ill-suited to the different techniques found in most multicenter investigations. More recently, Lesperance et. al. [28] suggested that in the absence of adequate visualization in orthogonal planes, single plane geometric evaluations may provide analogous data if it fulfills the criteria of narrowest stenotic appearance. In concordance with these findings, when data from unpaired evaluations were added to data obtained from paired projection analyses (either averaged or the maximum/minimum of two), we observed little change in correlation coefficient or standard deviation. Figure 3 describes the effect of including single projection data of minimal lumen diameter with the average value from two projections. Inclusion of single plane points did not affect the overall standard deviation (averaged projection data alone $= \pm 0.29$ mm; averaged data with single projection points $= \pm 0.30$ mm). Moreover, the admission of single plane data points increased the overall total number of analyses from 65% to 80% of the total possible. These data suggest that core facilities should strive to obtain quantitative analysis data from paired orthogonal planes to optimize reproducibility. However, the inclusion of analyses limited by assessment in a single plane maximizes the analyses included in the data base without sacrificing reliability.

Operator dependant factors of core laboratory variability

Computer systems intrinsically vary in analysis technique. Institutional guidelines for performing film-based assessments are frequently individualized and factors which are necessarily a part of the technique such as, qualifications

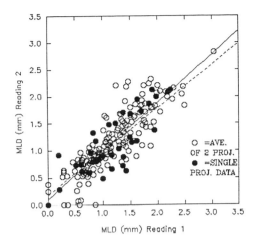

Figure 3. Reproducibility of minimal lumen diameters analyzed from externally controlled blinded readings. (MLD = minimal lumen diameter)

for image and analysis acceptability, the number of operators involved with the evaluations, and methods of defining reference segments have been shown to be variable among quantitative laboratories [21, 29]. Of all the methodologic differences noted between core quantitative laboratories, projection and frame selection has been suggested as the most likely source of significant variability.

Frame selection. Data describing the effects of differing frame selection schemes on quantitative results are limited and little consensus exits regarding the optimal method of frame selection. Currently, the three most widely used methods are: 1) selection of a frame at an end-diastolic timing, 2) selection of the frame indicating the sharpest luminal silhouette and greatest luminal narrowing independent of specific cardiac cycle timing, 3) averaging values from consecutive cardiac cycles. The basis for selection by the first method relies upon the relative lack of motion and "straightening" of the vessel segment during this timing. Reiber et al. investigated the variability in the measurements of the obstructive arterial dimensions when different frames are proposed for the quantitative analysis in the end-diastolic phase of the cardiac cycle [30, 31]. In a total of 38 patient films obtained at 25 frames/s they selected the frame φ demonstrating the severity of a lesion optimally as judged by a senior cardiologist, the three preceding frames, the three following frames, and one frame precisely one cycle prior to or following frame φ. Frame φ was always chosen in the end-diastolic phase. They concluded that there was no particular frame associated with smaller values in terms of mean difference or standard deviation than any other frame, and therefore, the selection of a cineframe in the end-diastolic phase of the cardiac cycle was not found to be very critical.

Contrasting these considerations, there is actually little assurance that any one specific timing in the R-R interval will provide adequate visualization of the target stenosis (free from vessel overlap or foreshortening). Vessels which lie in the atrio-ventricular groove for example, tend to move rapidly during the diastolic portion of the cardiac cycle leading to sub-optimal focusing. Selzer et al. [32], investigating the reproducibility and variability of frame sampling schemes in quantitative arteriography, reported that incomplete opacification was a major cause of variability in frame-to-frame analyses. Their findings suggest that schema using averaging techniques (end-diastolic frames from sequential cardiac cycles) yield the most reproducible estimates. Although reported to be superior with regards to precision, multiple frame averaging techniques (whether from sequential cycles or otherwise) can significantly lengthen the analysis process. Currently, only a few core laboratories find enough benefit over analysis schemes using single frames from opposing projections to warrant the extra expenditure of time.

We investigated the significance of frame selection methods in a small population (II) of randomly chosen cinefilms (eleven patient studies) from an ongoing clinical investigation. The films, which came from several different catheterization laboratories (participating V.A. Medical Centers), were baseline arteriographic studies describing varying degrees of obstructive coronary artery disease in the left anterior descending [5], circumflex [4], and right coronary arteries [3]. Of importance is to note that the image quality of the majority of these films, although of sufficient diagnostic quality, was not optimal for quantitative coronary arteriography, which certainly had an effect on the results obtained. Two observers from different quantitative core laboratories, experienced in both cineangiography and quantitative coronary analysis, performed independent reviews of each film identifying the most suitable projections for individual frame selection. From all the projections identified each observer independently selected frames thought to be optimal for analysis. Random frame selections were performed in accordance with the frame selection methodology specific to each core facility represented, as described earlier. One observer choose frames based on "sharpest-narrowest" criteria, without regard to cardiac cycle timing. The other investigator preferably choose frames by an "end-diastolic" method; if the end-diastolic frame was not optimal, e.g. due to vessel overlap, foreshortening, etc. another frame was chosen. Both observers sought to identify optimal frames early in each cine sequence following complete vessel opacification. Each observer also sought to identify frames from orthogonal (or near orthogonal) projections for the targeted segments. A total of twenty-seven (27) individual frames were selected by the two observers. In addition to each observer's selection, frames representing end-diastasis (EDS), end-diastole (ED), and end-systole (ES) were identified in two consecutive cardiac cycles by a consensus reading. The actual timing of each observers frame selections,

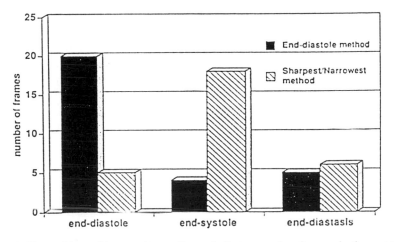

Figure 4. The position, with respect to cardiac cycle timing, random frame selections were made by independent observers using different methods.

with respect to the cardiac cycle, is described in Figure 4. For the most part, frames were selected from complete opposite timings in the cardiac cycle, with a small but equal number of selections by each observer occurring at a point in between.

Each observer completed an independent analysis of all randomly chosen frames using the quantitative angiographic system at the University of Maryland (ADAC 4100 Plus). Minimal lumen diameters (MLD), assessed from each respective frame selection method were compared with MLD measurements from specified timing in the cardiac cycle. The plots shown in Figure 5 describe this relationship. The linear regression lines on each plot are nearly identical. Table 2 summarizes the mean differences, standard deviations, and correlation coefficients for the 2 plots. No significant differences ($p < 0.05$) were observed between MLD values of each observer's random frame selection and specified cardiac cycle frames or between the frame selections of either observer (0.06 ± 0.23 mm). The blinded, analyses of all selected frames performed by each observer revealed no observer bias in the analysis of frames chosen by the respective methods in that mean differences were similar (0.08 ± 0.21 mm). The results of such comparisons indicate that computer calculated MLD values, when obtained from the analysis of frames identified by these selection schemes, will yield highly similar data.

Intra-observer variability. Assessment of temporal reproducibility for frames identified by each selection scheme was determined from a repeated analysis (intra-operator) of earlier digitized and stored cineframes conducted in

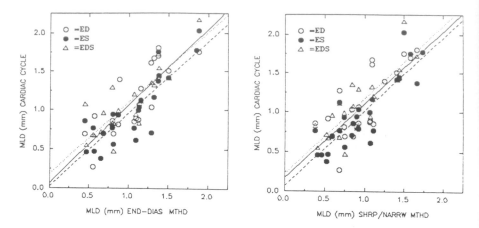

Figure 5. Comparison of correlations between minimal lumen diameter values determined from frames of static points in the cardiac cycle and frames of differing selection methods. (ED = end-diastole, ES = end-systole, EDS = end-diastasis, End-Dias Mthd = end-diastolic method, Shrp/narrw Mthd = Sharpest/Narrowest Method, MLD = minimal lumen diameter)

blinded fashion at a four month interval. Figure 6 shows the relationship of MLD calculations for each frame selection scheme at two readings. Average minimal lumen diameter differences between readings of either frame selection method were not found to be significantly different ($p < 0.05$). However, nearly a two-fold difference was noted in the variability (standard deviation) of repeated analyses between the two methods (±0.29 mm, end-diastolic versus ±0.16 mm, sharpest/narrowest). Similarly, substantial differences were noted in the reproducibility of each method ($r = 0.75$, end-diastole versus $r = 0.93$, sharpest/narrowest). These data suggest that arterial borders are more reproducibly determined from frames selected by schemes that emphasize visual determination of image clarity unrestricted to specific cardiac cycle timing. (This evaluation was assessed using the ADAC system only.)

Table 2. Mean differences ± standard deviations and correlation coefficients for minimal lumen diameter comparisons of differing frame selection method with static points of cardiac cycle

Static cardiac cycle	Random end-diastolic	Random sharpest/ narrowest
End-diastole	−0.06 ± 0.24 mm ($r = 0.82$)	−0.10 ± 0.27 mm ($r = 0.77$)
End-systole	0.05 ± 0.23 mm ($r = 0.85$)	−0.02 ± 0.23 mm ($r = 0.86$)
End-diastasis	−0.10 ± 0.23 mm ($r = 0.84$)	−0.09 ± 0.24 mm ($r = 0.82$)

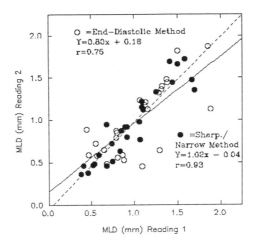

Figure 6. Intra-observer reproducibility of minimal lumen diameter values for frames frames selected by different methods. Blinded analysis was performed at a 4 month interval. (MLD = minimal lumen diameter)

Inter-laboratory and inter-system variability

The majority of commercially available automated quantitative coronary arteriographic analysis systems employ similar edge detection algorithms based on an densitometric examination of linear profiles through a contrast filled lumen and algorithms which differentiate pixel values (from 1st and 2nd derivative function analysis) between background and lumen. Beyond this general schema, final edge point determination and vessel contours are intricate methods of edge point determination, sampling intervals, spatial continuity of edge points, report generation and other programmable nuances specific to each system. Hypothetically, variation in the edge detection mechanisms of various quantitative systems could result in significant inter-laboratory (or inter-system) variability in the assessment of coronary anatomy. Unfortunately, while some data is available comparing automated quantitative methods with visual methods [7, 8, 33], no data is available comparing analysis results determined from differing automated quantitative systems.

Inter-laboratory comparisons were made in this study using the clinical images described in the preceding section (cinefilm population II). However, in contrast to the preceding comparison, this comparison of identical cine-frames included replication of the digitization process. The quantitative laboratories at the University of Maryland and the University of Leiden participated in the comparative analysis. Assessment methodology and system mechanics used by each laboratory were previously described.

Inter-laboratory variability. Inter-laboratory variability of reference segment diameters demonstrated the effect of methodologic differences between core laboratories. Reference segments subjectively defined by independent operators (U of Maryland) were compared with automated computer-interpolated reference segment calculations (U of Leiden). Differences between computerized reference definition and operator definition of reference segment was -0.04 ± 0.67 mm ($p = $ n.s.) (differences for subjective vs computer comparisons were identical for each of 2 independent operators). Although reference segment calculations, based on operator definition, were found to correlate poorly ($r = 0.66$) with values determined from automated methods, differences between the two were not found to be statistically significant ($p < 0.05$). Differences between subjectively determined reference segment values were also variable (inter-observer differences $= -0.04 \pm 0.56$ mm) and were indicative of the limited agreement (50%) between observers in designating a reference portion within each analyzed segment.

Although found to be more closely correlated than the reference diameter comparisons ($r = 0.75$ vs. $r = 0.66$), percent diameter stenosis variability was also greater between laboratories ($-6.35 \pm 12.6\%$) than between different observers (inter-observer variability was $2.96 \pm 8.3\%$). This is in part due to the effect of the variability of the constituent reference diameter factors.

Minimal lumen diameter (MLD) data (or the change in MLD) is a significant predictor of the physiologic consequence of occlusive coronary disease [34]. MLD values for all randomly selected clinical images (i.e. images selected by both observers) were determined by each laboratory and compared. Inter-laboratory differences (0.20 ± 0.35 mm) were found to be statistically significant ($p < 0.05$). However, the most relevant inter-laboratory comparison of MLD calculation, with respect to core laboratory variability, would compare MLD calculations based on each laboratories frame selection scheme, assessment methodology and system mechanics. This relationship is described in Figure 7, where MLD measurements determined from frames identified by the end-diastolic frame selection method and analyzed at the University of Leiden core laboratory (CMS system) are compared to MLD measurements determined from frames selected by the sharpest/narrowest frame selection method and analyzed at the University of Maryland (ADAC system). Average differences for this comparison were nearly identical to that found for the comparison of the entire clinical image cohort (0.23 ± 0.37 mm vs 0.20 ± 0.35 mm). As both laboratories use essentially the same assessment methods for this parameter (i.e. the single lumenal dimension of smallest diameter), this observation again suggests that frame selection methodology has little effect on core laboratory variability and indicates that the majority of core laboratory variability may be attributable to differences in system mechanisms. From Figure 6 it can be observed that in the majority of the cases the MLD-values from Leiden were larger than those assessed with the Baltimore system.

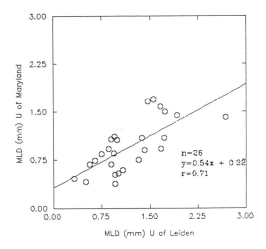

Figure 7. Comparison of minimal lumen diameter measurements determined from analyses performed at independent core quantitative facilities.(MLD = minimal lumen diameter)

Phantom analysis. To assess this possibility, cinefilm images of plexiglass arterial phantoms were obtained from an outside laboratory (Thomas Jefferson Memorial Hospital, Philadelphia, PA.) and independently analyzed by each respective laboratory. The precision drilled plexiglass phantoms were filmed over a patient's chest to incorporate clinically relevant radiographic parameters. A diagnostic catheter (7 Fr. Left Judkins) was present in the field for each of 12 separately filmed phantoms as a means of calibration. Each laboratory was provided with the actual dimension (determined by electronic caliper) of each corresponding catheter but was blinded to the actual phantom dimension. In addition, cinefilm images of a centimeter grid, acquired at corresponding image intensifier height and magnification, accompanied the phantom images. Phantoms dimensions ranged widely and included diameters of 0.4, 0.5, 0.8, 0.9, 1.0, 1.2, 1.5, 2.0, 2.5, 3.0, and 4.0 mm. Each laboratory assessed phantom dimensions based on calibrations by catheter and centimeter grid. These were compared against one another and against the actual diameter of the phantoms. Table 3 summarizes these inter-system comparisons. Overall, phantom diameter analyses between laboratories were highly correlated ($r > 0.95$). However, differences were noted based on the calibration method employed. Using a centimeter grid to calibrate, significant differences were noted between systems. Compared to the actual phantom diameters, the CMS quantitative system (University of Leiden), which was developed and initially validated against centimeter grid calibration techniques, assessed actual dimensions more accurately (mean difference = 0.06 ± 0.15 mm) than did the ADAC system (University of Maryland) (0.48 ± 0.34 mm), which is generally calibrated using a catheter. It

Table 3. Average difference and standard deviation between independent laboratory estimate and actual phantom diameters as well as inter-laboratory differences in phantom diameter estimates based on centimeter grid and catheter calibration techniques

	Leiden vs actual (mm)	Maryland vs actual (mm)	Leiden vs Maryland (mm)
Calibration by centimeter grid	0.06 ± 0.15	0.48 ± 0.34	−0.40 ± 0.26
Calibration by catheter	−0.34 ± 0.21	−0.27 ± 0.18	−0.07 ± 0.19

is clear from these data that in addition to variation in edge detection mechanisms, methods of calibration are also variables which affect core laboratory variability.

When edge detection algorithms were applied to the borders of contrast filled catheters, as a means of calibration, only small differences were observed in calculations of absolute diameters. Each system showed a tendency to overestimate actual dimensions across the range of phantom diameters. Mean differences for each laboratories estimate of actual diameters were essentially the same (−0.34 ± 0.21 mm-U of Leiden, − 0.27 ± 0.18 mm-U of Maryland). Differences in the calculation of diameters greater than 1.5 mm between labs were extremely small (averaging 6%). However, differences were greater (averaging 28%) for calculations of diameters smaller than 1.5 mm (differences were greatest for diameter less than 1.0 mm which were largely overestimated by the ADAC system). One of the obvious reasons for these large differences at the smallest sizes is the fact that the CMS edge detection algorithm corrects for the limited resolution of the entire X-ray imaging chain. It is well known that significant overestimations occur if such correction schemes are not applied. It is clear these factors impose significant limitations to reproducibility of quantitative assessments in this critical dimensional range and that such limitations may be of major consequence to core laboratory analysis of coronary anatomy.

Conclusion

We have investigated factors affecting the variability of core quantitative laboratory analyses of cine-arteriograms. Although quantitative analysis has become a necessity for objective evaluation of coronary artery disease treatment, little data are available describing truly blinded evaluations of laboratories. Most core facilities perform internally controlled evaluations of quantitative variability. These are often limited in scope and show little correlation to variability observed when evaluation is externally controlled and conducted in a randomized, blinded fashion.

Institutional guidelines for performing analyses and assessment methods are known to vary among facilities. However, the effect on core laboratory analysis variability is poorly understood. Frame selection criteria, perhaps the most common variable, was found to be of insignificant consequence. Although biplane analysis is theoretically advantageous, we found that restricting analysis inclusion to only biplane assessments significantly limited the number of data points and that inclusion of single plane data did not alter variability.

Comparative evaluations of clinical images between laboratories suggests that data derived from subjective operator determination (reference diameters or percent diameter stenosis) may be too variable. Although relatively unaffected by operator dependent factors, automated determinations of MLD are subject to differences in edge detection algorithms and system mechanics which can result in inter-laboratory variabilities for dimensions smaller than 1.5 mm.

QCA has matured over the past decade. As the use of this tool and the number of core quantitative laboratories increases, it is important that its limitations are not overlooked. Standardization of validation procedures, assessments of variability, and consistent methodological application remain as critical needs.

References

1. Detre KM, Wright E, Murphy ML, Takaro T. Observer agreement in evaluating coronary angiograms. Circulation 1975; **52**: 979–86.
2. Zir LM, Miller SW, Dinsmore RE, Gilbert JP, Harthorne JW. Interobserver variability in coronary angiography. Circulation 1976; **53**: 627–32.
3. DeRouen TA, Murray JA, Owen W. Variability in the analysis of coronary arteriograms. Circulation 1977; **55**: 324–8.
4. Sanmarco ME, Brooks SH, Blankenhorn DH. Reproducibility of a consensus panel in the interpretation of coronary angiograms. Am Heart J 1978; **96**: 430–7.
5. Fisher LD, Judkins MP, Lesperance J, et al. Reproducibility of coronary arteriographic reading in the coronary artery surgery study (CASS). Cathet Cardiovasc Diagn 1982; **8**: 565–75.
6. Meier B, Gruentzig AR, Goebel N, Pyle R, von Gosslar W, Schlumpf M. Assessment of stenoses in coronary angioplasty. Inter- and intraobserver variability. Int J Cardiol 1983; **3**: 159–69.
7. Kalbfleisch SJ, McGillem MJ, Pinto IMF, Kavanaugh KM, DeBoe SF, Mancini GBJ. Comparison of automated quantitative coronary angiography with caliper measurements of percent diameter stenosis. Am J Cardiol 1990; **65**: 1181–4.
8. Scoblionko DP, Brown BG, Mitten S, et al. A new digital electronic caliper for measurement of coronary arterial stenosis: comparison with visual estimates and computer-assisted measurements. Am J Cardiol 1984; **53**: 689–93.
9. Skelton TN, Kisslo KB, Mikat EM, Bashore TM. Accuracy of digital angiography for quantitation of normal coronary luminal segments in excised, perfused hearts. Am J Cardiol 1987; **59**: 1261–5.
10. Mancini GBJ, Simon SB, McGillem MJ, LeFree MT, Friedman HZ, Vogel RA. Automated

quantitative coronary arteriography: morphologic and physiologic validation in vivo of a rapid digital angiographic method. Circulation 1987; **75**: 452–60.

11. Rosenberg MC, Klein LW, Agarwal JB, Stets G, Hermann GA, Helfant RH. Quantification of absolute luminal diameter by computer-analyzed digital subtraction angiography: an assessment in human coronary arteries. Circulation 1988; **77**: 484–90.

12. Popma JJ, Eichorn EJ, Dehmer GJ. In vivo assessment of a digital angiographic method to measure absolute coronary artery diameters. Am J Cardiol 1989; **64**: 131–8.

13. Klein LW, Agarwal JB, Rosenberg MC, et al. Assessment of coronary artery stenoses by digital subtraction angiography: a patho-anatomic validation. Am Heart J 1987; **113**: 1011–7.

14. Katritsis D, Lythall DA, Anderson MH, Cooper IC, Webb-Peploe MM. Assessment of coronary angioplasty by an automated digital angiographic method. Am Heart J 1988; **116**: 1181–7.

15. Beauman GJ, Vogel RA. Accuracy of individual and panel visual interpretations of coronary arteriograms: implications for clinical decisions. J Am Coll Cardiol 1990; **16**: 108–13.

16. LeFree MT, Simon SB, Mancini GBJ, Bates ER, Vogel RA. A comparison of 35 mm cine film and digital radiographic image recording: implications for quantitative coronary arteriography. Film vs. digital coronary quantification. Invest Radiol 1988; **23**: 176–83.

17. LeFree MT, Simon SB, Mancini GBJ, Vogel RA. Digital radiographic assessment of coronary arterial diameter and videodensitometric cross sectional area. Proc SPIE 1986; **626**: 334–41.

18. Brown BG, Bolson E, Dodge HT. Quantitative computer techniques for analyzing coronary arteriograms. Prog Cardiovasc Dis 1986; **28**: 403–18.

19. Reiber JHC, Serruys PW, Kooijman CJ, et al. Assessment of short-, medium-, and long-term variations in arterial demensions from computer-assisted quantitation of coronary cineangiograms. Circulation 1985; **71**: 280–8.

20. Van der Zwet PMJ, Pinto IMF, Serruys PW, Reiber JHC. A new approach for the auto-mated definition of path lines in digitized coronary angiograms. Int J Card Imaging 1990; **5**: 75–83.

21. Reiber JHC. An overview of coronary quantitation techniques as of 1989. In: Reiber JHC, Serruys PW (Eds.), Quantitative coronary arteriography. Dordrecht: Kluwer Academic Publishers 1991: 55–132.

22. Van der Zwet PMJ, Von Land CD, Loois G, Gerbrands JJ, Reiber JHC. An on-line system for the quantitative analysis of coronary arterial segments. Comput Cardiol 1990: 157–60.

23. Brown BG, Bolson E, Frimer M, Dodge HT. Quantitative coronary arteriography. Esti-mation of dimensions, hemodynamic resistance, and atheroma mass of coronary artery lesions using the arteriogram and digital computation. Circulation 1977; **55**: 329–337.

24. Dehmer GJ, Popma JJ, van den Berg EK, et al. Reduction in the rate of early restenosis after coronary angioplasty by a diet supplemented with n-3 fatty acids. N Engl J Med 1988; **319**: 733–40.

25. Nichols AB, Gabrieli CFO, Fenoglio JJ Jr, Esser PD. Quantification of relative coronary arterial stenosis by cinevideodensitometric analysis of coronary arteriograms. Circulation 1984; **69**: 512–22.

26. Sanz ML, Mancini GBJ, LeFree MT, et al. Variability of quantitative digital subtraction coronary angiography before and after percutaneous transluminal coronary angioplasty. Am J Cardiol 1987; **60**: 55–60.

27. Tobis J, Nalcioglu O, Johnston WD, et al. Videodensitometric determination of minimum coronary artery luminal diameter before and after angioplasty. Am J Cardiol 1987; **59**: 38–44.

28. Lesperance J, Hudson G, White CW, Laurier J, Waters D. Comparison by quantitative angiographic assessment of coronary stenoses of one view showing the severest narrowing to two orthogonal views. Am J Cardiol 1989; **64**: 462–5.

29. Gurley JC, Nissen SE, Haynie D, Sublett K, Booth DC, DeMaria AN. Is routine automated quantitative analysis of coronary arteriography feasible? Evaluation of operator-dependent

variables inherent to the technique. J Am Coll Cardiol 1990, **15** (2 Suppl A): 115A (Abstract).

30. Reiber JHC, Van Eldik-Helleman P, Visser-Akkerman N, Kooijman CJ, Serruys PW. Variabilities in measurement of coronary arterial dimensions resulting from variations in cineframe selection. Cathet Cardiovasc Diagn 1988; **14**: 221–8.

31. Reiber JHC, Van Eldik-Helleman P, Kooijman CJ, Tijssen JGP, Serruys PW. How critical is the frame selection in quantitative coronary angiographic studies? Eur Heart J 10 (Suppl F), 1989: 54–59.

32. Selzer RH, Hagerty C, Azen SP, et al. Precision and reproducibility of quantitative coronary angiography with applications to controlled clinical trails. A sampling study. J Clin Invest 1989; **83**: 520–6.

33. Langer A, Wilson RF, Comparison of manual versus automated edge detection for determining degrees of luminal narrowing by quantitative coronary angiography. Am J Cardiol 1991; **67**: 885–8.

34. Harrison DG, White CW, Hiratzka LF, et al. The value of lesion cross-sectional area determined by quantitative coronary angiography in assessing the physiologic significance of proximal left anterior descending coronary arterial stenosis. Circulation 1984; **69**: 1111–29.

9. Automated physical assessment of image quality in digital cardiac imaging

ADAM WORKMAN, ARNOLD R. COWEN and
STUART VAUDIN

Summary

Image quality control is necessary in order to ensure a satisfactory level of
system performance and hence a reliable clinical diagnosis. Furthermore
where quantitative information is derived from clinical images, reproducible
and reliable imaging performance is crucial. The acquisition of data in a
digital format allows the derivation of quantitative information from test
images for the purposes of quality control. We have been developing methods
to automatically measure image quality parameters of a digital cardiac imaging system using specially designed test objects. Measures such as imaging
system dynamic range, image uniformity, run stability, contrast transfer function and Wiener spectrum can be derived. Also a contrast threshold detail
detectability measure can be derived using a computerised matched filter
technique to derive a measure of signal-to-noise ratio for details of varying
size. Subjective measurements are carried out along with these objective
measures to include the evaluation of the display of image information.
Preliminary results indicate that these measures can be used to ensure consistent and reliable imaging system performance.

Introduction

An image quality control regime plays an important part in monitoring and
maintaining the diagnostic efficiency and radiation safety of X-ray imaging
devices. Such a program can ensure that those properties which affect image
quality are optimized for a given imaging device and are maintained at this
level of optimization. In most cases diagnostic decisions are made by the
physician on the basis of subjective judgements as to the presence or absence
of pathology. However, there has been a growing movement in many areas
of diagnostic imaging towards using quantitative data from clinical images to
aid diagnosis. This has been aided somewhat in the last decade by the
availability of X-ray imaging systems which can directly acquire images in a

J.H.C. Reiber and P.W. Serruys (eds). Advances in Quantitative Coronary Arteriography, 161–176.
© 1993 Kluwer Academic Publishers. Printed in the Netherlands.

digital format, which can then be processed by computer. However, it seems that the derivation of reliable quantitative information from images requires the same if not a higher degree of technical quality control. The diagnosis will depend upon results obtained from the measurements which in turn depend upon the integrity of the data. The integrity of the data will obviously depend upon the inherent inaccuracies introduced by the imaging system. The degree of these inaccuracies depend on the quality of performance of the imaging system. Any significant deterioration in this level of performance will affect the integrity of the measurements made. Therefore, it is important in the case where quantitative measures are to be derived from a system that the imaging performance is regularly monitored for any deterioration in quality.

For many years FAXIL (Facility for the Assessment of X-ray Imaging at Leeds) has been involved in developing physical techniques to evaluate the image quality of clinical radiology systems. Through this work devices have been developed to aid testing and image quality measurement and to standardize such measurements [1, 2, 3]. These devices known as X-ray test objects can be used to test certain image quality parameters. In most cases these provide subjective or semi-quantitative measures of performance. As such they rely in part on the observers decision processes and consequently are subject to inter- and intra-observer variabilities and are sensitive to image viewing conditions.

Implementation of digital technology in imaging systems makes it possible to quantify image quality [4, 5]. Such measures would then be objective in nature and reproducible as they would be independent of any human observer. This also raises the possibility that an image quality control protocol could be carried out automatically on an appropriate set of test images.

In this paper we outline some methods of measuring physical image quality parameters and test objects designed for use with a Digital Cardiac Imaging system. Furthermore, some aspects of automating the image quality measurements are discussed.

X-ray Test Objects

We have developed a set of test objects appropriate for image quality monitoring of Digital Cardiac Imaging systems. The construction and design of each of these test objects will be discussed in turn:

*TO.TVF – (Figure 1). This test object was designed to assess aspects of the performance of the TV fluoroscopy system including:
1. High contrast spatial resolution – using a resolution grating with frequencies from $0.5 \rightarrow 5$ cycles per mm.
2. Contrast detectability – using an array of 11 mm diameter circular details of calibrated X-ray contrast ranging from 16% to 1.8%.
3. Display monitor set-up – a pair of squares representing 95% and 5% X-

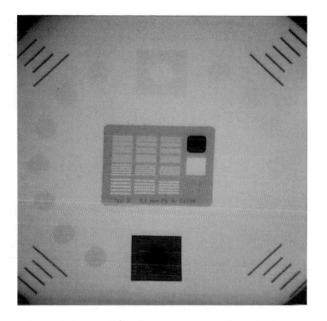

Figure 1. Image of TV fluoroscopy test object TO.TVF.

ray contrast with superimposed circles representing 99% and 0% X-ray contrast.

4. Field coverage – Diametrically opposed markers positioned at 15 to 22 cm diameter positions in 1 cm steps.

It can also be used to assess any of these features on the digital imaging system.

*TO.DR – (Figure 8). This test object was designed to measure system dynamic range, contrast rendition and signal-to-noise ratio(SNR). It comprises a uniform central region which allows correct automatic exposure stabilisation and around the periphery of the field a series of grey scale steps below and above the central level. These steps produce intensities which range up to approximately eight times greater than that of the background (average) level and ten times lower than the background. Superimposed upon these steps are sets of low contrast test details.

*TO.12 – This is the latest in a series of Leeds Threshold Contrast Detail Detectability (TCDD) test objects [6]. This test object consists of an array of circular low contrast details of varying and calibrated X-ray contrast and size. Details are presented in 12 sizes ranging from 11 mm to 0.25 mm in diameter. Each detail size is presented at nine contrast levels. A soft X-ray beam image producing a high contrast representation of the test object is shown in Figure 2.

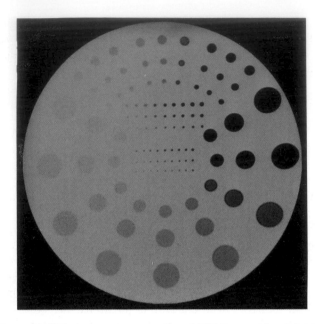

Figure 2. High contrast representation of TCDD test object TO.12.

Images of the test objects are normally acquired under calibrated beam conditions (viz 75kVp plus 1 mm copper pre-filtration).

Digital cardiac imaging system

It is appropriate at this stage to discuss some aspects of the design of the Philips DCI which influence the quality of the images produced by this system. The DCI is a digital fluorography system [7] designed as a digital replacement for cine-film cardiac-angiography. The DCI acquires images on a 512×512 pixel matrix with 8 bits (256 levels) of grey scale information. Images may be acquired at up to 50 frames per second. Exposure control is achieved by an average sensing method where the detector looks at a central circular area of the output phosphor. Typical entrance exposure levels for the 9″ image intensifier (II) field selection is 0.11 μGy per image frame.

Prior to digitization the video signal is processed by a nonlinear white crushing analogue circuit. The effect of this white crusher is to increase the contrast in lower signal levels (i.e. signals around the mean level) and reduce contrast in the highlight signals. This provides a mechanism for allowing a high dynamic range to prevent saturation from occurring and also to provide good contrast rendition in the heart region. Normal set-up of the DCI white compression stage maps the given average video level to a particular greyscale value. This is normally set such that 150 mV of video signal maps to a digital value of 96 within a small level of tolerance. The system should then have a dynamic range of approximately eight where the dynamic range is defined as the ratio between the average signal intensity and the peak signal intensity which the system can image.

Test object based subjective assessment of image quality

The Leeds DCI test objects were designed to enable the extraction of quantitative measurements of image quality parameters. Measurements which may be abstracted include system dynamic range, grey-scale rendition, high contrast resolution, geometric distortion and linearity, field sizing and low contrast detectability. Traditionally most of these measurements have relied upon subjective judgements of image quality.

TO.TVF enables an assessment to be undertaken of the image quality of the TV fluoroscopy system as well as addressing some aspects of DCI imaging performance. It contains a resolution test grating used to assess the limiting resolution of the imaging system. This is assessed from images of the test object acquired at a low peak kilovoltage ($\sim$50 kVp) with no metal prefiltration of the beam. These conditions maximize the contrast of the test grating bars. The finest spatial frequency grouping in which bars can be distinguished is taken as the limiting resolution.The limiting resolution corresponds to the high frequency limit of the imaging systems Modulation Transfer Function (MTF). Using the markers at the periphery of the test object it is possible to measure the image field size and visually assess the degree of geometrical distortion and any nonlinearity present in the system.

TO.DR enables the dynamic range of the imaging systems to be assessed. The filters around the periphery of the field address well defined levels within the systems operating dynamic range. Five low contrast details are superimposed upon each step to act as visual test probes. The positive going filters are calibrated to encompass a peak dynamic range greater than that of the acquisition device((8:1) with respect to the mean signal level). In a correctly adjusted system details in all but the highest filter square are reproduced. A reduction in the dynamic range results in a reduction in the number of positive filters in which details can be detected. Apart from verification of correct system adjustment this test object has been found useful in the development of image optimization strategies for various examinations and the correlation of image quality between the display monitor and the hard-copy film.

The threshold contrast detail detectability test object TO.12 has a contrast range matched to the sensitivity of grey-scale digital fluorography systems. Images of the test object are acquired under calibrated beam conditions (Figure 3). The observer then has the task of determining the minimum detectable contrast (threshold contrast) for details of different diameters. By determining the threshold contrast of each diameter of detail it is possible to make an overall assessment of image quality. Ideally, low contrast detect-

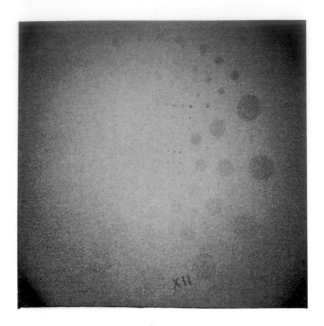

Figure 3. DCI Image of TO.12 acquired under calibrated beam conditions.

ability is determined by the image receptor entrance exposure levels [8]. In practice, TCDD image quality is evaluated subjectively by a human observer and therefore the efficiency with which the image is conveyed to the observer is included in the analysis. The results of Leeds TCDD tests are normally presented as a threshold detection index $H_T(A)$ curve, which is defined by the reciprocal product of the threshold contrast C_T and the square root of the test detail area, A,

$$H_T(A) = [C_T(A)A^{1/2}]^{-1}.$$

For an ideal imaging system the threshold detection index should assume a constant value set only by the square root of the X-ray quantum density at the image receptor entrance $[X_e.R]^{1/2}$ (where X_e is the entrance exposure and R is the conversion factor between exposure and quantum flux) and the subjective threshold criterion adopted by the observer (k_T). In practice, inherent technical deficiencies in the image acquisition process described by $[\eta.\phi < 1]$ and in the display/viewing process described by $[\psi < 1]$ degrade the perceived signal-to-noise ratio such that

$$H_T(A) = \frac{[X_e R \eta \phi \psi]^{1/2}}{k_T}.$$

These effects reduce the detectability of low contrast details and therefore

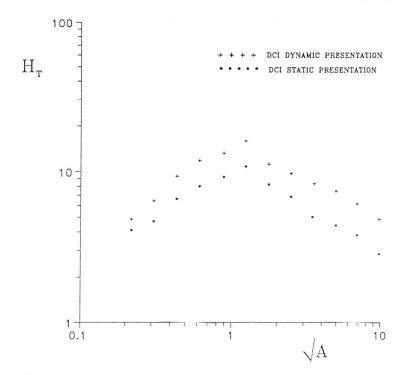

Figure 4. Detection index curves for DCI 9″ II field acquisition and static and dynamic display presentation.

reduce $H_T(A)$ below that predicted by X-ray quantum statistics alone. In practice, real systems also exhibit a progressive divergence in $H_T(A)$ from a constant value for both larger and smaller details. The former effect is believed to be due to visual processing mechanisms [9]. The latter is known to be due to the inherent unsharpness of the imaging system.

Detection index curves for the DCI system in 9″ II field selection are shown in Figure 4. Detection index curves are shown for both static and dynamic image presentation. The superior detection index values for the dynamic image presentation may be explained by the temporal integration effects of the eye reducing the apparent noise power in the image and thus improving the contrast sensitivity.

Physical assessment of image quality

The measurement of objective image quality parameters presents the obvious advantage that such measures could give absolute measures of imaging performance. Such measures would also allow reproducible and reliable performance monitoring. Furthermore these measures could be transportable and

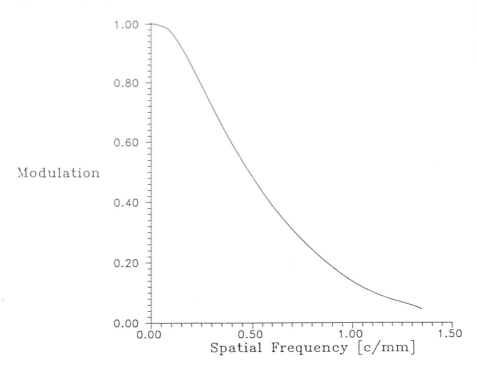

Figure 5. Modulation Transfer Function measured for 9″ II field DCI acquisition.

thus facilitate system intercomparison and allow more rigorous specification of performance parameters. The physical image quality of a DCI was determined by transferring the relevant test image data, via streamer tape, to a PC-based image workstation for analysis.

The physical performance of an imaging system can be characterized by its Modulation Transfer Function, Noise Power Spectrum and sensitometric response [10]. The MTF may be measured using either a slit or a resolution test grating. We have determined the MTF by measuring the modulation of the bars and spaces on a test grating and correcting for the nonlinear response of the system. The square wave response function is then corrected using the Coltman series to produce the sine wave response function(MTF). The MTF for the 9″ II field selection for the DCI system is shown in Figure 5. The method of measurement excludes measurement of the low frequency drop of the II tube. The Noise Power Spectrum may be measured directly from the digital images [5]. The Noise Power Spectrum measured from DCI images acquired with the 9″ II field selection is shown in Figure 6. The system sensitometric curve is measured using a highly collimated stepwedge of known X-ray transmission. These measurements may be combined to calculate a spatial frequency dependent measure known as the Noise Equivalent

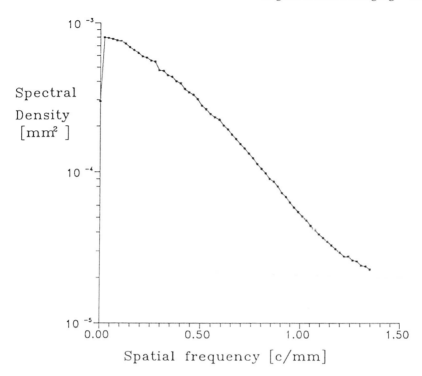

Figure 6. Noise Power Spectrum measured for 9″ II field DCI acquisition.

Quanta(NEQ). This expresses the apparent number of quanta recorded at a given spatial frequency and is an absolute measure of the systems performance as a photon detector. This is defined by

$$NEQ(f) = \frac{G^2 MTF(f)^2}{W(f)}.$$

In this equation G is the system macro transfer function and W is the Wiener or Noise power spectrum. We can also calculate the Detective Quantum Efficiency (DQE) which represents the proportion of exposing quanta which contribute information to the image. As such this determines the efficiency of the system as a photon detector and represents a SNR transfer function. DQE is defined by

$$DQE(f) = \frac{NEQ(f)}{Q_0},$$

where Q_0 is the density of exposing quanta incident on the image receptor. However, it must be emphasized that the measurement of physical image quality parameters is difficult to achieve in the clinical environment and is not practicable for the purposes of routine quality control.

Test object based objective assessment of image quality

An obvious extension of the present test object based image assessment which is facilitated by the availability of images in a digital form is to use a computer to make relevant measurements from the test objects. We have investigated the feasibility of making image quality measurements from test objects and have also considered some aspects of automating these measurements.

The design of TO.DR with the sub-details superimposed upon the greyscale steps allows a subjective assessment of dynamic range in that the observer assesses how many steps are imaged within the dynamic range by the number of steps in which details are visible. However, the dynamic range and contrast rendition can also be assessed by measuring the grey scale values in the test filter regions. This information is best presented in histogram form. In order to discriminate more easily the greyscale contribution of each step, data for histogram analysis is extracted from an annular region of the image corresponding to the position of the test filters. Regions corresponding to the positions of the filters are sampled and the greyscale histogram is constructed from the results of all twelve regions. Histograms are shown in Figure 7 for a system in correct adjustment whose TO.DR image is shown in Figure 8. The equivalent results produced by a system which is out of adjustment is shown in Figure 9 and displays the histogram shown in Figure 10. Using this method the histogram may be compared to a standard reference for the purpose of assuring consistent greyscale reproduction.

The unsharpness produced by an imaging system is best described by the system MTF. However in the field measurement of MTF is difficult to accomplish. A simple and easily implemented measure of unsharpness of digital imaging systems was proposed by Droege [11, 12]. This involved the measurement of the standard deviation of bar patterns of differing spatial frequencies. This was shown to be proportional to the modulation of the bars and as such could be used as a measure of modulation at different spatial frequency. The measure is, however, also sensitive to noise levels and contrast rendition (especially if the system is nonlinear); therefore, these parameters also have to be measured to ensure constancy and thus reliability of the unsharpness measure. Figure 11 shows the contrast transfer measure for the 9″ II field selection for DCI.

The detectability of details in an image is determined by the image signal-to-noise ratio, the contrast of the detail, and the efficiency of the display and the observers visual systems. The psychophysical processes associated with the detail detection process are subject to variation within the observers decision process. These intra-observer variabilities lead to variation in the response of the observer (determination of threshold contrast). Also inter- or

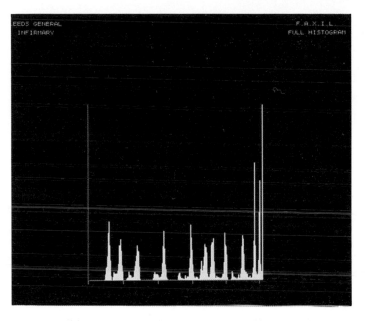

Figure 7. Histogram of greyscale steps of TO.DR for imaging system in correct adjustment.

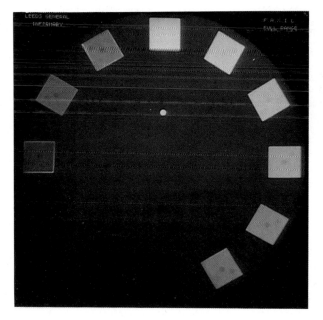

Figure 8. Image of TO.DR for imaging system in correct adjustment.

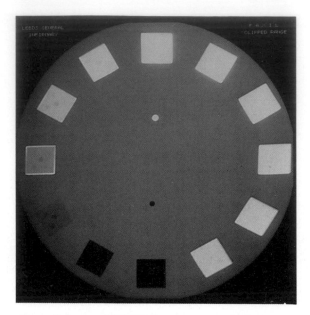

Figure 9. Image of TO.DR for system out of adjustment.

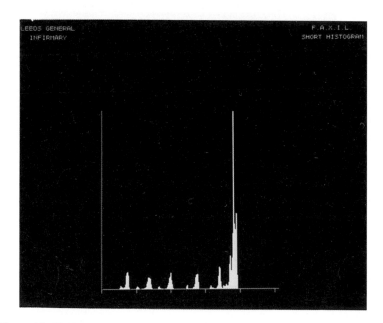

Figure 10. Histogram of greyscale steps of TO.DR for system out of adjustment.

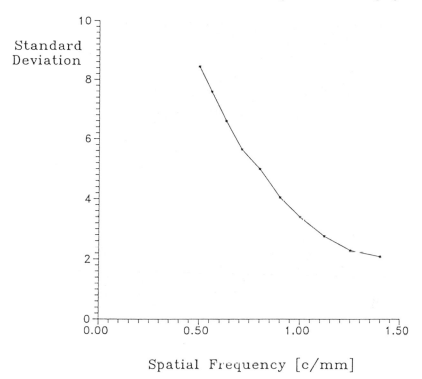

Spatial Frequency [c/mm]

Figure 11. Contrast Transfer Function measure for 9″ II field DCI acquisition.

between observer variabilities exist [13]. Subjective determination of contrast sensitivity also depends upon display conditions. All such variables can lead to a variation in the observers response when undertaking tests which are subjective in nature and unless the tests are carried out under controlled conditions the results of quality control constancy tests must be evaluated with great care. Furthermore, intercomparisons of system performance is impossible without reproducible test conditions. A computerized determination of contrast detectability from images would not be subject to such observer variabilities and would not depend upon display conditions.

In the detection task the observer has to decide whether a signal is present in an image or fluctuations are due to noise alone. The ideal observer [14] is one who will make optimal use of the information in the image i.e. maximize the signal-to-noise ratio for the given task. This SNR_{ideal} is given by

$$SNR_{ideal} = CG \left[\int \frac{|\Delta S(f)|^2 \, MTF(f)^2}{W(f)} \, df \right]^{1/2},$$

where $\Delta S(f)$ is the spectrum of the object and C is its subject contrast. This may be used to quantify the inherent performance characteristics of an imaging system and may be implemented by using $\Delta S^*(f)\text{MTF}(f)/W(f)$ as a matched filter. In practice, the derivation of $\text{SNR}_{\text{ideal}}$ is difficult as it requires full knowledge of fundamental physical measures as described before.

An alternative strategy is to implement a SNR measurement with an aperture matched to the known size of the input detail to be detected [15]. The application of this technique to images of low contrast detail test objects i.e. TO.12, can yield signal measurements for the different contrast details and noise measurements for the same size aperture. Given a certain criterion in terms of signal to noise ratio required for detection a threshold contrast can be derived for this observer. This observer signal-to-noise ratio which we call $\text{SNR}_{\text{detail}}$ is given by

$$\text{SNR}_{\text{ideal}} = CG \frac{\int \text{MTF}(f)|\Delta S(f)|^2 \, df}{[\int W(f)|\Delta S(f)|^2 \, df]^{1/2}}.$$

The measured threshold contrasts from a test object for the detail observer and the calculated threshold contrasts (from measured MTF, Wiener spectrum and sensitometric curve) for the ideal observer given the same decision criterion are shown plotted on a contrast detail curve in Figure 12. It is seen that these closely agree showing that for DCI both techniques provide similar results. However, $\text{SNR}_{\text{detail}}$ can be determined much more conveniently. Also shown in Figure 12 for comparison is the subjective threshold contrast detail detectability of the human observer.

The measurements outlined above can be used for quality control purposes to monitor system performance; however, it must be remembered that these measurements are performed upon the acquired image data and therefore do not take into account the efficiency with which it may subsequently be conveyed to the human observer. This aspect of performance may be assessed as detailed in the section on the subjective assessment of image quality.

Conclusions

We believe that a computerized image quality control regime represents an important development in monitoring the imaging performance of diagnostic X-ray imaging devices. Such schemes can provide useful data in the field and objective criteria against which image quality can be periodically monitored. The use of suitable test objects, analytical software and QC workstation should make it possible to assess image quality on a routine basis, conveniently and rigorously even by a non-specialist. Such systems will undoubtedly become increasingly necessary especially in areas where accurate quantitative anatomical/physiological measurements are to be made from image

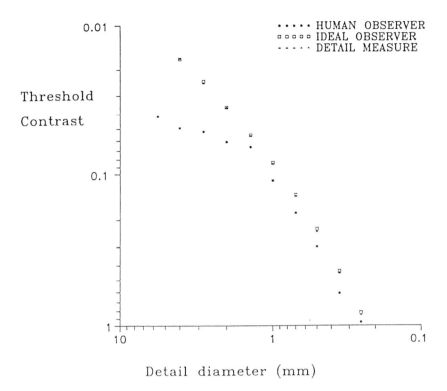

Figure 12. Contrast detail curves showing the performance of the ideal observer, the detail observer and the human observer for DCI 9″ II field acquisition.

data. It is also possible that eventually such automated QC routines, will be integrated into the imaging systems themselves as part of a self-verification package.

References

1. Hay GA, Clarke OF, Coleman NJ, Cowen AR. A set of X-ray test objects for quality control in television fluoroscopy. Br J Radiol 1985; **58**: 335–44.
2. Cowen AR, Haywood JM, Workman A, Clarke OF. A set of X-ray test objects for image quality control in digital subtraction fluorography. I: Design considerations. Br J Radiol 1987; **60**: 1001–9.
3. Cowen AR, Workman A, Haywood JM, Clarke OF. A set of X-ray test objects for image quality control in digital subtraction fluorography. II: Application and interpretation of results. Br J Radiol 1987; **60**: 1011–8.
4. Cowen AR, Workman A, Hartley PJ. The development of a computerised image quality control protocol for digital subtraction fluorography systems. In: Moores BM, Wall BF,

Eriskat H, Schibilla H, (Eds.), Optimization of image quality and patient exposure in diagnostic radiology. London: British Institute of Radiology 1989: 38–41.

5. Cowen AR, Workman A. A quantitative investigation of the noise processes in digital spot fluorography. In: Robertson J, Wankling P, Faulkner K, Holubinka MR, (Eds.), Computers in diagnostic radiology. York: Institute of Physical Sciences in Medicine 1990: 119–32.

6. Cowen AR. The physical evaluation of the imaging performance of television fluoroscopy and digital fluorography systems using the Leeds X-ray test objects: A UK approach to quality assurance in the diagnostic radiology department. In: Proceedings of AAPM Summer School 1991 (In press).

7. Verhoeven LA. Digital cardiac imaging. Medicamundi 1987; 32: 111–6.

8. Cowen AR. Digital X-ray-imaging. Meas Sci Technol 1991; 2: 691–707.

9. Chesters MS, Hay GA. Quantitative relation between detectability and noise power: Phys Med Biol 1983; 28: 1113–25. (Published erratum appears in Phys Med Biol 1984; 29: 602–4).

10. Sandrik JM, Wagner RF. Absolute measures of physical image quality: measurement and application to radiographic magnification. Med Phys 1982; 9: 540–9.

11. Droege RT, Morin RL. A practical method to measure the MTF of CT scanners. Med Phys 1982; 9: 758–60.

12. Droege RT. A practical method to routinely monitor resolution in digital images. Med Phys 1983; 10: 337–43.

13. Cohen G, McDaniel DL, Wagner LK. Analysis of variations in contrast-detail experiments. Med Phys 1984; 11: 469–73.

14. Wagner RF, Brown DG. Unified SNR analysis of medical imaging systems. Phys Med Biol 1985; 30: 489–518.

15. Workman A, Cowen AR. A method of quantitative image quality evaluation for digital radiographic systems. Med Phys 1990; 17: 740 (Abstract).

10. Experiences of a quantitative coronary angiographic core laboratory in restenosis prevention trials

WALTER RM HERMANS, BENNO J RENSING, JAAP PAMEYER and PATRICK W SERRUYS

Summary

Quantitative coronary angiography is increasingly being used as the method of analysis for defining the endpoint in restenosis prevention trials as it is more accurate and reproducible as compared to visual assessment. However, large variations in data acquisition and analyses are possible and they should be minimized. In this chapter our experiences in an angiographic core laboratory involved in four restenosis prevention trials with approaches toward standardized angiographic data acquisition and analysis procedure are presented.

Introduction

Since its introduction more than 14 years ago [1], percutaneous transluminal coronary angioplasty (PTCA) has been attended by a 17% to 40% incidence of restenosis, typically developing within 6 months of the procedure [2–5]. Each year the number of patients undergoing PTCA has increased and now approaches the number treated with coronary artery bypass grafting (CABG). In the last 10 years, experimental models have given us more insight into the restenosis phenomenon and pharmacological agents have been developed aming to prevent or reduce restenosis. Many of these "experimental" agents have been investigated in clinical restenosis prevention trials [4–7] and although these agents were able to reduce restenosis in the animal model, most of the clinical trials failed to demonstrate a convincing reduction in the incidence of restenosis in man. In these clinical trials, the primary endpoint has been either angiographic (change in minimal luminal diameter at follow-up; $> 50\%$ diameter stenosis at follow-up; loss $> 50\%$ of the initial gain) and/or clinical (death, nonfatal myocardial infarction; coronary revascularization; recurrence of angina requiring medical therapy, exercise test, quality of life). The use of an angiographic parameter as a primary endpoint provides the necessary objectively whereby the patient population

J.H.C. Reiber and P.W. Serruys (eds), Advances in Quantitative Coronary Arteriography, 177–192.

required for statistical analysis numbers between 500 and 700, whereas more than 2,000 patients are necessary if a clinical endpoint is used [6].

Despite the widespread and long-standing use of coronary angiography in clinical practice, as well as the outstanding improvement in image acquisition, the interpretation of the angiogram has changed very little and is still reviewed visually. However, visual assessment is a subjective evaluation with a large inter- and intra observer variability and can therefore not be used in important scientific studies for example restenosis prevention trials [8–9]. Quantitative coronary angiography has the advantage of being more accurate and reproducible in the assessment of lesion severity than visual or handheld caliper assessments. At the Thoraxcenter, the computer-assisted Cardiovascular Angiography Analysis System (CAAS) using an automated edge detection technique was developed and validated [8, 10]. A typical example of the quantitative analysis of a coronary obstruction is presented in Figure 1. Over the last 3 years, we have been the angiographic "core laboratory" (using the CAAS-system) in 4 restenosis prevention trials with recruitment of patients in Europe, United States and Canada (Table 1). In order to obtain reliable and reproducible quantitative measurements over time from coronary (cine)-angiograms, variations in data acquisition and analyses must be minimized.

In this chapter we present our experiences in the core laboratory with our approaches toward standardized angiographic data acquisition and analysis procedures as well as in qualitative or morphologic descriptions.

Potential problems with angiographic data acquisition and analysis (Table 2)

1. *Pincushion distortion*
Pincushion distortion of the image intensifier introduces a selective magnification of an object near the edges of the image as compared with its size in the center (Figure 2A). An inaccuracy in the measurement of the minimal lumen diameter of the stenosis over time could be introduced if, for example, the stenosis after the angioplasty procedure is filmed in the center and at follow-up near the edges of the image intensifier. To overcome this potential problem, a cm grid has to be filmed in each mode of the image intensifier in all the catheterization rooms to be used before the clinic can start to recruit and randomize patients for a restenosis prevention trial. With this cm grid film, the CAAS system calculates a correction factor for each intersection position of the grid wires so that the pincushion distortion can be corrected for (Figure 2B). Fortunately, the newer generations of image intensifiers introduce significantly less distortion than the older ones from the early and mid 80's; the degree of distortion is even less when the lower magnification modes are used with multi-mode image intensifiers.

At the present time there are in our database pincushion correction factors of 557 different modes of magnification (82 clinics with 207 angiorooms) from all over Europe, United States and Canada.

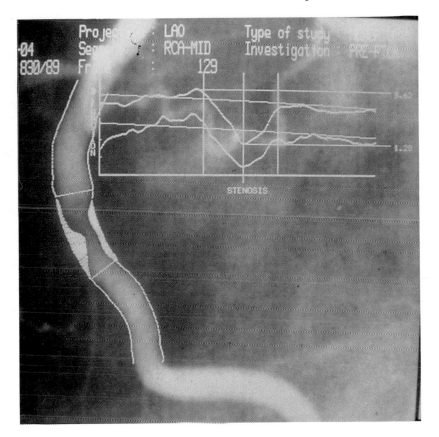

Figure 1a.

2. *Differences in angles and height levels of the X-ray gantry*

As it is absolute mandatory to repeat exactly the same (baseline) views of the coronary segments in studies to evaluate changes in lumen diameter over time, we have developed at the Thoraxcenter an on-line registration system of the X-ray system parameters such as parameters describing the geometry of the X-ray gantry for a particular cine film run (rotation of U-arm and object, as well as distances from isocenter to focus, table height) and also selected X-ray exposure factors (kV, mA). When repeat angiography is scheduled, the geometry of the X-ray system is set on the basis of the available data, so that approximately the same angiographic conditions are obtained. In a clinical study with repositioning of the X-ray system, it was found that the angular variability, defined by the standard deviation of the absolute differences of angular settings, was <4.2 degrees and that the variability in the various positions of image intensifier and X-ray source was

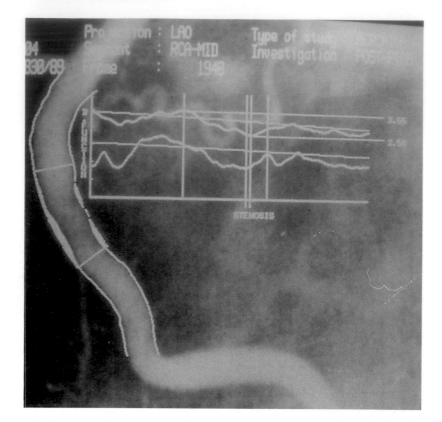

Figure 1b.

<3.0 cm [8, 11]. As on-line registration of the X-ray system settings is not available in all hospitals, we have developed a technician's worksheet that has to be completed during the PTCA procedure with detailed information of the procedure (view, catheter type, catheter size, balloon type, balloon size, balloon pressure, kV, mA, medication given) (Figure 3). In this way minimization of differences in X-ray settings at follow-up angiography is ensured. Furthermore, each center intending to participate in one of the trials is required to provide 2 sample cine-angiograms from each of its catheterization rooms for verification of their ability to comply to our standards.

3. *Differences in vasomotor tone of the coronary arteries*
As the vasomotor tone may differ widely during consecutive coronary angiographic studies, it should be controlled at all times. An optimal vasodilatative drug for controlling the vasomotor tone of the epicardial vessel should produce a quick and maximal response without influencing the hemodynamic state of the patient. Only nitrates and calcium antagonists satisfy these re-

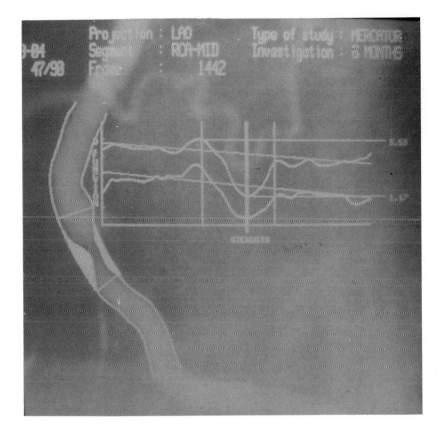

Figure 1C. Example of a quantitative analysis of a coronary obstruction of the mid portion of a right coronary artery: pre-PTCA (a), post-PTCA (b), follow-up (c). The upper curve represents the diameter function along the analyzed segment, the lower curve represents the densitometric function along the analyzed segment. The minimal lumen diameter is 1.28 mm pre-PTCA (a), 2.58 mm post-PTCA (b) and 1.17 mm (c) at follow-up.

quirements. On isolated human coronary arteries calcium antagonists are more vasoactive but they act more slowly; in the in-vivo situation, however, the nitrates are more vasoactive than the calcium antagonists [12–15].

We have measured in 202 patients the mean diameter of a normal segment of a non-dilated vessel in a single view pre-PTCA, post-PTCA and at follow-up angiography 6 months later. In cases where a stenosis of the left anterior descending artery (LAD) had been dilated, a non-diseased segment in the left circumflex artery (LCX) was analyzed and vice versa; where dilatation of a stenosis in the right coronary artery (RCA) was performed, a non-diseased segment proximal to the stenosis was used for analysis. All patients were given intracoronary (either 0.1 to 0.3 mg of nitroglycerin or 1 to 3 mg

Table 1. Angiographic Core Laboratory in 4 restenosis prevention trials between 1988 and 1991

CARPORT	Coronary Artery Restenosis Prevention On Repeated Thromboxane antagonism. Intake and analysis complete, 707 patients, published: Circulation Oct 1991.
MERCATOR	Multicenter European Research trial with Cilazapril after Angioplasty to prevent Transluminal coronary Obstruction and Restenosis. Intake and analysis complete, 735 patients, publication pending.
MARCATOR	Multicenter American Trial and Cilazpril after Angioplasty to prevent Transluminal coronary Obstruction and Restenosis. Intake complete, follow-up analysis pending, 1436 patients.
PARK	Post Angioplasty Restenosis Ketanserin trial. Intake complete, follow-up analysis pending, 703 patients

Table 2. Potential problems with angiographic data acquisition and analysis

1	Pincushion disortion of image intensifier
2	Differences in angles and height levels of X-ray system settings
3	Differences in vasomotor tone
4	Variation in quality of mixing of contrast agent with blood
5	Catheter used as scaling device (angiographic quality, influence of contrast in catheter tip on the calibration factor, size of catheter)
7	Variation in data analysis

isosorbide dinitrate (ISDN)) before PTCA and before follow-up and all but 34 received similar dosage before the angiogram immediately after PTCA. Table 3 summarizes the results of the analyses; a decrease in mean diameter of -0.11 ± 0.27 (mm) was observed in the segments of patients studied without intracoronary nitrates post-PTCA, whereas a small increase was seen of $+0.02 \pm 0.21$ (mm) in the group with intracoronary nitrates prior to post-PTCA angiography ($p < 0.001$). No difference in the mean diameter between pre-PTCA and follow-up angiography was measured.

In summary, the vasomotor tone should be controlled in quantitative coronary angiographic studies. This is only achieved by means of a vasodilator drug that produces fast and complete vasodilation without any peripheral effects. Therefore, we strongly advocate the use of 0.1 to 0.3 mg nitroglycerin or 1 to 3 mg of ISDN pre-PTCA, after the last balloon inflation before repeating the views used pre-PTCA and at follow-up angiography.

4. *Influence of contrast agent on vasomotor tone of epicardial coronary agents*

Jost et al. have clearly demonstrated that the vasodilative changes in vessel dimensions due to contrast medium administration are significantly smaller with the use of a nonionic rather than ionic contrast medium [16]. Therefore,

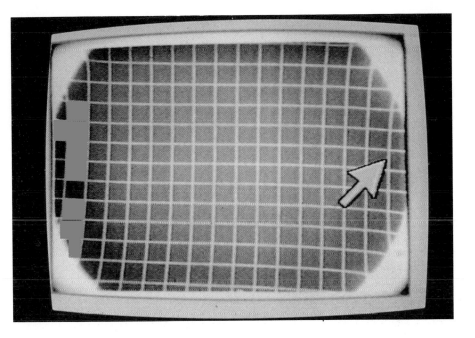

Figure 2a. Example of pincushion distortion introduced by the image intensifier (A, see arrow) and of the calculated correction factors with the use of the filmed cm-grid (B).

in quantitative coronary angiographic studies, nonionic contrast media with iso-osmolality should be applied.

It has been suggested to administer the contrast medium by an ECG triggered injection system. This is however not (yet) feasible during routine coronary angioplasty even in a setting of a clinical trial.

5. *Catheter used as scaling device for measurements of absolute diameters*

A. Angiographic versus microcaliper measured size of catheter. The image quality of the (X-ray radiated) catheter is dependent on the catheter material, concentration of the contrast agent in the catheter and kilovoltages of the X-ray source. Reiber et al. in 1985 showed that there was a difference of +9.8% in angiographically measured size as compared with the true size for catheters made from nylon. Smaller differences were measured for catheters made from woven dacron (+0.2%), polyvinylchloride (−3.2%) and poly-urethane (−3.5%) [17]. It was concluded that nylon catheters could not be used for quantitative studies.

B. Influence of variation in contrast filling of the catheter on calibration. It was also demonstrated that catheters made from woven dacron, poly-

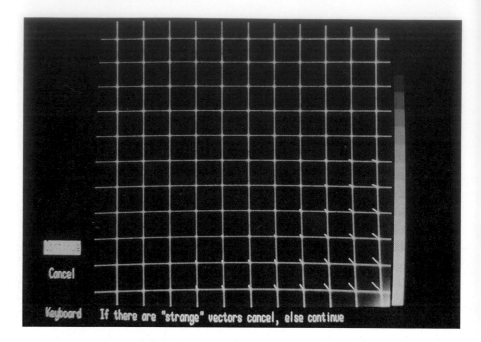

Cancel

Keyboard   If there are "strange" vectors cancel, else continue

Figure 2b.

vinylchloride and polyurethane when flushed with saline had, identical image contrast qualities whereas differences in image contrast at various fillings (air, contrast with 3 different concentrations (Urografin-76, Schering AG, Berlin, Germany; 100%–50%–25%)) of the catheters acquired at different kilovoltages was seen [17].

In addition, we measured the calibration factor in 95 catheters from 15 different clinics to compare contrast with filled saline catheter. Figure 4 summarizes our results. In a considerable number of cases, a difference in calibration factor was present with an average calibration factor of 0.143 ± 0.020 (mm/pixel) for the flushed (contrast empty) catheter versus 0.156 ± 0.030 (mm/pixel) for the catheters filled with contrast ($p < 0.001$). This means that with the use of a contrast filled catheter instead of a flushed catheter, the minimal luminal diameter will have an apparent increase in diameter value of ± 0.05 mm pre-PTCA, ± 0.15 mm post-PTCA and ± 0.20 mm for the reference diameter.

For this reason we strongly advise the clinics to flush the catheters before each cine-run to have an "identical flushed catheter" for calibration throughout the study period.

C. Size of the catheter. Until recently only 7F and 8F catheters have been used for follow-up angiography and from earlier studies it is known which

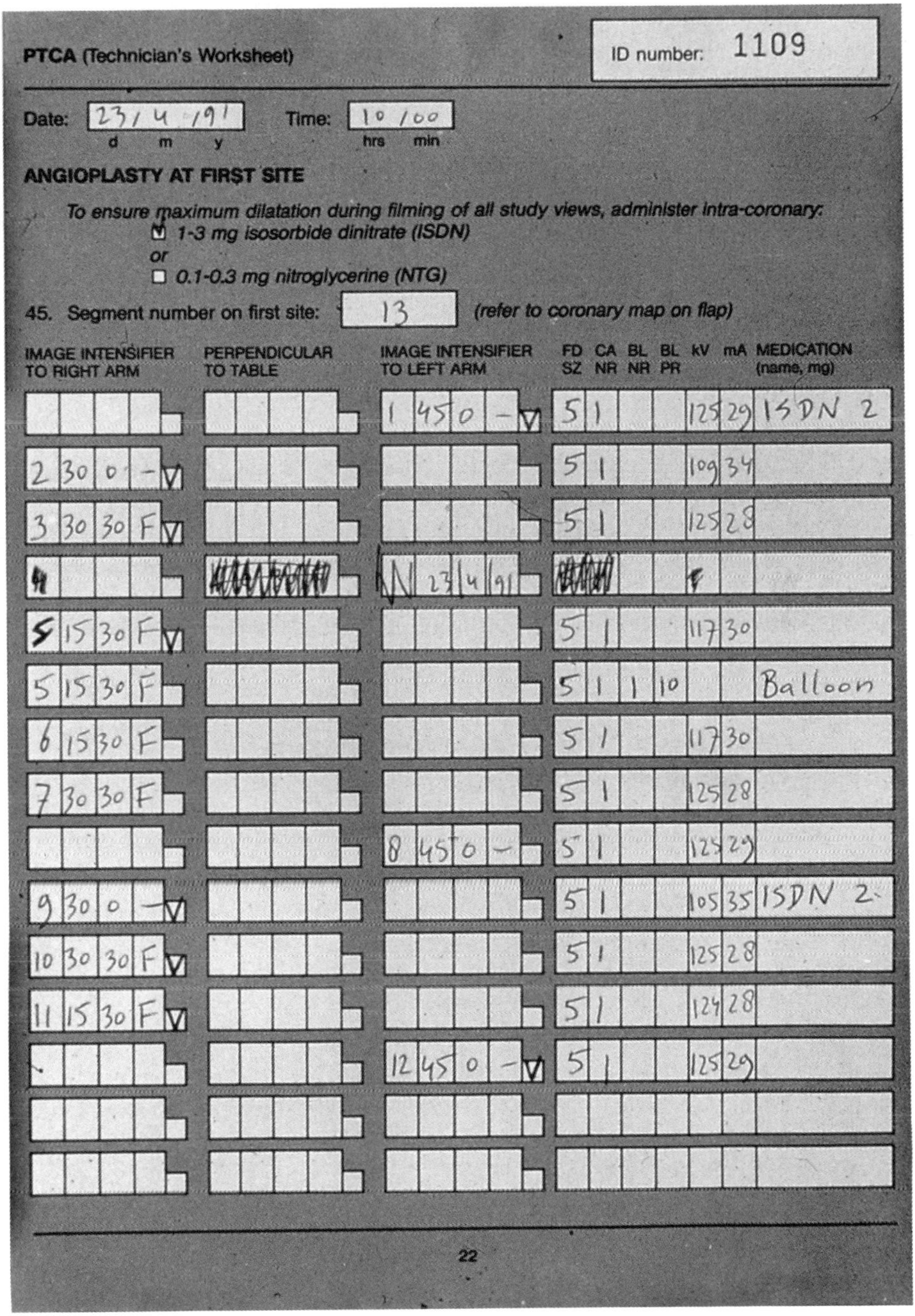

PTCA (Technician's Worksheet)

ID number: 1109

Date: 23 / 4 / 91   Time: 10 / 00
　　　d　　m　　y　　　　　　hrs　　min

ANGIOPLASTY AT FIRST SITE

To ensure maximum dilatation during filming of all study views, administer intra-coronary:
　☑ 1-3 mg isosorbide dinitrate (ISDN)
　or
　☐ 0.1-0.3 mg nitroglycerine (NTG)

45. Segment number on first site: ⟦ 13 ⟧ (refer to coronary map on flap)

IMAGE INTENSIFIER TO RIGHT ARM	PERPENDICULAR TO TABLE	IMAGE INTENSIFIER TO LEFT ARM	FD SZ	CA NR	BL NR	BL PR	kV	mA	MEDICATION (name, mg)
		1 45 0 − ▽	5	1			125	29	ISDN 2
2 30 0 − ▽			5	1			109	34	
3 30 30 F ▽			5	1			125	28	
4 ▨▨▨	▨▨▨▨	▨ 23 4 91	▨▨▨				F		
5 15 30 F ▽			5	1			117	30	
5 15 30 F			5	1	1	10			Balloon
6 15 30 F			5	1			117	30	
7 30 30 F			5	1			125	28	
		8 45 0 −	5	1			125	29	
9 30 0 − ▽			5	1			105	35	ISDN 2
10 30 30 F ▽			5	1			125	28	
11 15 30 F ▽			5	1			124	28	
		12 45 0 − ▽	5	1			125	29	

22

Figure 3. Example of a page of the technician's worksheet.

Table 3. Influence of nitroglycerin on the mean diameter of nondiseased segments in 202 patients in single projection

Mean diameter (mm)	Without Nitro Post-PTCA N = 34	With Nitro Post-PTCA N = 168	*t*-test
Pre-PTCA	3.12 ± 0.63	2.74 ± 0.63	
Post-PTCA	3.01 ± 0.64	2.75 ± 0.59	
Follow-up	3.18 ± 0.55	2.82 ± 0.63	
Delta (Post–Pre)	−0.11 ± 0.27	+0.02 ± 0.21	p < 0.001
Delta (Fup–Pre)	+0.06 ± 0.22	+0.07 ± 0.22	P = ns

ns = not statistically significant; p = probability value (*t*-test)(; Fup = follow-up.

of the catheters are preferred for quantitative analysis [17, 18]. However, 5F and 6F catheters are available and increasingly being used for follow-up angiography. Koning et al. have carried out a study to determine whether these catheters can be used for calibration purposes (Internal Report), (Table 4). They found that the differences between the true and angiographically measured diameters of the 5F and 6F catheters in all cases were lower for 6F than for the 5F catheters. Secondly, the Argon catheters showed the

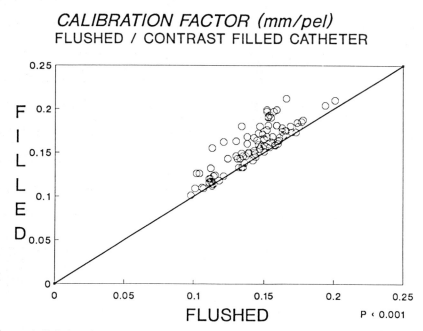

Figure 4. Relationship between the callibration factor calculated using an contrast empty (flushed) catheter versus a contrast filled catheter. A considerable number of measurements with the contrast filled catheter are above the line of identity.

Table 4. Comparison of the true sizes of the 5F and 6F catheter segments with angiographically measured dimensions (measurements were averaged over the three different fillings (water, contrast medium concentrations of 185 and 370 mg l/cc), each at two different kilovoltages (60 and 90 kV)

	True size (mm)	Angiographically measured size (mm)	Avg dif (%)
5F Catheters			
Argon	1.66	1.85 ± 0.09	11.3
Cordis	1.73	1.79 ± 0.15	3.2
Edwards	1.66	1.80 ± 0.08	8.5
Mallinckrodt	1.73	1.72 ± 0.14*	−0.8
Schneider	1.69	1.79 ± 0.07	6.1
USCI	1.61	1.75 ± 0.14	8.5
6F Catheters			
Argon	1.98	2.14 ± 0.07	8.1
Cordis	2.01	2.03 ± 0.11	1.1
Edwards	1.96	2.10 ± 0.07	7.1
Medicorp (left)	1.97	2.07 ± 0.04	5.1
Medicorp (right)	1.99	2.02 ± 0.10	1.6
Mallinckrodt	1.97	1.91 ± 0.15*	−2.9
Schneider	1.94	2.00 ± 0.09	3.0
USCI	1.99	2.06 ± 0.08	3.4

Mean value ± standard deviation, * measurements of the Softouch tip will be more favorable.

largest overall average difference, followed by the Edwards catheters and the 5F USCI catheter. The Cordis catheters, the 6F right Judkins Medicorp, the 6F Schneider and 6F USCI have the lowest average differences between the true and measured diameters. However, none of the catheters satisfy earlier established criteria [17], being that the average difference of the angiographically assessed and true diameter is lower than 3.5% and that the standard deviation of the measured diameters be smaller than 0.05 mm, under the following conditions: filled with 100% contrast concentration, filled with water, acquired at 60 kV and 90 kV. On the basis of these results, it was concluded that 5F or 6F catheters should not be used for QCA studies using the CAAS-system at the present time.

6. *Deviations in the size of the catheter as listed by the manufacturer*

In our experience, the size of the catheter as specified by the manufacturer often deviates from its actual size, especially disposable catheters. If the manufacturer cannot guarantee narrow ranges for the true size of the catheter, all catheters should be measured by a micrometer. Therefore, all catheters used during the angioplasty procedure and at follow-up are collected, labelled and sent to the angiographic core laboratory for actual measurement.

As the actual measurement can be hampered by individual variation, we have evaluated the inter- and intraobserver variability of catheter measure-

Table 5. Intra- and inter-observer variability of 96 catheter diameter measurements with an electronic microcaliper

Intra-observer variability

	n	Overall mean	Mean of diff	*p*-value	s.d. of diff
9F	30	2.75	0.008	NS	0.026
8F	114	2.56	0.009	NS	0.028
7F	132	2.25	0.001	NS	0.008
6F	12	1.94	−0.002	NS	0.006

Inter-observer variability

	N	1 vs 2		1 vs 3		2 vs 3	
		Mean Diff	s.d. Diff	Mean Diff	s.d. Diff	Mean Diff	s.d. Diff
9F	20	0.00	0.04	0.00	0.02	0.00	0.04
8F	76	0.00	0.03	0.00	0.02	0.00	0.03
7F	88	0.00	0.01	−0.01	0.02	0.00	0.02
6F	8	−0.02	0.03	−0.01	0.00	0.01	0.03

s.d. = standard deviation; diff = difference.

ments at the Core Laboratory. A total of 96 catheters with different sizes (6F to 9F) were measured by 3 different analysts independent of each other. One month later, all three analysts measured the same catheters for a second time, unaware of the results from the first time (Table 5). The intraobserver variability was excellent with a mean difference of less than 0.01 mm and a standard deviation of the difference of less than 0.03 mm for all catheter sizes. Similarly the interobserver variability between the 3 analysts showed a mean difference of less than 0.03 mm and a standard deviation depending on the size between 0.00 and 0.04 mm. We conclude that the catheter can be measured with an excellent accuracy and precision.

7. Variation in data analysis

Reference diameter. Although the absolute minimal luminal diameter is one of the preferred parameters for describing changes in the severity of an obstruction as a result of an intervention, percent diameter stenosis is a convenient parameter to work with in individual cases. The conventional method of determining the percent diameter stenosis of a coronary obstruction requires the user to indicate a reference position. This selection of the reference diameter is hampered by observer variation. In arteries with a focal obstructive lesion and a clearly normal proximal arterial segment, the choice of the reference diameter is straightforward and simple. However in cases where the proximal part of the arterial segment shows combination of stenotic and ectatic areas, the choice may be difficult. To minimize these variations, the CAAS-system uses an interpolated or computer defined reference technique.

Length of analyzed segment
Anatomic landmarks such as bifurcations are used for the manual definition of start and end points of arterial segments so as to minimize the problem of non identical analyses. For that purpose, drawings are made by the investigator of all different views suitable for quantitative analysis, pre-PTCA, post-PTCA and at follow-up. In addition, a hardcopy is made of every drawing, to enable analysis of the exact same segments at follow-up angiography.

Frame selection
Usually, an end-diastolic cineframe is selected for the quantitative analysis of a coronary obstruction to avoid blurring effect of motion. If the obstruction is not optimally visible in that particular frame (e.g. by overlap by another vessel) a neighboring frame in the sequence is selected. However, since a marker is not always present on the cinefilm, the visually selected cineframe may not be truly end-diastolic. Beside that, individual analysts may choose different frames even when the same selection criteria are followed. In addition, it is possible that the frames are selected from different cardiac cycles, in relation to the moment of contrast injection. Reiber et al. have critically assessed this problem in 38 films whether selection of the frame (3 frames preceding, 3 frames immediately following the frame and the same frame as chosen by the senior cardiologist as the reference end-diastolic frame, but one cardiac cycle earlier or later) resulted in a significant differences in the measurements. They found no significant difference in the mean and the standard deviation of the differences for the obstruction diameter, interpolated reference diameter, percent diameter stenosis, extent of the obstruction and area of atherosclerotic plaque obtained in various frames with respect to the "select reference frame". Therefore, it is concluded that the selection of a true end-diastolic cineframe for quantitative analysis is not very critical and that in case of overlap it is possible to select a neighboring frame [19].

Quality control in the Mercator trial

In the MERCATOR-trial – a restenosis prevention trial with a new angiotensin converting enzyme inhibitor cilazapril – in which 26 clinics have participated, quantitative coronary angiography was used to determine the primary endpoint as defined by the rate and extent of restenosis. Before the clinics could start to recruit patients for the study, they had to supply 2 sample cinefilms for analysis to demonstrate that they could comply with the required standards. Of all participating clinics 1 or more cm-grid films of all modes of all image intensifiers were received at the core laboratory to allow correction for pincushion distortion of the image intensifiers. All clinics received a set of radiopaque plates to be able to make it clear on the film whether nitroglycerin or isosorbide dinitrate was given before the contrast injection, which field size of the image intensifier was used, the balloon pressure and balloon size used etc. In a period of 5 months (June 1989–November 1989), a total of 735 patients were recruited with a minimum of 8 patients and a maximum of 56 patients per clinic. Five of the 735 patients were not included in the final analysis of the trial because their cinefilm could not be quantitative analyzed; in 1 patient the film developing machine broke down so that no post-PTCA film was available for analysis; in 2 patients analysis was not possible due to a large coronary artery dissection; in 1 patient no matching views were available and in 1 patient poor filling of the vessel had occurred (due to the use of a catheter with side holes) making comparison with the baseline film unreliable.

In 2 patients pre-PTCA, 34 patients post-PTCA and in 4 patients at follow-up angiography intracoronary nitroglycerin or isosorbide dinitrate had not been administered as assessed by the absence of the plate on the film and nothing had been recorded in the column "medication given during the procedure". In 26 patients, a 5 or 6 French catheter was used at the time of follow-up angiography. In 8% of the views pre-PTCA, 12% of the post-PTCA views and 12% of the follow-up views, the images had to be analyzed with a contrast-filled catheter because no flushed catheter was available. Figure 5 shows the average number of matched views available for QCA analysis per segment dilated.

Qualitative assessment

In addition to quantitative measurements, an angiographic core laboratory can assess qualitative or morphologic factors, such as type of lesion (according the AHA classification), description of the eccentricity of the lesion and type of dissection after the procedure, using modified NHLBI criteria, to establish the roles of these descriptors in the restenosis process. Recently, we have studied the interobserver variability for the description of the lesion and the type of dissection [20, 21]. Using the Ambrose classification there was an agreement of 80% between the two assessors of the core laboratory and for dissection there was an agreement of 87%. At the present time, no additional data is available; however, these will become available in the near future.

Conclusion

The use of quantitative coronary angiography is an objective and reliable method to evaluate changes in arterial dimensions over time. An angio-

AVERAGE NUMBER OF PROJECTIONS PER SEGMENT

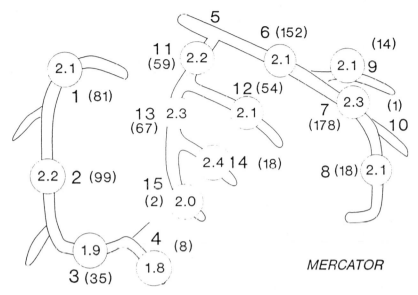

Figure 5. The average numer of matched projections (pre-PTCA, post-PTCA and at follow-up) that were used for quantitative analysis in the MERCATOR trial per segment are given in the circles. The numbers between the brackets are the total number of stenoses for that particular segment.

graphic core laboratory plays a crucial role in minimizing the problems of data acquisition and data analysis as well as the overall quality of the trial. Beside that an angiographic core laboratory may help demonstrating the reproducibility of qualitative factors and their role in the occurrence of acute and late complications of PTCA.

Furthermore, in our experience it has been possible to standardize angiographic data acquisition from 82 different clinics in Europe, the United States and Canada.

References

1. Gruntzig AR, Senning A, Siegenthaler WE. Nonoperative dilatation of coronary artery stenosis: percutaneous transluminal coronary angioplasty. N Engl J Med 1979; **301**: 61–8.
2. Serruys PW, Luijten HE, Beatt KJ, et al. Incidence of restenosis after successful coronary angioplasty: a time-related phenomenon. A quantitative angiographic study in 342 consecutive patients at 1, 2, 3, and 4 months. Circulation 1988; **77**: 361–71.
3. Nobuyoshi M, Kimura T, Nosaka H, et al. Restenosis after successful percutaneous transluminal coronary angioplasty: serial angiographic follow-up of 299 patients. J Am Coll Cardiol 1988; **12**: 616–23.
4. Serruys PW, Rensing BJ, Luijten HE, Hermans WRM, Beatt KJ. Restenosis following

coronary angioplasty. In: Meier B (Ed.), Interventional cardiology. Bern, Hogrefe and Huber publishers 1990: 79–115.

5. Califf RM, Ohman EM, Frid DJ, et al. Restenosis: the clinical issue. In: Topol E (Ed.), Textbook of interventional cardiology. New York, Saunders 1990: 363–94.

6. Popma JJ, Califf RM, Topol EJ. Clinical Trials of restenosis following coronary angioplasty. Circulation. (In press).

7. Hermans WR, Rensing BJ, Strauss BH, Serruys PW. Prevention of restenosis after percutaneous transluminal coronary angioplasty: the search for a "magic bullet". Am Heart J 1991; **122**: 171–87.

8. Reiber JH, Serruys PW. Quantitative coronary angiography. In: Marcus ML, Schelbert HR, Skorton DJ, Wolf GL (Eds.), Cardiac imaging: a companion to Braunwald's Heart Disease. Philadelphia: Saunders 1991: 211–80.

9. Beauman GJ, Vogel RA. Accuracy of individual and panel visual interpretation of coronary arteriograms: implications for clincal decisions. J Am Coll Cardiol 1990; **16**: 108–13. Comment in: J Am Coll Cardiol 1990; **16**: 114.

10. Reiber JH, Serruys PW, Kooyman CJ et al. Assessment of short-, medium-, and long-term variations in arterial dimensions from computer-asisted quantitation of coronary cineangiograms. Circulation 1985; **71**: 280–8.

11. Zijlstra F, den Boer A, Reiber JH, van Es GA, Lubsen J, Serruys PW. Assessment of immediate and long-term functional result of percutaneous transluminal coronary angioplasty. Circulation 1988; **78**: 15–24.

12. Feldman RL, Marx JD, Pepine CJ, Conti CR. Analysis of coronary responses to various doses of intracoronary nitroglycerin. Circulation 1982; **66**: 321–7.

13. Lablanche JM, Delforge MR, Tilmant PY, Thieuleux FA, Bertrand ME. Effects hemodynamiques et coronaries du dinitrate d'isosorbide: comparision entre les voies d'injection intracoronaire et intraveineuse. Arch Mal Coeur 1982; **75**: 303–15.

14. Rafflenbeul W, Lichtlen PR. Release of residual vascular tone in coronary artery stenoses with nifedipine and glyceryl trinitrate. In: Kaltenbach M, Neufeld HN (Eds.), New therapy of ischemic heart disease and hypertension: proceedings of the 5th international adalat symposium. Amsterdam, Excerpta Medica 1983: 300–8.

15. Jost S, Rafflenbeul W, Reil GH, et al. Reproducible uniform coronary vasomotor tone with nitrocompounds: prerequisite of quantitative coronary angiographic trials. Cathet Cardiovasc Diagn 1990; **20**: 168–73.

16. Jost S, Rafflenbeul W, Gerhardt U, et al. Influence of ionic and non-ionic radiographic contrast media on the vasomotor tone of epicardial coronary arteries. Eur Heart J 1989; **10**: (Suppl F): 60–5.

17. Reiber JH, Kooijman CJ, den Boer A, Serruys PW. Assessment of dimensions and image quality of coronary contrast catheters from cineangiograms. Cathet Cardiovasc Diagn 1985; **11**: 521–31.

18. Leung WH, Demopulos PA, Alderman EL, Sanders W, Stadius ML. Evaluation of catheters and metallic catheter markers as calibration standard for measurement of coronary dimension. Cathet Cardiovasc Diagn 1990; **21**: 148–53.

19. Reiber JH, van Eldik-Helleman P, Kooijman CJ, Tijssen JG, Serruys PW. How critical is frame selection in quantitative coronary angiographic studies? Eur Heart J 1989; **10**: (Suppl F): 54–9.

20. Dorros G, Cowley MJ, Simpson J, et al. Percutaneous transluminal coronary angioplasty: report of complications from the National Heart, Lung, and Blood Institute PTCA Registry. Circulation 1983; **67**: 723–30.

21. Ambrose JA, Winters SL, Stern A, et al. Angiographic morphology and the pathogenesis of unsTable angina pectoris. J Am Coll Cardiol 1985; 609–16.

PART FOUR

Coronary blood flow and flow reserve

11. Flow and flow reserve by parametric imaging

JOHN G.B. MANCINI

Summary

9 mongrel dogs were instrumented with electromagnetic flow probes (EMF) to measure coronary blood flow through the left anterior descending (LAD) and left circumflex (LCX) coronary arteries at rest and after maximal, adenosine induced coronary vasodilation. Relative coronary blood flow was determined by parametric imaging using digital subtraction angiography (DSA). Transmural myocardial perfusion of the LAD and LCX beds was determined with tracer-labeled microspheres. Coronary flow reserve (CFR, maximal coronary blood flow divided by resting blood flow) was calculated under control conditions and after constriction of the proximal LAD or LCX by a screw occluder. Coronary blood flow showed a good correlation between EMF and microspheres (correlation coefficient $r = 0.87$, $p < 0.001$) with a standard error of estimate (SEE) of 0.78 ml/gm/min. CFR also showed a good correlation between EMF and microspheres ($r = 0.82$, $p < 0.001$) with an SEE of 0.93. There was a moderate correlation between EMF and DSA ($r = 0.68$, $p < 0.001$) with a SEE of 1.35 ($=40\%$ of the mean CFR). The correlation coefficient between microspheres and DSA was 0.54 ($p < 0.01$) with an SEE of 1.46 ($=39\%$ of the mean CFR). Thus determination of CFR by parametric imaging is associated with large variations that are greater than variations also inherent in the two reference techniques. This low precision is probably due to the superposition of different cardiac structures in the two-dimensional display of a three-dimensional perfusion zone, potentially inhomogeneous contrast distribution, poor temporal resolution of the once-per-cycle imaging, inadequate displacement of blood by contrast material, and perturbations of flow caused by contrast material.

Introduction

Coronary arteriography determines the severity of a coronary stenosis solely in terms of anatomy. More recently, functional measurements reflecting the

J.H.C. Reiber and P.W. Serruys (eds), Advances in Quantitative Coronary Arteriography, 195–211.
© 1993 Kluwer Academic Publishers. Printed in the Netherlands.

physiologic significance of stenosed coronary arteries have become available. For example, digital subtraction angiography has been used successfully to determine coronary flow reserve (CFR) in patients with coronary artery disease [1–5] but the requirement for expensive and complex techniques has limited its clinical application. Intracoronary Doppler flow probes have also been used to measure CFR [6–7] but catheter positioning, changes in coronary luminal diameter, limited access to distal stenoses and inability to simultaneously measure flow velocities in different myocardial regions have restricted its use for assessing CFR in daily practice. Moreover, this technique measures only epicardial arterial flow reserve which may not reflect myocardial flow reserve in the presence of collateral recruitment and infarction. Positron emission tomography is another means for evaluating CFR in patients with coronary artery disease [7–9] and trials are underway to determine its suitability in the clinical setting.

The purpose of the present study was to determine the accuracy and reproducibility of a specific digital subtraction angiography method [1, 2] for measuring relative coronary blood flow and CFR in the experimental animal. We compared it to regional coronary arterial flow reserve measured with electromagnetic flowmeters and myocardial flow reserve measured with tracer-labelled microspheres.

Material and methods

Animal preparation. Mongrel dogs were anesthetized with 35 mg/kg pentobarbital iv. and were intubated and ventilated with a Harvard ventilator pump. A left thoracotomy was performed in the fifth intercostal space and the heart was exposed and supported in a pericardial cradle. The proximal left anterior descending (LAD) and the proximal left circumflex (LCX) coronary arteries were dissected free and an appropriately sized and calibrated electromagnetic flow probe (Carolina Medical Electronics, King, NC) was placed on each vessel. A screw occluder was placed distal to the flow probe either on the LAD ($n = 2$) or LCX ($n = 4$) or both ($n = 3$) arteries. Vascular sheaths were introduced into the left and right carotid artery and the left jugular vein for vascular access. A calibrated 5F micromanometer (Millar Instruments, Houston TX) was passed into the left ventricle via an apical stab wound and secured with a purse-string suture. A second 5F micromanometer was passed through the right carotid artery sheath into the ascending aorta.

A 7F Amplatz catheter was introduced through the left carotid artery into the ascending aorta and positioned into the ostium of the left coronary artery while being careful to avoid subselective placement. Six milliliters of a nonionic contrast medium (iohexol, Winthrop-Breon, New York, NY) were injected at a flow rate of 4 ml/s using a power injector with ECG gating (Medrad, Mark IV). Immediately after intracoronary injection of contrast

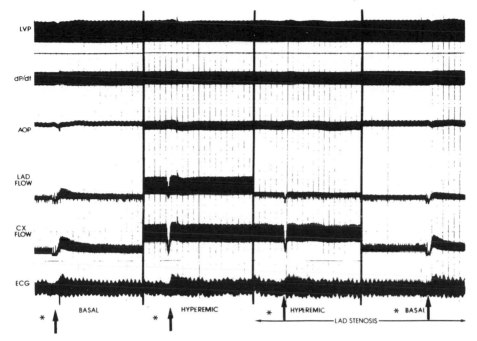

Figure 1. Original recordings of ventricular pressure (=LVP), its first derivative (=dP/dt), aortic pressure (=AOP), electromagnetic blood flow of the left anterior descending (=LAD FLOW) and left circumflex coronary artery (CX FLOW). Data are shown at rest (=basal), after adenosine infusion (=hyperemic), after coronary stenosis with (=hyperemic + LAD stenosis) and without adenosine infusion (=basal + LAD stenosis). Left ventricular pressure was kept constant by aortic constriction. Coronary blood flow increased three to five times after adenosine infusion and was decreased in the perfusion zone of the LAD after coronary constriction (=LAD stenosis). Microspheres were injected prior to coronary angiography under steady state conditions (crosses). Immediately following microsphere injection, coronary angiography was performed with a triggered power injector (arrows). (Reproduced from Reference 19, with permission.)

material cancellation of the flow signal was observed due to the nonionic nature of the contrast followed by a short hyperemic response which lasted usually up to 30 seconds in the control state (Figure 1). A polyethylene tube was placed in the left atrial appendage for injection of tracer-labelled microspheres; a second catheter was placed in the femoral artery for withdrawal of reference blood samples using a Harvard withdrawal pump. A Blalock clamp was placed around the descending aorta for constriction of the aorta to maintain peak systolic pressure constant during the experiment.

Coronary blood flow measurements

Electromagnetic flow probe. Coronary blood flow through the LAD and LCX arteries (Figure 1) were measured with electromagnetic flow meters.

Normalization of coronary blood flow was carried out at the conclusion of the experiment by dividing the electromagnetic flow data by the corresponding muscle mass of the LAD or LCX [10]. The perfusion beds of the two arteries were determined by selective intracoronary infusion with 2,3,5–triphenyltetrazolium chloride (TTC, Sigma Chemical) and Evan's blue (Sigma Chemical), respectively.

Parametric digital angiography. Two images per cardiac cycle (at 50 and 75% of the RR interval) were acquired in the left posterior oblique orientation on a Philips angiographic system (Optimus M200, Eindhoven, The Netherlands) which was interfaced directly to a digital radiographic computer (ADAC, DPS-4100C, Milpitas, CA). Radiographic parameters were kept constant (kVp, mA) for each image run. No correction of scatter or veiling glare was undertaken. Logarithmic analogue to digital conversion was employed. The images were stored on a digital disk with a matrix of $512 \times 512 \times 8$ bits. All images were processed by mask-mode subtraction, whereby the last image before contrast administration was chosen as the mask. Five to 8 consecutive images were selected as the image subset (only 1 image per cardiac cycle). A threshold generally less than or equal to 25% of the available grey levels was selected to minimize background noise. Pixel densities exceeding the threshold were used to generate a functional image. Red was assigned to pixels that had an intensity that surpassed the threshold in the first postinjection cycle, yellow for the second cycle, white for the third, green for the fourth and so on [10]. A region of interest was defined by two observers in the perfusion area of the LAD and LCX arteries. These regions contained between 500 and 1500 pixels and were placed carefully to exclude the large and middle-sized coronary arteries, the aortic root, the coronary sinus and areas which were perfused by both the LAD and LCX. The same pair of regions and the same threshold were used for baseline, hyperemia and stenosis images.

Mean arrival time (AT) and peak contrast density (CD) were calculated from the regions of interest. The mean AT obtained in cardiac cycle units was converted into seconds by multiplying the units by the true cycle time. Pixels appearing in the first cardiac cycle after contrast administration were assigned an AT of 0.5 cycle, those in the second cycle to have an AT of 1.5 cycles and so on. Peak CD was defined as the maximal density achieved during the entire series. From these measurements a relative coronary flow index (FI) was obtained as [1–4, 10]:

$$FI = CD/AT \ (1/\text{sec})$$

CFR was defined as hyperemia-to-baseline FI and was calculated as [1, 2, 7, 8]:

$$\frac{FI_{\text{hyper}}}{FI_{\text{basal}}} = \frac{CD_{\text{hyper}}}{CD_{\text{basal}}} \cdot \frac{AT_{\text{basal}}}{AT_{\text{hyper}}}$$

Microsphere technique. Myocardial perfusion was determined with the reference withdrawal technique using commercially available microspheres (15 micron diameter; New England Nuclear, Boston MA) labeled with Sn^{113}, Sc^{46}, Ce^{141} or Sr^{85}. The sample was carefully ultrasonicated and vortexed and then injected over 60 sec through the left atrial line. At the same time a reference arterial sample was withdrawn from the femoral artery (7.6 ml/min) using a Harvard withdrawal pump. Nine tissue samples were obtained from each perfusion bed (LAD and LCX perfusion areas) and transmural as well as subendocardial, midmyocardial, and subepicardial blood flows were determined. Radioactive counts were determined with a Tracor (model 1185) gamma scintillation counter and blood flow was calculated as [11]:

$$Q_m = (c_m Q_r)/c_r$$

where Q_m = myocardial blood flow in ml/min, c_m = counts in the tissue sample (counts/min), Q_r = withdrawal rate of the reference blood sample (ml/min) and c_r = counts in the reference blood sample (counts/min). Blood flow per gram of tissue was calculated by dividing Q_m by the weight of the tissue sample [10].

Study protocol

Left ventricular pressure, its first derivative (dP/dt), aortic pressure, electromagnetic coronary blood flow of the LAD and the LCX arteries and a standard lead of the electrocardiogram were recorded (Figure 1) on a Gould recorder (model 2800S, Gould Electronics, Cleveland OH) which was interfaced to an IBM-AT modified for on-line signal digitization at 200 Hz per channel. In each animal 10 beats were averaged and stored on disk for further analysis. Then, microspheres were injected over 60 sec and hemodynamic data of 10 cardiac cycles were digitized and averaged during the injection period. After completion of the microsphere injection, digital angiography was performed. The respirator pump was turned off during angiography and only sequences with good quality coronary angiograms and without premature beats were selected for further analysis.

Hyperemia was induced by infusion of 1 mg/kg/min adenosine (Sigma Chemical). Adenosine was dissolved in warmed saline and was heated during the infusion to prevent precipitation. Adenosine was infused through the jugular sheath. The infusion rate was 0.382 ml/min which was considered to cause maximal coronary vasodilation because contrast material injection had no further hyperemic effect during adenosine infusion (Figure 1). Since adenosine caused peripheral vasodilation with a significant drop in aortic pressure, constriction of the descending aorta was performed with a Blalock clamp to maintain peak aortic pressure constant during the experiment.

Coronary stenosis was induced by a screw occluder during adenosine infusion. This occluder was tightened until electromagnetically measured

Table 1. Coronary blood flow data

	n	EMF (ml/gm/min)	Spheres (ml/gm/min)	DSA (1/sec)
Control conditions:				
Baseline	17	1.08 ± 0.35	1.54 ± 0.58	0.41 ± 0.23
Hyperemia	17	3.90 ± 1.24	4.99 ± 1.48	1.40 ± 0.32
CFR	17	3.84 ± 1.59	3.71 ± 1.76	4.17 ± 1.75
Coronary stenosis:				
Baseline	7	0.98 ± 0.25	1.50 ± 0.36	0.33 ± 0.18
Hyperemia	7	1.83 ± 0.63***	2.25 ± 1.02***	0.78 ± 0.19***
CFR	7	1.93 ± 0.68**	1.53 ± 0.75**	2.63 ± 0.92**

Legend: Coronary blood data in 9 dogs under control conditions and after coronary constriction at rest (= baseline) and during adenosine infusion (=hyperemia). Flow data for electromagnetic flow probe are reported during microspheres injection. CFR = coronary flow reserve (hyperemia/rest), EMF = electromagnetic flow probe, DSA = digital subtraction angiography (=parametric imaging), **$p < 0.01$ (vs. control conditions), ***$p < 0.001$ (vs. control conditions). (Reproduced with permission from Reference 19.)

coronary blood flow had fallen to values approximating control flow values before adenosine infusion. After reaching a steady state pressure, flow data were recorded and stored on disk. Microspheres were then injected and digital angiography was carried out as described previously [12]. A second control run in the presence of coronary stenosis was obtained after turning off the adenosine infusion (Figure 1). Aortic constriction was usually released at this stage to maintain peak aortic pressure constant. Then pressure and flow data of 10 cardiac cycles were digitized, averaged and stored on disk. Microsphere injection and digital angiography were performed thereafter. The experiments were concluded by the administration of an overdose of pentobarbital and potassium chloride.

Thirty-four mongrel dogs were studied but the protocol was completed in only 22 (44 arterial beds). Of these, data from 24 beds were excluded due to greater than 10% changes in EMF blood flow measurements during microsphere injections. In 3 dogs (6 arterial beds), technical difficulties occurred with the withdrawal of a reference sample during microsphere injection. One dog (2 arterial beds) was excluded due to a technically inadequate parametric image. Thus, this report is based on 12 arterial beds from 9 dogs.

Results

Coronary Flow Measurements (Table 1)

Coronary blood flow in ml/gm/min increased significantly during adenosine infusion. Flow data were in the same range (NS) for the electromagnetic flow meter and microspheres. Absolute coronary blood flow cannot be mea-

Table 2. Accuracy and precision

	Mean difference	SD	MAD
Coronary blood flow:			
EMF vs. spheres	−20.68**	0.94	0.9010.73***
($n = 48$)			
Coronary flow reserve:			
EMF vs. spheres	0.22	1.04	0.71 + 0.78***
($n = 24$)			
EMF vs. DSA	−0.10	1.38	1.05 + 0.88***
($n = 24$)			
DSA vs. spheres	−0.64	1.70	1.39 + 1.14***
($n = 24$)			

Legend: Mean difference (=accuracy) and standard deviation (SD) of difference (=precision) for the comparison of coronary blood flow and coronary flow reserve between electromagnetic flow probe (=EMF), microspheres (=spheres) and digital angiography (=DSA). MAD = mean absolute difference ±1 standard deviation, ***$p < 0.001$ versus zero (paired t test). (Reproduced with permission from Reference 19).

sured with parametric imaging and, therefore, a coronary flow index (FI defined above) is reported for parametric imaging in Table 2. CFR on the average was similar (NS) with all 3 techniques, ranging from 3.71 (microspheres) to 4.17 (parametric imaging). Coronary constriction was associated with a significant reduction in hyperemic blood flow but resting coronary flow was not different from baseline. CFR was significantly reduced by all measurement methods after coronary constriction when compared to baseline.

Correlations between electromagnetic flow probe, microspheres and parametric imaging (Figures 2–5)

Coronary blood flow. Normalized coronary blood flow (electromagnetic flowmeter) and transmural myocardial blood flow (microspheres) showed a good correlation (Figure 2; correlation coefficient $r = 0.87$) with a standard error of 0.78 ml/gm/min (=36% of the mean blood flow). The correlation between the coronary flow index (parametric imaging) and transmural blood flow (microspheres) was good (Figure 2) but there was an underestimation of high blood flows by parametric imaging. When a semilogarithmic plot was used, the correlation coefficient between coronary flow index and the natural logarithm of transmural blood flow was 0.81 with a standard error of estimate of 0.32 (=40% of the mean blood flow).

Coronary flow reserve. There was a good correlation (Figure 3) between CFR measured with electromagnetic flow meter and microspheres (correlation coefficient $r = 0.82$) with a standard error of estimate of 0.93 (=28% of the mean flow reserve). The correlation of coronary flow reserve determined with parametric imaging and microspheres was only moderate (corre-

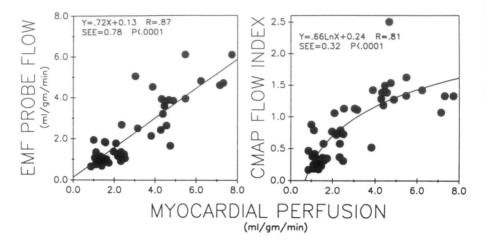

Figure 2. Correlation between normalized coronary blood flow (electromagnetic flow probe = EMF) and transmural blood flow (microspheres; left hand panel) and between coronary flow index (parametric imaging = CMAP) and transmural blood flow (microspheres; right hand panel). There was a fair correlation for both comparisons with a correlation coefficient of 0.87 and 0.81, respectively. Since large transmural blood flows were underestimated by parametric imaging, a semilogarithmic plot between parametric imaging and microsphere data was chosen. Standard errors of estimate (=SEE) amounted to 0.78 ml/min and 0.32 ml/gm/min, respectively. (Reproduced from Reference 19, with permission).

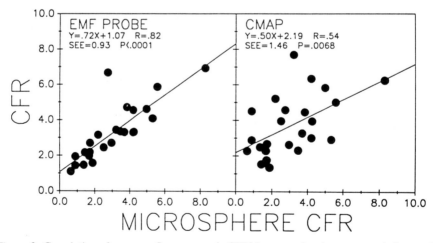

Figure 3. Correlation of coronary flow reserve (=CFR) between the electromagnetic flow probe (=EMF probe) and microspheres (left hand panel) and between parametric imaging (=CMAP) and microspheres (right hand panel). The correlation between EMF and microsphere data is clearly better (correlation coefficient $r = 0.82$) than between CMAP and microspheres (correlation coefficient $r = 0.54$). The standard errors of estimate are 0.93 and 1.46, respectively. (Reproduced from Reference 19, with permission.)

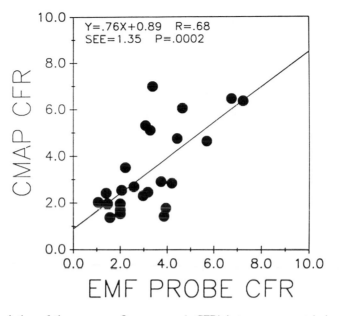

Figure 4. Correlation of the coronary flow reserve (=CFR) between parametric imaging (= CMAP) and electromagnetic flow probe (=EMF). There is a moderate correlation between these two measurements with a correlation coefficient of 0.68 and a standard error of estimate of 1.35. (Reproduced from Reference 19, with permission.)

lation coefficient $r = 0.54$) with a standard error of estimate of 1.46 (=39% of the mean flow reserve). The correlation of electromagnetically derived CFR and parametric imaging CFR was somewhat better (correlation coefficient $r = 0.68$) and was associated with a standard error of estimate of 1.35 (=40% of the mean flow reserve) (Figure 4).

The angiographic flow reserve parameters (Figure 5) such as contrast density ratio, arrival time ratio and flow index ratio (=CFR) also showed a weak correlation with the CFR estimates based on microsphere derived data; the correlation coefficient was 0.48 for the contrast density ratio, 0.47 for arrival time ratio and 0.54 for flow index ratio.

Accuracy and precision (Table 2)

Coronary blood flow was significantly less when it was determined by the flowmeter than by microspheres. The mean difference (accuracy) of coronary blood flow between the electromagnetic flow probe and microspheres was -0.68 ml/gm/min ($p < 0.001$ versus zero) with a standard deviation of difference (precision) of 0.94 ml/gm/min. The mean difference in CFR between the electromagnetic flow meter and parametric imaging measurements was smaller (-0.1) than between the flow meter and microspheres (0.22) or

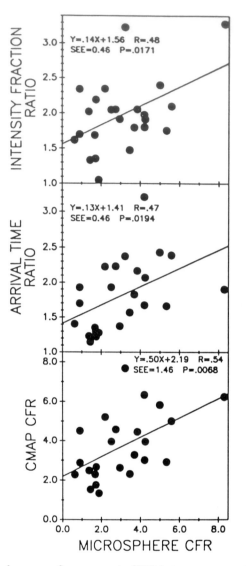

Figure 5. Correlations of coronary flow reserve (=CFR) between parametric imaging (=ordinate) and microspheres (=abscissa). Coronary flow reserve was determined from the intensity fraction ratio (upper panel), the arrival time ratio (middle panel) and from the ratio of the intensity fraction divided by the arrival time (=coronary flow reserve; lower panel). All three comparisons showed weak correlations. Abbreviations are as in Figures 3–5. (Reproduced from Reference 19, with permission.)

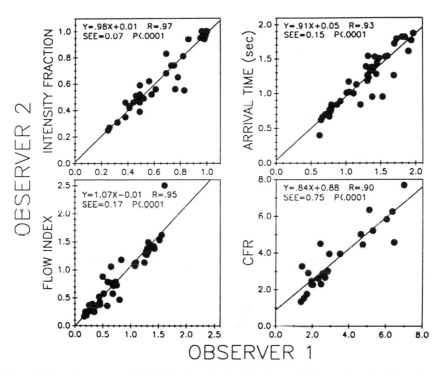

Figure 6. Interobserver variability for intensity fraction (upper left panel), arrival time (upper right panel), flow index (lower left panel) and coronary flow reserve (lower right panel) as measured with parametric imaging. Abbreviations are as in Figures 3–6. (Reproduced from Reference 19, with permission.)

microspheres and parametric imaging (-0.64) but none of these were significantly different from zero. That is, both the electromagnetic flow meter and the parametric images showed good accuracy. The standard deviation of difference or precision for CFR measurements was better between the electromagnetic flow meter and microsphere measurements (1.0) than between microspheres and parametric imaging (1.7).

Observer variability (Figure 6)

There were excellent correlations between observer 1 and 2 for intensity fraction (correlation coefficient $r = 0.97$), arrival time ($r = 0.93$), coronary flow index ($r = 0.95$) and CFR ($r = 0.90$) as assessed by parametric imaging. The standard error of estimate for CFR was 20% between observer 1 and 2, the mean difference was 0.34 and the standard deviation of difference 0.79.

Discussion

Estimates of stenosis severity using conventional coronary arteriography are based on anatomic criteria that may not reflect the physiologic significance of a coronary stenosis. The effect of diffuse atherosclerosis or eccentric lesions on CFR is difficult to estimate solely from the anatomic information derived from coronary arteriography. Several attempts have been made to directly quantify CFR in patients with coronary artery disease by gas clearance methods, thermodilution, digital angiography, Doppler flow techniques, positron emission tomography and newer approaches such as contrast echocardiography, ultrafast computed tomography and magnetic resonance imaging [7, 8]. Each technique is characterized by certain limitations and none have been used thus far to assess the functional significance of a coronary stenosis in daily clinical practice.

Use of parametric imaging to assess CFR is conceptually appealing because the same technique can be used to determine anatomy and the functional significance of a stenosis. Coronary arteriography remains the gold standard for determination of location and severity of coronary artery disease and provides the basic information necessary for performance of coronary bypass surgery. Thus, the combination of quantitative coronary arteriography and parametric imaging would seem to have considerable potential for widespread clinical application. There has been, however, some debate on the value and limitations of parametric imaging for the assessment of coronary flow reserve [7, 8, 12–14]. For example, Nishimura et al. [14] observed that videodensitometric measurements of CFR do not accurately reflect CFR measured by microspheres [14]. Accordingly, the purpose of the present study was to carefully re-evaluate the accuracy and precision of a specific parametric imaging method for the assessment of CFR in the experimental animal and to compare this method to two standard techniques, electromagnetic flow meters and microsphere measurements.

Coronary blood flow and coronary flow reserve

In the present study, coronary blood flow was examined over a wide range in normal and stenotic conditions both at rest and during hyperemia induced by adenosine. Radiographic measurements of coronary flow index and CFR were made during the first 1.5 to 5 sec of contrast material injection in an effort to minimize the effect of contrast medium on coronary flow [1].

There was some scatter between the electromagnetic flow meter and microsphere measurements of absolute flow (Figure 2) with a standard error of estimate of 0.8 ml/gm/min and a standard deviation of difference of 0.9 ml/gm/min. The scatter may be explained, at least in part, by the fact that muscle mass of the perfusion bed of the LAD and the LCX arteries had to be determined for normalization of electromagnetic flow data and by the fact that collateral blood flow is not taken into account by the electromagnetic flow meter. Some scatter was also reported between coronary blood flow measurements using the microsphere technique and flow measurements by collection of coronary venous return in dogs and sheep [15]. The comparison of coronary flow index (parametric imaging) and microsphere flow data also showed some variations with a standard error of estimate of 0.32. Perhaps most importantly, high coronary blood flows were underestimated by the flow index (Figure 2).

CFR estimates based on the electromagnetic flow meter data paralleled the microsphere derived data well but tended to underestimate CFR measured with microspheres at higher flow rates. The correlation coefficient was 0.82 with a standard error of estimate of 0.93 (Figure 3). The correlation between parametric imaging and microspheres was characterized by greater scatter (Figure 3) with a larger standard error of estimate (1.46). The correlation between parametric imaging and electromagnetic flow meter measurements was slightly better (Figure 4). The correlations are clearly not as strong as those that have been reported previously [2]. The mean difference (accuracy) was, however, good (−0.1) although the standard deviation of difference (precision) was poor (1.4) (Table 2). Interobserver variability was excellent and cannot explain the scatter in measuring CFR by parametric imaging.

Other angiographic flow reserve parameters such as intensity fraction ratio and arrival time ratio, were characterized by weaker correlations with the microsphere data (Figure 5) than the ratio of the two. Similarly poor correlations and wide scatter between videodensitometric measurements and microsphere data were reported by Nishimura and coworkers [14].

Limitations. The limitations of this study relate to three broad areas: the use of radiographic techniques, the unique limitations of the specific parametric imaging modality chosen for study, and the limitations imposed by the model and protocol that were necessary for the successful acquisition of adequate microsphere data and digital angiograms.

In general, some inaccuracy and imprecision results whenever radiographic techniques are used to analyze two-dimensional images of a three-dimensional perfusion bed. In the left posterior oblique projection used in most studies the area of interest for measuring coronary blood flow represents an integral of different perfusion areas in the posterolateral wall including subendocardial and subepicardial perfusion zones. Consequently, defining the precise three-dimensional location of the myocardial perfusion zone under investigation is difficult. Additionally, recirculation of contrast through the coronary sinus may cause difficulties with density measurements. Although it has been assumed that the inaccuracies of videodensitometry should cancel each other out when calculating density ratios (i.e. densities at baseline and hyperemia), this may not always be the case since the amount of contrast material in the myocardium during hyperemic images is likely to be greater.

Furthermore, the spill over can vary from injection to injection depending on absolute coronary blood flow and coronary vascular resistance. These factors will cause differences in the effects of scatter and beam hardening on the density values.

The specific parametric method we utilized is limited by the temporal imprecision inherent in once-per-cardiac-cycle image analysis of appearance time and density. This factor is probably most important in explaining the systematic underestimation of high flows noted in Figure 3. These errors would tend to cause overestimation of appearance time and underestimation of contrast density. Cusma et al. [4] suggested that improvement in the temporal resolution of the method could be achieved by interpolation methods and that this could simultaneously improve determination of actual appearance time and peak density. Such methods were not utilized in this study since we set out to examine the methodology originally proposed in an earlier report [2] in which this factor was taken into account only by assigning values of 0.5, 1.5, and 2.5 cycles to the first, second and third images, etc. The limitation imposed by this factor may be more notable in the current study than in prior studies since maximal flow was sustained by continuous infusion of adenosine and maintenance of perfusion pressure whereas prior validation attempts utilized submaximal stimuli such as atrial pacing [1] and graded contrast injections [2].

An underlying prerequisite for this method of parametric CFR imaging is that contrast material must virtually displace blood. The need for this was recognized in prior studies [2] and was explicitly elucidated by Cusma et al. [4]. While this prerequisite may be approximated, it is virtually impossible to guarantee it, especially during hyperemic flow, despite using maximally tolerable doses of contrast injected rapidly. Although studies with overt streaming and/or subselective contrast injection were omitted from analysis, the possibility of more subtle streaming or preferential flow of contrast into one or the other coronary arteries when contrast was injected into the main-stem of the arterial bed could not be completely eliminated. It is possible that this limitation might be overcome by relating the peak density in the myocardial bed to the peak density in the proximal coronary arteries so that the input of contrast and the actual degree of blood displacement achieved by the bolus injection can be taken into account. This approach would require more precise registration of the proximal arteries and avoidance of segments superimposed by reflux into the aortic root to avoid invalidating the intraluminal density values.

The experimental model and protocol we used also presented some unavoidable limitations. The microsphere technique requires a prolonged steady-state for injection and collection of samples. This precluded acquisition of the parametric images simultaneously with the microsphere injections. Moreover, the prolonged, systemic infusion of adenosine and the maximal hyperemia of the entire vascular bed may have promoted substantial collateral flow, a factor known to diminish the CFR value [16]. This possibility is supported by the general underestimation of microsphere-determined perfusion by flowmeter measurements. In theory, measurement of contrast density in the myocardium rather than the arteries should have reduced error due to collateral perfusion. The effects of the contrast agent on red cell morphology and the resultant effects on the rheologic characteristics of collateral flow, however, may have led to an under representation of collateral flow by the parametric imaging technique which was always performed after the microsphere determination of blood flow. In addition, though nonionic contrast was used, such agents can cause a diminution of blood flow that may have caused underestimation of maximal CFR [17]. Capillary solubility, uptake by myocardial cells, extravasation into the extracellular space and the effect of the high viscosity and osmotic pressure of the dye itself on the small vessels may all influence the densitometric assessment of perfusion [14]. Finally, although considered as the gold standard for measures of myocardial perfusion, the variability of microsphere measurements [11] and the regional heterogeneity of CFR measures by microspheres [18] cannot be ignored.

Comparison to prior validation studies

The initial clinical validation of the appearance time concept for measures of changes in flow were undertaken using atrial pacing as the hyperemic stimulus and coronary sinus blood flow as the reference measure [1]. Since atrial pacing does not induce maximal hyperemia, CFR estimates were probably not as adversely affected by the factors of high flow and collateralization that may have played a major role in the present study. On the other hand, the coronary sinus flow measurements cannot be considered a true gold standard for measurement of myocardial perfusion. Finally, since the study did not include an analysis of density, the inaccuracies of videodensitometry could not have affected the results.

Subsequently, another validation study was undertaken in dogs utilizing contrast material as the vasodilating substance [2]. A range of CFR values was created by graded doses of contrast material, whereas in our current study, flow was altered by imposing a stenosis on a fully vasodilated bed. This means that only submaximally dilated states were evaluated in the earlier study and that problems potentially related to high flow and collateralization were probably not critical. Furthermore, in the absence of maximal vasodilation, blood may have been more adequately displaced by contrast material thereby minimizing the errors of videodensitometry and the errors caused by potentially insufficient contrast injection.

In the study of Cusma et al. [4], electromagnetic flow meter measurements were used as the only reference standard. A curve interpolation method, discussed above, was used to improve density and temporal resolution [4]. Intracoronary boluses of adenosine were used and the transient hyperemia that resulted may have minimized difficulties attributable to collateral flow

[4]. In addition, contrast doses were injected more rapidly (5 to 10 ml/sec) than in the current study (4 ml/sec). Thus, methodological differences may explain part of the reason we failed to observe correlations similar to those previously reported.

Nishimura et al. [14] undertook a study comparing microsphere-derived blood flow estimates with parametric imaging. Differences from our methods include use of gamma variate curve fitting to construct time-density curves, use of the one half maximum density value to determine the time parameter, use of interpolation to determine peak density, use of highly disparate stimuli to induce changes in blood flow (intracoronary adenosine and vasopressin, rapid atrial pacing), post-processing from videotaped images and inclusion of a paucity of high flow reserve values (only 3 values greater than 2.0). Nonetheless, the conclusion of Nishimura et al. [14] is basically similar to our own. That is, parametric image analysis is reproducible but the CFR values correlate only moderately well with microsphere determined CFR ratios.

Clinical implications

Parametric imaging enables estimation of CFR that correlates with microsphere derived measure of flow reserve only moderately well over a wide range of values in this animal model. On the average, however, CFR results obtained by parametric imaging were not different from values measured by electromagnetic flowmeter and microspheres. The specific parametric technique has inherent limitations that lead to imprecision in the measurements. At the present time, only changes of 40% or greater in CFR can be expected to be demonstrated reproducibly with this specific parametric method. Efforts directed at improving the accuracy of both time and density measurements, minimizing the effects induced by contrast material and collateral flow and avoiding the need for full displacement of blood by contrast material will be required to make the methodology more precise [19].

Acknowledgements

This study was supported, in part, by funds from the Veterans Administration, Washington D.C.
This article summarizes a prior publication [19] which can be referred to for fuller details of the experimental protocol.

References

1. Vogel RA, LeFree MT, Bates ER, et al. Application of digital techniques to selective

coronary arteriography: Use of myocardial contrast appearance time to measure coronary flow reserve. Am Heart J 1984; **107**: 153–64.

2. Hodgson JMcB, LeGrand V, Bates ER, et al. Validation in dogs of a rapid digital angiographic technique to measure relative coronary blood flow during routine cardiac catheterization. Am J Cardiol 1985; **55**: 188–93.

3. LeGrand V, Aueron FM, Bates ER, et al. Value of exercise radionuclide ventriculography and thallium-201 scintigraphy in evaluating successful coronary angioplasty: Comparison with coronary flow reserve, translesional gradient and percent diameter stenosis. Eur Heart J 1987; **8**: 329–39.

4. Cusma JT, Toggart EJ, Folts JD, et al. Digital subtraction angiographic imaging of coronary flow reserve. Circulation 1987; **75**: 461–72.

5. Zijlstra F, van Ommeren J, Reiber JHC, Serruys PW. Does the quantitative assessment of coronary artery dimensions predict the physiologic significance of a coronary stenosis? Circulation 1987; **75**: 1154–61.

6. Wilson RF, Marcus ML, White CW. Prediction of the physiologic significance of coronary arterial lesions by quantitative lesion geometry in patients with limited coronary artery disease. Circulation 1987; **75**: 723–32.

7. Marcus ML, Wilson RF, White CW. Methods of measurement of myocardial blood flow in patients: a critical review. Circulation 1987; **76**: 245–53.

8. Klocke FJ. Measurements of coronary flow reserve: defining pathophysiology versus making decisions about patient care. Circulation 1987; **76**: 1183–9.

9. Gould KL, Goldstein RA, Mullani NA, et al. Noninvasive assessment of coronary stenoses by myocardial perfusion imaging during pharmacologic coronary vasodilation. VIII: Clinical feasibility of positron cardiac imaging without a cyclotron using generator-produced rubidium-82. J Am Coll Cardiol 1986; **7**: 775–8.

10. Mancini GBJ, McGillem MJ, DeBoe SF, Gallagher KP. The diastolic hyperemic flow versus pressure relation. A new index of coronary stenosis severity and flow reserve. Circulation, 1989; **80**: 941–50.

11. Heymann MA, Payne BD, Hoffman JIE, Rudolph AM. Blood flow measurements with radionuclide-labeled particles. Prog Cardiovasc Dis 1977; **20**: 55–79.

12. Mancini GBJ, Higgins CB. Digital subtraction angiography: a review of cardiac applications. Prog Cardiovasc Dis 1985; **18**: 111–41.

13. Nissen SE, Elion JL, Booth DC, Evans J, DeMaria AN. Value and limitations of computer analysis of digital subtraction angiography in the assessment of coronary flow reserve. Circulation 1986; **73**: 562–71.

14. Nishimura RA, Rogers PJ, Holmes DR Jr, Gehring DG, Bove AA. Assessment of myocardial perfusion by videodensitometry in the canine model. J Am Coll Cardiol 1987; **9**: 891–7.

15. Utley J, Carlson EL, Hoffmann JIE, Martinez HM, Buckberg GD. Total and regional myocardial blood flow measurements with 25 micron, 15 micron, 9 micron and filtered 1–10 micron diameter microspheres and antipyrine in dogs and sheep. Circ Res 1974; **34**: 391–405.

16. Legrand V, Mancini GBJ, Bates ER, Hodgson JMcB, Gross MD, Vogel RA. Comparative study of coronary flow reserve, coronary anatomy and results of radionuclide exercise tests in patients with coronary artery disease. J Am Coll Cardiol 1986; **8**: 1022–32.

17. Friedman HZ, DeBoe SF, McGillem MJ, Mancini GBJ. The immediate effects of iohexol on coronary blood flow and myocardial function in vivo. Circulation 1986; **74**: 1416–23.

18. Austin RE Jr, Aldea GS, Coggins DL, Flynn AE, Hoffman JIE. Profound variation of regional coronary flow reserve. Circulation 1988; **78** (Suppl 2): II-82 (Abstract).

19. Hess OM, McGillem MJ, DeBoe SF, Pinto IMF, Gallagher KP, Mancini GBJ. Determination of coronary flow reserve by parametric imaging. Circulation, 1990; **82**: 1438–48. Comment in: Circulation 1990; **82**: 1533–5.

12. Maximal myocardial perfusion as a measure of the functional significance of coronary artery disease

NICO H.J. PIJLS, JOOST DEN AREND,
KAREL VAN LEEUWEN, TRUUS PIJNENBURG,
EVERT LAMFERS, JACQUES D. BARTH,
GERARD J.H. UIJEN and TJEERD VAN DER WERF

Summary

Over the last decade it has become more and more obvious that, besides anatomic information about the severity of coronary artery stenoses, information about coronary and myocardial blood flow is necessary to completely understand the functional significance of these lesions. Methods to measure flow in clinical practice, however, have been disappointing until now.

Recently, we demonstrated in an animal study in dogs that at maximal vasodilation of the myocardial vascular bed maximally achievable blood flow through the myocardium is inversely proportional to mean transit time (T_{mn}) of contrast passage, determined by ECG-triggered digital radiography. In the present study the feasibility of this method was tested in men and applied in 50 patients with angina pectoris to compare maximal blood flow before and after a PTCA.

Maximal vasodilation was induced immediately before and 15 min after the PTCA by i.c. administration of 8 mg (RCA) or 12 mg (LCA) papaverine and corresponding digital angiographic studies were performed. Excellent quality subtraction images could be obtained and reliable determination of T_{mn} during maximal hyperemia was possible in 42 patients both before and after the PTCA.

The ratio between maximal flow after and before PTCA, called maximal flow ratio (MFR), was represented by the ratio between T_{mn} before and after the intervention and compared with the results of exercise testing 24–48 hours before and 7–10 days after the procedure. After correction for pressure changes, MFR was 2.2 ± 1.5 for the dilated vessels and 1.0 ± 0.2 for 30 normal vessels serving as a control. In all but two patients, an MFR value of > 1.6 or < 1.6 discriminated between presence or absence of reversal of exercise test result from positive to negative.

If on-line judgement of success was based upon angiographic parameters or measurement of transstenotic pressure gradient, the relation with noninvasive functional improvement was present only in 68% and 74% of all patients, respectively. At last, a definite range of what can be called normal

J.H.C. Reiber and P.W. Serruys (eds). Advances in Quantitative Coronary Arteriography. 213–233.

T_{mn} at maximal hyperemia could be distinguished and post-PTCA values for successfully dilated arteries returned to this normal range almost completely.

We conclude that accurate comparison of maximal myocardial perfusion before and after PTCA is possible in man, that improvement in maximal flow is highly related to functional improvement as indicated by exercise test results and therefore that this method provides a straightforward way for on-line evaluation of the result of the intervention.

Introduction

Since many years it has been widely recognized that the functional significance of coronary artery disease cannot be completely understood by mere anatomical data. Therefore, increasing need is present for methods, directly measuring the effect of these stenoses on coronary and myocardial blood flow [1–3]. One method for flow measurement which is applied in clinical practice nowadays, is ECG triggered digital radiography [2, 4].

Videodensitometry for coronary or myocardial flow assessment was already suggested by Rutishauser more than 20 years ago [5–7]. The basic principle of this method is that after injection of contrast agent into a coronary artery, time-density curves over myocardial regions of interest can be obtained. These time-density curves represent contrast density as a function of time and resemble dye-dilution curves. They contain useful information about myocardial perfusion.

Calculation of flow from these curves, however, has been complicated by a number of problems [8]. In the first place the only correct time parameter to be used from a physiologic point of view, is mean transit time (T_{mn}). Determination of T_{mn}, however, is demanding with respect to image quality because a large part of the time-density curve corresponding with up to 15 heart cycles has to be known. A second problem is that the vascular volume V is unknown and changing between different situations in which flow is compared. A third major problem is that flow itself is not constant, even not during the acquisition of the time-density curve, because of the hyperemic response to contrast agent. At last, contrast density is measured instead of contrast concentration and the relation between these two variables is unknown unless the vascular volume is constant.

In a recent animal study, we showed how these problems can be circumvented in dogs by performing all studies at maximal coronary hyperemia, corresponding with a maximal – and therefore constant – volume of the myocardial vascular bed [8]. If maximal coronary hyperemia is present, no additional hyperemic stimulus is provided by the contrast injection and flow remains constant during image acquisition. Moreover, comparison of maximal flow between different situations becomes possible because the vascular volume remains unchanged. The constancy of the vascular volume also guarantees that contrast concentration and contrast density are linearly pro-

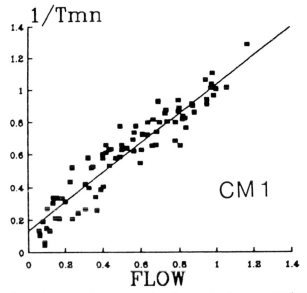

Figure 1. Normalized data from 8 dogs, showing the relation between maximal flow velocity, measured in the left circumflex (LCx) artery by an epicardial Doppler probe and inverse hyperemic mean transit time, corresponding with the myocardium supplied by that artery.

portional, which means that changes in density are representative for changes in contrast concentration.

We also demonstrated in that study that, at least in animals, image quality – and therefore time-density curve quality – can be improved in such a way that the physiologic correct time parameter mean transit time can be determined reliably from the time-density curve [8]. With all these precautions, an excellent relation proved to be present in these dogs between inverse mean transit time and real flow (Figure 1).

Apart from the pathophysiologic insights provided by this study, we considered what could be its value in the clinical situation. It should be clearly stated that only an index of maximal flow is provided by this method. No information about resting flow and therefore no coronary flow reserve (CFR) can be obtained. In this context, however, it should be realized that the majority of patients is not complaining about insufficient resting flow, but about inadequate maximal flow. The functional status of a patient with angina pectoris is determined by the maximally achievable flow through the myocardium, and therefore maximal flow is a clinically relevant parameter. As shown in Figure 1, this maximally achievable blood flow through the myocardium supplied by a coronary artery, is reliably reflected by hyperemic mean transit time, derived from a region of interest over the myocardium supplied by that particular artery.

If therefore the results of the animal study could be applied in man, this would provide a means to compare maximal flow between different situations, e.g. after and before a PTCA. In our opinion the increase in maximal flow would be the most direct and straightforward way to evaluate the result of such an intervention. Moreover, unlike CFR, the ratio between maximal flow after and before PTCA, is not dependent on heart rate, left ventricular hypertrophy, previous infarction in other segments, or the PTCA procedure itself. It is only dependent on pressure which can easily be measured and corrected for [9, 10, 11].

The specific aims of this clinical study were therefore:
1. to investigate if image quality in man could be improved in such a way that mean transit time could be determined reliably and reproducibly;
2. to investigate how increase in maximal flow obtained by a PTCA and reflected by decrease of T_{mn}, correlates with functional improvement of the patient, and
3. to investigate if a range of "normal values" for mean transit time at maximal hyperemia does exist.

Methods

All digital studies in our catheterization laboratory are performed in patients who have to be catheterized or have to undergo a PTCA anyhow. These patients, are seen at the outpatients' department 24–48 hours before the procedure. The aims of the study are explained to them at that time and this is followed by extensive training to hold breath at maximal inspiration, using a nose clamp. Careful attention is paid to avoid any motion of head, neck, shoulders and thorax during breath holding. The patients are asked to repeat this training in the evening and if possible the next day. Training and instruction of the patients takes about 30 minutes.

To evaluate the value of decrease of hyperemic mean transit time for determining PTCA success, we selected 50 consecutive patients with sinus rhythm, who had angina pectoris class III, a positive exercise test (ET) and single vessel disease at coronary arteriography less than 6 weeks before and who had been accepted for elective PTCA. When these patients were seen at the outpatient department 24–48 hours before the intervention, another exercise test was performed. The aim of the study was explained to the patient and thereafter training to hold breath at maximal inspiration was thoroughly performed, as described above. Exercise testing was repeated 7 to 10 days after the PTCA procedure. Reversal of exercise test result from positive (ischemia) to negative (no signs of ischemia) was considered as decisive for functionally successful PTCA.

In the search for normal values of T_{mn} at maximal hyperemia, it was postulated that such a value should be derived from an anatomically normal branch in a patient with a negative exercise test. In practice, in patients with single vessel disease after successful PTCA according to exercise test result, the values of the nondilated branches could be defined as normal [12].

Image acquisition

At the time of the PTCA, a 6 French stimulation catheter was positioned into the right atrium and the following protocol was applied: In case of a stenosis in the left circumflex (LCx) or left anterior descending (LAD) artery or one of its major branches, a diagnostic Judkins catheter was advanced into the right coronary artery and an ECG-triggered study of this artery was performed during maximal vasodilation in the RAO 30° projection. This was followed by a similar study of the left coronary artery (LCA) in the LAO 60° projection. Thereafter the regular PTCA procedure was performed, followed by another ECG-triggered study of the left coronary artery after 10–15 minutes.

In case of a right coronary artery (RCA) stenosis, RCA and LCA were interchanged in this protocol. By following this protocol, not only maximal flow in the diseased artery could be compared before and after the intervention, but also reference data for apparently normal coronary arteries, could be collected.

For all studies 6 ml Iohexol was injected using a power injector with an injection speed of 4 ml/sec in analogy to the former animal validation study [8]. One image was taken per heart cycle at exactly the same moment, just before onset of the QRS-complex and using synchronous X-ray pulses [12, 13, 14]. Contrast injections started 30 sec after i.c. administration of 8 mg papaverine in the RCA and 12 mg papaverine in the LCA to provide maximal hyperemia. It has been documented by the Iowa and Rotterdam groups that this dose of papaverine induces maximal vasodilation for about 25–60 seconds after its administration [15, 16]. Therefore, a maximal and constant vascular volume was assumed to be present during image acquisition. Image acquisition always started 7 seconds before contrast injection and the breathing command was given at the start of image acquisition. Generally it takes 3–4 seconds for a patient to achieve maximal inspiration. This time is utilized by the image acquisition equipment (Siemens Bicor and Digitron) to adapt the exposure parameters. Thereafter, the automatic brightness control is switched off and 3–5 more heart beats are available to indicate a stable baseline density. The sequence of these events is summarized in Figure 2.

During image acquisition, mean arterial pressure was continuously recorded in the iliac artery.

Processing of regions of interest and time-density curves

Regions of interest (ROIs) are chosen over the tip of the coronary catheter to record start of contrast injection and over the myocardium supplied by the respective arteries [12, 13]. For the left anterior descending artery, the

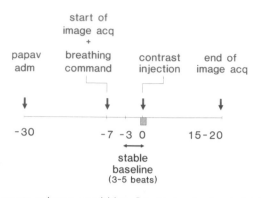

Figure 2. Sequence of events at image acquisition. I.c. papaverine is administered 30 seconds before contrast injection to ensure maximal vasodilation during image acquisition. The start of image acquisition as well as the breathing command are timed 7 seconds before contrast injection. Achieving deep inspiration and lying down motionless again, takes approximately 4 seconds and this time is utilized by the Digitron to adapt exposure parameters. Thereafter, the automatic brightness control is switched off and 3–5 more heart cycles are available to obtain a stable baseline density. The contrast injection is represented by a block-shaped input signal with a width of 1.5 seconds. Time $t = 0$ is defined halfway the injection, being the mean transit time of this input signal. Thereafter, 15–20 more images are acquired to study contrast passage and to delineate the time-density curve.

myocardial ROI is preferably chosen over the antero-apical region, for the left circumflex artery over the posterolateral area at the level of the posterom-edian papillary muscle and for the RCA over the central portion of the posterior septum (Figure 3). All myocardial ROIs are circular and of identical size within one patient. ROIs are chosen in such a way that overlap of LAD and LCx myocardium is avoided and care is taken to avoid overprojection of the large epicardial arteries and veins. Close to the myocardial ROIs, background ROIs are chosen for analysis of changes in background density [8, 12]. This analysis is performed because the background always shows slight variations in density over time, predominantly a slight increase. This is caused by instability of the X-ray chain, small motion artifacts, and some-times overlap of extramyocardial structures such as the descending aorta or the right atrium, which are faintly stained by contrast agent during the latter phase of image acquisition. Once chosen, position and size of the ROIs are kept constant within each patient. This procedure is fundamentally similar to the former animal validation study [8].

Time-density curves are obtained by sampling the average pixel density within a ROI in the consecutive images and corrected by subtraction of the sampled average density in the corresponding background ROI. A gamma function is fitted to the remaining data according to the Marquardt method, using all samples between $t = 0$ and the instant at which the descending part of the curve becomes less than 60% of the peak value [17, 18, 19]. The

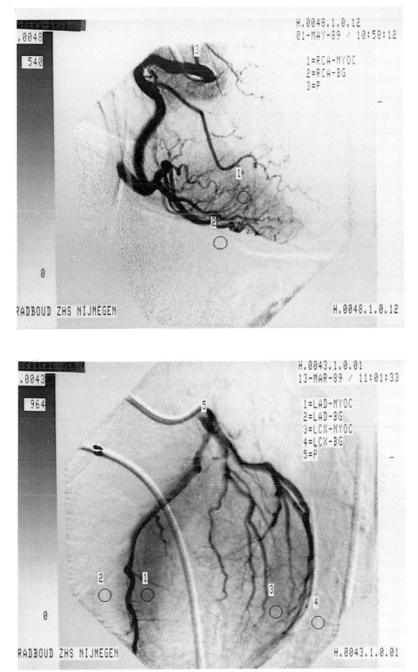

Figure 3. Representative examples of location of regions of interest (ROIs) over the parts of the myocardium supplied by the right coronary artery (top), the left anterior descending artery and the left circumflex artery (bottom), as well as the corresponding background ROIs.

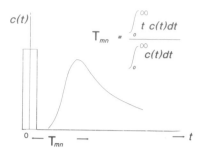

Figure 4. Temporal relations and definition of time $t = 0$. Contrast injection is considered as a block pulse with a width of 1.5 s. Therefore, $t = 0$ is defined as the moment 0.75 s after start of contrast injection, which is registered in a ROI at the tip of the coronary catheter. Mean transit time (T_{mn}) of the contrast agent from the injection site to the myocardial ROI is defined according to theory.

quality of the curve is judged by calculating the relative error (E_r) between sampled data and the fit.

A 10% value of E_r is considered as the upper limit for acceptance of the fit as being representative for the sampled data. This is also in analogy with the former animal validation study [8]. Mean transit time (T_{mn}) is calculated from the fit function d(t) according to theory by the equation [20]:

$$T_{mm} = \frac{\int_0^\infty t \cdot d(t)\, dt}{\int_0^\infty d(t)\, dt},$$

where $t = 0$ is defined as in Figure 4 and where $d(t)$ represents the gammafit and is defined as:

$$d(t) = a_0 + D_{max} \cdot \Theta a \cdot e^{-} a(\Theta - 1) \qquad (t \geq t_0)$$
$$d(t) = a_0 \qquad (t < t_0)$$

with:

D_{max} = maximal value for contrast density of the sampled data
$\Theta = (t - t_0)/(t_{max} - t_0)$
t_{max} = time of maximal contrast density
a is a shaping factor

T_{mn} can be calculated from the parameters of the gamma function as follows.

$$T_{mm} = \frac{(a+1)}{a} \cdot (t_{max} - t_0) + t_0$$

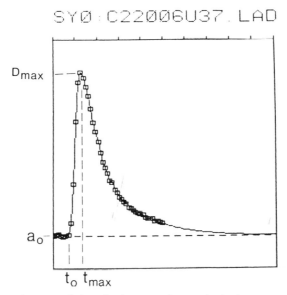

SYØ C22006U37 LAD

Figure 5. Background corrected time-density curve (squares), the best gammafit (drawn line) and the parameters necessary to obtain this fit. a_0 = baseline density level, t_0 = time at which the ascending part of the curve starts, D_{max} = maximal contrast intensity, t_{max} – time corresponding with D_{max}.

where t_0, t_{max} and a_0 are defined as in Figure 5 and a is a shaping factor of the gamma function.

One kind of manual correction of the fit is permitted in the human studies: contrast injection in these studies always starts about 6.25 seconds after the inspiration command (Figure 2). Mostly a deep inspiration lasts less than 4 seconds, which means that, at an average heart rate of 80/min, at least 4 motionless images are available before start of contrast injection to provide a stable baseline level. Sometimes, however, inspiration takes longer and in that case problems may be encountered in determination of the baseline density (zero level). If the baseline is clearly discernible by the remaining sample points, manual correction of the baseline is permitted by indicating the parameter a_0. If any doubt remains, the curves are rejected [21].

Data Processing and Statistical Analysis

The ratio between maximal coronary blood flow after and before the PTCA was called the maximal flow ratio (MFR) for the respective ROI and calculated as

$$MFR = \frac{T_{mn} \text{ at maximal hyperemia before PTCA}}{T_{mn} \text{ at maximal hyperemia after PTCA}}.$$

Because of the pressure dependency of flow during maximal vasodilation, MFR was corrected for changes in mean arterial pressure in the studies before and after PTCA. This was performed by multiplying MFR by the ratio $Pa(1)/Pa(2)$ where $Pa(1)$ and $Pa(2)$ represent the mean arterial pressures at the studies before and after PTCA, respectively. The corrected value was called MFR_c.

In testing reproducibility of calculation of T_{mn}, in 2×10 patients one study of either the LCA or the RCA was performed twice during maximal vasodilation under identical circumstances with an interval of 10 minutes. In these paired studies, image processing and ROI processing were performed in exactly identical way [22]. Correction for possible pressure changes between the paired studies, was performed by multiplying T_{mn} at the second measurement by the ratio $Pa(2)/Pa(1)$ where $Pa(1)$ and $Pa(2)$ represent the mean arterial pressures at the first and the second of the paired studies, respectively. Linear regression plots were drawn and the correlation coefficients between the first and the second measurement were calculated for the ROIs corresponding with the LAD, LCx and RCA respectively.

Angiographic success of PTCA was defined as a reduction of the area stenosis of at least 20% by densitometry and a residual area stenosis of less than 50% compared to the size of a nearby normal segment [23]. Success according to pressure measurements was considered to be present if the mean transstenotic pressure gradient after the PTCA was $\leqslant 15 \, mmHg$ [23, 24]. The PTCA was considered to have been functionally successful if a positive ET 1–2 days before the PTCA, reversed to negative 7 days after the procedure.

To determine separation between MFR_c values indicative for successful or unsuccessful PTCA according to ET results, linear discriminant analysis was performed on the logarithmic data. The performance of the angiographic criterion, transstenotic pressure gradient and MFR_c for classification of PTCA results was calculated and was expressed as percentage of correct classification. Furthermore, the relations between the result of exercise testing and result of the PTCA according to angiographic stenosis reduction, transstenotic pressure gradient, and MFR_c were evaluated by Chi-square tests. Statistical analysis was performed using the SAS-software package (SAS institute Inc, Cary, NC). Hemodynamic data are presented as mean ± s.d.

Results

Quality and reproducibility of image acquisition and time-density curves

The average image quality in man was surprisingly good. Adequate fits to the sampled time-density curves could be obtained in 91% of all studies, the relative error E_r being less than 10%. Some representative examples of

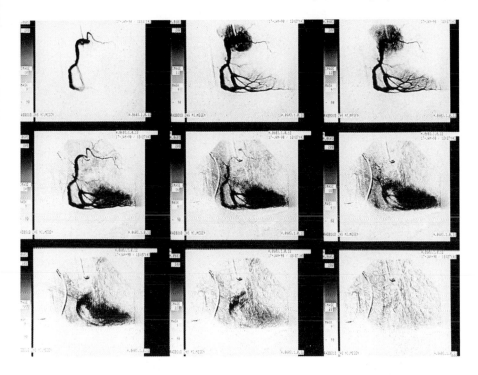

Figure 6. Example of a sequence of mask-mode subtracted images of the right coronary of a 63–year-old male. Contrast injection starts at the 10th heart cycle after start of image acquisition. Image 9, therefore, has been chosen as mask. Filling of the capillary bed of the posterior septum by contrast agent and the subsequent washout can be clearly distinguished and even at the last image, corresponding with the 28th heart cycle after start of image acquisition, motion artifacts are only mild.

images are shown in Figures 6 and 7. Some examples of background corrected time-density curves and the corresponding fits are also presented in Figure 7. Reproducibility of T_{mn}, obtained from 2 identical studies with an interval of 10 min, was excellent. After correction for the small changes in mean arterial pressure in the paired studies as outlined in the methods section, the correlation coefficients between the first and second measurement were 0.97, 0.95, 0.95, for the LAD, LCx and RCA, respectively (Figure 8).

Value of the maximal flow ratio to predict PTCA result

For validating the value of increase of maximal flow to predict the functional improvement of the patient correctly, the ratio between mean transit time at maximal hyperemia before and after PTCA was correlated in these patients to exercise test results. Some important data and results are summarized in Table 1. The ratio between T_{mn} after and before PTCA was called the

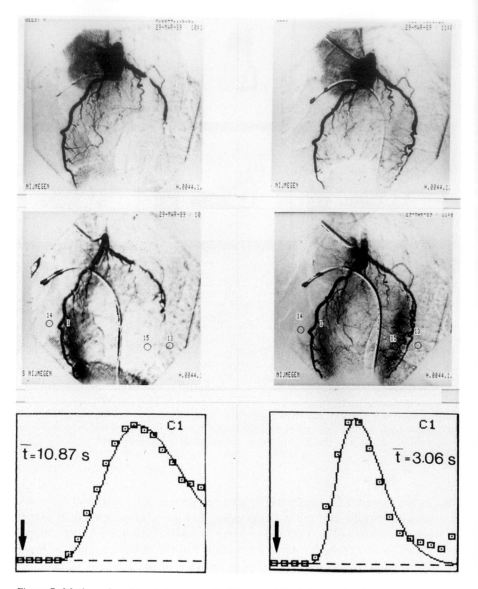

Figure 7. Mask mode subtracted images of a 69–year-old lady before (left) and after successful PTCA (right) of the left circumflex artery. The coronary artery itself, the filling of the myocardium by contrast agent, and the time-density curve over the indicated region of interest (#15) are shown. The ratio between mean transit time at maximal hyperemia after and before PTCA was 10.87: 3.06 which means that, as a result of the PTCA, maximally achievable flow through the LCx myocardium increased by 356%. The arrow indicates the start of contrast injection.

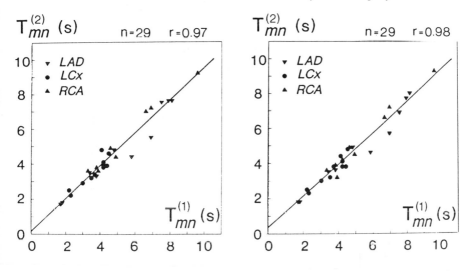

Figure 8. Relation between mean transit time at maximal hyperemia at the first ($T^{(1)}_{min}$) and the second ($T^{(2)}_{min}$) measurement, before (left) and after (right) correction for pressure changes. The line represents the line of identity. Values, derived from the myocardium of the left anterior descending, left circumflex and right coronary artery are indicated by the inverse triangles, circles, and upright triangles, respectively.

maximal flow ratio and, as explained, constitutes a direct measure for improvement of maximal flow. After correction for pressure changes, this maximal flow ratio averaged 2.2. Exercise time before and after the PTCA is also displayed and correlated well with the MFR (Table 1).

Next, pressure corrected maximal flow ratio of more or less than 1.6 was correlated to presence of absence of reversal of exercise test result. In Table 2 it can be seen that MFRc determined from studies just before and 10 minutes after PTCA is highly predictive for functional success or failure of the intervention as indicated by exercise testing. A correct classification was made in 95% of all cases. MFR was at least 1.6 in all but one patients who had reversal of exercise test result from positive to negative. On the other hand, in 9 patients MFR was less than 1.6 and in 8 of these 9 patients no reversal of ET result was present.

Table 1. Area stenosis severity (determined by quantitative densitometry), transstenotic pressure gradient (ΔP), mean transit time at maximal hyperemia (T_{mn}) and exercise time before and after PTCA (mean ± s.d.)

	Pre-PTCA	Post-PTCA	n
% Area stenosis	81 ± 12	39 ± 18	48
Transstenotic ΔP (mm Hg)	45 ± 10	14 ± 9	27
T_{mn} at max hyperemia (s)	6.8 ± 2.0	3.4 ± 1.2	42
Exercise time (s)	370 ± 184	535 ± 86	48

Table 2. Relations between maximal flow ratio after correction for pressure changes (MFR$_c$), angiographic success, and transstenotic pressure gradient as measured 5 minutes after the last balloon inflation (ΔP), and presence or absence of reversal of exercise test (ET) result (+indicates positive ET; – indicates negative ET). Angiographic success was defined as ≥20% area stenosis reduction and residual stenosis <50%, calculated by quantitative coronary arteriography

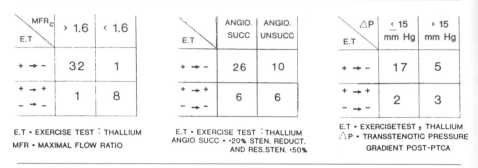

MFR$_c$ / E.T	> 1.6	< 1.6
+ → –	32	1
+ → + / – → –	1	8

E.T • EXERCISE TEST ∶ THALLIUM
MFR • MAXIMAL FLOW RATIO

/ E.T	ANGIO. SUCC	ANGIO. UNSUCC
+ → –	26	10
+ → + / – → –	6	6

E.T • EXERCISE TEST ∶ THALLIUM
ANGIO SUCC • >20% STEN. REDUCT.
AND RES.STEN. <50%

ΔP / E.T	< 15 mm Hg	> 15 mm Hg
+ → –	17	5
+ → + / – → –	2	3

E.T • EXERCISETEST ± THALLIUM
$\triangle$P • TRANSSTENOTIC PRESSURE
GRADIENT POST-PTCA

Despite their limitations, some other methods have been used to date for on-line evaluation of the PTCA, such as assessment of angiographic stenosis severity or measurement of transstenotic pressure gradients [23, 24]. Therefore we also investigated the relation between these on-line parameters and ET results. From Table 2, it is clear that both relations are significantly less reliable than is the case for MFR.

In those 30 patients with one diseased and one normal branch of the LCA, T_{mn} at maximal hyperemia of the normal vessel could be compared before and after PTCA of the diseased branch. MFR$_c$ for these control arteries was 1.0 ± 0.2 which confirms the intrinsic correctness of our method (Figure 9).

ONE STENOTIC BRANCH OF LCA ⎤
ONE NORMAL BRANCH OF LCA ⎦ N = 30

MFR = 2.5 ± 0.7

MFR = 1.0 ± 0.2

Tmn DISEASED BRANCH
─────────────────── : 2.2 ± 0.3 --> 0.9 ± 0.3
Tmn NORMAL BRANCH

Figure 9. Maximal Flow Ratio for the dilated branch of the left coronary artery and for the normal branch which served as a control vessel (mean value ± s.d.).

We also investigated the ratio between mean transit time at maximal hyperemia corresponding with the diseased vessel of the left coronary artery and the normal branch of the left coronary artery. This ratio decreased from 2.2 ± 0.3 to 0.9 ± 0.3 after PTCA.

Mean transit time at maximal hyperemia of apparently normal
coronary arteries

At last, we collected the values of mean transit time derived from the myocardium supplied by apparently normal coronary arteries. These values were compared with the data of the corresponding diseased arteries before and after PTCA. The results are displayed in Figure 10. It can be seen that there is a definite range of what can be called a normal mean transit time during maximal hyperemia. For the RCA these values seem to be larger than for the LAD and LCx and are more scattered. In the diseased arteries before PTCA a large range of values was found as expected. After PTCA, however, the values return to normal with minimal scatter. For the LAD and LCx artery, almost complete separation was present between normal and pathologic data.

Discussion

The videodensitometric approach for flow measurement as used in this clinical study, was very similar to the method validated in animal experiments before [8, 12]. In that validation study it was proved, that comparison of maximal myocardial flow between situations with different degrees of stenosis can be accurately performed by calculating ratios of hyperemic mean transit time.

In this clinical study, after extensive breath holding training and using synchronous X-ray pulses, image quality was so good that passage of contrast agent through the myocardium could be studied long enough to allow reliable determination of T_{mn} in about 90% of the patients. Reproducibility of T_{mn} in paired studies under identical circumstances was excellent [22]. Therefore, it can be concluded that this videodensitometric approach is applicable in clinical practice, at least in stable patients, and our first aim has been achieved by that.

A difference between the previously mentioned experimental study and these clinical studies is the different method to induce maximal hyperemia. In the validation study, continuous infusion of dipyridamole was applied for this purpose [8, 12]. For practical reasons, such as its short time of action, intracoronary papaverine was used in the present study. It has been proved by former investigators that for approximately 25 to 60 seconds after i.c. administration of 8–12 mg of papaverine, maximal vasodilation of the myocardial vascular bed is achieved [15, 16]. Therefore, we assumed that during acquisition of the time-density curve, the vascular volume remained maximal and constant and flow was not influenced by contrast injection.

In the clinical study in the PTCA patients, exercise testing 24–48 hours before and 7–10 days after the PTCA was the method of choice for noninvasive functional evaluation of the result of the procedure. Because in all patients the combination of anginal complaints NYHA class III, a positive ET and proved single vessel disease had been present less than 6 weeks before the PTCA, exercise testing can discriminate accurately between presence or absence of (residual) ischemia in this particular group of patients [25, 26]. Moreover, because of the presence of just single vessel disease, it is justified in this group to assume that ischemia, if present at exercise testing, is actually caused by the affected artery [25]. Therefore, ET results could be used in this study as the gold standard for PTCA success. MFR_c, angiographic result, and final transstenotic pressure gradient were correlated to this gold standard.

Because exercise testing after the PTCA was performed several days after the flow measurements, changes in coronary anatomy and physiology could have occurred in the meantime. The 95% agreement between MFR_c and ET seems to be very high in this respect. If, however, PTCA result in this study was judged by classical anatomical criteria, a previously positive ET remained positive despite an angiographically successful intervention in 12% of the patients within one week which is in accordance with current literature [27, 28]. One may speculate whether this finding merely reflects the hypothesis that insufficient increase in maximal flow after PTCA is a better predictor for restenosis than coronary anatomy.

The approach used in this study for calculation of flow is only valid in situations of maximal vasodilation to guarantee constant vascular volume. It should be emphasized that no information about resting flow can be obtained and therefore no coronary flow reserve can be calculated. This approach, however, offers the possibility to compare maximal blood flow before and after an appropriate intervention, such as angioplasty in this study but possibly also long-lasting lipid lowering therapy. Unlike coronary flow reserve, this maximal flow ratio is independent of resting flow which is in turn influenced by heart rate, left ventricular hypertrophy, previous infarction in other segments, prolonged ischemia and the PTCA procedure itself [10, 11, 29, 30, 31]. At maximal vasodilation, flow is only dependent on pressure which can easily be measured and corrected for as was done in this study. In fact, MFR_c as defined in this study can be considered as the improvement of relative coronary flow reserve as recently defined by Gould et al. [32]. It should be realized in this context that anginal complaints in the majority of patients are due to inadequate maximal flow. Therefore, increase in maximal flow is a clinically relevant parameter and is expected to reflect improved exercise tolerance.

In the practice of interventional cardiology, parameters for on-line evaluation of the result of the intervention are essential. Because T_{mn} can be calculated within minutes after image acquisition and decrease of this value correlates well with the functional result of the PTCA, determination of MFR_c can be used for this purpose and proved to be superior to other parameters used to date for on-line evaluation of the PTCA, such as assessment of angiographic stenosis severity or measurement of transstenotic pressure gradients (Table 2) [25, 26, 33, 34].

In many former videodensitometric approaches, flow has been represented by maximal contrast density divided by a certain time parameter such as appearance time [4, 35, 36, 37]. Because maximal contrast density, expressed in arbitrary units, is dependent on many factors not related to flow, and differs more than thousand percent between different patients, it has been regarded as impossible to indicate normal values in these studies. Because in the present study merely a time parameter was used as an index of flow, it made sense to look whether a range of normal values for T_{mn} at maximal hyperemia did exist. Most of the patients in this study provided 2 apparently normal coronary arteries and a definite range for T_{mn} of these normal vessels during maximal hyperemia could be distinguished. This means that also in diagnostic catheterization one single determination of T_{mn} at maximal coronary hyperemia may provide useful information about the functional significance of a coronary artery stenosis.

In our studies, after successful PTCA according to exercise testing, T_{mn} completely returned to the normal range (Figure 10). In previous studies using digital radiography for evaluation of CFR improvement after PTCA, it was observed that CFR immediately after the intervention did not return to normal [37]. It has been hypothesized that this phenomenon could be caused by the fact that resting flow after PTCA would still be elevated due to prolonged ischemia and to the procedure itself [2, 37]. Our results are in favor of this explanation because T_{mn} at maximal flow in the dilated vessel was not longer than T_{mn} at maximal flow in apparently normal coronary arteries. Furthermore, in those 34 patients with one diseased and one normal branch of the left coronary artery, the ratio (T_{mn} diseased artery)/(T_{mn} normal artery) decreased from 1.9 ± 0.3 before PTCA to 0.9 ± 0.3 after PTCA, which provides further support to that explanation. This last observation also suggests that the ratio between T_{mn} of a stenotic and of a normal branch can help to assess the functional significance of the stenosis. Finally, it was observed in this group that the MFR_c of normal control vessels was 1.0 ± 0.2, which argues for the intrinsic correctness of this method (Figure 9).

A limitation of this approach is that acquisition of well interpretable time-density curves is highly dependent on sufficient image quality. In the present study adequate image acquisition was possible in about 90% of all patients but one can doubt on this point in case of emergency situations where no chance for previous training to hold breath is present. In that case, motion artifacts serious enough to interfere with reliable image processing, may be present more often.

Another factor which may restrict the clinical value of the MFR, is the

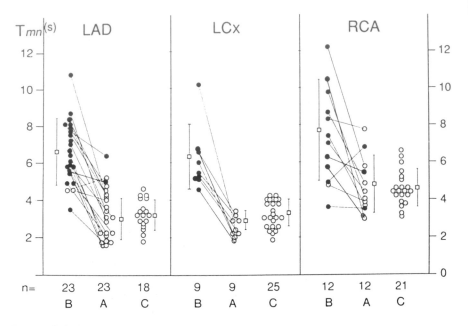

Figure 10. Values for mean transit time (s) at maximal myocardial hyperemia belonging to stenotic vessels before (B) and after (A) successful PTCA and to normal control vessels (C). LAD = left anterior descending artery; LCx = left circumflex artery; RCA = right coronary artery. The closed points correspond with a positive exercise test and the open points with a negative exercise test. The mean value ± s.d. is indicated in the figure.

presence of collateral circulation, excluded in this study. In that case, transport of contrast agent injected into the vessel itself can be slowed down by collateral blood supply [12]. This also holds true for patients with bypass grafts in whom the native vessel is not completely occluded.

Next, it is necessary that overprojection of the myocardium supplied by the analyzed artery can be avoided while nevertheless its thickness in the chosen projection should be large enough to ensure sufficient staining after contrast injection. This can be hard to obtain for diagonal and intermediate branches of the LAD artery and for posterolateral branches of the LCx artery.

Further applications and future developments

At the moment, this method for flow measurement is applied in some placebo-controlled trials about the influence of long-lasting lipid lowering therapy on the coronary arterial tree. Cardiac catheterization is performed in these trials at the beginning and at the end of a 2–year treatment period, which is considered as the intervention. In this kind of studies, sophisticated anatomic methods have been developed to score progression or regression of the atherosclerotic lesions. A final evaluation, however, often remains hazardous: especially in the case of multiple lesions within one vessel, some placques may either show regression or progression, which makes it hard to estimate the net effect of the therapy. If, on the contrary, one studies the maximal flow achievable by the distal myocardium supplied by such a vessel, one integral measure is obtained for the summed effect of all lesions which unambiguously and accurately reflects functional improvement or impairment at the end of the study period.

In a collaborative study with the division of Cardiology of the University of Texas, changes in hyperemic mean transit time obtained by PTCA are correlated to improvement of stenosis geometry, reflected by changes in stenosis flow reserve as defined by Kirkeeide and Gould [3, 32]. Thus, geometrical and functional properties of a stenosis can be studied in a combined way and contribute to a more complete understanding of coronary artery disease [38]. Other present studies are directed to define ranges of hyperemic T_{mn} under different pathologic conditions and to unravel the complex relation between myocardial perfusion disturbance and abnormalities of contractile state. From these studies, we hope to acquire more insight into the sequence of coronary anatomy, myocardial perfusion, and contractile function.

Conclusion

Despite some limitations, this study shows that excellent digital subtraction images of the coronary arteries can be obtained and that functional information about flow can be derived from these images in a theoretically sound way during both diagnostic and therapeutic cardiac catheterization. This study illustrates how a more complete understanding of coronary disease has become possible by integration of both anatomic and physiologic data obtained by digital radiography and enables on-line evaluation of PTCA results.

References

1. White CW, Wright CB, Doty DB, et al. Does visual interpretation of the coronary arteriogram predict the physiologic importance of a coronary stenosis? N Engl J Med 1984; **310**: 819–24.
2. Nissen SE, Elion JL, Booth DC, Evans J, DeMaria AN. Value and limitations of computer analysis of digital subtraction angiography in the assessment of coronary flow reserve. Circulation 1986; **73**: 562–71.
3. Kirkeeide RL, Gould KL, Parsel L. Assessment of coronary stenoses by myocardial perfusion imaging during pharmacologic coronary vasodilation. VII. Validation of coronary flow reserve as a single integrated functional measure of stenosis severity reflecting all its geometric dimensions. J Am Coll Cardiol 1986; **7**: 103–13.
4. Vogel RA. The radiographic assessment of coronary blood flow parameters. Circulation 1985; **72**: 460–5.

5. Rutishauser W, Simon H, Stucky JP, Schad N, Noseda G, Wellauer J. Evaluation of Roentgen cinedensitometry for flow measurement in models and in the intact circulation. Circulation 1967; **36**: 951–63.
6. Rutishauser W, Bussmann WD, Noseda G, Meier W, Wellauer J. Blood flow measurement through single coronary arteries by roentgen densitometry. A comparison of flow measured by a radiologic technique applicable in the intact organism and by electromagnetic flow-meter. Radium Ther Nucl Med 1970; **109**: 12–20.
7. Rutishauser W, Noseda G, Bussman WD, Preter B. Blood flow measurement through single coronary arteries by roentgen densitometry. Right coronary artery flow in conscious man. Radium Ther Nucl Med 1970; **109**: 21–4.
8. Pijls NH, Uijen GJ, Hoevelaken A, et al. Mean transit time for the assessment of myocardial perfusion by videodensitometry. Circulation 1990; **81**: 1331–40. Comment in: Circulation 1990; **81**: 1431–5.
9. Hoffman JI. Maximal coronary flow and the concept of coronary vascular reserve. Circulation 1984; **70**: 153–9.
10. Marcus M, Wright C, Doty D, et al. Measurements of coronary velocity and reactive hyperemia in the coronary circulation of humans. Circ Res 1981; **49**: 877–91.
11. Klocke FJ. Measurements of coronary flow reserve: defining pathophysiology versus making decisions about patient care. Circulation 1987; **76**: 1183–9.
12. Pijls NH, Uijen GJ, Hoevelaken A, et al. Mean transit time for videodensitometric assessment of myocardial perfusion and the concept of maximal flow ratio: a validation study in the intact dog and a pilot study in man. Int J Card Imaging 1990, **5**: 191–202.
13. Pijls NH, Aengevaeren WR, Uijen GJ, et. al. Concept of maximal flow ratio for immediate evaluation of percutaneous transluminal coronary angioplasty result by videodensitometry. Circulation 1991; **83**: 854–65.
14. Van der Werf T, Heethaar RM, Stegehuis H, Meijler FL. The concept of apparent cardiac arrest as a prerequisite for coronary digital subtraction angiography. J Am Coll Cardiol 1984; **4**: 239–44.
15. Wilson RF, White CW. Intracoronary papaverine: an ideal coronary vasodilator for studies of the coronary circulation in conscious humans. Circulation 1986; **73**: 444–51.
16. Zijlstra F, Serruys PW, Hugenholtz PG. Papaverine: the ideal coronary vasodilator for investigating coronary flow reserve? A study of timing, magnitude, reproducibility and safety of the coronary hyperemic response after intracoronary papaverine. Cathet Cardiovasc Diagn 1986; **12**: 298–303.
17. Bevington PR. Data reduction and error analysis for the physical sciences. New York: McGraw-Hill 1969: 204–46.
18. Press WH, Flannery BP, Tenkolsky SA, Vettering WT. Numerical recipes: the art of scientific computing. Cambridge: Cambridge University Press 1986: 523–8.
19. Uijen GJ, Pijls NH, Hoevelaken A, Van der Werf T. The accuracy of densitometric time parameters in the analysis of myocardial perfusion. Comp Cardiol 1988: 215–8.
20. Zierler KL. Circulation times and the theory of indicator-dilution methods for determining blood flow and volume. In: Hamilton WF (Section Ed.), Circulation: volume 1 (Handbook of Physiology: Section 2). Washington: American Physiological Society 1962: 585–615.
21. Pijls NH. Maximal myocardial perfusion as a measure of the functional significance of coronary artery disease. Dordrecht: Kluwer Academic Publishers 1992 (in press).
22. Pijls NH, Uijen GJ, Pijnenburg T, et al. Reproducibility of mean transit time for maximal myocardial flow assessment by videodensitometry. Int J Cardiac Imaging 1991; **6**: 101–8.
23. Kent KM, Bentivoglio LG, Block PC, et al. Percutaneous transluminal coronary angioplasty: report from the Registry of the National Heart, Lung, and Blood Institute. Am J Cardiol 1982; **49**: 2011–20.
24. MacIsaac HC, Knudtson ML, Robinson VJ, Manyari DE. Is the residual translesional pressure gradient useful to predict regional myocardial perfusion after percutaneous transluminal coronary angioplasty? Am Heart J 1989; **117**: 783–90.
25. Hamilton GW, Trobaugh GB, Ritchie JL, Gould KL, DeRouen TA, Williams DL. My-

ocardial imaging with [201]Thallium: an analysis of clinical usefulness based on Bayes' theorem. Semin Nucl Med 1978; **8**: 358–64.
26. Melin JA, Piret LJ, Vanbutsele RJM, et al. Diagnostic value of exercise electrocardiography and thallium myocardial scintigraphy in patients without previous myocardial infarction: a Bayesian approach. Circulation 1981; **63**: 1019–24.
27. Nobuyoshi M, Kimura T, Nosaka H, et al. Restenosis after successful percutaneous transluminal coronary angioplasty: serial angiographic follow-up of 299 patients. J Am Coll Cardiol 1988; **12**: 616–23.
28. Serruys PW, Rensing BF, Luyten HE, Hermans WR, Beatt KJ. Restenosis following coronary angioplasty. In: Meier B (Ed.), Interventional cardiology. Göttingen: Hogreve & Huber Publishers 1990: 79–115.
29. Klein LW, Agarwal JB, Schneider RM, Hermann G, Weintraub WS, Helfant RH. Effects of previous myocardial infarction on measurements of reactive hyperemia and the coronary vascular reserve. J Am Coll Cardiol 1986; **8**: 357–63.
30. Serruys PW, Juilliere Y, Zijlstra F, et al. Coronary blood flow velocity during percutaneous transluminal coronary angioplasty as a guide for the assessment of the functional result. Am J Cardiol 1988; **61**: 253–59.
31. Vogel RA, Mancini GBJ. Assessment of coronary flow and myocardial perfusion with digital radiography. In: Mancini GBJ (Ed.), Clinical applications of cardiac digital angiography. New York, Raven Press 1988: 281–90.
32. Gould KL, Kirkeeide RL, Buchi M. Coronary flow reserve as a physiologic measure of stenosis severity. J Am Coll Cardiol 1990; **15**: 459–74.
33. Chokshi SK, Meyers S, Abi-Mansour P. Percutaneous transluminal coronary angioplasty: ten years' experience. Prog Cardiovasc Dis 1987; **30**: 147–210.
34. Rothman MT, Baim DS, Simpson JB, Harrison DC. Coronary hemodynamics during percutaneous transluminal coronary angioplasty. Am J Cardiol 1982; **49**: 1615–22.
34. Hodgson JM, Legrand V, Bates ER, et al. Validation in dogs of a rapid digital angiographic technique to measure relative coronary blood flow during routine cardiac catheterization. Am J Cardiol 1985; **55**: 188–93.
36. Bates ER, Aueron FM, Legrand V, et al. Comparative long-term effects of coronary artery bypass graft surgery and percutaneous transluminal coronary angioplasty on regional coronary flow reserve. Circulation 1985; **72**: 833–9.
37. Zijlstra F, Reiber JC, Juilliere Y, Serruys PW. Normalization of coronary flow reserve by percutaneous transluminal coronary angioplasty. Am J Cardiol 1988; **61**: 55–60.
38. Pijls NH, Kirkeeide RL, Van Leeuwen K, Lamfers E, Stuart YM, Gould KL. Increases in maximal coronary blood flow by PTCA: correlation of stenosis flow reserve and mean transit times. Circulation. (in press).

13. Angiographic measurement of coronary blood flow

JACK T. CUSMA, KENNETH G. MORRIS and THOMAS M. BASHORE

Summary

The need for an accurate method of assessing the physiological significance of coronary artery stenoses has led to a number of efforts utilizing angiographic image data to measure coronary blood flow. Most of these methods, applied to either digitized cinefilm or digital angiographic image sequences, have as their objective relative measures of flow such as determination of coronary flow reserve (CFR). Others have attempted to measure absolute coronary blood flow using similar processing techniques. No single method for the determination of even the relative measurement of CFR has yet to meet with widespread acceptance. This is due in part to the additional technical demands of these measurements and the fact that they require a more thorough understanding of the physiological and physical processes which can lead to inaccurate results. These methods, in general, require relatively complicated algorithms to correctly measure the time parameters and contrast volumes needed to calculate parameters of relative flow as well as absolute mean and phasic blood flow. The two main classes of angiographic methods are: (a) those utilizing contrast and time measurements in the proximal coronary arteries; (b) those employing measurements in the myocardial perfusion bed. The rationale for each class and the relative advantages of the two is discussed along with a review of a number of efforts. Furthermore, more general techniques require accurate measurement of blood volumes through densitometric measurement of contrast volume, in turn requiring implementation of correction techniques for the effects of radiation scatter, veiling glare and beam hardening, all sources of potentially large errors in such measurements. With the appropriate use of such correction methods, it will be possible to provide coronary blood flow measurements during routine catheterization.

J.H.C. Reiber and P.W. Serruys (eds), Advances in Quantitative Coronary Arteriography, 235–252.
© 1993 Kluwer Academic Publishers. Printed in the Netherlands.

Introduction

The primary technique used to assess the extent and severity of coronary artery disease today remains selective coronary arteriography using 35 mm cinefilm as the recording medium. This remains the case even in the face of a well-documented limitation of visual assessment of disease in general, and of anatomical measurements of coronary stenosis geometry in particular. The limitations of visual assessment include inter- and intra-observer variability [1–3], poor correlation with postmortem measurements of coronary stenoses [4], and poor correlation with physiologic measures of the significance of coronary lesions [5, 6]. The introduction of quantitative coronary angiography (QCA) techniques has resulted in substantial success with regard to reduction of the variability of stenosis assessment but a method which accurately provides a reproducible measurement of physiological significance remains lacking.

One measurement proposed for the assessment of physiological significance is coronary flow reserve (CFR), the ratio of maximal coronary blood flow to baseline blood flow. A measurement of CFR theoretically provides an assessment of the effect of a coronary stenosis on coronary blood flow by measuring the extent of the compensatory vasodilation of the perfusion bed in response to the pressure drop across the stenosis [7]. A number of problems exist, however, with the use of CFR as an indicator of stenosis severity. As has been pointed out by Klocke [8], factors that may affect CFR other than the presence of a stenosis include changes in aortic pressure, abnormal basal flow, left ventricular hypertrophy, tachycardia, collateral flow, and other disease processes. One alternative, proposed by Gould [9] is the calculation of stenosis flow reserve for a specific lesion using QCA measurements of artery geometry and assumptions regarding normal flow reserve, baseline blood velocity and mean aortic pressure. Another alternative, the measurement of absolute coronary blood flow would provide a measurement of physiological significance that is not subject to the same sources of error affecting CFR and could be used as an independent measure of lesion significance.

Methods for measuring both relative and absolute coronary blood flow include those utilizing the image data acquired as part of the catheterization procedure and those which require additional instrumentation or procedures. In this latter category are the recently developed intracoronary Doppler catheter which measure relative changes in coronary blood velocity [10] and an impedance angioplasty catheter [11] which measures absolute coronary blood flow using indicator dilution principles. Other types of imaging modalities which have shown potential for the measurement of relative or absolute coronary and regional myocardial blood flow include positron emission tomography (PET), ultra-fast computed tomography (cine-CT) and magnetic resonance imaging (MRI) [12].

The purpose of this paper is to review methods for measuring coronary

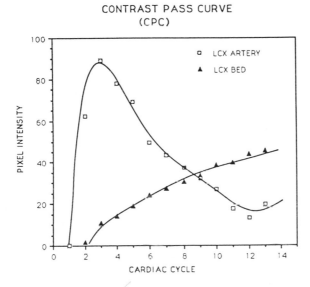

Figure 1. Examples of contrast pass curves measured in the proximal coronary artery and in the perfusion bed from a sequence of DSA images acquired in a dog following selective contrast injection into the left circumflex (LCx) coronary artery.

blood flow during the catheterization procedure using the angiographic images acquired as part of the procedure. Such methods have an advantage since they do not require an additional diagnostic procedure and they more fully utilize the information available in the angiographic image data. In general, they require the application of image processing techniques to either digitized cinefilm images or to images acquired directly in digital format. The basis for all the methods is analysis of the contrast pass curve (Figure 1), the change in intensity as a function of time following the introduction of contrast material. The complexity of the required image processing varies greatly from one method to another but the algorithms can in general be broken down into two classes. The first class utilizes intensity-time measurements in the proximal coronary arteries following injection of contrast material to arrive at flow parameters. The second major class employs contrast intensity-time information in the myocardial perfusion bed or the entire heart rather than only the epicardial vessels. Arterial methods for measuring relative and absolute blood flow have used indicator dilution theory, mean transit time analysis or videodensitometry. These methods, described below in further detail, are complicated by factors which include the frequent requirement for subselective contrast injection, the presence of misregistration artifacts, sensitivity to changes in vessel diameter, and a requirement for high framing rates. The methods based on myocardial region analysis have been based on indicator dilution theory, parametric imaging, and videodensitometric

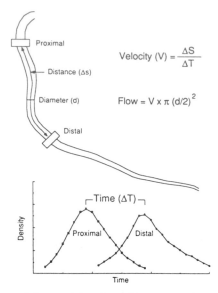

Figure 2. Schematic diagram of the arterial regions of interest used to calculate absolute coronary blood flow with the transit time method. (From Nissen SE, et al. Methods for the calculation of coronary flow reserve by computer processing of digital angiograms. In: Heintzen PH, Bürsch JH (Eds.), Progress in Digital Angiocardiography, 1988, p. 237.)

techniques. The specific methods, along with their relative advantages will be discussed in further detail below.

Arterial methods for measurement of coronary blood flow

Transit time analysis

The earliest efforts to measure coronary blood flow from angiographic data sets applied transit time theory to cineangiographic images acquired following the injection of contrast material into the coronary arteries. Among these were efforts by Rutishauser [13] and Smith [14] which reported the use of a densitometric method to measure absolute coronary blood flow. As shown in Figure 2, the mean transit time Δt between two fixed regions of interest along the coronary artery was calculated and combined with a distance measurement Δl between the two points and the vessel area A to determine volume flow Q as a function of time:

$$Q = \frac{\Delta l}{\Delta t} \cdot A. \tag{1}$$

While these were referred to as densitometric methods, there was not an explicit calculation of the relationship between the signal due to contrast and the vessel geometry. The use of densitometric analysis is discussed further below. The transit-time approach was modified by Spiller [15] to use the leading edge of the contrast intensity curve rather than the mean arrival time of the density curves at a fixed location. The motivation for the use of the wavefront lies partly in the assumption that this reduced the errors due to the alterations in flow resulting from the contrast material itself. Using this approach they were able to measure phasic blood flow in coronary artery bypass grafts and coronary arteries from cineangiograms using the time interval between two arterial sampling points along with vessel geometry as described above. While these methods have demonstrated promise for the calculation of absolute coronary blood flow their acceptance has been restricted due to technical and theoretical difficulties. Due to the complex motion of the coronary arteries, it is difficult to reproduce regions of interest on the arteries, unlike the situation with the straighter, stationary femoral or carotid arteries where such methods have met with greater success. A need for accurate measurements of distance and vessel geometry is also complicated by the motion of the arteries. It is likewise necessary that the artery be perpendicular to the X-ray beam along its axis for the measurements to be accurate. Due to these technical factors measurements are restricted to larger proximal sections of the coronary arteries, reducing their applicability. In addition, the assumptions of circular geometry used to calculate artery dimensions are often not valid in many clinical situations.

Indicator dilution analysis

A different approach for the measurement of relative changes in coronary blood flow which did not require accurate measurements of vessel geometry was pursued by Foerster [16] using a video dilution technique. Changes in coronary blood flow from baseline to maximal conditions were measured from videotapes acquired during sequential injections of contrast into the coronary arteries. The integral of the contrast density in a fixed arterial region of interest was calculated for the two flow conditions and the ratio of flows was calculated as:

$$\frac{Q_2}{Q_1} = \frac{A_1}{A_2} \cdot \frac{M_2}{M_1} \tag{2}$$

where A_1 and A_2 are the values of the integrated contrast density and M_1 and M_2 are the amounts of contrast material injected for the two flow conditions. The use of selective injections avoided the background variations in contrast signal present following injections into the aortic root or left ventricle which was proposed by Lantz [17] and later modified by Kruger [18] as part of a method which calculated coronary blood flow as a fraction of the cardiac output. The video dilution technique was validated in phantom and canine experiments and was used to measure reactive hyperemia during clinical angiography, the first method to attempt to measure coronary flow reserve from angiographic data. This approach has been extended in order to utilize digital angiographic techniques by Nissen [19] in an effort to measure coronary flow reserve as part of the clinical procedure. Following subselective injection of a known quantity of contrast material into the coronary artery, contrast intensity curves were integrated and corrected for background signal. Measurement of the curve areas for the two flow states were then combined to produce a ratio of flows. As in the earlier approaches using video images, good correlation was found in animal studies and the feasibility of clinical implementation was demonstrated. As an example of the potential of the method, coronary flow reserve was encoded in different colors to form a parametric image of flow reserve values [20].

There are several drawbacks to the indicator dilution approach to the measurement of CFR, both technical and theoretical. As is the case with all such techniques, the amount of contrast material, expressed as M in Equation (2), must be known or at least the ratio of masses must be known. This is difficult to achieve in general and the injection procedures often lead to reflux of contrast material or problems with streaming and non-uniform mixing. The method is also limited by the fact that, at best, only measurements in proximal locations can meet the assumptions of known contrast masses and measurements for branches are not possible. Like the transit-time approach the motion of the coronary arteries can further complicate the analysis of the indicator dilution curves. Foreshortening of the arteries is also a problem.

Videodensitometry

Numerous efforts have attempted to take advantage of the theoretical relationship between the thickness of contrast material present in the path of an incident X-ray beam and the detected intensity signal. As described by the Beer-Lambert Law, the transmitted intensity of X-rays is an exponential function of the thickness of absorbing material. In other words, the logarithm of the detected intensity I_t is linearly proportional to the thickness of material

$$\log I_t = -\mu x + \text{constant} \qquad (3)$$

where μ is the attenuation coefficient. Theoretically, an integration of the contrast intensity in a logarithmically transformed image results in a measurement of vessel volume which is independent of geometrical assumptions. The application of this method to cineangiograms, referred to as cinedensitometry, and to television based imaging systems – videodensitometry – includes several efforts at measuring absolute blood flow. The majority of efforts which have applied densitometric techniques to coronary arteriography have focused on the measurement of vessel geometry but, with the recent development of digital angiographic methods, several investigators have attempted to incorporate the temporal variations along with the geometrical measurements. Parker [21] has combined 3D reconstruction of the coronary artery tree from multiple view digital coronary angiograms with videodensitometry to calculate blood flow. While density information could be used to calculate volume directly, in first reports the density curves are used only to generate mean transit times rather than absolute volume. In a similar approach, Swanson [22] has used a videodensitometric method to calculate absolute flow in coronary artery bypass grafts from digital subtraction angiograms by tracking the movement of contrast down the vessel to calculate transit times. The further application of "true" densitometric techniques is complicated by factors described above for other transit time methods, including vessel motion and foreshortening. In addition, the presence of radiation scatter, image intensifier veiling glare and X-ray beam hardening introduces errors [23] making Equation (3) invalid. The routine implementation of videodensitometric techniques requires the use of correction methods [24] as well as the precautions required in the arterial transit time methods.

Myocardial methods for measurement of coronary blood flow

Indicator dilution methods

The indicator dilution principle described above in the description of arterial methods for angiographic determination of coronary blood flow has also been applied to methods which utilize myocardial regions to make flow measurements. A number of variations on the indicator dilution principle have been investigated, most often for the extraction of transit time parameters and relative rather than absolute coronary blood flow measurements. In general, these methods make use of the contrast pass curve measured in a myocardial region-of-interest from angiographic images (Figure 3). The particular type of image data used has included digitized cinefilm, digitized videotape and both subtracted and unsubtracted digital angiograms. The methods also differ with regard to whether a hypothetical model is fit to the measured data or whether the actual data itself is used to calculate one of a variety of temporal parameters, e.g. washout time, time to peak contrast, or mean transit time. In one class of experiments, the falloff of the myocardial contrast pass curve is modeled as a monoexponential and a characteristic falloff time is measured to determine the flow/unit volume for a given flow state. Whiting [25] investigated such a model in dog studies where sequences of digital angiograms were acquired following selective injection of contrast material. Myocardial contrast intensity curves were calculated following temporal filtering and correction for scatter and veiling glare, from which an exponential decay constant k was determined. This in turn was interpreted as the flow per unit volume of contrast material distribu-

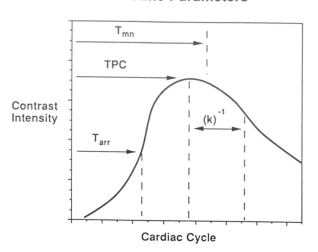

**Indicator Dilution Theory
Time Parameters**

Figure 3. Schematic diagram of the contrast pass curve measured in the myocardium and the various time parameters calculated in indicator dilution methods. The different parameters, described further in the text: the time-to-peak contrast (TPC); the arrival time T_{arr}; the mean transit time T_{mn}; the washout decay constant k.

tion. From the same data set, a second index of myocardial perfusion was determined by using the leading edge of the contrast intensity curve to calculate the time to peak contrast (TPC). A comparison of the relationships between 1/TPC, 1/k, and actual measured flow demonstrated that both showed a modest correlation with actual flow.

The concept of washout decay time as an estimate of myocardial blood flow was also investigated by Ikeda [26], who calculated the contrast disappearance half-life from time-density curves measured in digital subtraction coronary angiograms. Following the drawing of an epicardial outline of the left ventricle, the myocardium was divided into 8 45°C sectors and sectorial time-density curves were used to extract the appearance time T_{peak} and the disappearance half-life $T_{1/2}$. Comparison of values for the $T_{1/2}$ parameter between a group of patients with coronary artery disease and a group of normals showed a significant increase in $T_{1/2}$ in the presence of disease.

Nissen [19] evaluated several myocardial approaches along with arterial methods using myocardial density curves. Time to peak contrast (TPC) as well as decay rate were calculated and compared to EMF measurements of coronary flow reserve. They found moderate correlation between flow ratios calculated from TPC and EMF values ($r = .68$, slope $= .16$) and worse results for washout decay rate ($r = .34$).

Eigler [27] extended the methods reported by Whiting by applying a mathematical approach, utilizing general theories of linear systems analysis to calculate the general transfer function for contrast material in the heart. By modelling the coronary circulation as a two compartment system, a mathematical model was derived for the way that a bolus of contrast injected into the coronary artery is transformed as it progresses through the heart. This model could then be applied to a sampled input function for an actual injection to predict the shape as it entered the myocardium and from the predicted function, temporal parameters could be calculated. For example, time to peak contrast (TPC), washout rate k, and mean transit time T_{sys} were calculated from the predicted transfer function and compared to actual flow/volume in phantom and animal studies. The inverse of the system mean transit time $(T_{sys})^{-1}$ showed much better correlation with actual flow per volume than the other temporal parameters. The advantages of this approach were that it was relatively insensitive to injection parameters and specific hyperemic stimulus. The results indicated that alterations in T_{sys}^{-1} measured during resting flow could be used to characterize stenotic vessels from normals.

The impulse response method of Eigler described above demonstrated promise for the detection of compensatory vasodilation of the microcirculation in the presence of a stenosis even in the absence of a hyperemic state. In contrast, an alternative method reported by Pijls [28] uses an indicator dilution measurement of mean transit time during maximum flow conditions to assess myocardial perfusion. In validation studies performed in dogs, digital subtraction angiograms were acquired during maximal flow following selective contrast injection. Contrast intensity curves were measured in myocardial regions-of-interest over periods of 20–25 cardiac cycles and corrected for background intensity. A number of temporal parameters were calculated such as appearance time T_{app}, and time to peak T_{max} along with T_{mn}, the mean transit time calculated from a fit of the intensity curve to a gamma variate. Their results indicated that $(T_{mn})^{-1}$ correlated better with absolute coronary flow under conditions of fixed perfusion volume. While this method is not suitable for calculations of coronary flow reserve it may provide a measurement of maximal flow before and after PTCA [29] or bypass surgery.

A major difficulty in all of the above myocardial indicator dilution methods is a need for good quality contrast intensity curves lasting as long as 15–25 seconds. This in turn makes the methods susceptible to misregistration artifacts (in the case of subtraction images) and, most often, a significant contribution from overlying structures as the contrast recirculates following the first venous phase. The presence of this significant background signal makes it difficult to obtain an ideal representation for the curve such as a gamma variate and an adequate background correction is often not possible. Methods that only measure temporal parameters without providing an estimate of perfusion volume will not result in a measurement related to blood flow since the volume of the microcirculation is variable as a function of flow.

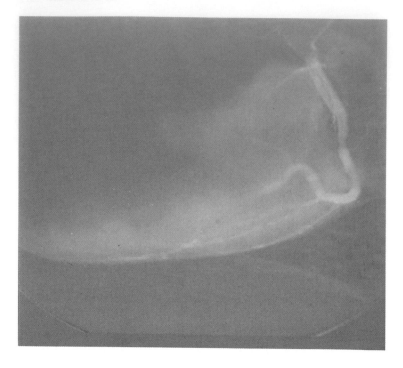

Figure 4a.

Parametric imaging

The development of digital radiography has led to the introduction of power-ful image processing methods which produce images of physiological pa-rameters in addition to anatomical features. Among the first to utilize digital radiographic methods were Bürsch and Heintzen and colleagues who investi-gated the use of such *parametric imaging* methods in non-cardiology as well as cardiology applications [30]. One example of the types of images that can be produced is a transit time *image*, i.e. a two-dimensional representation of the time required for contrast material to reach different areas of the heart. Such temporal images were used to assess coronary blood flow under varying physiological conditions. Another form of processing, for example, produces images of maximum contrast intensity acquired during a sequence of images and reflects the vascular volume filled by the contrast material. One class of these parametric imaging methods has been employed to mea-sure coronary flow reserve from digital subtraction coronary angiograms. Among the first efforts was the work by Vogel and associates [31] who used a modified transit time method to produce an image of the time of arrival of contrast material to regions of the heart under baseline and during hypere-mia. This appearance time approach was found to underestimate coronary

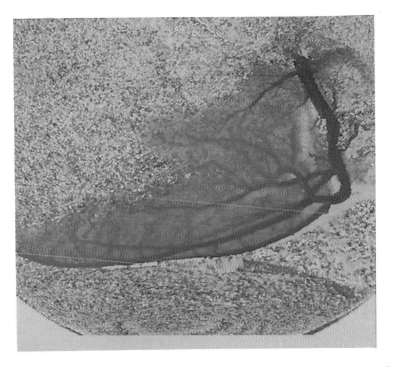

Figure 4. Examples of parametric images used to calculate the coronary flow reserve from a sequence of end-diastolic DSA images acquired in a dog: (a) an image of maximum contrast intensity; (b) an image of arrival time.

flow reserve due to the fact it did not reflect changes in the regional vascular volume filled by the contrast material. Incorporation of density information by Hodgson [32] to measure changes in volume resulted in improved correlation with actual values for CFR. While the general approach is similar to the indicator dilution methods described above, the parametric imaging method differs in several significant ways. By using the leading edge of the contrast pass curve, the method avoids the later portions of the curve which take place during changes in blood flow and are subject to significant background contributions to the contrast signal. This latter factor is a particular problem for those indicator dilution methods which assume a specific theoretical shape for the contrast pass curve. While one criticism of the parametric imaging method is the fact that it is not based on traditional indicator dilution theory, its empirical foundation has resulted in a method which shows good results when properly implemented. The technical aspects of the parametric imaging approach were investigated by Cusma [33] where the Vogel approach was modified in several ways. Temporal resolution was improved through the use of a linear interpolation algorithm for the determination of contrast arrival time and parametric images of "flow" acquired for baseline and hyperemia were combined to produce a composite ratio image which resulted in a pixel by pixel representation of relative flow. Examples of the parametric images are shown in Figure 4.

As with all angiographic methods for determining coronary and myocardial blood flow, the parametric imaging method suffers from the fact that the two dimensional measurement cannot differentiate between flow contributions arising from tissues at different positions orthogonal to the image plane. Several studies have investigated whether flow measurements derived from angiographic images agree with radioactive microsphere measurements of myocardial blood flow. A study by Nishimura [34] investigated the correlation of microsphere measurements in dogs with several videodensitometric parameters used to calculate flow reserve from digitized videotape. Two temporal parameters and peak density were calculated from a γ variate fit to the contrast intensity curves measured in myocardial regions of interest and compared to the microsphere measurements of myocardial blood flow. Ratio of peak density values correlated fairly well ($r = 0.81$) with microsphere flow ratios but neither time to one-half peak density nor washout time showed good correlation with microsphere results. The investigators did not attempt to combine parameters in a manner similar to that used in the parametric imaging method so that a direct comparison was not possible. Hess [35] attempted to validate the Vogel method with microsphere flow measurements in a series of dog studies. Using the algorithm described above to generate parametric images, coronary flow reserve was calculated using the image measurements and compared to electromagnetic flow (EMF) probe measurements and microsphere measurements of myocardial blood flow. Results indicated only moderate correlation between parametric imaging and microspheres ($r = 0.54$) and a slightly better correlation between parametric imaging and EMF ($r = 0.68$). They also reported a relatively high standard error for the parametric imaging (1.0–1.7 CFR units). The inaccuracy and imprecision were attributed to several factors including the fact that a two-dimensional image cannot differentiate overlapping perfusion areas and because the procedure used to define three-dimensional locations relative to their image location is difficult to implement. In addition, this particular parametric imaging method is limited by the low temporal resolution inherent in the calculation of contrast appearance time, leading to potentially large errors at high flow values. The method introduced by Cusma which attempts to improve upon the temporal resolution through the use of an interpolation technique has also been validated versus microsphere measurements in a canine model [36]. In order to carefully identify tissue samples with image regions of interest, the heart was fixed at physiologic pressure at the conclusion of the imaging study and the coronary arteries were injected with a radio-opaque mixture to delineate the epicardial vessels along with the intramyocardial vessels. The heart was sectioned into 8 slices, and X-ray films were acquired of each slice and were then used to identify myocardial regions supplied by corresponding opacified vessels. Regions of interest in

MICROSPHERE VALIDATION OF
PARAMETRIC IMAGING

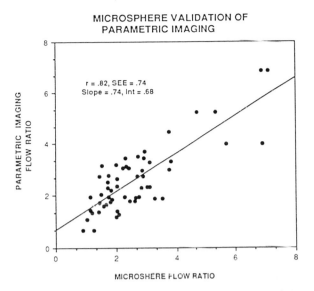

Figure 5. Results of microsphere validation study in dogs of the parametric imaging method for determining myocardial flow reserve. A plot of the parametric image-derived flow ratios is plotted against the microsphere flow ratios along with the results of a linear regression analysis.

the two-dimensional flow parameter images were correlated with the corresponding tissue samples with the aid of the radiograph of the sectioned heart. Figure 5 shows a plot of the parametric image measurements of CFR plotted along with the tissue sample microsphere flow measurements. A fairly good correlation was found with $r = 0.82$, accuracy $= -0.02$, precision $= 0.82$ CFR units. It should be noted that the variation between the image-derived values and microsphere results is due in part to the difficulty involved in identifying corresponding tissue samples with image ROI's along with any inaccuracies due to the theoretical model.

In summary, the parametric imaging approach has shown promise but the method requires careful attention paid to image acquisition protocols in order to assure good results.

Videodensitometry

The videodensitometric principle described above in the description of arterial methods has also been extended to angiographic methods using contrast intensity information in the myocardial regions of the heart. Marinus [37] has reported the development of a method for the measurement of absolute coronary artery blood flow using digital subtraction angiography. The method actually integrates density values over the entire heart following a selective

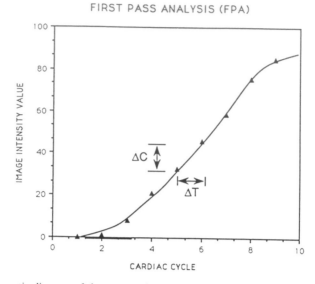

Figure 6. Schematic diagram of the myocardial contrast pass curve and the parameters used in the First Pass Analysis (FPA) algorithm for calculation of absolute coronary blood flow.

injection into the coronary artery to calculate the cyclic blood flow. In this approach the change in integrated density is converted to an incremental change in iodine volume through a videodensitometric calibration from a proximal segment of the coronary artery. Assumptions of the model lead to the requirement that the measurement period is limited to several cardiac cycles but preliminary phantom and animal studies showed good agreement between the angiographic determination and actual flow values. One potential problem with their investigation was the fact that no correction method for radiation scatter and veiling glare was used, leading to potential errors in the calibration of the relationship between iodine-filled blood volume and contrast signal in digital subtraction images. In a similar approach Hangiandreou [38] has developed a first pass distribution analysis (FPA) approach to measure coronary blood flow from digital subtraction image sequences. This method also requires the integration of intensity values over the entire heart and, therefore, requires the application of a scatter and glare correction technique along with a measurement of the iodine attenuation coefficient under the specific acquisition conditions. As shown in Figure 6, the FPA method requires a measurement of the incremental change in contrast ΔC and the time interval ΔT. Following the application of a videodensitometric correction method, the incremental volume ΔV and the absolute flow Q are calculated. Results from phantom studies showed good agreement between image flow measurements and known values over a range of 30–280 ml/min with $r = 0.99$, slope = 1.05 and SEE = 19.2 ml/min. Shown in Figure 7 is a

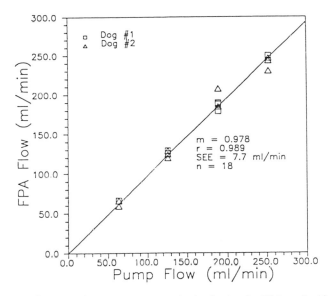

Figure 7. Results of absolute flow measurements obtained using the FPA method in dogs plotted against the known flow values (from Ref. 38).

plot of FPA results from studies in dogs using EMF probes for validation, showing fairly good agreement as well with $r = 0.94$, slope $= 0.98$ and SEE $=$ 12.7 ml/min over a range from 60–260 ml/min. The results of these studies indicated that a limiting factor in accuracy of the FPA flow measurement may actually be residual camera lag, resulting in an error in the detected intensity signal. The results of the experiment also validated the first pass assumptions used in the development of the model. These two recent approaches again demonstrate the potential for videodensitometric determination of absolute coronary blood flow under appropriate conditions and with adequate correction techniques. Whether these conditions can be met in typical clinical situations remains to be determined.

Conclusions

The clinical desire and need for measurements that more accurately reflect the extent and severity of coronary artery disease, combined with the development of new imaging methods and image analysis, methods, has resulted in an array of approaches for measuring coronary blood flow from angiographic images. The various methods include the application of traditional principles to cineangiographic and digital angiographic images, along with the development of new approaches made possible by the advent of new imaging technologies. Despite the fact that all the methods have shown promising results in their initial validations, no single method has met with sufficiently widespread acceptance and therefore no one approach has entered the routine diagnostic repertoire. Among the principle reasons is the fact that all of these methods demand a procedure significantly more complex than required for the acquisition of anatomical images, a level of complexity often difficult to achieve in the clinical environment. With the application of proper technique and attention to potential sources of errors, a thorough clinical evaluation may lead to a more complete understanding of the relative advantages and limitations of the different approaches. As a result, one or more methods may indeed provide the long desired direct measurement of the physiological significance of a coronary artery stenosis in patients.

References

1. Detre KM, Wright E, Murphy ML, Takaro T. Observer agreement in evaluating coronary angiograms. Circulation 1975; **52**: 979–86.
2. Zir LM, Miller SW, Dinsmore RE, Gilbert JP, Harthorne JW. Interobserver variability in coronary angiography. Circulation 1976; **53**: 627–32.
3. Galbraith JE, Murphy ML, de Soyza N. Coronary angiogram interpretation. Interobserver variability. JAMA 1978; **240**: 2053–6.
4. Grondin CM, Dyrda I, Pasternac A, Campeau L, Bourassa MG, Lesperance J. Discrepancies between cineangiographic and postmortem findings in patients with coronary artery disease and recent myocardial revascularization. Circulation 1974; **49**: 703–8.
5. White CW, Wright CB, Doty DB, et al. Does visual interpretation of the coronary arteriogram predict the physiologic importance of a coronary stenosis? N Engl J Med 1984; **310**: 819–24.
6. Harrison DG, White CW, Hiratza LF, et al. The value of lesion cross-sectional area determined by quantitative coronary angiography in assessing the physiologic significance of proximal left anterior descending coronary arterial stenoses. Circulation 1984; **69**: 1111–9.
7. Gould KL, Lipscomb K. Effects of coronary stenoses on coronary flow reserve and resistance. Am J Cardiol 1974; **34**: 48–55.
8. Klocke FJ. Measurements of coronary flow reserve: defining pathophysiology versus making decisions about patient care. Circulation 1987; **76**: 1183–9.
9. Gould KL, Kirkeeide RL, Buchi M. Coronary flow reserve as a physiologic measure of stenosis severity. J Am Coll Cardiol 1990; **15**: 459–74.
10. Wilson RF, Laughlin DE, Ackel PH, et al. Transluminal subselective measurement of coronary artery blood flow velocity and vasodilator reserve in man. Circulation 1985; **72**: 82–92.
11. Martin LW, Johnson RA, Scott H, et al. Impedance measurement of absolute blood flow using an angioplasty catheter: a validation study. Am Heart J 1991; **121**: 745–52.
12. White CW, Wilson RF, Marcus ML. Methods of measuring myocardial blood flow in humans. Prog Cardiovasc Dis 1988; **31**: 79–94.
13. Rutishauser W, Bassmann WD, Noseda G, Meier W, Wellauer J. Blood flow measurment through single coronary arteries by roentgen densitometry. I. A comparison of flow measured by a radiologic technique applicable in the intact organism and by electromagnetic flowmeter. Am J Roentgenol Radium Ther Nucl Med 1970; **109**: 12–20.
14. Smith HC, Sturm RE, Wood EH. Videodensitometric system for measurement of vessel blood flow, particularly in the coronary arteries, in man. Am J Cardiol 1973; **32**: 144–50.

15. Spiller P, Schmiel FK, Politz B, et al. Measurement of systolic and diastolic flow rates in the coronary artery system by X-ray densitometry. Circulation 1983; **68**: 337–47.
16. Foerster JM, Link DP, Lantz BM, Lee G, Holcroft JW, Mason DT. Measurement of reactive hyperemia during clinical angiography by video dilution technique. Acta Radiol [Diagn] (Stockh) 1981; **22**: 209–16.
17. Lantz BMT. Relative flow measured by roentgen videodensitometry. In: Heintzen PH, Bürsch JH (Eds.), Roentgen-video-techniques for dynamic studies of structure and function of the heart and circulation: 2nd international workshop conference, April 1976. Stuttgart: Georg Thieme Verlag 1978: 69.
18. Kruger RA, Anderson RE, Koehler PR, Nelson JA, Sorenson JA, Morgan T. A method for the noninvasive evaluation of cardiovascular dynamics using a digital radiographic device. Radiology 1981; **139**: 301–5.
19. Nissen SE, Elion JL, Booth DC, Evans J, DeMaria AN. Value and limitations of computer analysis of digital subtraction angiography in the assessment of coronary flow reserve. Circulation 1986; **73**: 562–71.
20. Elion JL, Nissen SE, DeMaria AN. Functional imaging of coronary artery flow reserve. Am J Card Imaging 1987; **1**: 103–7.
21. Parker DL, Pope DL, van Bree RE, Marshall H. Blood flow measurements in digital cardiac angiography using 3D coronary artery reconstructions. In: Heintzen PH, Bürsch JH (Eds.), Progress in digital angiocardiography. Dordrecht: Kluwer Academic Publishers 1988: 215–21.
22. Swanson DK, Myerowitz PD, Hegge JO, Watson KM. Arterial blood-flow waveform measurement in intact animals: new digital radiographic technique. Radiology 1986; **161**: 323 8.
23. Nalcioglu O, Roeck W, Seibert JA, Lando AV, Tobis JM, Henry WL. Quantitative aspects of image – intensifier based digital x-ray imaging. In: Kereiakes JG, Thomas SR, Orton CG (Eds.), Digital Radiology: selected topics. New York: Plenum Press 1986.
24. Naimuddin S, Hasegawa B, Mistretta CA. Scatter-glare correction using a convolution algorithm with variable weighting. Med Phys 1987; **14**: 330–4.
25. Whiting JS, Drury JK, Pfaff JM, et al. Digital angiographic measurement of radiographic contrast material kinetics for estimation of myocardial perfusion. Circulation 1986; **73**: 789–98.
26. Ikeda H, Koga Y, Utsu F, Toshima H. Quantitative evaluation of regional myocardial blood flow by videodensitometric analysis of digital subtraction coronary arteriography in humans. J Am Coll Cardiol 1986; **8**: 809–16.
27. Eigler NL, Pfaff JM, Zeiher A, Whiting JS, Forrester JS. Digital angiographic impulse response analysis of regional myocardial perfusion: linearity, reproducibility, accuracy and comparison with conventional indicator dilution curve parameters in phantom and canine models. Circ Res 1989; **64**: 853–66.
28. Pijls NH, Uijen GJ, Hoevelaken A, et al. Mean transit time for the assessment of myocardial perfusion by videodensitometry. Circulation 1990; 81: 1331–40. Comment in: Circulation 1990; **81**: 1431–5.
29. Pijls NH, Aengevaeren WR, Uijen GJ, et al. Concept of maximal flow ratio for immediate evaluation of percutaneous transluminal coronary angioplasty result by videodensitometry. Circulation 1991; **83**: 854–65.
30. Bürsch JH, Heintzen PH. Parametric imaging. Radiol Clin North Am 1985; **23**: 321–33.
31. Vogel R, LeFree M, Bates E, et al. Application of digital techniques to selective coronary arteriography: use of myocardial contrast appearance time to measure coronary flow reserve. Am Heart J 1984; **107**: 153–64.
32. Hodgson J McB, LeGrand V, Bates ER, et al. Validation in dogs of a rapid digital angiographic technique to measure relative coronary blood flow during routine cardiac catheterization. Am J Cardiol 1985; **55**: 188–93.
33. Cusma JT, Toggart EJ, Folts JD et al. Digital subtraction angiographic imaging of coronary flow reserve. Circulation 1987; **75**: 461–72.

34. Nishimura RA, Rogers PJ, Holmes DR Jr., Gehring DG, Bove AA. Assessment of myocardial perfusion by videodensitometry in the canine model. J Am Coll Cardiol 1987; **9**: 891–7.
34. Hess OM, McGillem MJ, DeBoe SF, Pinto IM, Gallagher KP, Mancini GB. Determination of coronary flow reserve by parametric imaging. Circulation 1990; 82: 1438–48. Comment in: Circulation 1990; **82**: 1533–5.
36. Cusma JT, Morris KG, Chu A, Spero LA, Bashore TM. An image processing algorithm for the determination of changes in coronary blood flow from digital coronary angiograms. Comp Cardiol 1990: 125–8.
37. Marinus H, Buis B, van Benthem A. Pulsatile coronary flow determination by digital angiography. Int J Card Imaging 1990; **5**: 173–82.
38. Hangiandreou NJ. Coronary blood flow measurement using digital subtraction angiography and first pass distribution analysis [dissertation]. Wisconsin: University of Wisconsin 1990.

PART FIVE

QCA in regression/progression of atherosclerotic disease

14. Value and limitations of quantitative coronary angiography to assess progression or regression of coronary atherosclerosis

PIM J. DE FEYTER, JEROEN VOS, JOHAN H.C. REIBER and PATRICK W. SERRUYS

Summary

Coronary angiography has its inherent limitations to assess extent and severity of coronary atherosclerosis. Angiography is a two-dimensional shadowgram of an opacified vessel. It demonstrates only the lumen of the artery and disease of the arterial wall can only be inferred when the disease encroaches upon the lumen. Early stages of coronary artery disease, which do not affect the arterial lumen, because of remodeling of the coronary artery wall (early compensatory enlargement and medial thinning) are not appreciated by coronary angiography. Diffuseness of atherosclerosis tends to underestimate the angiographic assessment of the severity of the disease.

However, serial coronary angiography is currently the most powerful tool to assess progression or regression of coronary artery disease induced by different treatments. Visual interpretation of coronary angiograms has its acknowledged limitations because assessment of stenosis severity is associated with: a) a large intra- and interobserver variability (8–37%); b) only relative stenosis measurements are provided; and c) severity of diffuse atherosclerosis is difficult to estimate by eye.

Until now trials studying the effects of intervention on progression of coronary atherosclerosis have focussed only on lesion changes, and have not accounted for diffuse atherosclerosis; thus many changes in the coronary artery tree will proceed unnoticed. Quantitative coronary angiography allows assessment of focal and diffuse atherosclerosis and provides us with: a) relative measurements (diameter stenosis, area stenosis); b) absolute measurements, both from the lesion and segments of the coronary tree: mean width of segment (mm), minimal luminal diameter of the stenosis (mm). Relative measurements, although widely used for clinical purposes, may misinterpret progression or regression and are unable to measure "diffuse atherosclerosis". The mean width of a segment of a vessel is the only variable able to assess changes of progression of diffuse atherosclerosis as well as changes of focal atherosclerosis. It offers the opportunity to account for all changes in the coronary tree to provide a global coronary atherosclerosis

J.H.C. Reiber and P.W. Serruys (eds). Advances in Quantitative Coronary Arteriography, 255–271.
© *1993 Kluwer Academic Publishers. Printed in the Netherlands.*

score per patient. Absolute stenosis measurements appear to be the best markers of progression or regression of lesions.

Conclusion: Different measurements obtained with quantitative coronary angiography should be performed to provide the reader with sufficient data to gain insight into the benefit of an intervention. Both local and diffuse atherosclerotic changes should be taken into account. The most important measurement is the mean width of a segment of a vessel (mm). In addition, other absolute, and relative measurements also should be presented to allow for further clinical and pathophysiologic insights.

Introduction

To angiographically assess progression or regression of coronary artery disease after intervention with cholesterol lowering drugs, Ca-antagonists, intensive diet or life style changes, various approaches with different degrees of sophistication have been used employing: a) cardiologists viewing the angiograms alone [1–3], or as panel members [4–7]; b) cardiologists or trained technicians tracing vessel edges by hand for later computer analysis [8, 9]; and c) more recently quantitative angiography using computerized edge-finding techniques [10–13]. All these studies have emphasized focal atherosclerosis i.e. on progression or regression of pre-existing lesions or the development of new lesions. The observed changes have been expressed in terms of percent diameter stenosis or absolute measurement of the minimal luminal diameter of a stenosis. However, progression, and possibly regression, of coronary atherosclerosis is a complex process that involves the entire arterial wall. This is angiographically reflected not only in focal but also in diffuse encroachment upon the arterial lumen of the opacified vessel. Progression or regression should result in an decrease or increase of the volume of the lumen of the entire epicardial coronary artery tree. Therefore, ideally changes in the total volume of the coronary artery lumen and ensuing physiological consequences on coronary blood flow and myocardial perfusion should be assessed. However, due to the complex coronary anatomy, the varying course of the coronary arteries in a three-dimensional plane and the cyclic changing caliber of the coronary arteries, complicated by the beating heart, it is impossible to measure accurately the volume of the coronary artery tree in man with current angiographic techniques. Therefore, other approaches have to be employed to assess changes of coronary atherosclerosis, which take into account both focal and diffuse progression or regression of disease to provide better insights into the dynamics of coronary artery disease.

Quantitative coronary angiography has emerged as a useful technique and its value as both a clinical and a research tool has now been firmly established [14]. In this report we describe a new approach to assess both focal and diffuse atherosclerosis by using a quantitative method of angiographic analysis.

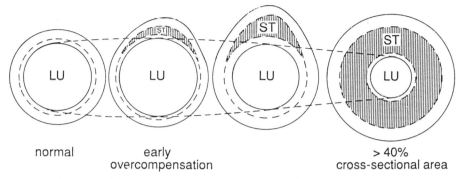

normal   early   > 40%
overcompensation   cross-sectional area

Figure 1. Diagrammatic representation of the sequence of luminal changes during the development of an early lesion to a severe atherosclerotic plaque. LU − lumen vessel, ST = stenosis, = internal elastic lamina. (adopted from Glagov et al.; N Engl J Med 1987; 316: 1371–75 and Stiel et al.; Circulation 1989; 80: 1603–09).

Limitations of angiography for the assessment of progression or regression of coronary artery disease

Coronary angiography is the production of a two-dimensional shadowgram of an opacified vessel. It demonstrates the effect of arterial wall disease on the contour of the arterial lumen and the underlying pathologic process can be identified only by inference. The use of coronary angiography to measure progression or regression of atherosclerosis is based on the assumption that a change in volume of the atherosclerotic plaque will have an effect on the size and shape of the contrast-filled lumen. However, atherosclerotic changes of the arterial wall are not reflected accurately enough by changes in the lumen. Many studies [15–25] have shown that coronary angiography frequently underestimates the severity of coronary artery lesions or even misses significant narrowings. The major reason appears to be the diffuseness of the atherosclerotic process. Diffuse atherosclerotic disease may narrow the entire lumen of a segment of a vessel smoothly so that angiography is unable to detect its existence. Only when the caliber of the arteries is unexpectedly small, diffuse coronary atherosclerosis can be inferred. Furthermore, underestimation and serious overestimation of coronary arterial stenosis at clinical arteriography also has been explained by the use of inadequate radiological views to visualize elliptical or D-shaped lumens [19, 26–28].

A complicating factor in evaluating coronary atherosclerosis is the occurrence of compensatory mechanisms that involve coronary artery remodeling.

Recently, it has been shown that compensatory enlargement of human atherosclerotic coronary arteries occurs during the early stages of plaque formation [29–32]. This compensatory enlargement results in preservation of a nearly normal lumen cross-sectional area so that an atherosclerotic plaque would have less hemodynamic effect (Figure 1). However, this implicates that angiography severely underestimates or is unable to detect early stages of coronary atherosclerosis. This problem is worsened by the finding that small plaques (early lesions) were associated with a larger than normal lumen area suggesting that in the very early phase of disease overcompensation of the artery may have occurred [30]. Angiographically this compensatory widening of the lumen would be misinterpreted as regression of atherosclerotic disease. Finally, it has been shown that in advanced atherosclerosis, beneath atheromatous plaques the media undergoes thinning, another form of compensation, so that the vascular lumen tends to be preserved [20, 33].

Furthermore, processes other than atherosclerotic changes such as arterial spasm, intimal dissection, thrombosis or embolism, which may cause abnormalities on the angiogram, cannot always be distinguished angiographically from atherosclerosis.

Limitations of assessing progression or regression from the changes in severity of local narrowing

Many trials studying the effects of an intervention on the progression or regression of coronary artery disease only have focussed on the changes of the severity of local encroachment of coronary artery disease on the opacified arterial lumen in terms of luminal diameter stenosis or minimal luminal diameter of the stenosis. This approach is based on our traditional clinical view that stenosis severity is directly associated with morbidity and mortality. However, progression or regression can not adequately be assessed only in terms of severity of stenosis because atherosclerosis of the coronary arteries occurs in a complex manner. Parts of the vessel wall may be entirely disease free, parts may be diffusely diseased, without apparent local encroachment of the arterial lumen, or the disease is limited to local areas of the vessel wall, with ensuing local encroachment on the lumen of the artery. Therefore, measurement only of stenosis severity to assess progression or regression has several limitations:

First: Obviously, measurement of only the stenosis does not take into account the process of diffuse atherosclerosis, so that progression or regression will go unnoticed if atherosclerosis is predominantly diffuse in nature (Figure 2). *Second*: Diffuseness of progression or regression may have unexpected effects on the measurement of the severity of a narrowing. Progression or regression may occur in a diffuse manner involving only the "normal" diameter used as reference to determine severity of stenosis. This may result in a calculated less severe lesion (Figure 2), suggesting regression, whereas actually progression has occurred, and therefore this should be regarded as pseudoregression. *Third*: The same volume of increase of a new local atheroma in different vessel sizes would result in substantial differences in the calculated percent diameter stenosis severity (Figure 3). *Fourth*: The same volume of progression or conversely regression of coronary artery disease, will, depending on the location and the three-dimensional orientation within

Mean width segm. (mm)	3.75	2.9
Min. lum. diam. (mm)	3.0	2.5
DS %	25	17

Figure 2. Progression of diffuse coronary atherosclerosis in a segment with pre-existing stenosis. Relative measurement (DS% = % diameter stenosis) suggests regression of severity of lesion, whereas, in reality absolute measurements mean width and minimal luminal diameter (mm) show progression of disease.

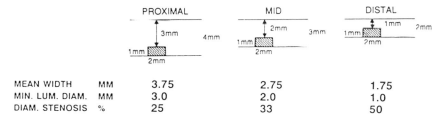

		PROXIMAL	MID	DISTAL
MEAN WIDTH	MM	3.75	2.75	1.75
MIN. LUM. DIAM.	MM	3.0	2.0	1.0
DIAM. STENOSIS	%	25	33	50

Figure 3. Impact of equal volume of atheroma on absolute and relative measurements in different vessel sizes.

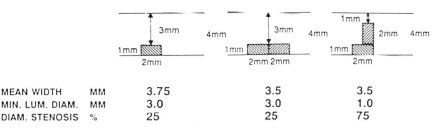

MEAN WIDTH	MM	3.75	3.5	3.5
MIN. LUM. DIAM.	MM	3.0	3.0	1.0
DIAM. STENOSIS	%	25	25	75

Figure 4. Diagrammatic representation of progression of the same "volume" of atherosclerosis with a different distribution within the vessel lumen to demonstrate the significant differences in stenosis measurements.

the vessel, have profound differences in calculated percent diameter stenosis severity (Figure 4). *Fifth*: Percent diameter stenosis does not accurately reflect the functional significance of a coronary lesion because it fails to account for other geometric-anatomic lesion characteristics such as lesion length, absolute diameters of diseased and normal segments, and hemodynamic behavior for different magnitudes of coronary blood flow [15, 16, 34–

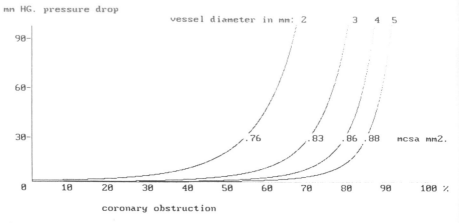

obstruction length= 5.0 mm coronary flow= 2.0 ml/s. blood viscosity=.030 g/cm s.

Figure 5a.

41]. For instance a 50% narrowing in a vessel with a diameter of 4 mm has a totally different haemodynamic impact than a 50% narrowing of a vessel with a 2 mm diameter (Figures 5a & b). *Sixth*: The relative diameter is usually determined by comparing the diameter at the site of maximal reduction with the diameter in adjacent areas that appear either normal or only minimally diseased. Therefore these measurements are highly dependent on the diameter of the reference area. In cases with focal obstructive disease and a proximal angiographic non-diseased area, the determination of a reference area is simple and straightforward. However, the nearby "normal" portion of the vessel lumen, the diameter of which forms the denominator of the percent stenosis estimate, may be dilated by the aging process [42–44] or by poststenotic turbulence [45, 46] or it may be narrowed by diffuse atherosclerotic narrowings [47–49] so that these segments show combinations of stenotic and ectatic areas and determination of a "normal" reference diameter poses important problems (Figure 6).

Simplified approach to assess progression or regression of coronary artery disease using quantitative coronary angiography

Conceptually angiographical assessment of progression or regression should be viewed as an increment or decrement of volume intruding on the arterial lumen of the entire coronary tree. Progression is defined as the occurrence of: a) increase of degree and extent of focal atherosclerosis; b) development of a new lesion; c) increase of degree and extent of diffuse atherosclerosis; and d) the combination of a, b and c. This implies that we should measure changes in the luminal volume of the opacified coronary artery tree. This is

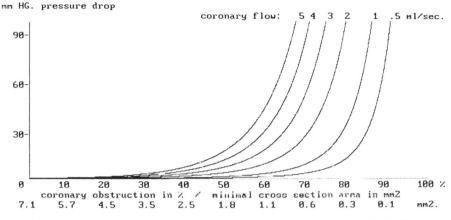

mm HG. pressure drop

coronary flow: 5 4 3 2 1 .5 ml/sec.

coronary obstruction in % / minimal cross section area in mm2

vessel diameter= 3.0 mm.   length stenosc= 5.0 mm.   blood viscosity=.030 g/cm s.

Figure 5b. An example of a computer-derived functional estimate, using quantitative angio-graphy to measure dimensions of percent narrowing, absolute diameter and lesion length. These were combined into a fluid dynamic equation to provide a single integrated measure of haemodynamic severity i.e. pressure gradient over the lesion. The following equation was used: $\triangle P = fQ + sQ^2$ (Kirkeeide et al. JACC 1986; 7: 102–13). MCSA mm^2: minimal cross-sectional area.

$$Where\ f = \frac{8\pi\mu L}{A_s^2}\ and\ s = \frac{\rho}{2} \times \left[\frac{1}{A_s} - \frac{1}{A_n}\right]^2$$

When $\triangle P$ is pressure loss across the stenosis, μ is absolute blood viscosity, L is stenosis length, A_n is the cross-sectional area of the normal artery, A_s is the cross-sectional area of the stenotic segment, Q is volume flow and ρ is blood density. From the available morphologic data of the obstruction, the Poiseuille and turbulent resistances at different flows ranging from 0.5 ml to 5 ml (simulating conditions at rest or maximal exercise) and thus the resulting transstenotic pressure gradients can be computed. A) Relation between pressure drop, varying degrees of severity of stenosis and varying vessel size (2, 3, 4 and 5 mm in diameter) with fixed coronary flow. B) Relation between pressure drop, varying coronary flow (0, 5, 1, 2, 3, 4, 5 ml/sec), and varying degrees of severity of stenosis in fixed vessel diameter.

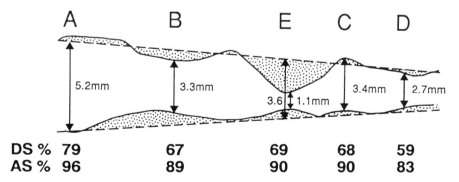

Figure 6. Influence of determination of reference area in a tapering vessel with diffuse athero-sclerosis on relative percent diameter and area stenosis (assuming circular cross sections).

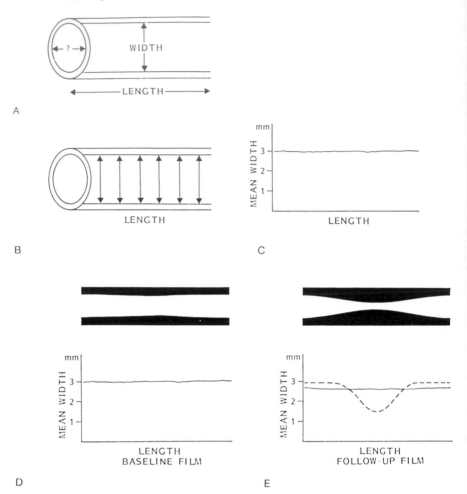

Figure 7. a) Measurement of width and length of a segment in a two-dimensional plane. The diameter of the segment perpendicular to that plane is unknown. b) Determination of diameter at different sample points. c) Construction of the diameter function along the length of the segment. The average of all diameters is the mean width. d) Determination of mean width in baseline film. e) Reflection of progression of disease on mean width (decrease) in follow-up film. For details: see text.

impossible with angiographic techniques and therefore, when using angiography, a simplified approach must be employed.

A segment of the coronary tree, not foreshortened in that projection, is taken and the length and diameter (in two-dimensional plane) is determined (Figure 7a). The diameter of the segment in the plane perpendicular to this two-dimensional plane is unknown. The diameter is determined at many sampling points along the entire segment from proximal to distal (Figure 7b) to derive a diameter function over that entire segment (Figure 7c). The mean width (mm) is the averaged value of all these diameters that were obtained at multiple sampling points.

The area under the diameter function represents a two-dimensional vessel area of the "lumen" of that segment, which can be approximated by the summation of the individual diameter values multiplied by the distance to the following sampling point, or in formula:

$$\text{vessel area} = \sum_{i=0}^{N} d_1 . \blacktriangle L_1, \tag{1}$$

where d_i are the individual diameter values and $\blacktriangle L_i$ the sampling distance for $i = 0$ from the proximal end to $i = n$ to the distal end. If all sampling distances $\blacktriangle L_i$ are constant and equal to $\blacktriangle L$, which is not always the case in practice, equation (1) simplifies to:

$$\text{vessel area} = \blacktriangle L . \sum_{i=0}^{N} d_i. \tag{2}$$

On the other hand, the mean diameter $\bar{D}$ of such vessel segment is defined by:

$$\bar{D} = \frac{\sum_{i=0}^{N} d_i}{\sum_{i=0}^{N} \blacktriangle L_i} \tag{3}$$

which again can be simplified to:

$$\bar{D} = \frac{\sum_{i=0}^{N} d_i}{N . \blacktriangle L} \tag{4}$$

if all sampling distances are equal to $\blacktriangle L$.

From equations (2) and (4) it becomes clear that vessel area = $\bar{D} . N . (\blacktriangle L)^2$.

If we make sure during the analysis of the baseline and post-intervention angiogram that the lengths of the corresponding segment in both frames are identical (within a practical limit of say 0.2–0.3 mm), then any change in vessel area will also be found in the mean diameter value, a parameter which is directly available on the CAAS systems (Figure 7d and 7e).

Therefore, the derived mean width (in mm) can be considered as a measure that does assess to a first approximation in a two-dimensional plane changes, either focal or diffuse, independent of shape and location in that plane. Progression of disease, focal or diffuse, in that segment will result in a change in the diameter at the diseased area and this will be reflected in a change in the mean width of the entire segment.

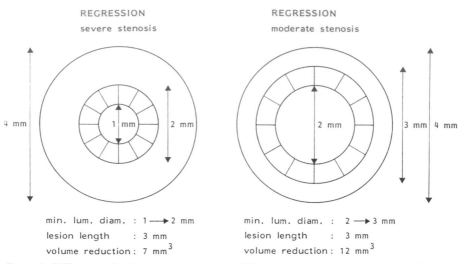

Figure 8. Difference of volume of regression of different degrees of severity of stenosis both resulting in 1 mm increase in luminal diameter.

Limitations of this simplified approach

Obviously, a two-dimensional assessment of an in principle three-dimensional process has its inherent limitations. Under and overestimation of progression or regression of coronary artery disease will likely occur, but can be limited to a certain extent by using orthogonal angiographic projections of the same coronary segment and subsequently averaging the measurements. Inability to measure changes of volume in a three-dimensional plane may potentially lead to erroneous conclusions. For instance, severe stenosis may show greater regression than milder ones, because removal of the same amount of cholesterol from a severe stenosis having a small circumference would cause more improvement and a larger increase in a minimum diameter than the same amount of cholesterol removed from a mild stenosis having a larger circumference (Figure 8). This cannot be assessed by measuring in a two-dimensional plane. Finally, as discussed under the preceding section the mean diameter approach suffers from the fact that all sampling distances need to be constant, both per frame and in the corresponding pre- and post-intervention frames. Although this will not be the case in practice, the resulting error will likely be acceptably small. A better approach would be to assess the actual vessel area by the summation of all pixels between the contours. This approach has been implemented in the new Cardiovascular Measurement System (CMS) [50].

Value of quantitative coronary angiography

Quantitative coronary angiography provides us with relative measurements of stenosis (percent diameter stenosis), with absolute measurements of stenosis (minimal luminal diameter in mm) and "functional" estimates of stenosis (pressure drop across stenosis), and in addition with absolute measurements of non-diseased or diffuse diseased segments (mean width of entire segment in mm). Therefore quantitative coronary angiography allows us to assess both diffuse and focal atherosclerosis in the coronary tree and therefore enables us to more accurately assess the complex processes of progression, and possibly regression, of coronary artery disease.

Absolute measurements to assess focal atherosclerosis
Recent reports have shown that absolute measurements such as mean coronary diameter, minimal luminal diameter or minimal cross-sectional area of narrowings, provide more information than percentage of stenosis with regard to hemodynamic significance of a stenosis and are better markers of progression or regression of coronary atherosclerosis [11, 12, 14–15, 34, 39, 40, 51]. The absolute value of the minimum lumen diameter is the greatest single determinant of the hemodynamic impact of a coronary narrowing, because the luminal stenosis diameter affects flow by a fourth power term [35–41, 52–54].

Absolute measurement to assess diffuse atherosclerosis
The mean width (mm) is an absolute measurement of a particular segment which is independent of a reference diameter. It is the only parameter that is able to measure progression or regression of diffuse atherosclerosis in angiographically "normal" appearing segments or of diffuse atherosclerosis in combination with focal atherosclerosis (Figure 2).

How to assess progression or regression of atherosclerosis

In line with our foregoing reasoning we believe that progression or regression of disease should be assessed first by measuring the change of volume of the lumen of the coronary artery tree, indirectly measured by for instance our simplified method: the mean width in mm of an entire segment. Second, the impact of a change of volume at the level of the lesions will be assessed by measuring the change of severity of pre-existing lesions or the severity of newly developed lesions.

In Table 1 we propose a set of measurements derived from quantitative coronary angiography which may be used to assess progression or regression of disease. The mean width of segment (mm) is the most important measurement, because it is able to assess progression or regression of diffuse atherosclerotic disease. It is also able to measure changes of focal atherosclerotic disease and it is the single measurement able to assess the combination of diffuse and focal atherosclerosis.

The absolute measurement, (minimal luminal diameter in mm) of lesions is extremely valuable to assess changes of focal atherosclerosis. Although relative measurements are subject to many drawbacks it may be useful to

Table 1. Significance of measurements used to assess progression or regression of coronary atherosclerosis

	Diffuse atherosclerosis	Focal atherosclerosis	Combination of diffuse and focal atherosclerosis
Coronary segment score			
1. Mean width per vessel segment (mm)	+ +	+	+ +
Coronary lesion score			
1. ABSOLUTE MEASUREMENTS: Minimal luminal diameter (mm)	±	+ +	+
2. Relative Stenosis Measurements: Diameter stenosis %	– – – –	+	±

present these to meet the traditional clinical practice of grading stenoses as percent stenosis.

It is common clinical practise to present the efficacy of an intervention on a per patient-oriented basis. However, in trials studying the effect of an intervention on progression or regression of coronary artery disease a patient-oriented progression assessment only can be ambivalent, since one lesion may worsen, while another may improve in the same patient.

From the clinical point of view it is important not only to be informed of the response of an individual patient, but also on the response of an individual lesion or segment. A trial should address the following questions. Which patient will respond favourably to an intervention and to what extent? Which lesion or segment will progress, regress or is immutable? Therefore, individual patients, lesions or segments (either with or without a lesion) should be classified as progressing, regressing or non-responding. This categorical approach requires definition of a clinical significant threshold level which may for instance be set at a level of a 10% change [8].

Since progression or regression is expected to occur in a continuous fashion and quantitative angiography enables discrimination of more subtle changes analysis should also be performed with a continuous approach.

To provide the reader with sufficient data to gain appropriate insights into the potential efficacy of an intervention we belief that data should be presented on a patient based assessment as well as on lesion/segment based assessment (Tables 1, 2). Patient-based analysis should include: a) a coronary tree score which measures all analyzable segments (including those with lesions) and serves as a total score to assess diffuse and focal atherosclerosis; b) a coronary lesion score to assess focal atherosclerosis; and c) a coronary segment score (segments without lesions) to assess changes in diffuse atherosclerosis.

Table 2. Assessment of progression or regression of coronary atherosclerosis

Patient based	
Coronary tree score	1) Mean width (mm) of all segments
Coronary lesion score	1) Minimal luminal diameter (mm)
	2) Diameter stenosis (%)
Coronary segment score	1) Mean width (mm)
Lesion based	
Coronary lesion score	1) Minimal luminal diameter (mm)
	2) Diameter stenosis (%)
Segment based	
Coronary segment score	1) Mean width (mm)

Future developments

"*Functional*" estimates of focal atherosclerosis
Transstenotic pressure losses can be estimated by applying Newtonian fluid dynamic equations to computer-estimated angiographic stenosis in man [37–39, 41, 53, 54]. The calculated transstenotic pressure gradient over a particular stenosis derived from quantitative coronary angiography describes the hemodynamic impact which that particular lesion would have under a range of different flow conditions, within the range of "normal" aortic pressures (Figure 5B). This calculation represents merely an approximation because the formula used is based on non-pulsatile flow in a rigid, and straight tube. It does not account for the effects of pulsatile flow or of curved and tapered vessels, more than 1 lesion in a vessel, the collateral circulation or perfusion of areas of non-viable myocardium; and it assumes a noncompliant stenosis. It would be erroneous to extrapolate from these equations an absolute hemodynamic impact on the global perfusion in an effort to evaluate the significance of a coronary artery lesion in a specific patient. But, it enables us to estimate the relative hemodynamic impact of a stenosis between patients and it enables us to estimate the hemodynamic impact of progression or regression of a particular lesion, assuming certain conditions.

Because of the relation between resistance and degree of stenosis, an important change in clinical status can result from a small increment in severity of an established stenosis. Conversely a small decrease in stenosis severity, could have important therapeutic benefit (Figure 5A, B).

Videodensitometry
Basically, two techniques are currently available for quantitative coronary angiography: edge-detection algorithms and densitometric computer-aided analysis.

Theoretically, densitometry seems the ultimate solution for the computation of the vessel's cross-sectional area from a single angiographic view

[55–62]. Perspex phantom studies have shown that densitometry is a very attractive, precise and accurate technique for the assessment of the severity of coronary obstructions from only a single view. However, the reality in routine clinical practice is different [53–58]. This is due to various error sources. Densitometry is much more sensitive than edge detection to densitometric non-linearities (X-ray scatter, veiling glare and beam hardening), orthogonality of vessel beam (foreshortening of the vessel), overlapping with other structures (arterial branches), patient structure noise (background noise) and inaccurate contrast filling of vessels. This is also demonstrated by the fact that only few investigators have demonstrated a very close agreement of densitometric results from different views taken from the same vessel [56, 59].

In the future, videodensitometry may play an important role in measuring cross-sectional areas from a single view provided that important technical problems have been solved. Potentially, densitometry should be able to measure the "volume" of a coronary segment from a single view. If repeated studies are anticipated, then the same view must be utilized to avoid large errors due to potential differences in foreshortening, background, veiling glare and scatter [56, 60, 62].

Intravascular coronary echocardiography
Intravascular coronary echocardiography holds great promise to study progression or regression of disease. It provides insights into the disease processes of the vessel wall, also in the earlier stages of coronary artery disease, it has potential to characterise and quantify the disease, and it may predict which lesion has potential for regression.

Acknowledgements

We thank Claudia Sprenger de Rover for preparation of the manuscript.

References

1. Kuo PT, Hayase K, Kostis JB, Moreyra AE. Use of combined diet and colestipol in longterm (7–7½ years) treatment of patients with type II hyperlipoproteinemia. Circulation 1979; **59**: 199–211.
2. Nash DT, Gensini G, Esente P. Effect of lipid-lowering therapy on the progression of coronary atherosclerosis assessed by scheduled repetitive coronary arteriography. Int J Cardiol 1982; **2**: 43–55.
3. Nikkilä EA, Viikinkoski P, Valle M, Frick MH. Prevention of progression of coronary atherosclerosis by treatment of hyperlipidaemia: a seven year prospective angiographic study. Br Med J 1984; **289**: 220–3.
4. Cohn K, Sakai FJ, Langston MF Jr. Effect of clofibrate on progression of coronary disease: a prospective angiographic study in man. Am Heart J 1975; **89**: 591–8.
5. Brensike JF, Levy RI, Kelsey SF, et al. Effects of therapy with cholestyramine on progres-

sion of coronary arteriosclerosis: results of the NHLBI Type II Coronary Intervention Study. Circulation 1984; **69**: 313–24.

6. Blankenhorn DH, Nessim SA, Johnson RL, Sanmarco ME, Azen SP, Cashin-Hemphill L. Beneficial effects of combined colestipol-niacin therapy on coronary atherosclerosis and coronary venous bypass grafts. JAMA 1987; **257**: 3233–40 [published erratum appears in JAMA 1988; **259**: 2698].

7. Buchwald H, Varco RL, Matts JP, et al. Effect of partial ileal bypass surgery on mortality and morbidity from coronary heart disease in patients with hypercholesterolemia. Report of the Program on the Surgical Control of the Hypercholesterolemia (POSCH). N Engl J Med 1990; **323**: 946–55. Comment in: N Engl J Med 1991; **324**: 562–4.

8. Brown G, Albers JJ, Fisher LD, et al. Regression of coronary artery disease as a result of intensive lipid-lowering therapy in men with high levels of apolipoprotein B. N Engl J Med 1990; **323**: 1289–98. Comment in: N Engl J Med 1990; **323**: 1337–9.

9. Kane JP, Malloy MJ, Ports TA, Philips NR, Diehl JC, Havel RJ. Regression of coronary atherosclerosis during treatment of familial hypercholesterolemia with combined drug regimens. JAMA 1990; **264**: 3007–12.

10. Arntzenius AC, Kromhout D, Barth JD, et al. Diet, lipoproteins, and the progression of coronary atherosclerosis The Leiden Intervention Trial. N Engl J Med 1985; **312**: 805–11.

11. Lichtlen PR, Hugenholtz PG, Rafflenbeul W, Hecker H, Jost S, Deckers JW. Retardation of angiographic progression of coronary artery disease by nifedipine. Results of the International Nifedipine Trial on Antiatherosclerotic Therapy (INTACT). INTACT Group Investigators: Lancet 1990; **335**: 1109–13. Comment in: Lancet 1990; **336**: 172–4.

12. Waters D, Lespérance J, Francetich M, et al. A controlled clinical trial to assess the effect of a calcium channel blocker on the progression of coronary atherosclerosis. Circulation 1990; **82**: 1940–53. Comment in: Circulation 1990; **82**: 2251–3.

13. Ornish D, Brown SE, Scherwitz LW, et al. Can lifestyle changes reverse coronary heart disease? The Lifestyle Heart Trial. Lancet 1990; **336**: 129–33. Comment in: Lancet 1990; **336**: 624–6.

14. de Feyter PJ, Serruys PW, Davies MJ, Lubsen J, Richardson P, Oliver M. Quantitative coronary angiography to measure progression or regression of coronary atherosclerosis: value, limitations and implications for clinical trials. Circulation 1991; **84**: 412–23.

15. Harrison DG, White CW, Hiratzka LF, et al. The value of lesion cross-sectional area determined by quantitative coronary angiography in assessing the physiologic significance of proximal left anterior descending coronary arterial stenoses. Circulation 1984; **69**: 1111–9.

16. Rosenberg MC, Klein LW, Agarwal JB, Stets G, Hermann GA, Helfant RH. Quantification of absolute luminal diameter by computer-analyzed digital subtraction angiography: an assessment in human coronary arteries. Circulation 1988; **77**: 484–90.

17. Tobis J, Sato D, Nalcioglu O, et al. Correlation of minimum coronary lumen diameter with left ventricular functional impairment induced by atrial pacing. Am J Cardiol 1988; **61**: 697–703.

18. Marcus ML, Armstrong ML, Heistad DD, Eastham CL, Mark AL. Comparison of three methods of evaluating coronary obstructive lesions: postmortem arteriography, pathologic examination and measurement of regional myocardial perfusion during maximal vasodilation. Am J Cardiol 1982; **49**: 1699–706.

19. Schwartz JN, Kong Y, Hackel DB, Bartel AG. Comparison of angiographic and postmortem finds in patients with coronary artery disease. Am J Cardiol 1975; **36**: 174–8.

20. Hutchins GM, Bulkley GH, Ridolfi RL, Griffith LS, Lohr FT, Piasio MA. Correlation of coronary arteriograms and left ventriculograms with postmortem studies. Circulation 1977; **56**: 32–7.

21. Thomas AC, Davies MJ, Dilly S, Dilly N, Franc F. Potential errors in the estimation of coronary arterial stenosis from clinical arteriography with reference to the shape of the coronary arterial lumen. Br Heart J 1986; **55**: 129–39.

22. Arnett EN, Isner JM, Redwood DR, et al. Coronary artery narrowing in coronary heart

disease: comparison of cineangiographic and necropsy findings. Ann Intern Med 1979; **91**: 350–6.
23. Kemp HG, Evans H, Elliott WC, Gorlin R. Diagnostic accuracy of selective coronary cinearteriography. Circulation 1967; **36**: 526–33.
24. Vlodaver Z, Frech R, Van Tassel RA, Edwards JE. Correlation of the antemortem coronary arteriogram and the postmortem specimen. Circulation 1973; **47**: 162–9.
25. Grondin CM, Dyrda I, Pasternac A, Campeau L, Bourassa MG, Lesperance J. Discrepancies between cineangiographic and postmortem findings in patients with coronary artery disease and recent myocardial revascularization. Circulation 1974; **49**: 703–8.
26. Vlodaver Z, Edwards JE. Pathology of coronary atherosclerosis. Prog Cardiovasc Dis 1971; **14**: 256–74.
27. Isner JM, Kishel J, Kent KM, Ronan JA Jr, Ross AM, Roberts WC. Accuracy of angiographic determination of left main coronary artery narrowing. Angiographic – histologic correlative analysis in 28 patients. Circulation 1981; **63**: 1056–64.
28. Freudenberg H, Lichtlen PR. Das normale Wandsegment bei Koronarstenosen – eine postmortale Studie. Z Kardiol 1981; **70**: 863–9.
29. Glagov S, Weisenberg E, Zarins CK, Stankunavicius R, Kolettis GJ. Compensatory enlargement of human atherosclerotic coronary arteries. N Engl J Med 1987; **316**: 1371–5.
30. Zarins CK, Weisenberg E, Kolettis G, Stankunavicius R, Glagov S. Differential enlargement of artery segments in response to enlarging atherosclerotic plaques. J Vasc Surg 1988; **7**: 386–94.
31. Stiel GM, Stiel LS, Schofer J, Donath K, Mathey DG. Impact of compensatory enlargement of atherosclerotic coronary arteries on angiographic assessment of coronary artery disease. Circulation 1989; **80**: 1603–9.
32. McPherson DD, Sirna SJ, Hiratzka LF, et al. Coronary arterial remodeling studied by high-frequency epicardial echocardiography: an early compensatory mechanism in patients with obstructive coronary atherosclerosis. J Am Coll Cardiol 1991; **17**: 79–86.
33. Isner JM, Donaldson RF, Fortin AH, Tischler A, Clarke RH. Attenuation of the media of coronary arteries in advanced atherosclerosis. Am J Cardiol 1986; **58**: 937–9.
34. White CW, Wright CB, Doty DB, et al. Does visual interpretation of the coronary arteriogram predict the physiologic importance of a coronary stenosis? N Engl J Med 1984; **310**: 819–24.
34. Brown BG, Bolson E, Frimer M, Dodge HT. Quantitative coronary arteriography: estimation of dimensions, hemodynamic resistance and atheroma mass of coronary artery lesions using the arteriogram and digital computation. Circulation 1977; **53**: 329–37.
36. Feldman RL, Nichols WM, Pepine CJ, Conti CR. Hemodynamic significance of the length of a coronary arterial narrowing. Am J Cardiol 1978; **41**: 865–71.
37. Klocke FJ. Measurements of coronary blood flow and degree of stenosis: current clinical implications and continuing uncertainties. J Am Coll Cardiol 1983; **1**: 31–41.
38. Gould KL. Identifying and measuring severity of coronary artery stenosis. Quantitative coronary arteriography and positron emission tomography. Circulation 1988; **78**: 237–45.
39. Zijlstra F, van Ommeren J, Reiber JH, Serruys PW. Does quantitative assessment of coronary artery dimensions predict the physiologic significance of a coronary stenosis? Circulation 1987; **75**: 1154–61.
40. McMahon MM, Brown BG, Cukingnan R, et al. Quantitative coronary angiography: measurement of the "critical" stenosis in patients with unstable angina and single-vessel disease without collaterals. Circulation 1979; **60**: 106–13.
41. Kirkeeide RL, Gould KL, Parsel L. Assessment of coronary stenoses by myocardial perfusion imaging during pharmacologic coronary vasodilation VII. Validition of coronary flow reserve as a single integrated functional measure of stenosis severity reflecting all its geometric dimensions. J Am Coll Cardiol 1986; **7**: 103–13.
42. Learoyd BM, Taylor MG. Alterations with age in the viscoelastic properties of human arterial walls. Circ Res 1966; **18**: 278–92.

43. Bader H. Dependence of wall stress in the human thoracic aorta on age and pressure. Circ Res 1967; **20**: 354–61.
44. Roberts CS, Roberts WC. Cross-sectional area of the proximal portions of the three major epicardial coronary arteries in 98 necropsy patients with different coronary events. Relationship to heart weight, age and sex. Circulation 1980; **62**: 953–9.
45. Roach MR. Reversibility of poststenotic dilatation in the femoral arteries of dogs. Circ Res 1970; **27**: 985–93.
46. Roach MR. Changes in arterial distensibility as a cause of poststenotic dilatation. Am J Cardiol 1963; **12**: 802–15.
47. Roberts WC. The coronary arteries and left ventricle in clinically isolated angina pectoris: a necropsy analysis. Circulation 1976; **54**: 388–90.
48. Svindland A. The localization of sudanophilic and fibrous plaques in the main left coronary bifurcation. Atherosclerosis 1983; **48**: 139–45.
49. McPherson DD, Hiratzka LF, Lamberth WC, et al. Delineation of the extent of coronary artherosclerosis by high-frequency epicardial echocardiography. N Engl J Med 1987; **316**: 304–9.
50. Reiber JHC, van der Zwet PMJ, Koning G, von Land CD, Padmos I, Buis B, van Benthem AC, van Meurs B. Quantitative coronary measurements from cine and digital arteriograms; methodology and validation results. Abstract book 4th Intern. Symp. on Coronary Arteriography, Rotterdam, June 23–25, 1991; 36.
51. Ellis S, Sanders W, Goulet C, et al. Optimal detection of the progression of coronary artery disease: comparison of methods suitable for risk factor intervention trials. Circulation 1986; **76**: 1235–42.
52. Wijns W, Serruys PW, Reiber JH, et al. Quantitative angiography of the left anterior descending coronary artery: correlations with pressure gradient and exercise thallium scinitigraphy. Circulation 1985; **71**: 273–9.
53. Gould KL. Dynamic coronary stenosis. Am J Cardiol 1980; **45**: 286–92.
54. Young DF, Cholvin NR, Roth AC. Pressure drop across artificially induced stenoses in the femoral arteries of dogs. Circ Res 1975; **36**: 735–43.
55. Reiber JH, Serruys PW, Kooijman CJ, et al. Assessment of short-, medium-, and long-term variations in arterial dimensions from computer-assisted quantitation of coronary cineangiograms. Circulation 1985; **71**: 280–8.
56. Reiber JH. An overview of coronary quantitation techniques as of 1989. In: Reiber JH, Serruys PW (Eds.), Quantitative coronary angiography. Dordrecht: Kluwer Academic Publishers 1991: 55–132.
57. Whiting JS, Pfaff JM, Eigler NL. Advantages and limitations of videodensitometry in quantitative coronary angiography. In: Reiber JH, Serruys PW (Eds.), Quantitative coronary angiography. Dordrecht: Kluwer Academic Publishers 1991: 43–54.
58. Mancini GB, Simon SB, McGillem MJ, LeFree MT, Friedman HZ, Vogel RA. Automated quantitative coronary arteriography: morphologic and physiologic validation in vivo of a rapid digital angiographic method. Circulation 1987; **75**: 452–60. [published erratum appears in Circulation 1987; **75**: 1199].
59. Sanz ML, Mancini J, LeFree MT, et al. Variability of quantitative digital subtraction coronary angiography before and after percutaneous transluminal coronary angiography. Am J Cardiol 1987; **60**: 55–60.
60. Herrold EM, Goldberg HL, Borer JS, Wong K, Moses JW. Relative insensitivity of densitometric stenosis measurement to lumen edge detection. J Am Coll Cardiol 1990; **15**: 1570–7.
61. Serruys PW, Reiber JH, Wijns W, et al. Assessment of percutaneous transluminal coronary angioplasty by quantitative coronary angiography: diameter versus densitometric area measurements. Am J Cardiol 1984; **54**: 482–8.
62. Mancini GB. Digital coronary angiography: advantages and limitations. In: Reiber JH, Serruys PW (Eds.), Quantitative coronary angiography. Dordrecht: Kluwer Academic Publishers 1991: 23–42.

15. The impact of the calcium antagonist nifedipine on the angiographic progression of coronary artery disease: Results of the INTACT (international nifedipine trial on antiatherosclerotic therapy)

PAUL R. LICHTLEN, WOLFGANG RAFFLENBEUL,
STEFAN JOST, PETER NIKUTTA, PAUL HUGENHOLTZ,
JAAP DECKERS, BIRGITT WIESE and the INTACT study group

Summary

INTACT is a study on the progression of coronary artery disease based on quantitated coronary angiography, applying the CAAS-system to assess the diameters of segments and stenoses and their changes over time. 348 of 425 patients (82%) underwent 2 angiograms after 3 years (175 on placebo, 173 on nifedipine, 80 mg per day). The analysis followed the intention to treat principle, as 66 patients stopped the trial medication for the last 12–18 months. Progression was defined either as an increase in the degree of stenosis by $\geqslant 20\%$ or transition to occlusion, or as development of new stenoses (narrowings $\geqslant 20\%$) or new occlusions in coronary segments or sections previously angiographically normal. New lesions were selected both visually and by computer assessment. After 3 years no differences were found between groups with regard to pro- and regression of existing stenoses; however, there were fewer new lesions on nifedipine (144 on placebo versus 103 on nifedipine, -28%, $p = 0.034$) and also a trend to fewer patients with new lesions on nifedipine (-17%, n.s.). Hence, the calcium-antagonist significantly reduced the appearance of new stenoses and occlusions. There were interesting insights into the progression of CAD in general. Only 11.3% of existing stenoses showed progression and even fewer (4.3%) regression over 3 years, only few stenoses went into occlusion (2% of existing and 7.7% of new stenoses) ($p = 0.000$). Altogether, 56% of patients showed progression, 30.5% only in new stenoses, 11.8% only in old ones, and 14.1% in both. Hence, the strongest manifestation of progression of CAD was found in the development of new lesions (44.6% of all patients or 79% of all progressing patients showed new lesions). Conclusions: Repeated coronary angiography on a quantitative basis offers an excellent opportunity to study the progression of coronary artery disease, especially also during preventive interventions. A limitation is the angiographic definition of progression, which has to be based on sound statistical criteria as data from direct comparisons with the abnormal anatomy are not available as of yet.

J.H.C. Reiber and P.W. Serruys (eds), Advances in Quantitative Coronary Arteriography, 273–284.

Introduction

INTACT represents the first prospective study on the angiographic progression of coronary artery disease (CAD) including not only existing but also the development of new stenoses, extending over a relatively long period of time (3 years), and based on computer analysis (CAAS-system). The primary aim of the study was to demonstrate the impact of the calcium antagonist nifedipine on the progression of CAD in patients with angiographically proven disease [1–3]. The study is based on numerous animal experiments demonstrating a significant retardation of the formation of atherosclerotic plaques in animals fed with a diet rich in cholesterol, when nifedipine is simultaneously administered [4–7]. As the results of INTACT were already published extensively [1–3], this article will, in addition to summarize briefly the INTACT data, also present data on the experience on the progression of coronary artery disease in man as found by computer-assisted angiographic analysis in general.

Methods

425 patients were included from 6 German and 3 Dutch cardiology centers (see annex). For inclusion patients had to be below 65 years of age, presenting mild to moderate CAD at coronary angiograms, i.e. demonstrate rather few lesions (approximately 3–4 per patient) (for details, see [1, 2]). All patients received 80 mg nifedipine/day; 348 could be followed over 3 years (1090 ± 149 days for placebo, 1097 ± 144 days for nifedipine) (175 patients on placebo, 173 on nifedipine). Sixty-six% of patients were on the full dose over the entire interval, 34% reduced or stopped treatment before the second angiogram; the data presented include all patients with a second angiogram after 3 years, following the intention to treat principle. There were no clinical differences between groups both with regard to risk factors (levels of total cholesterol, LDL- and HDL-cholesterol throughout the study, smoking, hypertension), or class of angina, percent of patients with positive exercise tests, with old myocardial infarctions or undergoing PTCA or CABG (for details see [1–3]).

Angiographic analysis

Angiograms of the RCA and LAD were carried out in several projections, the 2–3 best ones, preferably in orthogonal positions, being selected for computer processing; the angles and projections of all scenes were exactly recorded to allow repetition in identical positions after 3 years. Coronary arteries were dilated with 10 mg isosorbide dinitrate sublingually, 10 minutes prior to angiography. Calibration for diameter measurements was done by comparing the true diameter of the angiographically visible part of the shaft or tip of the catheter, measured immediately after angiography by a precision caliper (precision 0.05 mm) with the mean diameter as assessed by computer analysis in the cineframe; pincushion distortion was assessed and corrected for by a filmed grid (line distances 1 cm).

Optimal cineframes were selected by 2 experienced cardiologists on the Tagarno projector, identifying for the operator the segments and stenoses to be analyzed by CAAS. The inclusion of segments followed the recommendations of the American Heart Association [8]; segments with diameters of < 1 mm or distal to occlusions were excluded.

Altogether 9,533 segments were analyzed in 2 projections by CAAS (amounting to 19107 segment measurements). *Definition of progression and regression of existing stenoses* as well as of new stenoses was based on previously obtained statistical criteria for CAAS, where the single standard deviation of 2 cineframes in identical projections from 2 different movies 90 days apart amounted to 6.52% [9]. Hence, a stenosis was defined as localized diameter reduction of a normal segment by more than 3 times the standard deviation, i.e. ≥20%. Similar changes were asked for pro- and regression of existing stenoses (f.i. an increase from 20 to 40% or a vice versa decrease). The aim of these arbitrary definitions (together with coronary dilation by isosorbide dinitrate) was to reduce false positive findings to a minimum (see also [3]). Minimal diameter changes had to reach at least 0.4 mm to be accepted as biologically valid; this corresponded to twice the standard deviation of repeated measurements after 90 days [9]; in addition, this somewhat arbitrary value corresponded to 1/4 of the average minimal diameter (0.6 mm, range 0.47–3.8 mm). Special algorithms of CAAS were applied both for segment contour analysis as well as calculation of percent stenosis [9, 10]. Thus, the angiographic endpoints were as follows: for progression of existing stenoses, an increase in the degree of stenoses by ≥20% diameter stenosis or ≥0.4 mm in absolute minimal diameter, or transition to occlusion; for regression a similar decrease; for the appearance of new lesions, narrowings ≥20% or new occlusions in segments with normal appearance at the first angiogram (visual estimate of normality). Hence, new lesions were detected either by the computer, based on changes in the diameter function curve or visually, with subsequent confirmation by the computer.

Results

First angiogram (Table 1)

The 348 patients followed over 3 years, at entrance showed a total of 1,255 lesions (3.61 lesions/patient). No differences were observed between groups (3.754 lesions/patient on placebo and 3.457 lesions/patient on nifedipine;

Table 1. Angiographic baseline data

No. of lesions	Total n	Lesions/ patient	Placebo n	Lesions/pat.	Nifedipine n	Lesions/pat.	p-value PL/NIF
Stenoses >20%	1105	3.175	581	3.32	524	3.029	0.3848
Occlusions	150	0.43	76	0.434	74	0.428	0.913
Total	1255	3.61	657	3.754	598	3.457	0.3850

Table 2. Pro- and regression of existing stenoses over 3 years (INTACT); changes of the degree of stenoses >20%

Degree of stenosis at 1st angio	No changes	Progression >20%	Regression >20%	Total
<40%	400	81 (16.7%)	5 (1.0%)	486
40–59%	436	34 (6.8%)	32 (6.4%)	502
>60%	62	5 (4.2%)	8 (10.7%)	75
Total	898	120 (incl. 20 occlusions)	45	1063
	84.5%	11.3%	4.2%	

$p = 0.385$) (Table 1). The minimal diameter of stenoses averaged 1.65 ± 0.52 mm for placebo and 1.64 ± 0.52 mm for nifedipine ($p =$ n.s.). Interestingly, 80% of stenoses had a degree of less than 60%, i.e. were clinically asymptomatic, i.e. not detectable by noninvasive means.

Second Angiogram

a) Changes in preexisting lesions (Table 2)

A progression (increase in degree of stenoses by ≥20%) was observed in 120 (11.3%) of the 1063 existing stenoses (20 going into occlusion; 2.1% of all stenoses) being analyzable in the second angiogram (a small number of stenoses was lost due to new occlusions or insufficient quality). Regression (a decrease of degree of stenoses by ≥20%) was observed in 4.2%. Hence, the majority of stenoses (more than 85%) had remained unchanged over 3 years. As expected, there were significantly more stenoses progressing in the low grade (<40%) and more regression in the high grade range (>60%) ($p < 0.05$). Concerning differences between the 2 groups, there was no discernable influence of nifedipine on pro- or regression: in the placebo group 16% of stenoses progressed, 6% regressed, in the nifedipine group 13% progressed and 5% regressed. Ten stenoses on placebo and 12 on nifedipine went into occlusion. When changes of stenoses were analyzed per patient, 20 and 25% showed progression, and 15 and 17% regression, respectively. A similar behavior was seen with regard to minimal diameter changes.

Table 3. Angiographic progression of CAD, progression/patient

Existing stenoses progression by >20% or to occlusion	New lesions		Total
	No	Yes	
No	152	106	258
Yes	41	49	90
Total	193	155	348

196 patients progressing (56.3%, 18.8%/year)	100%
41 patients only in existing lesions	20.9%
106 patients only in new lesions	54.1%
49 patients both in old and new lesions	25.0%

b) New lesions
Altogether there were 247 new lesions (228 new stenoses $\geqslant 20\%$, average degree $39.4 \pm 10.2\%$, range 20 to 70%, and 19 new occlusions) in coronary segments previously angiographically normal. These new lesions occurred in 155 patients (44.5% of all patients) (Table 3), i.e. there were 0.71 new lesions/patient or 1.26 lesions/progressive patient. Ninety-seven patients presented with one, 34 with two, 15 with three, 8 with four and one patient with five new lesions. One hundred and six patients progressed only in new lesions (30.5% of all, or 68.4% of those with progression), 41 only in old ones (11.8% of all or 26.4% of those with progression) and 49 both in old and new ones.
    The following observations were made regarding progression in general:
1. Applying rather strict criteria, 44% of patients showed no progression over 3 years; or vice versa only 18.7% of patients progressed/year. This was considerably less than the 33% estimated from previous retrospective, quantitative angiographic studies [11, 12].
2. The strongest progression concerned the formation of new lesions (79% of all progressing patients); furthermore, new lesions showed an almost identical average degree of stenoses (39.4%) as those existing at first angiography, thus, were mostly without clinical manifestation.
3. New lesions had a higher incidence of occlusions (7.7%) than old ones (1.9%) ($p < 0.05$), i.e. a higher tendency to plaque rupture and thrombotic occlusion [13, 14].

c) Influence of nifedipine on new lesion formation (Figure 1)
Nifedipine significantly reduced the number of new lesions: after 3 years there were 103 new lesions in patients on nifedipine (0.59/patient) versus 144 new lesions in patients on placebo (0.82/patient), a difference of -28%, $p = 0.03$ (Cochran's linear trend test, 2–sided). Interestingly, there was a close correlation between the number of existing lesions/patient at entrance and the number of new lesions/patient after 3 years (Figure 1). Patients with higher numbers of lesions at entrance also presented higher numbers of new lesions; this correlation was significant both for placebo ($r = 0.192$, $p =$

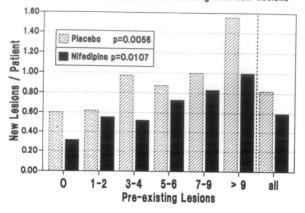

Figure 1. Correlation of the number of preexisting lesions/patient with the number of newly formed lesions/patient. There is a significant correlation insofar as patients with higher number of existing lesions also produced more new lesions; this was significantly influenced by nifedipine.

0.0056) as well as for nifedipine ($r = 0.175$, $p = 0.011$). However, for all groups (patients with no lesions up to patients with >9 lesions at first angiography) there were more new lesions on placebo than on nifedipine. Hence, nifedipine was equally successful to suppress new lesions both in patients with mild as well as advanced progression.

Discussion

a) Limitations of the study

The study shows interesting aspects not only on the preventive effect of nifedipine with regard to the progression of CAD in man, but also on the computerized angiographic analysis of the progression of CAD in man in general. However, this new angiographic approach has some limitations. Although INTACT and a few additional prospective studies [15, 16, 17] confirmed the applicability of computer-assisted techniques for the angiographic follow-up of CAD in man, especially in the control of the efficacy of calcium antagonists, it is still open to which extent the observed anatomical changes translate into clinical events [14]. Nevertheless, in view of the encouraging results of the POSCH-study [18], demonstrating a close correlation between early angiographic and late clinical improvements in preventive treatment, followed over 10 years, angiography could represent a "shortcut" in testing the effects of preventive measures against atherosclerosis. In this context one has to remember, that due to the relative slow angiographic progression of CAD (low incidence of number of stenoses/patient, less than

20% of patients progressing/year) [19], large numbers of patients and a relatively long follow-up are necessary to reach significance [20].

A major problem lies in the *angiographic definition of progression*. It is relatively easy with regard to the recognition of new stenoses or occlusions in previously angiographically normal coronary segments; however, when it concerns the further pro- or regression of already existing stenoses, definition is difficult especially with regard to the lower limit. This is due to several reasons: 1) the variability of the different computer-assisted systems in measuring the degree of stenoses over longer intervals is quite large [9]; 2) there are problems in the assessment of the so-called "normal" reference segment, when calculating the degree of stenosis; 3) there is considerable variation in minimal diameters between different projections and angles, 4) changes in vasomotor tone in the free relatively undiseased wall segment of eccentric stenoses influence morphology.

Thus, so far the decision on a lower limit for progression of stenoses remains somewhat arbitrary. Nevertheless, the 20% limit chosen in this study for pro- or regression is probably too high [19]; a comparison between the increase and decrease of the degree of stenosis in the more than 1,000 stenoses included in this study suggests a lower limit of approximately 15% to be still above the variability of the system; between 0 and 15% no differences were found in the number of pro- or regressing stenoses, whereas above 15%, the number for pro- and regressing stenoses started to diverge [19]. To further analyze the limit for angiographic recognition of pro- or regressing stenoses one would need either more in vivo studies f.i. gathered by intravascular ECHO-probes or from postmortem comparisons with histologic specimens. It should, however, always be remembered that angiography can only demonstrate localized changes in the coronary lumen diameters above a certain size; the angiographic sensitivity certainly does not include the visualization of fatty streaks and also not of plaques growing primarily within the intima [21, 22]. On the other hand, if angiography is understood as a tool indicating those processes which eventually might become clinically detrimental, such as plaque rupture and coronary occlusion leading to myocardial infarction [23], its sensitivity is sufficient. This includes the recognition of fresh, low grade plaques, clinically not yet manifest, but possible candidates for plaque rupture and acute myocardial infarction as well as high grade, stenosing plaques leading to impairment of coronary blood flow. Thus, if f.i. INTACT is not able to provide any data on the number of fatty streaks inhibited by nifedipine, this is clinically irrelevant; important is that angiography showed that the number of those fatty streaks later developing into plaques were significantly reduced, because these are the clinically potentially dangerous ones.

Finally, the study also supports the experience that computerized analysis of angiographic progression of CAD is superior to a qualitative judgment f.e. by scoring systems, where independent viewers compare the 2 subsequent movies and decide on pro- or regression. Unfortunately many of these qualitative studies [18, 24, 25] did not analyze the new lesions, which would have provided "hard" endpoints; they also do not indicate the size or degree of stenosis and of minimal diameters and therefore render judgments on their results rather difficult. One has therefore to conclude that without exact, precise measurements the data on pro- or regression are considerably more doubtful than when these analyses are quantitated by computer assistance.

b) The role of calcium antagonists in the prevention of CAD in man
In addition to INTACT 3 other studies confirmed the retarding effect of calcium antagonists on the angiographic progression of CAD, especially with regard to the development of new lesions [15, 16, 17] (Table 4). Hence, this effect is now well established, however, still needs clinical confirmation. The latter, being more problematic (see above) as it will ask for a longer follow up (6 to 10 years) and has to include more patients. It will also ask for further characterization of the optimal drug (its galenic form, efficacy, side effects) as well as its clinical profile. Further studies are necessary and are on their way.

c) General aspects of the angiographic progression of CAD based on this prospective, long-term study
As INTACT is the first 3 year follow-up study based on a computerized, prospective analysis of atherosclerosis, it was to be expected that a host of new aspects on the progression of CAD in man would be revealed. A special aspect is the analysis of the *development of new coronary lesions.* To us, their importance was first evidenced in a retrospective study with an interval of 6 years [26]; although this was still a qualitative angiographic analysis, it showed that 70% of total progression came from the newly formed stenoses and occlusions and not from changes in existing stenoses. This observation was now confirmed by INTACT. Also here 79% of the progression concerned new lesions; in addition, new lesions also showed a significantly higher tendency for plaque rupture (7% over 3 years) than old stenoses (2%), probably due their still fragile fibrous cap [23]. Interestingly, their degree of stenosis was rather low (approximately 40%); hence, the majority was recognizable only by angiographic means.

Old plaques seemed to be rather consolidated; only 2% ruptured and occluded over 3 years. Interestingly, their average degree was also low, approximately 40%, similar as for new ones. This suggests that most plaques, after developing from fatty streaks, remain unchanged for a long period of time. Further "growth" is due to complications, plaque rupture, platelet adhesion and integration [23]. Our observation, demonstrating for the first time in a prospective manner that the majority of stenoses going into occlusion and leading to myocardial infarctions is of low grade, between 30 and 60%, not recognizable by noninvasive means and also not leading to angina or silent ischemia long before the event, is sustained by recent studies in patients with acute myocardial infarction; they analyzed the degree of

Table 4. Angiographic studies with calcium antagonists

Study	Medication	No. patients with 2 angios			New lesions/patient		Percent reduction of new lesions	P-value	Lower limit for percent degree of stenosis
		Total	PL	Ca-Ant.	PL	Ca-Ant.			
Gottlieb et al. 1989, 1 year CABG	Nifedipine 3 × 20 mg per day	64	37	27	65/37 1.75/pat. 48% of CABG diseased	31/27 1.15/pat. 33%	-35%	<0.04	-
Loaldi et al. 1989, 2 years	4 × 20 mg Nifedipine vs Propranolol 320 mg vs ISDN 80 mg	113	36 38	39	12/36 0.333/pat. 11/38 0.289/pat.	4/39 0.102/pat.	-57%	<0.05	20%
Waters et al. 1990, 2 years	Nicardipine 3 × 20 mg	217	118	99	38/118 0.32/pat.	16/99 0.16/pat.	-50%	<0.046	10%
Lichtlen et al. 1990, 3 years	Nifedipine 4 × 20 mg	348	175	173	144/175 0.82/pat.	103/173 0.59/pat.	-28%	<0.034	20%

PL = Placebo; Ca-Ant = Calcium-Antagonist.

stenosis after thrombolysis and demonstrated in the majority of cases also a pre-infarction degree of stenoses of approximately 50–60% [27, 28, 29, 30].

Finally, the *correlation to risk factors* is of special interest. There was a very close relation between the generation of new lesions and *cigarette smoking*. Non-smokers had the lowest number of new lesions (0.45/patient), in ex-smokers it increased by + 42% (0.64/patient), in moderate smokers by 82.2% (0.82/patient) and in heavy smokers by + 155% (1.15/patient). Hence, the effect of cigarette smoking on the formation of new lesions was highly significant ($p = 0.0001$); however, there was also a significant reduction of this type of new lesion by nifedipine [27].

Total cholesterol as a risk factor was less impressive over the short interval of 3 years. There was no relation between total cholesterol and the evolution of new lesions ($p = 0.937$), whereas high cholesterol levels ($> 256\,mg/dl$) were associated with more progressing old lesions/patient ($p = 0.0197$). Cholesterol obviously exerts its influence over a longer period of time.

Appendix

The following centres and physicians participated in the study:

Division of Cardiology, Hannover Medical School, FRG (Central office of the study), Paul R. Lichtlen, M.D., study director; Wolfgang Rafflenbeul, M.D., co-director; Ulrich Nellessen, M.D., Stefan Jost, M.D., Peter Nikutta, M.D., Ivo Amende, M.D.

Division of Cardiology, University Hospital Hamburg, FRG; Walter Bleifeld, M.D., Christian Hamm, M.D.

Division of Cardiology, University Hospital Frankfurt, FRG; Martin Kaltenbach, M.D., Harald Klepzig, M.D., Gisbert Kober, M.D.

Division of Cardiology, University Hospital Erlangen, FRG; Kurt Bachmann, M.D., Siegfried Haetinger, M.D.

City Hospital Links der Weser, Bremen, FRG; Hans-Jürgen Engel, M.D., Holger Werner, M.D.

Division of Cardiology, University Hospital Berlin, FRG; Horst Schmutzler, M.D., Harald Bias, M.D.

Erasmus Universiteit Rotterdam, The Netherlands; Paul Hugenholtz, M.D., co-director of the study, Jaap Deckers, M.D., study assistant; Patrick Serruys, M.D., Hans Reiber, Ph.D.

Department of Cardiology, Catharina Hospital, Eindhoven, The Netherlands; Hans Bonnier, M.D., Rolf Michels, M.D., Rael Troquay, M.D.

Academic Ziekenhuis Groningen, The Netherlands; K. Lie, M.D., E.D. de Muinck, M.D.

Division of Biomedics, Hannover Medical School,FRG; B. Schneider, Ph.D., Hartmut Hecker, Ph.D., Birgitt Wiese, Ph.D.

References

1. Lichtlen PR, Hugenholtz PG, Rafflenbeul W, Hecker H, Jost S, Deckers JW. Retardation of angiographic progression of coronary artery disease by nifedipine. Results of the International Nifedipine Trial on Antiatherosclerotic Therapy (INTACT) Lancet 1990; **335**: 1109–13. Comments in: Lancet 1990; **336**: 172–4.

2. Lichtlen PR, Hugenholtz PG, Rafflenbeul W, et al. Retardation of coronary artery disease in humans by the calcium-channel blocker nifedipine: results of the INTACT study (International Nifedipine Trial on Antiatherosclerotic Therapy). Cardiovasc Drugs Ther 1990; **4** (Suppl 5): 1047–68.

3. Lichtlen PR, Rafflenbeul W, Nikutta P, Jost S, Wiese B and the INTACT-study group. The influence of nifedipine on the progression of coronary artery disease in man: the INTACT study. In: Lichtlen PR, Reale A (Eds.), Adalat: a comprehensive review. Berlin: Springer Verlag 1991: 203–25.

4. Henry PD. Calcium antagonists as antiatherogenic agents. Ann N Y Acad Sci 1988; **522**: 411–9.

5. Henry PD, Bently KI. Suppression of atherogenesis in cholesterol-fed rabbit treated with nifedipine. J Clin Invest 1981; **68**: 1366–9.

6. Henry PD. Antiatherogenic effects of calcium channel blockers: possible mechanisms of action. Cardiovasc Drugs Ther 1990; **4** (Suppl 5): 1015–20.

7. Nayler W, Dillon J, Panagiotopoulos S. Dihydropyridines and the ischemic myocardium. In: Lichtlen P (Ed.), 6th International Adalat Symposium. Amsterdam: Excerpta Medica 1985: 386–98.

8. Austen WG, Edwards JE, Frye RL, et al. A reporting system on patients evaluated for coronary artery disease. Report of the Ad Hoc Committee for Grading of Coronary Artery Disease, Council on Cardiovascular Surgery, American Heart Association. Circulation 1975; **51** (4 Suppl): 5–40.

9. Reiber JHC, Serruys PW, Kooijman CJ, et al. Assessment of short-, medium-, and long-term variations in arterial dimensions from computer-assisted quantitation of coronary cineangiograms. Circulation 1985; **71**: 280–8.

10. Reiber JH, Kooijman JC, Slager CJ, Gerbrands JJ, Schuurbiers JC. Computer-assisted analysis of the severity of obstructions from coronary cineangiograms: a methodological review. Automedica 1984; **5**: 219–38.

11. Bruschke AV, Wijers TS, Kolsters W, Landmann J. The anatomic evolution of coronary artery disease demonstrated by coronary angiography in 256 nonoperated patients. Circulation 1981; **63**: 527–36.

12. Rafflenbeul W, Nellessen U, Galvao P, Kreft M, Peters S, Lichtlen P. Progression und Regression der Koronarsklerose im angiographischen Bild. Z Kardiol 1984; **73** (Suppl 2): 33–40.

13. Davies MJ, Thomas AC. Plaque fissuring – the cause of acute myocardial infarction, sudden ischaemic death and crescendo angina. Br Heart J 1985; **53**: 363–73.

14. Davies MJ, Krikler DM, Katz D. Atherosclerosis: Inhibition or regression as therapeutic possibilities. Br Heart J 1991; **65**: 302–10.

15. Gottlieb SO, Brinker JA, Mellits ED et al. Effect of nifedipine on the development of coronary bypass graft stenoses in high-risk patients: a randomized, double-blind, placebo-controlled trial. Circulation 1988; **80** (4 Suppl II): II–228 (Abstract).

16. Loaldi A, Polese A, Montorsi P, et al. Comparison of nifedipine, propranolol and isosorbide dinitrate on angiographic progression and regression of coronary arterial narrowings in angina pectoris. Am J Cardiol 1989; **64**: 433–9.

17. Waters D, Lespérance J, Francetich M, et al. A controlled clinical trial to assess the effect of a calcium channel blocker on the progression of coronary atherosclerosis. Circulation 1990; **82**: 1940–53. Comment in: Circulation 1990; **82**: 2251–3.

18. Buchwald H, Varco RL, Matts JP et al. Effect of partial ileal bypass surgery on mortality and morbidity from coronary heart disease in patients with hypercholesterolemia. Report of the Program on the Surgical Control of the Hyperlipidemias (POSCH). N Engl J Med 1990, **323**: 946–55. Comment in: N Engl J Med 1991; **324**: 562–4.

19. Lichtlen PR, Nikutta P, Jost S, Rafflenbeul W, Wiese B. Anatomical progression of coronary artery disease in man, as seen by prospective, repeated, quantitated coronary angiography. Relation to clinical events and risk factors. (In press).

20. Ellis S, Sanders W, Goulet C, et al. Optimal detection of the progression of coronary artery

disease: comparison of methods suitable for risk factor intervention trials. Circulation 1986; **74**: 1235–42.

21. Glagov S, Weisenberg E, Zarins CK, Stankunavicius R, Colettis GJ. Compensatory enlargement of human atherosclerotic coronary arteries. N Engl J Med 1987; **316**: 1371–5.

22. Stiel GM, Stiel LS, Schofer J, Donath K, Matey DG. Impact of compensatory enlargement of atherosclerotic coronary arteries on angiographic assessment of coronary artery disease. Circulation 1989; **80**: 1603–9.

23. Davies MJ. A macro and micro view of coronary vascular insult in ischemic heart disease. Circulation 1990; **82** (3 Suppl): II 38–46.

24. Blankenhorn DH, Nessim SA, Johnson RL, Sanmarco ME, Azen SP, Cashin-Hemphill L. Beneficial effects of combined cholestipol niacin therapy on coronary atherosclerosis and coronary venous bypass grafts. JAMA 1987; **257**: 3233–40. (Published erratum appears in JAMA 1988; **259**: 2698).

25. Levy RI, Brensike JF, Epstein SE, et al. The influence of changes in lipid values induced by cholestyramine and diet on progression of coronary artery disease: results of NHLBI Type II Coronary Intervention Study. Circulation 1984; **69**: 325–37.

26. Nellessen U, Rafflenbeul W, Hecker H, Lichtlen P. Zur Progression der Koronarsklerose. Untersuchungen bei 19 Patienten über 6 Jahre mittels quantitativer Koronarangiographie. Z Kardiol 1984; **73**: 760–7.

27. Nikutta P, Jost S, Deckers J, et al. The beneficial effect of smoking cessation on angiographic progression of coronary disease. Results of the INTACT study. Circulation 1990; **82** (4 Suppl III): III–299 (Abstract).

28. Hackett D, Davies G, Maseri A. Pre-existing coronary stenoses in patients with first myocardial infarction are not necessarily severe. Eur Heart J 1988; **9**: 1317–23.

29. Serruys PW, Arnold AE, Brower RW, et al. Effects of continued rt-PA administration on the residual stenosis after initially successful recanalization in acute myocardial infarction – a quantitative coronary angiography study of a randomized trial. Eur Heart J 1987; **8**: 1172–81.

30. Ambrose JA, Tannenbaum MA, Alexopoulous D et al. Angiographic progression of coronary artery disease and the development of myocardial infarction. J Am Coll Cardiol 1988; **12**: 56–62.

16. Progression and regression of coronary atherosclerosis: data from a controlled clinical trial with nicardipine

DAVID WATERS and JACQUES LESPÉRANCE

Summary

Interventions that may influence the evolution of coronary atherosclerosis can be evaluated more rapidly and efficiently in clinical trials with angiographic endpoints as opposed to using coronary events as endpoints. Quantitative coronary arteriography provides precise and reproducible measurements of coronary artery dimensions. Variability of repeat measurement of minimum diameter, expressed as 1 standard deviation of the mean, increased from 0.088 mm (same frame) to 0.197 mm (films 1 to 6 months apart) as conditions decreased from optimal to those encountered in clinical studies. A change in minimum diameter ≥ 0.4 mm is more than 2 standard deviations of the midterm variability and therefore represents a true change, either progression or regression, with greater than 95% probability.

To determine whether the calcium channel blocker nicardipine influences the progression of coronary atherosclerosis, 383 patients with stenoses $\leq 75\%$ in at least 4 coronary segments were randomized to 2 years of treatment with placebo or nicardipine 30 mg 3 times per day. Repeat coronary arteriography in 335 patients revealed progression of at least one lesion (using the ≥ 0.4 mm minimum diameter criterion) in 44% of nicardipine and 43% of placebo patients. Regression at one or more sites was seen in 23% of nicardipine and 19% of placebo patients. These differences were not statistically significant. However, minimal lesions, defined as those $\leq 20\%$ at the first study, progressed in 15 of 99 nicardipine patients compared to 32 of 118 placebo patients (15% versus 27%, $p = 0.046$).

These results suggest that nicardipine has no effect on advanced coronary atherosclerosis but may retard the progression of early lesions. This type of study, with quantitative coronary measurements as endpoints, is an excellent tool to assess the effect of an intervention upon the evolution of coronary atherosclerosis.

J.H.C. Reiber and P.W. Serruys (eds), Advances in Quantitative Coronary Arteriography, 285–298.

Introduction

Progression of coronary atherosclerosis causes angina and leads to myocardial infarction, heart failure and sudden death. Therapy that might stabilize coronary atherosclerosis or even induce regression would obviously have a major impact by reducing these complications. Based upon clinical trials reported to date, the most promising interventions are lipid-lowering therapy [1–5], calcium channel blockers [6, 7] and aspirin [8]. However, more studies are required before any of these drugs can be approved for use for an antiatherosclerosis indication.

Clinical trials that use coronary arteriographic endpoints instead of tabulating coronary events have the obvious advantage of being smaller, shorter and thus much less costly. Quantitative coronary arteriography is by far the most developed technique for assessing changes in the extent and severity of coronary atherosclerosis. Nevertheless, this methodology has important limitations as well as advantages, and no standard format has yet evolved for presenting results. The first part of this paper will discuss some of the issues related to the measurement of changes in coronary atherosclerosis that are relevant to clinical trials. In the remainder of the paper, a clinical trial using quantitative coronary arteriography to assess the effect of a calcium channel blocker upon the evolution of coronary atherosclerosis will be described.

Reproducibility of quantitative coronary measurements

The primary aim of measurements from coronary arteriograms is to detect changes in the extent and severity of coronary atherosclerosis reliably and accurately. Sample size requirements escalate as the sensitivity or specificity to detect progression or regression decrease [9]. Ideally, the measurements that are reported should be simple, so that their relevance can be quickly grasped, and comprehensive, so that they convey all of the important findings. Different trials could be more accurately compared if their results were reported using a standardized format.

Some investigators have also compared the extent and severity of inducible myocardial ischemia at the time of the two arteriograms. This strategy provides additional evidence that may bolster their conclusions, but has several limitations. Only a small minority of coronary stenoses cause myocardial ischemia and most patients with coronary atherosclerosis do not have such stenoses. Severe stenoses cause angina and are the target of revascularization procedures but their importance is overestimated; recent evidence indicates that most stenoses that occlude and produce myocardial infarction are less than 70%, and often less than 50% in stenosis diameter [10, 11]. An assessment of endothelial function with acetylcholine [12] would be more relevant to the pathogenesis of coronary progression and regression.

Table 1. Standard deviations for differences in repeat measurements under different conditions

Conditions of repeat measurement	Minimum diameter (mm)	Diameter stenosis		Reference diameter* (interpolated, mm)
		User-defined (%)	Interpolated (%)	
(1) Same frame (n = 54)	0.088	3.5	3.2	0.148
(2) Different frames, same film (n = 54)	0.141	5.3	4.7	0.129
(3) Films less than 1 mo. apart (n = 26)	0.143	5.0	5.6	0.219
(4) Films 1 to 6 mo. apart (n = 28)	0.197	8.0	6.7	0.279

* $n = 51$ because an interpolated reference diameter could not be calculated in 3 cases.

Several quantitative coronary arteriographic systems have been validated by measuring objects of known dimension and by repeat measurements to assess reproducibility [13–17]. The input to these systems varies from magnified traced images from cinefilm [13] to digital angiographic images [14] to digitized cinefilms [16, 17]. No system has established itself as clearly superior to the others because detailed comparisons have not yet been done and because other factors such as speed and ease of operation need to be taken into account.

It is important to assess variability under conditions similar to those of the clinical trials where the system will be applied. Accordingly, we assessed the variability of quantitative coronary arteriographic measurements in 21 patients who had two arteriograms 3 to 189 days (mean 72 days) apart. The Cardiovascular Angiographic Analysis System (CAAS) developed by Reiber et al. [16] was used and great care was taken to control the factors that increase variability. All angulations and gantry positions were carefully replicated and nitroglycerin was administered before all coronary injections to optimize coronary vasodilation. Diastolic cine frames with identical angulation that best displayed the stenosis, with maximum sharpness and no vessel overlap were selected.

Reproducibility was assessed in 54 target lesions under 4 different conditions: (1) same film, same frame, (2) same film, same view, different frame, (3) same view from different films obtained within one month, and (4) same view from different films obtained one to 6 months apart. The first of these comparisons measures the intrinsic variability of the computer system alone; the second adds the effect of different mixing of contrast material and slightly different positioning of the artery from one frame to another. The third and fourth comparisons measure short and mid-term variability respectively.

As shown in Table 1, variability, expressed as the standard deviation for

Table 2. Standard deviations for differences in repeated measurements according to stenosis severity and arterial diameter

	n	Minimum diameter (1 SD)			Diameter stenosis (%, 1 SD)		
		Same frame	Different frame	Different film	Same frame	Different frame	Different film
Minimum diameter							
<1 mm	15	0.069	0.134	0.103	2.6	5.1	4.4
1–1.5 mm	24	0.090	0.128	0.181	3.2	4.4	6.7
≥1.5 mm	15	0.085	0.112	0.124	3.1	3.2	6.6
Reference diameter							
<2.5 mm	13	0.085	0.127	0.159	4.0	5.9	7.6
2.5–3 mm	22	0.083	0.123	0.166	3.0	4.4	5.8
≥3 mm	16	0.074	0.160	0.187	2.6	4.1	5.6

differences in repeat measurements, increases progressively from condition (1) to condition (4). When minimum diameter is remeasured from the same frame, reproducibility is excellent with a standard deviation of less than 0.1 mm. This value increases substantially, to 0.141 mm, when repeat measurements are done from different frames of the same film. Variability does not increase further when the frames are taken from different arteriograms filmed within one month, but does increase again when the films are obtained from one to 6 months apart. Some of the increase between short and mid-term variability could be due to changes in the lesions over the mid-term.

The measurement of reference diameter was less reproducible than minimum diameter. Diameter stenosis, the ratio of minimum diameter/reference diameter, exhibited less variability with the interpolated as opposed to the user-defined method of measuring reference diameter. The standard deviation for diameter stenosis increased from 3.2% for same frame comparisons to 6.7% for mid-term variability.

Our results for same-frame measurements are similar to those of Brown et al. (0.1 mm for minimum diameter and 3% for diameter stenosis) [18] and Reiber et al. (0.1 mm and 3.9% respectively) [19]. Reiber et al. also assessed variability from 26 stenoses filmed 3 months apart: the standard deviation for diameter stenosis was 6.5% and for minimum diameter, 0.36 mm [19]. The former value is almost identical to the 6.7% found in our study; however, the latter is almost double the 0.197 mm that we report. The "worst-case" conditions in the study of Reiber et al. probably account for this difference; in particular, they did not rigorously control variables such as the administration of vasodilators before coronary injections.

To determine whether stenosis severity influenced the reproducibility of measurements, the lesions in our study were stratified into those with a minimum diameter >1 mm, those ≥1 mm but < 1.5 mm and those ≥1.5 mm. As shown in Table 2, variability was similar for the 3 categories for both minimum diameter and diameter stenosis measurements. Lesions were also stratified according to the diameter of the artery in the segment containing the stenosis. As shown in Table 2, variability for the measurement of minimum diameter was independent of arterial size. However, for the measurement of diameter stenosis, variability decreased as the size of the vessel increased from <2.5 mm to 2.5–3.0 mm to ⩾3 mm. This finding is not surprising because the arterial diameter is the denominator of diameter stenosis, but minimum diameter is independent of arterial size.

The study of variability is important to establish criteria for progression and regression for trials with repeat arteriography. A difference greater than twice the standard deviation for repeat measurements of mid-term variability will represent a true change with a greater than 95% probability. Thus, the minimum diameter criterion for change of 0.4 mm and the diameter stenosis criterion of ⩾15% appear both reasonable and sufficiently conservative. Indeed, the minimum diameter criterion used in angiographic trials has been 0.4 mm [6, 7], while both 10% [2, 5, 7] and 20% [6] have been used as diameter stenosis criteria.

Selection of specific lesion-related endpoints

The standard of measurement used to define progression and regression could be minimum diameter, stenosis diameter, minimum area, stenosis area, plaque area or plaque volume. Minimum diameter and minimum area are more reproducible than the other potential endpoints because they do not depend upon a measurement of the "normal" arterial dimension. Their major limitation is that they do not take into account the size of the vessel; a 0.4 mm change in a 3 mm artery is functionally much less relevant than a 0.4 mm change in a 1 mm artery. Stenosis diameter is clinically relevant and more widely appreciated but is less reproducible than minimum diameter. In addition, stenosis diameter can falsely underestimate progression: when the arterial lumen narrows diffusely and the minimum diameter remains unchanged, percent diameter stenosis will actually improve. In practice, minimum diameter and stenosis diameter measurements usually yield concordant results.

Plaque area, represented in the figures by the white areas between the stenosis and the interpolated arterial boundary, can be calculated automatically by quantitative systems. Plaque area and its three dimensional derivative, plaque volume, are appealing as endpoints because they seem most directly relevant to regression and also take into account the length of the lesion. However, the measurement of lesion length is not very reproducible [19]. The variability of plaque area measurements has not been reported but is likely to be high because of their dependence on interpolated diameter and lesion length. An intervention that induces a small change in plaque volume would have a major influence upon a severe stenosis and almost none at all upon a very mild lesion.

In summary, no single measurement is ideal. Minimum diameter has the advantage of being simple and highly reproducible. Although less reproducible, stenosis diameter is in wide clinical use and its relevance is well understood.

Patient-based versus lesion-based analyses

The most conservative approach to data analysis is categorical and patient-based; for example, classifying patients as either progressors or non-progressors. Those who experience a coronary event but do not undergo repeat arteriography can be counted as progressors. Using the patient as the unit of analysis yields results that are clinically relevant and statistically sound. With this method, patients who progress at one site and regress at another present a minor problem. They can be grouped with "unchanged" patients (a poor solution), placed in a separate category, or progression and regression can be assessed separately; i.e. analyzing the results for progression while ignoring regression and then doing the opposite.

A lesion-based approach to data analysis is statistically much more powerful. The change in all lesions in the treatment group between the two arteriograms can be compared to the change in all lesions in the control group. Sample size thus increases from the number of patients to the number of lesions. An advantage of this approach is that criteria for progression and regression are not needed. Furthermore, because the endpoint is not categorical, the analysis takes into account both the number of sites with change and the amount of change.

The statistical validity of this method is questionable because lesions are not completely independent of each other; for example, a stenosis that totally occludes will reduce flow in an artery and thus favour progression at other sites. Also, treatment is allocated on a per patient basis but patients contribute varying numbers of lesions to the analysis. A per lesion analysis introduces bias because a patient with 8 stenoses will contribute twice as much data as a patient with only 4. Patients with coronary events who do not undergo repeat arteriography present a problem; in some trials progression has been assumed to occur at all stenoses; however, this conclusion is unjustified and may skew the analysis.

The calculation of a score for each patient combines the patient-based and the lesion-based methods. Using this approach, Brown et al. [2] averaged the most severe stenosis in each of 9 proximal coronary segments to obtain a score for each arteriogram; the change in score for each patient is then compared between groups. Either minimum diameter or stenosis diameter can be meaned for the score. The advantage of this method is that each lesion contributes to the score but the patient remains the unit of analysis. Statistical power is preserved. A minor limitation is that progression and regression tend to cancel each other out so that the score does not distinguish between this circumstance and a patient with no change.

In the clinical trial described in the remainder of this paper, results will be presented as the number of patients with progression or regression of coronary atherosclerosis. A change in minimum lumen diameter of $\geqslant 0.4$ mm is used as the criterion to define a significant change in either direction. Patients with progression at one site and regression at another will be counted both as progressors and as regressors.

The Montreal Heart Institute nicardipine trial

The purpose of this study was to determine whether chronic treatment with nicardipine could influence the progression of coronary atherosclerosis [7, 20]. Patients age 65 or less with stenoses less than 75% in at least 4 coronary artery segments were randomized within one month of baseline coronary arteriography to double-blind therapy with placebo or nicardipine 30 mg 3 times per day. Excluded were those with previous or planned bypass surgery or angioplasty, those with an ejection fraction less than 0.40, severe triple vessel disease or left main stenosis and those requiring a calcium channel blocker. Of the 383 patients enrolled, 335 (87%) underwent repeat coronary arteriography at 24 months with coronary lesions measured quantitatively.

Coronary events (5 deaths, 22 myocardial infarctions and 28 episodes of unstable angina) occurred in 28 of 192 nicardipine patients and 23 of 191 placebo patients ($p = $ NS). The angiographic results of the trial are depicted

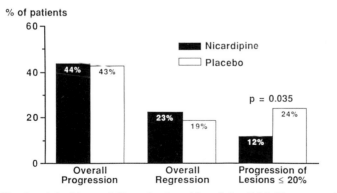

Figure 1. Results of the Montreal Heart Institute Nicardipine Trial. The proportion of patients with progression and the proportion with regression did not differ between nicardipine and placebo groups. Progression and regression were defined as a minimum diameter changes of $\geqslant 0.4$ mm. A patient with one or more progressing lesions was defined as a progressor; a regressor had one or more lesions that regressed. Progression of minimal lesions, defined as those $\leqslant 20\%$ on the first arteriogram, occurred significantly less frequently in nicardipine-treated patients.

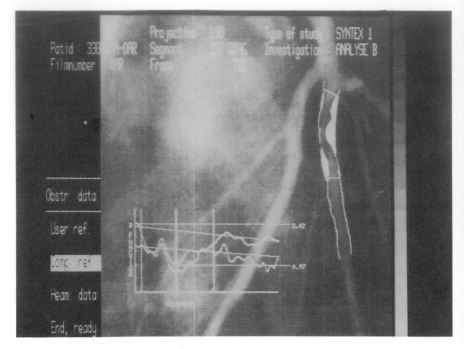

Figure 2a. Left panel.

in Figure 1. Progression, defined as a worsening of minimum diameter by at least 0.4 mm, was detected in 44% of nicardipine and 43% of placebo patients; 23% of nicardipine and 19% of placebo patients experienced regression of one or more lesions. None of these differences approach statistical significance. An example of a coronary stenosis that regressed is shown in Figure 2.

Among the 217 patients with 411 stenoses of 20% or less at the first arteriogram, such minimal lesions progressed in only 15 of 99 nicardipine patients compared to 32 of 118 placebo patients (15 versus 27%, $p = 0.046$). In this subgroup, 16 of 178 minimal lesions in nicardipine patients and 38 of 233 minimal lesions in placebo patients progressed ($p = 0.038$). An example of a minimal lesion that progressed is shown in Figure 3. By stepwise logistic regression analysis, baseline systolic blood pressure ($p = 0.04$) and the change in systolic blood pressure between baseline and 6 months ($p = 0.002$) correlated with progression of minimal lesions. This finding suggests that blood pressure reduction might account for the beneficial effect of nicardipine upon minimal lesions.

Overall, the results of this trial indicate that nicardipine has no effect upon advanced coronary atherosclerosis but may retard the progression of minimal lesions, defined as those less than 20% in stenosis diameter on the first arteriogram.

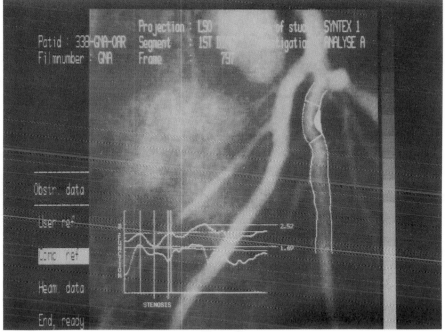

Figure 2b.

Figures 2a–b. Regression of coronary atherosclerosis. This lesion in the first diagonal branch of the left anterior descending coronary artery decreased in severity from a 56% diameter stenosis (left panel) to 23% (right panel) at the second arteriogram. The minimum diameter increased from 0.97 to 1.69 mm.

Other clinical trials of calcium channel blockers and coronary atherosclerosis

The purpose of the International Nifedipine Trial on Antiatherosclerotic Therapy (INTACT) was to assess whether treatment with nifedipine retarded the angiographic progression of coronary atherosclerosis [6]. In 9 European centres, 425 patients with "mild" coronary artery disease were randomly allocated to double-blind therapy with placebo or nifedipine 80 mg per day in divided doses.

The two groups were well matched for clinical variables and 282 of the patients (82%) had repeat arteriography at 3 years. Progression, defined as a decrease of at least 0.4 mm in minimum diameter, was seen in 35% of placebo and 29% of nifedipine-treated patients; 21% of placebo and 16% of nifedipine patients had regression; these differences were not statistically significant.

New coronary lesions, defined as stenoses of less than 20% on the first arteriogram and greater than 20% on the second, developed in 49% of placebo and 40% of nifedipine-treated patients. This difference was not

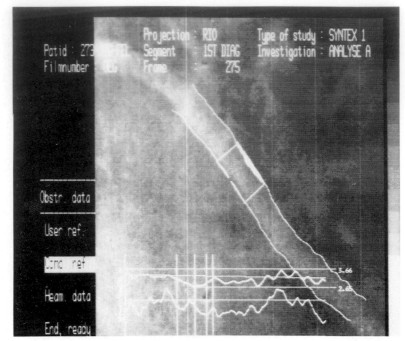

Figure 3a. Left panel.

statistically significant, but new lesions per patient, 0.82 in the placebo and 0.59 in the nifedipine group, represented a 28% reduction with active treatment ($p = 0.034$). Thus, the results of INTACT and of our trial with nicardipine yield concordant results, both with respect to established lesions, which were not influenced by dihydropyridine calcium channel blocker therapy, and for early lesions, where drug therapy reduced progression.

Loaldi et al. [21] compared the evolution of coronary atherosclerosis over 2 years in patients taking nifedipine to those taking isosorbide dinitrate or propranolol. Progression occurred less commonly in nifedipine patients compared to the other two groups and on a per lesion basis, nifedipine was associated with significantly more regression. This study was neither randomized nor blinded and the number of patients in each of the treatment groups was small. The results were not confirmed either by INTACT or by our trial with nicardipine.

Coronary atherosclerosis developing after cardiac transplantation is a major clinical problem that limits the long-term prognosis of these patients. The pathological appearance of these lesions differs from ordinary coronary atherosclerosis and the causative mechanisms may also be different. A preliminary report from an ongoing randomized study indicates that diltiazem may prevent the development of this type of atherosclerosis [22].

The effect of nifedipine upon the development of atherosclerosis in coron-

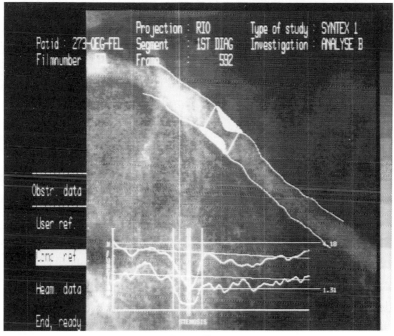

Figure 3b.

Figures 3a–b. Progression of a minimal coronary stenosis. The first arteriogram (left panel) revealed a minimal lesion in a diagonal branch of the left anterior descending coronary artery. Repeat arteriography at 2 years showed progression; the diameter stenosis has increased from 19% to 64% and the minimum diameter has decreased from 2.65 to 1.31 mm.

ary bypass grafts is being assessed in a randomized, double-blind, placebo-controlled trial. A preliminary report [23] suggests that nifedipine has a beneficial effect on graft lesions: 52% of placebo grafts and 67% of grafts in nifedipine-treated patients were free of lesions at one year in the first 64 patients with follow-up angiography ($p = 0.04$).

Calcium entry blockers and coronary atherosclerosis in perspective

The clinical trials completed to date demonstrate that calcium entry blockers do not influence the evolution of established coronary atherosclerosis but appear to prevent the progression of early lesions. This conclusion is tentative because it is based on only two studies. Whether this beneficial effect is a feature of all calcium entry blockers or only dihydropyridines is as yet unknown. The combined effect of lipid-lowering therapy and a calcium entry blocker upon human coronary atherosclerosis has not yet been investigated.

A major limitation of this type of clinical trial is that coronary arteriography provides limited information. Although quantitative techniques can accurately assess changes in the severity of arterial narrowings [24], the arterial wall and its pathology are not directly visualized. Newer techniques, specifically angioscopy [25, 26] and intravascular ultrasound [27, 28], circumvent this limitation and will eventually yield data on lesion changes to complement coronary arteriography. Although both of these techniques are now in their infancy, intravascular ultrasound is theoretically superior to angioscopy because it does not require a blood-free field of vision and displays the entire thickness of the vessel wall, not just the surface.

Progression and regression of coronary atherosclerosis are complex processes that are oversimplified by coronary arteriographic images. Progression may be initiated by rupture of a plaque with rapid accretion of thrombus onto the exposed surface, followed by lesion remodelling. How often progression is due to this type of event, as opposed to slow plaque growth by accumulation of lipids and cellular components, is unknown. Analogously, regression may result from the disappearance or remodelling of thrombus, or from the removal of plaque lipid and cellular elements. These processes could be influenced at many points by different interventions. For example, a drug that promotes stability of the fibrous cap of the atherosclerotic plaque and thus prevents plaque rupture might provide more benefit than a drug that induces regression. The ability of beta-adrenergic blockers to reduce the rate of reinfarction in infarct survivors by approximately 25% may be the consequence of a reduction in shear forces on the fibrous cap. Further studies are likely to yield on array of drugs that exert a favourable influence upon the evolution of coronary atherosclerosis, by acting upon different components of the atherosclerotic process.

References

1. Brensike JF, Levy RI, Kelsey SF, et al. Effects of therapy with cholestyramine on progression of coronary arteriosclerosis: results of the NHLBI Type II Coronary Intervention Study. Circulation 1984; **69**: 313–24.
2. Brown G, Albers JJ, Fisher LD, et al. Regression of coronary artery disease as a result of intensive lipid-lowering therapy in men with high levels of apolipoprotein B. N Engl J Med 1990; **323**: 1289–98.
3. Buchwald H, Varco RL, Matts JP, et al. Effect of partial ileal bypass surgery on mortality and morbidity from coronary heart disease in patients with hypercholesterolemia. N Engl J Med 1990; **323**: 946–55.
4. Cashin-Hemphill L, Mack WJ, Pogoda JM, Sanmarco ME, Azen SP, Blankenhorn DH. Beneficial effects of colestipol-niacin on coronary atherosclerosis. JAMA 1990; **264**: 3013–7.
5. Kane JP, Malloy MJ, Ports TA, Phillips NR, Diehl JC, Havel RJ. Regression of coronary atherosclerosis during treatment of familial hypercholesterolemia with combined drug regimens. JAMA 1990; **264**: 3007–12.
6. Lichtlen PR, Hugenholtz PG, Rafflenbeul W, Hecker H, Jost S, Deckers JW on behalf of the INTACT group investigators. Retardation of angiographic progression of coronary artery disease by nifedipine. Lancet 1990; **335**: 1109–13.

7. Waters D, Lespérance J, Francetich M, et al. A controlled clinical trial to assess the effect of a calcium channel blocker on the progression of coronary atherosclerosis. Circulation 1990; **82**: 1940–53.

8. Chesebro JH, Webster MWI, Smith HC, et al. Antiplatelet therapy in coronary disease progression reduced infarction and new lesion formation. Circulation 1989; **80** (Suppl II): II–266 (Abstract).

9. Blankenhorn DH, Brooks SH. Angiographic trials of lipid-lowering therapy. Arteriosclerosis 1981; **1**: 242–9.

10. Little WC, Constantinescu M, Applegate RJ, et al. Can coronary angiography predict the site of a subsequent myocardial infarction in patients with mild-to-moderate coronary artery disease? Circulation 1988; **78**: 1157–66.

11. Taeymans Y, Théroux P, Lespérance J, Waters D. Quantitative angiographic morphology of the coronary artery lesions at risk of thrombotic occlusion. Circulation 1992; **85**: 78–85.

12. Zeiher AM, Drexler H, Wollschlager H, Just H. Modulation of coronary vasomotor tone in humans. Circulation 1991; **83**: 391–401.

13. Brown BG, Bolson EL, Dodge HT. Arteriographic assessment of coronary atherosclerosis. Review of current methods, their limitations, and clinical applications. Arteriosclerosis 1982; **2**: 1–15.

14. Mancini GBJ, Simon SB, McGillem MJ, LeFree MT, Friedman HZ, Vogel RA. Automated quantitative coronary arteriography: morphologic and physiologic validation in vivo of a rapid digital angiographic method. Circulation 1987; **75**: 452–60.

15. Nichols AB, Gabrieli CFO, Fenoglio JJ, Esser PD. Quantification of relative coronary arterial stenosis by cinevideodensitometric analysis of coronary arteriograms. Circulation 1984; **69**: 512–22.

16. Reiber JHC, Kooijman CJ, Slager CJ, et al. Coronary artery dimensions from cineangiograms – methodology and validation of a computer-assisted analysis procedure. IEEE Transactions on Medical Imaging 1984; **MI–3**: 131–40.

17. Ellis S, Sanders W, Goulet C, et al. Optimal detection of the progression of coronary artery disease: comparison of methods suitable for risk factor intervention trials. Circulation 1986; **74**: 1235–42.

18. Brown BG, Bolson E, Frimer M, Dodge HT. Quantitative coronary arteriography. Estimation of dimensions, hemodynamic resistance, and atheroma mass of coronary artery lesions using the arteriogram and digital computation. Circulation 1977; **55**: 329–37.

19. Reiber JHC, Serruys PW, Kooijman CJ, et al. Assessment of short-, medium-, and long-term variations in arterial dimensions from computer-assisted quantitation of coronary cineangiograms. Circulation 1985; **71**: 280–88.

20. Waters D, Freedman D, Lespérance J, et al. Design features of a controlled clinical trial to assess the effect of a calcium entry blocker upon the progression of coronary artery disease. Contr Clin Trials 1987; **8**: 216–42.

21. Loaldi A, Polese A, Montorsi P, et al. Comparison of nifedipine, propranolol and isosorbide dinitrate on angiographic progression and regression of coronary arterial narrowings in angina pectoris. Am J Cardiol 1989; **64**: 433–9.

22. Schroeder JS, Gao SZ, Alderman EL, Hunt SA, Stinson E. Diltiazem inhibits development of early accelerated transplant coronary disease. An interim report. Circulation 1990; **82** (Suppl III): III–257 (Abstract).

23. Gottlieb SO, Brinker JA, Mellits ED, et al. Effect of nifedipine on the development of coronary bypass graft stenoses in high-risk patients: A randomized, double-blind, placebo-controlled trial. Circulation 1989; **80** (Suppl II): II–228 (Abstract).

24. Waters D, Lespérance J, Hudon G, Craven TE. Advantages and limitations of serial coronary arteriography for the assessment of progression and regression of coronary atherosclerosis: Implications for clinical trials. Circulation (in press).

25. Ramee SR, White CJ, Collins TJ, Mesa JE, Murgo JP. Percutaneous angioscopy during coronary angioplasty using a steerable microangioscope. J Am Coll Cardiol 1991; **17**: 100–5.

26. Mizuno K, Miyamoto A, Satomura K, et al. Angioscopic coronary macromorphology in patients with acute coronary disorders. Lancet 1991; **337**: 809–12.
27. Gussenhoven EJ, Essed CE, Lancée CT, et al. Arterial wall characteristics determined by intravascular ultrasound imaging: An in vitro study. J Am Coll Cardiol 1989; **14**: 947–52.
28. Potkin BN, Bartorelli AL, Gessert JM, et al. Coronary artery imaging with intravascular high-frequency ultrasound. Circulation 1990; **81**: 1575–85.

17. Computer quantitative measurements of CLAS coronary angiograms compared to evaluation by panels of human angiographers

ROBERT H. SELZER, DAVID H. BLANKENHORN,
ANNE M. SHIRCORE, PAUL L. LEE, JANICE M. PAGODA,
WENDY J. MACK, and STANLEY P. AZEN

Summary

CLAS, a placebo controlled trial of Colestipol/Niacin therapy in men with previous coronary artery bypass surgery, obtained 188 baseline, 162 two year and 103 four year angiograms. Human panel readers evaluated all films with treatment assignment and film order masked. All lesions in native arteries and grafts were identified, assigned percent stenosis estimates, lesion change estimates and an overall change score. In a 50% random sample, all processable segments have been computer evaluated with multiple lesion and segment based algorithms derived by the USC-Caltech/JPL method. Among nonocclusive lesions, 350 were evaluated for percent stenosis by panel and computer methods with correlation between the two methods of 0.70 $p < 0.0001$). Four hundred forty-two lesions (principally more severe) could only be evaluated by humans. Seventy-nine early lesions could be evaluated only by computer. Seven hundred thirty-one native coronary segments were analyzed by QCA including 302 segments without discrete lesions in addition to the 429 segments with discrete lesions that were compared with the panel evaluation. After accounting for baseline effects, position relative to grafts and within subject correlation, significant therapy effects were demonstrated by computer measures of both stenosis and vessel edge roughness. These data confirm that computer analsis of angiograms can reduce subject numbers compared to human panel reading and offer different endpoint measures.

Introduction

The Cholesterol Lowering Atherosclerosis Study (CLAS) was a randomized, controlled clinical trial testing niacin/colestipol plus diet therapy in non-smoking men with previous coronary bypass surgery. Coronary arteries were visualized in 162 patients at baseline and after two treatment years (CLAS-I). Biplane films at 60 frames/second were obtained using standardized 30 degree RAO and 60 degree LAO views and additional views as needed.

J.H.C. Reiber and P.W. Serruys (eds), Advances in Quantitative Coronary Arteriography, 299–310.
© 1993 *Kluwer Academic Publishers. Printed in the Netherlands.*

A coronary endpoint determination by a panel of human readers, used for safety monitoring during conduct of CLAS-I, was the first endpoint reported [1]. Quantitative Coronary Angiography (QCA) has been applied to all processable segments of a in a 50% random sample of the 162 angiogram pairs using multiple lesion and segment based algorithms derived by the USC-Caltech/JPL method [2].

In this paper, we compare human panel reading and QCA measurements of stenosis in 85 film pairs evaluated by both methods. We show that film evaluation by human panel readers and QCA are complementary procedures assessing information in different but overlapping sets of coronary lesions. In addition, the application of a QCA segment-based analysis is described.

Methods

Panel evaluation of angiograms

The CLAS panel reading method has been previously described. [3, 4] In brief, a panel consisted of a moderator and two readers who evaluated paired coronary films (Film A mounted on the left projector and Film B mounted on the right projector as set by predetermined randomization). Each reader (masked to treatment assignment and to the true temporal order of films) independently identified and estimated lesion size (percent stenosis) of all lesions on Film A. Visible lesions believed to be <20% were recorded as 20%. Next, a consensus diagram of Film A was created after open discussion by the two readers with the moderator. Using the Film A consensus diagram as a guide, the readers then independently viewed Film B to evaluate changes in lesion size as well as to identify and estimate additional lesions, if any, not apparent on Film A. Another open discussion took place and a consensus diagram of changes observed in Film B was created. All lesions were uniquely labeled on this diagram for subsequent analyses with QCA.

Quantitative Coronary Angiography

Details of the methods for QCA have been previously described [2]. QCA employs dual projectors as seen in Figure 1. The baseline film is mounted on the left projector and the two year angiogram on the right projector. Each projector is equipped with a 1024 line vidicon camera whose video output is fed to an image digitizer contained in a Megavision 1024C image processing system. The angiographic view of each segment was matched on both films for orientation and degree of contrast filling. Arterial segments were defined from branch to branch. Three sequential frames exposed during end-diastole were digitized unless unobstructed, matched end-diastolic frames could not be found; in that case, three sequential frames from other phases of the cardiac cycle were used.

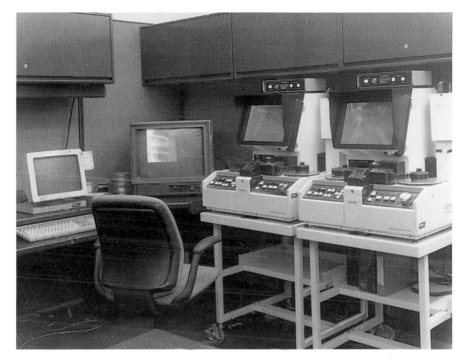

Figure 1. Projector system used for QCA.

To find the edges of a vessel, the computer operator first identified the approximate vessel midline with a cursor. The computer algorithm then searched perpendicular to this midline to find points of maximum intensity gradient. The search was restricted to a window of pixel values centered on the prior detected edge point.

All edge coordinates were corrected for pincushion distortion with a one centimeter grid filmed at the beginning of each angiogram. Since the grid was filmed in the A-P view with the X-ray system used to obtain RAO views, images from this system were selected for QCA processing whenever possible. Ninty-three percent of the processed frames came RAO 15, 30 and 45 degree views and 7% from the corresponding LAO views obtained with the orthogonal X-ray cine system.

To avoid over-estimation of narrow points within segments the number of pixels used to calculate intensity gradients was adjusted from 5 to 13 according to the average width of the previous five vessel diameters. Computed intensity gradients for edge location were smoothed over 3 to 7 pixels, depending on the size of the moving window. To reduce the effect of multiple gradient maxima/minima in a single scan line (typically due to branches or nearby vessels), an exponential weighting function, centered at a distance from the midline corresponding to the prior edge location, was applied to

CORONARY ROUGHNESS

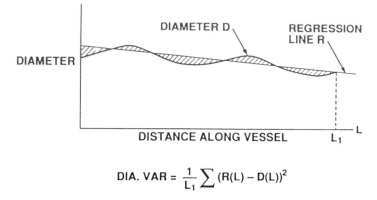

$$\text{DIA. VAR} = \frac{1}{L_1} \sum (R(L) - D(L))^2$$

Figure 2. Coronary roughness definition.

the smoothed gradient values. The coordinates of the maximum weighted gradient was selected as the edge point. To reduce technician-associated variability in selecting the initial midline, each edge search was repeated using a new computer-generated midline derived from initially detected edges. All diameters were converted to mm by a scaling factor using the known diameter of the catheter and corrections from a radiographic grid.

QCA measurements

For each film, all processable segments were tracked and evaluated. A series of measurements derived from diameter information was obtained for each segment and averaged over the three sequential frames. The major measurements are described below:

Percent Stenosis
Segment stenosis was measured using the 3rd and 90th percentile of the diameter profile as estimates of minimum and reference diameter. That is, Percent Stenosis = $(1-D3/D90) \times 100$.

Roughness
As shown in Figure 2, roughness was defined as the root-mean-square difference between the diameter profile and a minimum least square straight line fit to the profile.

CORONARY DISEASE LENGTH AND PERCENT DISEASE INVOLVEMENT

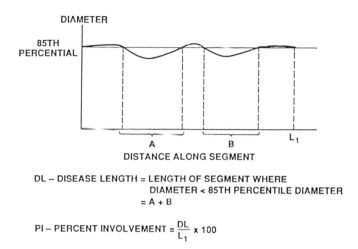

DL – DISEASE LENGTH = LENGTH OF SEGMENT WHERE
               DIAMETER < 85TH PERCENTILE DIAMETER
               = A + B

PI – PERCENT INVOLVEMENT = $\frac{DL}{L_1}$ x 100

Figure 3. Definition of coronary disease length and percent disease involvement.

Diseased roughness
Roughness restricted to segments with an identified lesion of 20% or more.

Percent involvement
As shown in Figure 3, Disease Length, DL, was defined and the length of a segment whose diameter values were less than the 85th percentile of all diameters measured over the entire segment of length L_1. Percent Involvement, PI, was defined as $D_L/L_1 \times 100$.

Average diameter
Average of all measured diameters within a segment.

Measurement acceptance criteria

The coefficient of variation of the three sequential frame measurements of average and minimum diameter was calculated for every segment and used to monitor image and edge tracking quality. When the coefficient of variation of the average diameter exceeded 5 percent or that of the minimum diameter exceeded 13 percent, the computer indicated to the operator that questionable data had been generated. At this point, the operator reviewed the edge tracking of the frames in question and corrected detectable errors such as overlooked crossing vessel shadows. If the edge tracking problems could not be corrected, for example if the segment was not uniformly opacified, was

COMPARISON OF LESION SIZE
BY PANEL AND QCA

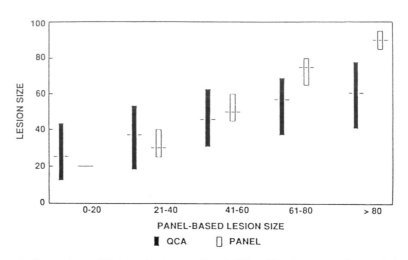

Figure 4. Comparison of lesion size by panel and QCA. The bottom and top of the bar represents the 5th to 95th percentile, the horizontal line through the bar represents the median.

too small or the film contrast was too poor, the operator decided the segment was not measurable and marked the entry in the database as unacceptable.

Comparison of QCA and panel evaluation

Of the 731 native segments analyzed by QCA, 429 segments had nonocclusive discrete lesions and a measurable reference diameter that made it possible to calculate percent stenosis. The values of QCA for these segments were compared with stenosis values obtained by the human panel. The conditions under which percent stenosis could not be measured are discussed below.

Of the 429 lesions measured with QCA, 350 were also recognized and measured by the panel and 79 were not identified or measured by the panel. An additional 442 lesions were measured by the panel but could not be measured by QCA.

Lesions measured by both QCA and the panel

A comparison of the panel and QCA measurement of lesion size for the 350 lesions measured by both is shown in Figure 4. As seen in this figure, there is reasonably good agreement for lesions with stenosis less than 60% but for panel estimate of stenosis greater than 60%, QCA stenosis measures are

COMPARISON OF CHANGE IN LESION
SIZE BY PANEL AND QCA

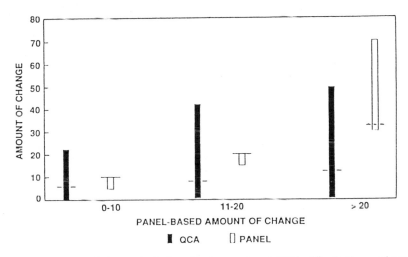

Figure 5. Comparison of change in lesion size by panel and QCA. The bottom and top of the bar represents the 5th to 95th percentile, the horizontal line through the bar represents the median.

consistently lower than that of the panel. Panel estimates of stenosis change are also generally higher than those for QCA, as seen in Figure 5.

A categorical comparison of the QCA and panel methods was carried out by defining lesion progression from baseline to the year 02 angiogram as a stenosis increase of at least 10% (ex. from 40% to 50%) and regression as decrease of at least 10%. For 56 lesions the panel classified as regressing, QCA classified 54 as regressing and 2 as progressing. For 53 lesions the panel found as progressing, QCA classified 50 as progressing and 3 as regressing.

Lesions measured by the panel but not by QC
There are a number of reasons why lesions identified by the panel were not QCA measurable. A major reason was the inability of the computer to measure lesions with greater than 90% stenosis because of the difficulty of reliably tracking the edge of the vessel image when the width of the vessel image was only a few pixels. As discussed above, the edge finding algorithm required computation of intensity adients over 5 to 13 pixels. Thus vessels narrower than 0.2–0.3 mm (about 3–4 pixels) could not be measured.

Another important difference between the QCA and panel method relates to identification of the "normal" reference used to compute stenosis. In 46 of the total of 731 segments processed by QCA, measurement of the reference diameter was designated invalid by the operator because the segments were

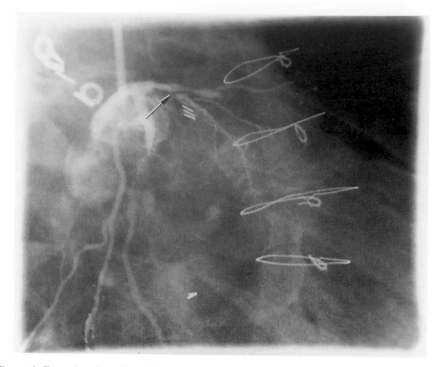

Figure 6. Example of angiographic image illustrating tight stenosis and diffuse disease that cannot be reliably measured by QCA (see arrow.)

ectatic or has severe diffuse disease that left no portion of the segment normal. Stenosis was not computed for these segments although other measures not dependent on the reference diameter such as average diameter and roughness were computed. It is not clear how the panel estimated the reference diameter for segments such as those described above but one possibility is they utilized information from segments proximal or distal to the one being analyzed. Figure 6 illustrates a case where the lumen is too narrow to track and in addition, a meaningful reference diameter is not evident.

Other factors that prevented a lesion from being analyzed by QCA included crossing vessels or other overlapping artifacts such as sternum clips, incomplete mixing of the contrast media or poor segment visualization due to low image contrast. In general, this type of problem made edge tracking difficult or impossible but did not create as much of a problem for the human panel members since the panel could compensate by "seeing through" the artifacts or by mentally integrating information from a sequence of images.

Lesions measured by QCA but not by the panel

The 79 lesions evaluated by QCA but not recognized by the panel were significantly different from lesions evaluated by both QCA and panel with

QCA MEANS (SD), BY-SEGMENT
PARAMETERS – NATIVE ARTERIES

PARAMETER	DRUG			PLACEBO			
	BASELINE	TWO-YEAR	WITHIN	BASELINE	TWO-YEAR	WITHIN	BETWEEN
3rd PCT. DIAMETER (mm)	1.76 (0.76)	1.77 (0.82)	NS	1.76 (0.71)	1.75 (0.73)	NS	NS
PERCENT STENOSIS (%)	34.50 (14.82)	32.71 (14.30)	0.003	32.52 (13.45)	34.12 (16.47)	0.055	0.002
PERCENT INVOLVEMENT (%)	39.95 (19.68)	37.37 (20.83)	0.009	39.08 (20.92)	37.54 (20.01)	NS	NS
ROUGHNESS x 10 (mm^2)	2.34 (1.33)	2.26 (1.27)	0.03	2.19 (1.22)	2.23 (1.28)	NS	NS
DISEASED ROUGHNESS x 10 (mm^2)	2.45 (1.28)	2.34 (1.26)	0.02	2.31 (1.15)	2.34 (1.22)	NS	0.02

SEGMENTS MEASURED: 281 TO 364
SUBJECTS: 41-44

Figure 7. Per-segment change, baseline-2 year, for native arteries. Means (standard deviations) shown. P-values shown in columns labeled WITHIN and BETWEEN.

regard to size ($p < 0.001$) and location ($p < 0.001$). Lesions located by QCA but not by the panel were smaller in size and were more prevalent in branches of the right coronary. In addition, there were a number of cases where the panel found small lesions (20–40%) to have regressed to zero while the QCA found these lesions to be unchanged and to have stenosis.

QCA as a endpoint in the CLAS study

A total of 731 native coronary artery segments and 349 graft segments were processed from the baseline and year 02 films of 85 subjects. Analysis of change in five QCA measures shown in Figure 7 indicates that for the drug group, percent stenosis, percent involvement, roughness and diseased roughness show significant changes in the direction of decreased disease while for the placebo group, percent stenosis shows a significant change in the direction of increasing disease. Further, a significant difference between the drug and placebo group is shown for percent stenosis and diseased roughness. Note that percent involvement and minumum diameter (3rd percent diameter) did not show significant change within or between groups. As seen in Figure 8, no significant measured changes were observed for bypass grafts.

A regression analysis was carried out to identify segment characteristics such as segment type, location and graft status predictive of the two-year outcome regardless of treatment assignment. For each significant segment

QCA MEANS (SD), BY-SEGMENT
PARAMETERS – GRAFTS

PARAMETER	DRUG BASELINE	DRUG TWO-YEAR	DRUG WITHIN	PLACEBO BASELINE	PLACEBO TWO-YEAR	PLACEBO WITHIN	BETWEEN
3rd PCT. DIAMETER (mm)	(3.32 (0.92)	3.38 (0.92)	NS	3.05 (1.00)	3.11 (1.01)	NS	NS
PERCENT STENOSIS (%)	24.46 (10.93)	25.13 (12.89)	NS	25.88 (13.57)	27.37 (16.36)	0.04	NS
PERCENT INVOLVEMENT (%)	26.03 (22.15)	26.37 (22.71)	NS	24.82 (22.18)	27.03 (23.48)	0.01	NS
ROUGHNESS x 10 (mm^2)	2.90 (1.64)	2.93 (1.75)	NS	2.80 (2.06)	2.94 (2.01)	0.02	NS
DISEASED ROUGHNESS x 10 (mm^2)	3.39 (1.48)	3.45 (1.63)	NS	3.41 (1.88)	3.58 (1.94)	NS	NS

SEGMENTS MEASURED: 84-184
SUBJECTS: 32-42

Figure 8. Per-segment change, baseline-2 year, for bypass grafts. Means (standard deviations) shown. P-values shown in columns labeled WITHIN and BETWEEN. Each graft was divided into 3 equal lengths for analysis.

characteristic, a treatment effect size was calculated as the absolute difference in mean change over two years divided by the pooled variance. As shown in Figure 9, drug treatment was most strongly reflected by percent stenosis in vessels proximal to grafts and hemodynamically related (HR). A segment was defined as being hemodynamically related to a graft if it carried blood that mixed with blood from the graft. Drug treatment was also significantly reflected in the minimum diameter and roughness of segments proximal to grafts and HR. Percent stenosis and roughness of native coronary artery segments were also predictive of treatment.

Discussion

If percent stenosis is used as a measure of coronary atherosclerosis in clinical trials, film evaluation by panel readers tends to be more effective than QCA for high grade stenosis where a normal reference diameter cannot be measured or where the vessel is narrowed to the point where edge tracking cannot be accomplished. Conversely, the 79 lesions identified and evaluated by QCA but not by the panel were principally early lesions. This suggests that the two methods derive information from different but overlapping sets of coronary lesions and that the best available estimate of segment stenosis

TREATMENT EFFECT SIZE FOR
QCA MEASURES

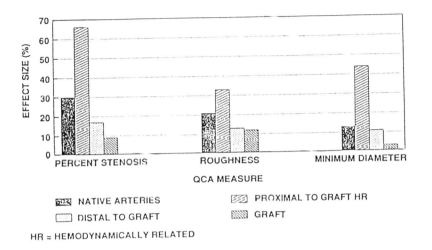

Figure 9. Treatment effect size for QCA measures.

in a population under study in a clinical trial might be obtained using both methods.

Percent stenosis is the most commonly used measure of coronary disease for both panel evaluation and QCA and has the advantages of being essentially independent of image magnification and allowing comparison of the two methods. On the other hand, there are some limitations to percent stenosis that may be important. In particular, if compensatory dilation of coronary arteries and accompanying wall thickening occurs in early stages of atherosclerosis, as described by Glagov [5], percent stenosis will not be sensitive to disease until the ratio of lumen area to lumen plus wall area is less than 60%. If this pre-stenotic early wall thickening does not occur uniformly along the artery, which is a reasonable assumption given the appearance of stenotic lesions, a wall roughness measurement similar to that described in this paper may provide a means to assess early disease not detectable with percent stenosis.

The fact that substantial numbers of segments could be evaluated by the panel but not by QCA is on first inspection rather disturbing. However, it should be pointed out that the segments rejected for QCA were generally poor quality images that would result in high variability for any derived measurements. To state the argument in reverse, imposing acceptance criteria, as described above, results in QCA measurements that are more reliable than would be the case if poor quality images were allowed to be analyzed.

The value of QCA measurements in clinical trials may be enhanced by greater ability to measure changes in small lesions. Although angiographic trials are conducted in subjects with symptomatic coronary disease (who have relatively advanced lesions), a bonus which should be exploited is the chance to study formation and growth in early lesions because this might lead to more effective primary atherosclerosis prevention. As shown by the ability of QCA measurements to detect significant drug effects in CLAS from a sample of half of the study population, QCA may make it possible to reduce the required sample size in clinical trials.

Acknowledgment

The research described in this paper was carried out by the Jet Propulsion Laboratory, California Institute of Technology and the University of Southern California School of Medicine and was sponsored in part by the National Heart, Blood and Lung Institute Program Project Grant HL 23619, through an agreement with the National Aeronautics and Space Administration.

References

1. Blankenhorn DH, Nessim SA, Johnson RL, Sanmarco ME, Azen SP, Cashin-Hemphill L. Beneficial effects of combined colestipol-niacin therapy on coronary atherosclerosis and coronary venous bypass grafts. JAMA 1987; 257: 3233–3240. [published erratum appears in JAMA 1988; **259**: 12698].
2. Selzer RH, Hagerty C, Azen SP, et al. Precision and reproducibility of quantitative coronary angiography with applications to controlled clinical trials: A sampling study. J Clin Invest 1989; **83**: 520–6.
3. Blankenhorn DH, Johnson RL, Nessim SA, Azen SP, Sanmarco ME, Selzer RH. The Cholesterol Lowering Atherosclerosis Study (CLAS): design, methods, and baseline results. Controlled Clin Trials 1987; **8**: 354–87.
4. Azen SP, Cashin-Hemphill L, Pogoda JM, et al. An evaluation of human panelists in assessing coronary atherosclerosis. Arterioscler Thromb 1991; **11**: 385–94.
5. Glagov S, Weisenberg E, Zarins CK, Stankunavicius R, Kolettis GJ. Compensatory enlargement of human atherosclerotic coronary arteries. N Engl J Med 1987; **316**: 1371–5.

18. A maximum confidence strategy for measuring progression and regression of coronary artery disease in clinical trials

B. GREG BROWN, LYNN A. HILLGER, XUE-QIAO ZHAO, DIANNE SACCO, BRAD BISSON and LLOYD FISHER

Supported in part by grants (P01 HL 30086 and R01 HL 19451) from the National Heart, Lung, and Blood Institute and by a grant from the John L. Locke, Jr. Charitable Trust, Seattle, WA

Summary

The FATS trial compared three lipid-lowering strategies in 120 patients having atherosclerotic lesions of varying severity in 1034 proximal coronary segments. Film pairs (2.5 year interval) were viewed together in a dual projection system at five-fold magnification by two observers blinded to identity, treatment, and film sequence. Two frames per film were selected from comparable views as representative images of each lesion. Lesions were visually classified by consensus as "not-," "definitely-," or "possibly-changed" and then rapidly calipered (nearest 5% S(tenosis)). For "possibly changed" lesions, a third frame was selected. The borders of each selected lesion image and the catheter were traced by a technician (two techs each traced the 3 "possible" frames), reviewed for accuracy, and the tracings measured (QCA) for minimum diameter and percent stenosis. For 16 lesions, major discrepancies between the two methods dictated a fully blinded repeat analysis.

In the comparison of semi-quantitative visual (SQ-VIS) versus QCA estimates of change, lesions classified as "not-," "possibly-," or "definitely-changed" were measured to change by $\geq 10\%$ stenosis in 0.3%, 11%, and 81% of cases, respectively. By a logistic regression analysis, 9.3% stenosis (we use 10%) was identified as the "best" measured value for distinguishing "definite" from "no" change.

The primary outcome analysis of the FATS trial, employing a continuous variable estimate of %S change, gave virtually the same favorable result whether the assessment of disease change was by QCA ($p = 0.0028$) or by the SQ-VIS method ($p = 0.0033$). A secondary outcome analysis, categorizing patients as showing "progression only" or "regression only" also gave vir-

J.H.C. Reiber and P.W. Serruys (eds), Advances in Quantitative Coronary Arteriography, 311–326.
© 1993 *Kluwer Academic Publishers. Printed in the Netherlands.*

tually the same results using, as a criterion for true change, either $\geq 10\%$ S change, $\geq 9.3\%$ S change, or "definite" change. Frequency of clinical cardiovascular events was reduced by 73% among the intensively treated patients.

The excellent agreement between these two fundamentally different methods of disease change assessment (after reconciliation of occasional major discrepancies), and the concordance between disease change and clinical outcomes, serves to greatly strengthen the confidence in these measurement techniques and in the overall findings of this study. These observations have important implications for the design of clinical trials with arteriographic end-points.

Quantitative analysis of atherosclerosis change

Arterial imaging trials, commonly using arteriography, have been shown to be effective alternatives to clinical endpoint studies for determining the natural history of, and the effect of therapy upon atherosclerotic vascular disease [1–13]. This approach is particularly attractive, because it permits studies which require only 100-to-200 patients to determine a treatment benefit to arterial obstruction, instead of the several thousand needed in order to demonstrate a substantial clinical benefit [14–16]. Furthermore, arteriographic approaches permit a more direct assessment of the mechanisms of benefit. While the arteriogram does not visualize the components of the atherosclerotic plaque (collagen, lipid, macrophage, smooth muscle, and thrombus) changes in arteriographic lumen dimensions are a reflection of change in these components.

Certain morphologic clues regarding the mechanisms of abrupt disease progression are also provided by the arteriogram. For example, thrombus can be visualized, or its presence inferred from the arteriogram [12, 17], as well as plaque ulceration and hemorrhage into the plaque. Responsiveness to vasoactive agents can be determined as an indication of the adequacy of "vascular function." Thus, these morphologic features and vasomotor responsiveness add mechanistic information beyond that provided simply by changes in measured lumen caliber.

One problem with quantitative arteriographic approaches to the study of disease progression is the lack of consensus on what endpoint measure(s) constitutes a meaningful change in arterial disease. Whereas clinical endpoints are usually straightforward in their definition (there is seldom a question that a patient has died of a cardiac event or has had an acute myocardial infarction) we have yet to establish standardized approaches to the QCA studies; and there is relatively little carefully obtained data on disease progression to provide a clear basis for judging studies. Quantitative arteriography is now performed by a number of centers, many of which have different standards for disease progression and many of which have different technical approaches to making these measurements. How, then, should we interpret a statement that "15% of all lesions (or patients) worsened" in a given treatment group? The gold standard for disease change is the pathology; but it is impossible to conduct serial pathological studies of atherosclerosis progression or regression. Intravascular ultrasound [18-20] may provide some of these answers, but it is presently not widely-used or well-standardized. Despite its limitations, arteriography is presently the most widely-used imaging technique and is the most accurate method for defining lumen caliber. It appears to be the natural medium by which to study the course of obstructive atherosclerosis in man. Our group has spent the past 15 years developing approaches to certain of the thorny issues which must be addressed in the performance of disease progression trials. The culmination of these efforts was the analysis performed in the FATS trial [8], a clinical study in which aggressive lipid-lowering therapy has been shown to reduce the frequency of disease progression per patient, and increase the frequency of observed regression, in comparison with a conventionally treated patient group. In this report, we detail the strategy used for arteriographic analysis in FATS. With it, we attempted to address most of the important methodologic and outcome questions in at least two different ways which, together, provide internal checks on the accuracy of the analysis. Thus the strength of the analysis described is its *consistency* in obtaining essentially the same answer by more than one approach to a given question. This internal consistency assures us of the robustness of the analysis and provides maximum confidence that the observations described are, indeed, correct.

Familial atherosclerosis treatment study (FATS)

Patients. The study has been described in detail elsewhere [8]. Briefly, 146 men, 62 years of age or younger, with elevated apolipoprotein B levels and a family history of premature cardiovascular disease were assigned randomly to one of three therapeutic strategies. For entry, patients must have evidence of coronary atherosclerosis on arteriogram, a family history of premature cardiovascular disease, and an apolipoprotein B level of 125 mg/dl or greater. This is approximately the 88th population percentile for a 47 year old man [21]. Between January 1984 and September 1989, 120 patients were enrolled and completed the protocol, including an arteriogram done at baseline and again 2.5 years later. Patients were treated with niacin and colestipol or with lovastatin and colestipol; these two treatment groups were called, "intensive" lipid-lowering therapy. A "conventionally" treated control group was given placebos unless the LDL-cholesterol was above the 90th percentile for age, in which case, active colestipol was given. Patients were seen monthly and were professionally counseled in the AHA Step I, or II, diet at the Northwest Lipid Research Clinic during the first year of follow-up, and were subsequently seen bi-monthly. Lipid and lipoprotein response to these three forms of therapy were determined in detail.

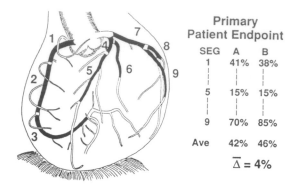

Figure 1. Location of nine standard proximal segments of the coronary anatomy. The lesion causing the worst stenosis in each of these segments was measured; the average percent stenosis among these segments was computed, and the mean change in this value between the two studies (time points A and B) was determined ($\Delta\% S_{prox}$). This estimate of the mean change in the severity of proximal stenosis (here 4 percent) was made for each patient.

Coronary arteriography. At the baseline catheterization, five views of the left coronary artery (10° RAO, 45° LAO with 30° cranial angulation, 80° LAO, 10° RAO with 40° cranial angulation, and 35° RAO with 15° caudal angulation), and two views of the right (40° LAO with 10° cranial angulation and 45° RAO) were obtained. These views gave at least one clear image of each coronary segment, and they formed four suitable, perpendicular view-pairs for biplane quantitative analysis [22]. The use of nitrates and other vasoactive drugs, and the sequence of arteriographic projections, catheters, and x-ray field size were recorded; these conditions were duplicated as nearly as possible in the second study 30 months later.

Location of Disease. At the time of the initial catheterization, a careful review of the cinefilm was performed. The dominance of the anatomic vessel distribution was characterized as *right, small right, balanced,* or *left.* An appropriate "*map,*" of the sort illustrated in Figure 1, was selected for each patient. The branch size and site of origin of various vessels were redrawn, as needed, according to the patient's actual anatomy. Once the vessel anatomy was accurately displayed, lesions of any degree of severity were drawn in at their best estimated locations. This mapping step is a particularly important one for defining the location of visible lesions found in each patient; it often consumes the better part of an hour.

Lesion location within the standard coronary anatomy was specified in terms consistent with the AHA reporting scheme [23], described in detail by Dodge et al. [22] as illustrated in Figure 1. "Proximal" segments include the first three segments of the right coronary artery (RCA), the first two segments of the left anterior descending (LAD) and a major diagonal branch, and the first two segments of the circumflex (LCx) and a major obtuse marginal branch. When a large trifurcation marginal branch was present, it was substituted for a diagonal or marginal branch, as appropriate. When two diagonals or two marginals were of comparable size, the one with the most severe lesion at baseline was called the proximal segment. When the anatomic dominance *was balanced* or *left*, three or four LCx segments and two or one RCA segments were specified as proximal. The worst lesion (%S) identified visually in each of these nine proximal segments was coded as the "proximal" lesion for that segment. Other, less severe, lesions in these proximal segments and lesions located more distally were identified and measured, and were included in secondary disease progression analyses. Lesions in the proximal RCA and in the left main which were in direct contact with the catheter in either of the two studies were called "catheter" lesions and measured, but excluded from the analysis for reasons to be provided below. If a given proximal coronary segment appeared entirely free of disease, it was coded as "normal." An entirely normal segment was found at at least one of the two time points (films) in 90 segments in 55 patients.

Disease change assessment

For purposes of this study, change in the severity of these coronary lesions, so identified, was assessed both visually and quantitatively. In both assessments, two experienced observers were blinded to the patient's identity and treatment group and to the sequence of films. Each of the two films, obtained 2.5 years apart, had its leader cut off and was labeled only with a study code. Each pair of films was viewed simultaneously side-by-side, at fivefold magnification, in a dual overhead-projector system (Vanguard Instrument Corp., Melville, N.Y.). A reference frame was marked so that specific frames could be re-located.

Visual assessment. Two cineframes taken at the same point in the cardiac cycle were selected from each film as good-quality, representative images of each lesion; whenever possible, two frames were chosen from each of two perpendicular views of the lesion. On the basis of direct side-by-side visual comparison of these representative frames, lesions were classified by consensus as "unchanged," "definitely changed," or "possibly changed". For "possibly changed" lesions, a third frame was selected from each view for each film. In addition, for "possibly changed" lesions an effort was made to identify good lesion images in perpendicular views for biplane analysis. After this classification, a quick "paper caliper" estimate of the severity of one representative lesion image in each view from each film was performed. This was done by tracing the lesion minimum diameter as two parallel 1–2 mm long lines on a scrap of paper and, using one of these lines as a border, tracing another short, parallel line(s) for the opposite border(s) of the specified normal reference segment(s). The percentage of the traced normal diameter that the minimum diameter represents was visually estimated, rounded to the nearest 5% stenosis, and recorded. This visual estimate was aided by drawing a final parallel line midway between the lines representing the normal diameter estimate. Films were then removed from the projector.

Quantitative assessment. After all 120 film pairs had been evaluated by the above semi-quantitative visual approach, they were evaluated by the presumably more precise quantitative methods. At an average of 3.5 months after the SQ-VIS assessment, film pairs were remounted in the projectors, and the borders of each lesion and the catheter were manually traced from the selected frames onto a standard form. For lesions classified as unchanged or definitely changed, the two frames selected from each view were traced from each film by one of two technicians. For "possibly changed" lesions, the three frames selected for each view were traced by *each* of two technicians. As a result, an average of 2.4 frames per film were traced for "unchanged" and "definitely changed" lesions (22% biplane), as compared to 7.6 frames (26% biplane) per film for lesions felt to be possibly changed. Thus we made a substantially greater effort to obtain accurate estimates for these lesions felt to be marginally changed. All tracings were reviewed for accuracy by an experienced technician and were then processed with use of the most precise of the techniques developed and validated in our laboratory [16]. The diameter of the lumen at the point of greatest local narrowing (minimum diameter, or DM), and nearby normal diameter (or diameters if the average of a proximal and distal normal diameter was judged the appropriate reference (DN) were measured, in millimeters, with the catheter used as a scaling factor. The two principal measures of disease were DM and the percent stenosis ($\%S = 100 (1 - DM/DN)$). Each final lesion estimate was an average of the estimates for all tracings measured, which averaged 3.1 per film (range, 2 to 12).

Reconciliation of major disagreements. As a rule (see below), lesions which were classified as "unchanged" were seldom measured to change by more than 5% stenosis. Similarly, those classified as "possibly changed" were usually found to differ by ±5%-to-10% stenosis at the two time points; and those classed as "definitely changed," usually did so by more than 10%S. Occasionally a lesion was classified as "unchanged" and yet measured to change by more than 10%, or was classed as definitely changed, and yet measured to change by less than 5%; we regarded this as a *major disagreement* between QCA and the semiquantitative visual assessment of change (SQ-VIS). There were 8 instances of the first kind and 8 of the latter among 1034 proximal lesions measured. Lesions for which disagreement was this great were again completely re-read without knowledge of the previous assessment. This re-reading was controlled by a study coordinator who set up the films and views and specified the lesions to be re-read. Fully blinded technicians again selected frames, visually assessed lesion change and estimated stenosis severity by the semi-quantitative method. At a later time, lesions were re-traced from the selected frames and measured by QCA. This was the final attempt to reconcile disagreements between the two methods. In fact, 12/16 (75%) of the major disagreements were resolved by this approach.

Lesion measurement variability

Intrinsic measurement variability for selected frames. One hundred thirty-two of these lesion images were classified as "possibly changed" and were traced and measured by two observers using three frames selected from each view used at each of the two time-points. These six estimates of disease severity were averaged to provide the final estimate for that view. The standard deviation of these six estimates of % stenosis is termed the intrinsic variability for measurement of selected images in a given injection and reflects, in part, the frame-to-frame variation of lesion images judged to be "representative." This index of variability for %S was determined as a function of its actual measured mean values.

Repeat variability. A subset of 6 randomly selected patients had all their lesions ($n = 49$) remeasured, as above, in an entirely blinded fashion, without knowledge of the prior measurements. In each case, the repeat lesion measurements were made from the same angiographic projection(s) as the original ones, which had been selected as the best view(s) of the given lesion. These lesions ranged in severity from 6% to 93% stenosis. The original and repeat measurements were compared statistically.

Short term variability. Thirty-nine lesions were measured from a given view (or pair of views) and again from the same views repeated later during the same catheterization [16]. The mean time interval between these injections in a given patient was 21 minutes. During this interval the x-ray equipment was routinely rotated and the patient moved, to a limited extent on the table. The patient and x-ray equipment were returned to the original position for the repeat injections. Vasoactive drugs were not given in this time interval. The original and the repeat measurement were compared statistically.

Variability results. Table 1 provides data on the intrinsic, the repeat and the short-term QCA measurement variabilities for lesions classified as mildly (0–40%S), moderately (40–70%S), or severely (70–95%S) narrowed. As can be seen, variability was small, of the order of ±3%–5%S and ±0.10–0.20 mm, and was not strongly influenced by lesion severity. The blinded repeat measurements appeared to have a greater variability, largely because somewhat different locations for the operator-specified normal diameters

Table 1. Summary of various types of measurement variability for estimation of proximal coronary lesion severity

Type of variability	Severity of disease (% Stenosis)							
	Mild (0–40%S)		Moderate (40–70%S)		Severe (70–95%)		All lesions	
	n	SD	n	SD	n	SD	n	SD
Intrinsic* (QCA)	90	3.4%	33	3.8%	9	3.2%	132	3.4%
Repeat[†] (QCA)	35	5.4% (0.21 mm)	10	4.0% (0.22 mm)	3	7.2% (0.17 mm)	49	5.1% (0.20 mm)
Repeat[††] (SQ–VIS)	35	4.3% –	10	5.5%	3	5.0%	49	4.5%
Short-term‡ (QCA)	–	–	–	–	–	–	39	3.4%

* Average variability (SD) of six measurements of 3 frames by two observers in a given coronary injection.
[†] Variability (SD) of the difference distribution comparing the initial measurement of "% Stenosis" and "minimum diameter" (mm) with fully blinded repeat measurements using the same angiographic views.
[††] Similarly defined variability as in [†] above, but using the semi-quantitative visual estimate of "% Stenosis" (paper caliper to nearest 5%).
‡ Previously reported value [see ref. 16] of the variance (SD) of the difference distribution comparing the initial measurement of "% Stenosis" with a fully blinded second measurement made from a comparable angiographic projection performed 21 minutes later in the same catheterization.

were sometimes used in the repeat analysis. Thus this represents an overestimate of variability for the usual measurements using direct side-by-side comparison. Three standard deviations of the short-term variation in %S is 10.2%S. Because the distribution of differences between the initial and the short-term repeat measures does not differ significantly from Gaussian, a 10% change in measured stenosis severity approximates a 99% confidence criterion for "true" lesion change.

Comparison of two methods for measurement of change:

Correlation between paper caliper and QCA. For the 1034 proximal lesions, there was a strong correlation between the QCA estimates of disease severity (%S) and the paper caliper estimates (SQ-VIS):

$$SQ\text{-}VIS = 0.99 \; QCA + 0.1$$
$$r = 0.98; \; SEE = 4.8\%S$$

The %S difference (SQ-VIS-%S_{QCA}) between measurements made by these two methods is defined as the error of the crude caliper approach, using

Table 2. Characteristics of the error distribution and absolute error for the difference betweeen lesion %S measured by SQ–VIS and by QCA (the reference method)

| | QCA stenosis severity (%S) | | | |
	Mild (0–40%S) (n = 727)	Moderate (40–70%S) (n = 214)	Severe (70–95%) (n = 56)	All lesions* (n = 1034)
Group mean stenosis severity (%S)	21.3	51.1	78.7	33.4
Mean error (%S)[†]	0.0	−0.6	0.0	−0.1
Standard deviation (%S)	±4.5	±5.5	±7.0	±4.8
Mean absolute error (%S)	3.4	4.1	5.4	3.5

* Includes 37 lesions with total occlusion, for which error was zero.
[†] Error of SQ–VIS is defined as the difference between %S measured by SQ–VIS and by QCA.

QCA as the gold standard. This difference averages -0.1 ± 4.8 (SD) for all lesions. Table 2 shows that the mean error and absolute error, and their variances, are not strongly influenced by actual stenosis severity.

Relationship between visual classification and QCA. Figure 2 plots the frequency distribution of actual absolute measured lesion %S changes for each of the three visual classifications of disease change: "no," "possible," or "definite." As seen in Table 3, the average absolute change was 2.6, 5.1, and 19.1%S, respectively, for each of these three categories. Those classified as "no change" were rarely (2/756) measured to change by more than 10%S; and those classified as "definitely" changing usually (117/146) changed by that amount, or more. The sensitivity, and specificity, and predictive accuracy of various criterion levels of measured %S change for detecting visually appreciable change in these high-quality, magnified arterial images is plotted in Figure 3. A logistic discriminant analysis [24] identified 9.3%S measured change as the *best* value for distinguishing between "definite" and "no" lesion change as assessed by direct visual comparison.

FATS trial outcomes: comparison of methods

The SQ-VIS estimates of %S directly from the projected lesion images are in good agreement with the QCA measurements from their tracings. Therefore the *study outcomes* should also be comparable by either of these two independent, partly reconciled, approaches.

Continuous variable outcome comparison. Proximal disease severity, in FATS, was defined as the average %S value for the most severe lesion found

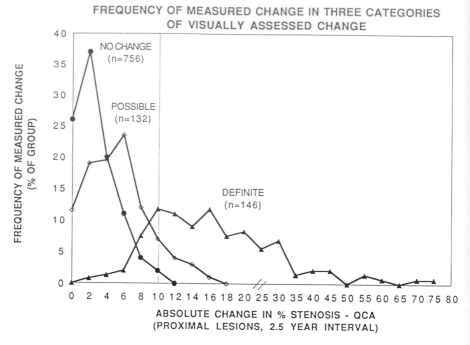

Figure 2. Frequency distribution of absolute measured coronary lesion *change* in three categories of visually assessed *change*, using a pair of highly magnified, simultaneously viewed, high quality coronary arteriograms separated, in time, by 2.5 years. The visual estimate (SQ-VIS) were performed initially. The quantitative determinations (QCA) were made independently, without knowledge of the initial estimates, about 3.5 months later. Major discrepancies between the two methods were largely resolved for 16 lesions by means of a blinded repeat analysis with both methods. A change of 9.3% S points was found to be the best discriminant between "definite change" and "no change." Based on this and short-term variability data (see Table 1) we have used a change of $\geq 10\%\,S$ as a criterion for "true" change.

Table 3. Comparison of proximal coronary lesion change measurements, over 2.5 years, in 3 different lesion groups classified by a semi-quantitative visual method

Visual lesion change classification	n	Average absolute change (%S ± SD)	Median absolute change (%S)	Range of changes (%S) change	Percent of group with ≥10%S change
No change	756	2.6 ± 2.4	2.0	0–18	0.3%
Possible change	132	5.1 ± 3.5	5.0	0–15	11.4%
Definite change	146	19.1 ± 12.4	16.0	2–83	80.1%
	1034				

ASSESSMENT OF CORONARY LESION CHANGE
(DETECTION OF "DEFINITE" CHANGE)

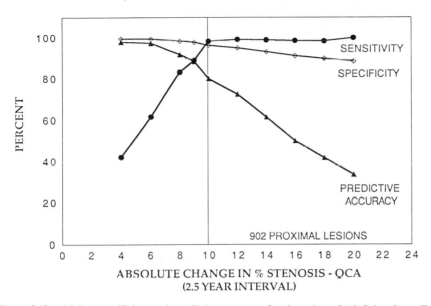

Figure 3. Sensitivity, specificity, and predictive accuracy for detection of "definite change" in coronary lesion severity, as assessed visually. The measurement method is quantitative coronary arteriography (QCA). Among the varying criterion levels of measured change, the most effective for detecting visually convincing change appear to lie in the 9%S-to-10%S change interval in which sensitivity is 0.89–to-0.98 and specificity is 0.98–to-0.96.

in each of the nine proximal coronary segments described above. Its change between the initial and final cineangiogram, a single index of proximal disease change, per patient, was the primary patient endpoint. The average change in mean, per patient proximal disease severity, as estimated by SQ-VIS and QCA, are given in Table 4 for each of the three treatment groups. The study outcome is here seen to be virtually identical by either of these methods of disease change assessment. The conventionally treated group (CONV), on average, worsened their proximal disease severity by about 2%S points during the 2.5–year interval, while the two intensively treated groups improved by nearly one percentage point. The QCA approach provided a slightly, but insignificantly smaller *p*-value by ANOVA [25] than the SQ-VIS.

Categorical variable outcome comparison. A secondary outcome analysis categorizes a patient as having certain combinations of change among the nine individual proximal lesions. In FATS, a patient was categorized as having shown *progression only* if at least one of the nine proximal segments worsened by at least 10%S points, and none of the other segments improved

Table 4. Comparison of two change assessment approaches for %S; continuous variables, per-patient analysis. Analysis of separate group of "catheter-tip" lesions

Rx	N[†]	n[‡]	Semiquantitative visual Average change in proximal %S	ANOVA	QCA Average change in proximal %S	ANOVA
Conv	46	402 (37)	$+2.0 \pm 3.2$		$+2.1 \pm 3.9$ (-2.2 ± 13.1)*	
L + C	38	325 (27)	-0.5 ± 4.8	$p = 0.0033$	-0.7 ± 5.2 $(+0.5 \pm 9.8)$	$p = 0.0028$
N + C	36	307 (27)	-0.8 ± 4.0		-0.9 ± 3.9 (-0.8 ± 10.8)	

* Numbers in parentheses give mean change ($\pm$SD) in catheter-tip lesions, in each group, as measured by QCA.
[†] Number of patients in group.
[‡] Total number of lesions in these patients.

by that amount; *regression only* was the converse of this. A patient showed *mixed change* if at least one proximal lesion worsened and at least one lesion improved by $\geqslant 10\%$S; *no change* occurred if none of the patient's nine proximal segments was measured to change by $\pm \geqslant 10\%$S points. Obviously, this classification scheme could be adapted to use "definite" progression or "definite" regression instead of the $\pm 10\%$S change criterion. Or, it could be adapted to use the $\geqslant 9.3\%$S change criterion shown above to be the best measured (QCA) change value for discriminating visually appreciable "definite change" from "no" change. The results of the FATS trial, as expressed in terms of these three variants of the categorical analysis, are shown in Table 5. As can be seen, the study outcome was, again, virtually identical by any of these three approaches. A slightly greater statistical confidence in the treatment benefit came from the QCA analysis using $\geqslant 9.3\%$S as the criterion for "true" change. There was, however, no significant difference in statistical power among these methods.

Catheter tip lesions: exclusion from analysis

There is a well-known potential for catheter-induced coronary spasm, particularly in the proximal right coronary artery, and also in the left anterior descending artery if the left main coronary is short. We therefore excluded any lesion from the "proximal" classification if, at any time during either of the two catheterizations, it was touched (entered) by the catheter tip. However, these lesions were measured by the methods outlined above and were separately classified as "catheter tip" lesions. As seen in Table 4, there were 91 of these lesions equitably distributed among the three treatment groups. Among these lesions, the variability of measured change was about three

Table 5. Comparison of three change assessment approaches, categorical variables, per-patient analysis.

(N)	Progression only	≥10% Measured change Mixed change	No change	Regression only	χ^{2*}
Conv (46)	21	2	18	5	
L + C (38)	8	4	14	12	$p = 0.017$
N + C (36)	9	1	12	14	

(N)	Progression Only	≥9.3%S Measured change Mixed Change	No Change	Regression Only	χ^2
Conv (46)	23	3	16	4	
L + C (38)	9	4	13	12	$p = 0.004$
N + C (36)	7	3	12	14	

(N)	Progression only	"Definite" change Mixed change	No change	Regression only	χ^2
Conv (46)	21	1	20	4	
L + C (38)	11	3	11	13	$p = 0.008$
N + C (36)	8	3	10	15	

* For the standard χ^2 test on the collapsed 3 × 3 contingency table in which "no change" and "mixed change" are combined.

times greater than for other proximal lesions, and the benefit from lipid lowering therapy was not observed.

Implications

For iterpretation of the FATS trial. The excellent agreement between these two fundamentally different, and partially reconciled methods for disease change assessment, and the concordance between disease change and clinical event outcomes of the trial serve to greatly strengthen the confidence in this dual measurement approach, and in the overall findings of the study.

For design of clinical arteriographic trials. The question of whether to analyze disease and its change by visual panel or by traditional quantitative arteriography is *not* effectively addressed by this study. Indeed, the use of both approaches served to strengthen the overall quality of each analysis. First, our visual analysis (SQ-VIS) was considerably more structured and detailed than other reported approaches [1, 2, 4, 26]. It included a semiquantitative paper-caliper approximation of the severity of disease found in each of nine specified proximal coronary segments, as seen in selected, representative cineframes. Second, lesions for which there were major discrepancies in the assessment of disease change between these two methods were re-evaluated in a fully blinded fashion. Thus each method benefitted from a comparison with the other. Each of these two data sets was improved in its credibility by this attempt to resolve major discrepancies.

The analysis of a single patient film pair, using these approaches, required an accumulated time of about 19 man hours. A team of three observers working nearly exclusively on this project completed the analysis of 146 baseline films and 120 completed film pairs in 9 months.

In this study, a per-patient *continuous* variable ($\Delta\%S$) approach confirmed the postulated treatment benefit with the greatest level of statistical confidence ($p = 0.0028$). However, the per patient *categorical* approach, using a $\geq 9.3\%S$ criterion level for "true" lesion change was not significantly less effective in resolving that benefit ($p = 0.004$).

While the ability to visually resolve a definite change in disease severity, and to perform three measurements, are acquired skills, one of the three technicians performing this assessment began with less than one year's experience in our laboratory. And one of the three technicians performing arterial border tracing actually had very little previous experience, but acquired these skills during a closely observed two month training period. In each phase of this dual analysis, at least one of the technicians judging change visually or checking the quality of the tracings had at least three year's experience in these techniques.

Acknowledgements

Skillful assistance in preparation of this manuscript was provided by Leslie Wilkins, BA.

References

1. Brensike JF, Levy RI, Kelsey SF, et al. Effects of therapy with cholestyramine on progression of coronary arteriosclerosis: results of the NHLBI Type II Coronary Intervention Study. Circulation 1984; **69**: 313–24.
2. Levy RI, Brensike JF, Epstein SE, et al. The influence of changes in lipid values induced by cholestyramine and diet on progression of coronary artery disease: results of the NHLBI Type II Coronary Intervention Study. Circulation 1984; **69**: 325–37.
3. Brown BG, Bolson EL, Pierce CD, Peterson RB, Wong M, Dodge HT. The progression of native coronary atherosclerosis is not altered by aspirin plus dipyridamole. Circulation 1983; **68** (Suppl 3): III–398 (Abstract).
4. Blankenhorn DH, Nessim SA, Johnson RL, Sanmarco ME, Azen SP, Cashin-Hemphill L. Beneficial effects of combined colestipol-niacin therapy on coronary athrosclerosis and coronary venous bypass grafts. JAMA 1987: **257**: 3233–40 (published erratum appears in JAMA 1988; **259**: 2698).
5. Buchwald H, Varco RL, Matts JP, et al. Effect of partial ileal bypass surgery on mortality and morbidity from coronary heart disease in patients with hypercholesterolemia. Report

of the Program on Surgical Control of the Hyperlipidemias (POSCH). N Engl J Med 1990; **323**: 946–55.

6. Ornish D, Brown SE, Scherwitz LW. Can lifestyle changes reverse coronary heart disease? The Lifestyle Heart Trial. Lancet 1990; **33-6**: 129–33. Comment in: Lancet 1990; **336**: 624–6.

7. Brown BG, Lin JT, Kelsey S, et al. Progression of coronary atherosclerosis in patients with probable familial hypercholesterolemia. Quantitative arteriographic assessment of patients in NHLBI type II study. Arteriosclerosis 1989; **9** (1 Suppl): I81–90.

8. Brown G, Albers JJ, Fisher LD, et al. Regression of coronary artery disease as a result of intensive lipid-lowering therapy in men with high levels of apolipoprotein B. N Engl J Med 1990; **323**: 1289–98. Comment in: N Engl J Med 1990; **323**; 1337–9.

9. Kane JP, Malloy MJ, Ports TA, Phillips NR, Diehl JC, Havel RJ. Regression of coronary atherosclerosis during treatment of famial hypercholesterolemia with combined drug regimens. JAMA 1990; **264**: 3007–12.

10. Brown BG, Adams WA, Albers JJ, Lin J, Bolson EL, Dodge HT. Quantitative arteriography in coronary intervention trials: rationale, study design and lipid response in the University of Washington Familial Atherosclerosis Treatment Study (FATS). In: Glagor S, Newman WP 3d, Schaffer SA (Eds.), Pathobiology of the human atherosclerotic plaque. New York: Springer-Verlag 1990: 535–50.

11. Waters D, LespÄrance J, Francetich M, et al. A controlled clinical trial to assess the effect of a calcium channel blocker on the progression of coronary atherosclerosis. Circulation 1990; **82**: 1940–53. Comments in: Circulation 1990; **82**: 2251–3.

12. Brown BG, Gallery CA, Badger RS, et al. Incomplete lysis of thrombus in the moderate underlying atherosclerotic lesion during intracoronary infusion of streptokinase for acute myocardial infarction: quantitative angiographic observations. Circulation 1986; **73**: 653–61.

13. Serruys PW, Wijns W, van den Brand M, et al. Is transluminal coronary angioplasty mandatory after successful thrombolysis? Quantitative coronary angiographic study. Br Heart J 1983; **50**: 257–65.

14. Brown BG, Pierce CD, Peterson RB, Bolson EL, Dodge HT. A new approach to clinical investigation of progressive coronary atherosclerosis (PCA). Circulation 1979; **60** (Suppl 2): II 66 (Abstract).

15. Reiber JH, Serruys PW, Kooijman CJ, et al. Assessment of short-, medium-, and long-term variations in arterial dimensions from computer-assisted quantitation of coronary cineangiograms. Circulation 1985; **71**: 280–8.

16. Brown BG, Bolson EL, Dodge HT. Quantitative computer techniques for analyzing coronary arteriograms. Prog Cardiovasc Dis 1986; **28**: 403–18.

17. Ambrose JA, Winters SL, Arora RR, et al. Angiographic evolution of coronary artery morphology in unstable angina. J Am Coll Cardiol 1986; **7**: 472–8.

18. Tobis JM, Mallery J, Mahon D, et al. Intravascular ultrasound imaging of human coronary arteries in vivo. Analysis of tissue characterizations with comparison to in vitro histological specimens. Circulation 1991; **83**: 913–26.

19. Yock PG, Johnson EL, Linker DT. Intravascular ultrasound: development and clinical potential. Am J Card Imaging 1988; **2**: 185–93.

20. Nissen SE, Grimes CL, Gurley JC, et al. Application of a new phased-array ultrasound imaging catheter in the assessment of vascular dimensions. In vivo comparison to cineangiography. Circulation 1990; **81**: 660–6.

21. Albers JJ, Brunzell JD, Knopp RH. Apoprotein measurements and their clinical application. Clin Lab Med 1989; **9**: 137–52.

22. Dodge JT Jr, Brown BG, Bolson EL, Dodge HT. Intrathoracic spatial location of specified coronary segments on the normal human heart. Applications in quantitative arteriography, assessment of regional risk and contraction, and anatomic display. Circulation 1988; **78**: 1167–80.

23. Austen WG, Edwards JE, Frye RL, et al. A reporting system on patients evaluated for

coronary artery disease. Report of the Ad Hoc Committee for Grading of Coronary Artery
Disease, Council on Cardiovascular Surgery, American Heart Association. Circulation 1975;
51 (P Suppl): 5–40.
24. BMDP Statistical Software Manual, Vol 2. University of California Press, Berkeley, 1990.
25. SAS Institute Inc. SAS user's guide: statistics; version 5 edition. Cary, N.C.: SAS Institute,
1985: 607–14.

PART SIX

QCA in restenosis studies

19. Pharmacological prevention of restenosis after percutaneous transluminal coronary angioplasty [PTCA]: overview and methodological considerations

PATRICK W. SERRUYS, WALTER R.M. HERMANS,
BENNO J. RENSING and PIM J. DE FEYTER

Summary

Despite 13 years of clinical experience and research in the field of restenosis after PTCA, there have been no major breakthroughs in pharmacologic interventions. Assessment of the value of drug trials that have been performed is extremely difficult because of differences in selection of patients, methods of analysis and definition of restenosis. Restenosis is now seen as an intimal proliferation of smooth muscle cells together with an abundant matrix production. This (re)growth is measured as a change in minimal luminal diameter between post-PTCA and follow-up angiography by quantitative coronary angiography, the only reliable technique that at the present time can be applied to large populations. This continuous measurement is now used in restenosis prevention trials as the primary endpoint and is a reflexion of how the lesion behaves after PTCA. Besides that, only one third of the number of patients are needed compared to the use of an arbitrarily defined categorial outcome in restenosis prevention trials.

Introduction

Despite the therapeutic success of coronary angioplasty, the exact mechanisms of dilatation remain speculative and involve multiple processes, including endothelial denudation, with rapid accumulation of platelet and fibrin; cracking, splitting or disruption of the intima and atherosclerotic plaque; dehiscence of the intima and plaque from the underlying media; and stretching or tearing of the media, with persistent aneurysmal dilatation of the media and adventitia [1, 2]. The major limitation of PTCA has been the high incidence of restenosis which has remained much the same over the last 13 years despite diverse pharmacological therapies and all kinds of new interventions [3]. Lack of a practical animal restenosis model has limited the ability to investigate potential therapies although recently a model of human

J.H.C. Reiber and P.W. Serruys (eds), Advances in Quantitative Coronary Arteriography, 329–350.
© 1993 Kluwer Academic Publishers. Printed in the Netherlands.

restenosis was developed in the domestic crossbred swine, fed a standard, nonatherogenic diet [4].

Possible mechanism of restenosis after PTCA

Beside the pathology of the dilated vessels of patients who died shortly or later on after PTCA [5–7], it has become possible, with the use of the transluminal atherectomy device, to remove and examine primary and restenotic lesions [8–10]. Primary stenotic lesions consisted in the majority of the cases out of atherosclerotic plaque (composed of dense fibrous tissue and variable amounts of fatty atheromatous debris); however, in a small group only intimal hyperplasia was seen, histological identical to restenotic lesions. Restenotic lesions showed in most cases intimal hyperplasia (characterized by proliferation of smooth muscle cells of the synthetic type with abundant extracellular matrix chiefly composed of proteoglycans) and in a minority, only atherosclerotic plaque was seen. Therefore, smooth muscle cell proliferation seems to play a pivotal role in the restenosis process.

The process that results in restenosis is initiated at the time the disruptive action of the inflated balloon on the intima (endothelium) and/or media takes place. As intact endothelium prevents platelet aggregation, a superficial endothelial injury leads to local platelet and leucocyte adhesion, but most of the platelets do not undergo a release action. However, in case of a deep endothelial injury (as with a successful angioplasty) the hemostatic system is activated. Blood is exposed to collagen and other substances of the subintima which are potent stimuli for platelet aggregation mediated by the release of adenosine diphosphate (ADP), serotonin, thromboxane A2 (TXA2), fibrinogen, fibronectin, thrombospondin and von Willebrand Factor (Figure 1). These substances activate neighboring platelets via different metabolic pathways (thromboxane A2, ADP and by a platelet activating factor) and promote intramural thrombus formation which could cause restenosis [11, 12] (Figure 1).

Concommitantly several growth factors including platelet derived growth factor (PDGF), epidermal growth factor (EGF) and transforming growth factor beta (TGF-β) are released from thrombocytes, smooth muscle cells, endothelium and macrophages. In this way they stimulate smooth muscle cells and fibroblasts to proliferate and migrate from the medial layer into the intima of the vessel wall. In some patients this response is excessive and is associated with abundant amounts of connective tissue formation. This results in hyperplasia of the intima with a reduction of luminal diameter and causes angiographic and or clinical restenosis [13–15] (Figure 1). Each of these steps could be sites of intervention that may halt the restenosis process [16] (Figure 2). Table 1 summarizies the results of the reported pharmacolgical trials in PTCA patients until now [17]. Assessment of the value of most of these trials is extremely difficult because of differences in selection of patients, methods of analysis and definition of restenosis [18]. Although there is no

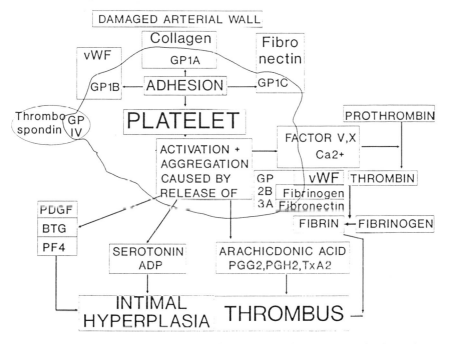

Figure 1. Simplified schematic presentation of platelet adhesion, platelet activation and aggregation. Vascular injury with endothelial denudation exposes subendothelial collagen to circulating blood and induces platelets to adhere using glycoprotein receptors (GP). This adhesion is stimulated by von Willebrand Factor (vWF), fibronectin, thrombospondin bind to other glycoprotein receptors of the platelets. This adhesion leads to activation and aggregation with release of adenosine diphosphate (ADP), serotonin, Ca^{2+} thromboxane A2, PDGF (platelet derived growth factor), BTG (betathromboglobulin), PF4 (platelet factor 4) which could lead to intimal hyperplasia and thrombus formation.

scientific proof that the tested drugs are effective, many clinicians continue to prescribe some of them to "prevent restenosis". Some positive results were found in highly selected patients that used fish oil, trapidil, verapamil and lovastatin. In the near future the results will be known of ongoing multicenter trials with ACE-inhibition, serotonin antagonist, hirudin, LMWH, angiopeptin and other promising drugs such as inhibitors of thrombin production, growth factor blockers, prostacyclin analogues and monoclonal antibodies against the platelet membrane receptors (GP IIb/IIIa) and the von Willebrand factor will be tested and the outcome of these trials may bring us closer to the pharmacological solution of the restenosis problem.

Symptoms, function or anatomy as criteria of restenosis?

Primary success and restenosis after PTCA may be defined by symptomatic criteria such as frequency and severity of anginal episodes, by functional

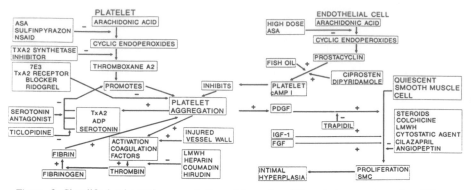

Figure 2. Simplified schematic presentation of how the different drugs act on the different processes involved in the restenosis process:
ASA = Acetyl salicylic Acid; NSAID = Non Steroidal Anti-inflammatory Drugs; TxA2 = Thromboxane A2; 7E3 = Antiplatelet glycoprotein receptor 2b/3a; ADP = Adenosine diphosphate; LMWH = Low Molecular Weight Heparin; cAMP = Cyclic Adenosine Mono Phosphate; PDGF = Platelet Derived Growth Factor; IGF = Insulin-like Growth Factor; FGF = Fibroblastic Growth Factor; SMC = Smooth Muscle Cell.

criteria such as pressure flow characteristic of the dilated vessel, coronary flow reserve and various noninvasive diagnostic tests, or may be defined by anatomic criteria using postmortem histology, angiography or intravascular ultrasound. These 3 criteria may be considered separately or may be interrelated so that the definition of restenosis becomes a complex issue. About the symptomatic criteria, it is fair to emphasize the five following points. First – Although the subjective improvement of symptoms after PTCA is probably the most desirable endpoint, it is also the least objective evaluation [19]. Second – The frequency of symptomatic improvement appears to be lower than that of angiographic success: only 80–85% of the patients with a satisfactory angiography result immediately post-PTCA exhibit such an improvement [20]. Third – The reappearance of angina as a sole criterion of restenosis underestimates the angiographic rate of restenosis. The reported incidence of silent restenosis may be as high as 33%. Fourth – However, the elapsed time from PTCA to recurrence of symptoms has shown to be clinically useful in identifying the most probable cause of recurrent angina:
– Within one month: incomplete revascularization from additional coronary artery disease and/or incomplete dilatation should be suspected.
– Within 1 to 6 months: restenosis, that is to say, lesion recurrence is most likely.
– After 6 months: new significant atherosclerosis disease should be considered [21].
  The value of recurrent anginal symptoms as a marker of restenosis is

Table 1(A). The effect of drug therapy on restenosis per patients after successful coronary angioplasty with follow-up angiography and/or clinical follow-up (I).

Author	Year	Drug	Dose	Patients Total	Fup	Time	Definition restenosis	Restenosis (%) drug vs placebo	Risk ratio	95% CI
Hirshfeld	1987	Heparin	Different duration	209	NR	4–12 mth	>50% DS Fup (visual)	Longer heparin less restenosis		
Ellis	1989	Heparin (18–24 h) Dextrose	<2.5 norm PTT	416	61%	3–9 mth	>50% DS Fup (visual)	41% 37%	1.1	0.8 to 1.5
Lehmann	1991	Heparin (daily)	10,000 units/day	50	77%	NR	NR	82%	2.5	0.8 to 7.8
Thornton	1984	ASA Coumadin	325 mg/day 2–2.5 norm PTT	248	72%	6–9 mth	loss > 50% gain stress test → +	27% 36%	0.7	0.5 to 1.1
Urban	1988	Coumadin + Verapamil Verapamil	≥2.5 nor PTT Not reported	110	77%	5 mth	>50% DS Fup	29%	0.8	0.4 to 1.4
Dyckmans	1988	ASA	1500 mg/day 320 mg/day	203	40%	6 mth	>50% DS Fup	21% 31%	0.7	0.4 to 1.5
Mufson	1988	ASA ASA	1500 mg/day 80 mg/day	453	37%	3–8 mth	>50% DS Fup (visual)	51% 47%		
Schanzenbacher	1988	ASA ASA	1000 mg/day 100 mg/day	79	100%	6 mth	Clinical (re-PTCA, CABG)	21% 17%	1.2	0.5 to 2.9
Kadel	1990	ASA ASA	1400 mg/day 350 mg/day	188	92%	4–6 mth	NR	31% 21%	1.5	0.9 to 2.5
Finci	1988	ASA Placebo	100 mg/day	40	73%	6 mth (visual)	>50% DS Fup	33% 14%	2.3	0.5 to 10.1
Schwartz	1988	ASA + Dipyridamol Placebo	990–225 mg/day	249	100%	4–7 mth (QCA)	>50% DS Fup	38% 39%	1.0	0.7 to 1.3
Chesebro	1989	ASA + Dipyridamol Placebo	975–225 mg/day	207	85% (QCA)	5 mth	Δ MLD (Post-PTCA) – (Fup)	0.18 mm P 0.14 mm ASA + D		
White	1987	ASA – Dipyridamol Ticlopidine Placebo	650–225 mg/day 750 mg/day	236	75%	6 mth	>70% DS Fup (visual)	18% 29% 20%	0.9 1.4	0.4 to 1.9 0.8 to 12.8
Yabe	1989	TxA2 synth inhibitor Placebo	600 mg/day	33	100%	>3 mth	loss > 50% gain	22% 53%	0.3	0.0 to 1.4*
Serruys	1991	TxA2 receptor blocker Placebo	40 mg/day	650	89%	6 mth	Δ MLD (post-PTCA) – MLD (Fup)	0.31 ± 0.53 TxA2 0.30 ± 0.54 P		

Table 1(B)

Author	Year	Drug	Dose	Patients Total	Fup	Time	Definition restenosis	Restenosis (%) drug vs placebo		Risk ratio	95% CI
Kitazume	1988	ASA ASA + Ticlopidine(Tic) ASA + Tic + Nicorandil	300 mg/day +200 mg/day +30 mg/day	280	100%	6 mth	>50% DS Fup	38% 27% 16%			
Bertrand	1990	Ticlopidine Placebo	500 mg/day	266	93%	6 mth	loss > 50% gain	50%	41:	1.3	1.0 to 1.8
Knudtson	1990	Prostacyclin + ASA + D ASA + Dipyridamol(D)	5 ng/kg/min 325+225 mg/day	270	93%	6 mth (caliper)	>50% DS Fup loss > 50% gain	27%	32%	0.9	0.6 to 1.3
Gershlick	1990	Prostacyclin Placebo	4 hg/kg/min	132	80%	5–7 mth	loss > 50% gain	31%	34%	0.8	0.5 to 1.4
Raizner	1988	Ciprostene Placebo	120 ng/kg/min max. 48 hours	311	80%	6 mth	>50% DS Fup (visual) Clinical (MI, re-PTCA, CABG, Death)	41% 17%	53% 34%	0.8 0.5	0.6 to 1.0 0.3 to 0.8
Okamoto	1990	Trapidil ASA + D	600 mg/day 300 + 150 mg/day	64	NR	6 mth	loss > 50% gain	20%	33%	0.6	0.3 to 1.5
Klein	1989	Ketanserin	0.1 mg/min for 24 hours	43	100%	4-6 mths	NR (QCA)	33%	29%	1.1	0.4 to 2.8
O'Keefe	1991	Colchicine Placebo	1.2 mg/day	197	74%	NR	return ≥ 70% DS and loss of ≥ 50% gain	22%	22%		
Corcos	1985	Diltiazem + ASA + D ASA + D	270 mg/day 650–225 mg/day	92	100%	5–10 mth	>70% DS Fup (visual)	15%	22%	0.7	0.3 to 1.7
O'Keefe	1991	Diltiazem+ ASA + D ASA + D	240+360 mg/day 325–225 mg/day	201	60%	12 mth	≥70% AS and loss of ≥50% gain	36%	32%	1.1	0.7 to 1.9
Whitworth	1986	Nifedipine + ASA ASA	40 mg/day	241	82%	6 mth	loss ≥ 50% of gain >50% DS Fup	29%	33%	0.9	0.5 to 1.4
Horberg	1990	Verapamil + ASA + D ASA + D	480 mg/day 660 + 330 mg/day	196	88%	5 mth	loss of ≥50% gain	56% 38%	62% 63%	unstable 0.9 stable 0.6	0.6 to 1.3 0.4 to 1.0

Table 1(C)

Author	Year	Drug	Dose	Patients Total	Fup	Time	Definition restenosis	Restenosis (%) drug	vs placebo	Risk ratio	95% CI
Slack	1987	Fish oil	2.4 g/day	162	85%	6 mth	Clinical	16%	33%*	0.5	0.2 to 1.0
		Placebo					Stress test → +	67%	58%**	1.2	0.7 to 1.8
Reis	1989	Fish oil	6.0 g/day	186	30%	6 mth	>70% DS Fup	34%	23%	1.5	0.9 to 2.5
		Placebo									
Milner	1989	Fish oil	4.5 g/day	194	23%	6 mth	>50% DS Fup	18%	27%		
		Placebo			100%	Clinical	Stress test → +	19%	35%	0.6	0.4 to 1.0
Dehmer	1988	Fish oil	3.2 g/day	82	100%	6 mth	>50% DS Fup (visual)	19%	46%	0.4	0.2 to 0.8
		Placebo									
Grigg	1989	Fish oil	3.0 g/day	103	94%	3–5 mth	loss > 50% of gain (caliper)	34%	33%	1.1	0.6 to 1.8
		Placebo									
Sahni	1989	Lovastatin	20–40 mg/day	157	50%	2–10 mth	>50% DS Fup	14%	47%	0.3	0.2 to 0.6
		Placebo									
Rose	1987	Steroid	48 mg/day	65	88%	3 mth	>50% DS Fup	33%	33%		
		Placebo									
Stone	1989	Steroid for restenosis	125 mg mp/day 240 mg p/week	102	53%	6 mth	>50% DS Fup	59%	56%	1.1	0.7 to 1.7
Pepine	1990	Steroid	1.0 g mp	722	71%	4–8 mth	>50% DS Fup (caliper)	43%	43%	1.0	0.8 to 1.2
		Placebo									

Fup = Follow up (% of successful PTCA); Sign = Significance; NR = Not Reported; mth = months; DS = Diameter stenosis; AS = Area stenosis; nor PTT = normal prothrombin time; ns = not significant; ASA = Acetylsalicylic Acid; pt = patient; TXA2 = Thromboxane A2 synthetase inhibitor; tic = ticlopidine; mp = methylprednisolene; D = Dipyridamole.

Risk ratio with 95% confidence intervals (CI). Risk ratio of <1 means that a lower restenosis rate is seen among the patients treated with the new drug compared with those who received placebo. A statistical significant (p < 0.05) lower restenosis rate is seen in those studies where the 95% confidence intervals do not cross risk ratio of 1. Risk ratio of more than 1 indicates a higher restenosis rate among the patients treated with the new drug.

336 P.W. Serruys et al.

Table 2. Detection of restenosis by symptoms.

Author	Year	Angiographic follow-up %	Restenosis %	Symptoms PPV %	NPV %
Simonton	'88	90	35	48	75
Caldiff	'90	100	38	60	85
Zaidi	'85	100	49	66	70
Mabin	'85	55	32	71	86
Levine	'85	92	40	76	96
Jutzy	'82	88	47	92	83
Gruentzig	'87	93	31	92	98

Modified from Califf et al. [22].
PPV: positive predictive value.
NPV: negative predictive value.

difficult to assess in many studies because the timing and completeness of angiographic followup often have been determined by symptomatic status. In studies with a high rate of angiographic follow-up, the probability that patients with symptoms had restenosis (i.e the positive predictive value of symptoms) ranged from 48% to 92%, whereas the probability that patients without symptoms were free of restenosis (i.e, the negative predictive value of symptoms) ranged from 70 to 98% (Table 2) [22].

The low positive predictive value found in many of these studies may be explained by the presence of other mechanism for angina, such as incomplete revascularization or progression of disease in other vessels.

Several studies have examined the ability of the exercise treadmill test to detect restenosis after PTCA. These studies have generally found that the presence of exercise-induced angina or ST segment depression or both is not highly predictive of restenosis whether the test is performed early or late after angioplasty. The positive predictive values of early treadmill testing range from 29 to 60%, whereas the corresponding values for late treadmill testing are ranging from 39 to 64 percent (Table 3). The low positive predictive value is most likely a consequence of incomplete revascularization: that is either a totally occluded vessel, or a significant stenosis at a site other than dilated by angioplasty. It is also possible that the noninvasive test is accurately demonstrating a functionally inadequate dilatation, despite the appearance of success on angiography.

Table 4 shows the accuracy of thallium scintigraphy for detection of restenosis in series which have a reasonable angiographic follow-up ranging from 55 to 100%. Since cardiac catherization remains "the gold standard" for detection of restenosis, the reported value of a noninvasive test is determined not only by the actual accuracy of the test, but also by the completeness of angiographic follow-up.

Table 3. Detection of restenosis by exercise treadmill testing.

Author	Angiographic follow-up %	Restenosis %	PPV %	NPV %	Timing of test
O'Keefe	100	13	29	73	<1 mth
Scholl	83	12	40	27	1 mth
Wijns*	74	35	50	65	3–7 wks
Wijns*	89	40	60	52	3–8 wks
Bengston	96	51	39	84	6 mths
Rosing	100	34	47	76	8 mths
Ernst	100	4	50	95	4–8 mths
Honan	88	58	57	64	6 mths
Scholl	83	12	64	50	6 mths

*Thoraxcenter.
Modified from Califf et al. [22].
PPV: positive predictive value.
NPV: negative predictive value.

Table 4. Detection of restenosis by thallium-201 scintigraphy.

Author	Angiographic follow-up %	Restenosis %	PPV %	NPV %	Timing of test
Jain	55	14	79	88	0–6 days
Miller	76	39	76	94	2wks
Lam	100	9	89	96	2 wks
Wijns*	74	35	74	83	3–7 wks
Wijns*	89	40	82	72	3–8 wks
Scholl	83	12	56	42	1 mth
Ernst	100	4	50	100	4–8 mths
Rosing	100	21	37	83	8 mths
Lefkowitz	Planar thallium		62	80	6mths
	Thonographic thallium		80	93	

*Thoraxcenter.
Modified from Califf et al. [22].
PPV: positive predictive value.
NPV: negative predictive value.

In these studies with a high rate of angiographic follow-up the positive predictive value of thallium scintigraphy is ranging between 56 and 89%.

Recently, Lefkowitz et al. have shown that the positive and negative predictive values for tomographic imaging in detection of restenosis were superior to the predictive values observed with planar imaging. In addition, the specific vascular territory was correctly localized to the PTCA territory in 77% of the tomographic studies [23].

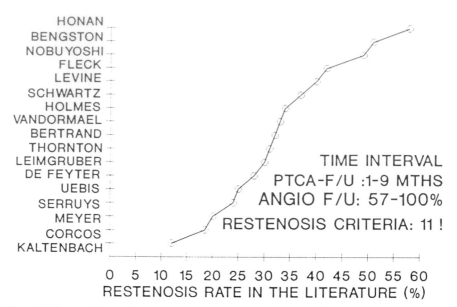

HONAN
BENGSTON
NOBUYOSHI
FLECK
LEVINE
SCHWARTZ
HOLMES
VANDORMAEL
BERTRAND
THORNTON
LEIMGRUBER
DE FEYTER
UEBIS
SERRUYS
MEYER
CORCOS
KALTENBACH

TIME INTERVAL
PTCA-F/U :1-9 MTHS
ANGIO F/U: 57-100%
RESTENOSIS CRITERIA: 11 !

0   5   10 15 20 25 30 35 40 45 50 55 60
RESTENOSIS RATE IN THE LITERATURE (%)

Figure 3. Restenosis rates found by different authors, applying 11 different restenosis criteria, different angiographic follow-up times (1–9 months) and different analysis techniques (visual or quantitative).

Coronary angiography still the "Gold Standard"

In view of the above, coronary angiography still is the most reliable method of judging the late results. Unfortunately, there are many studies on coronary restenosis reported that are distinguished by their lack of consistency in their methodologic approach and their definitions of restenosis. Figure 3 illustrates this point. On the vertical axis of this "nonscientific" figure, we have listed the names of the investigators, who have studied the restenosis problem, while along the horizontal axis the restenosis rates observed in their studies have been plotted. A restenosis rate ranging between 25 and 35% seems to emerge. However we have to emphasize the following facts: the angiographic follow-up in these patients range between 57 and 100%, the time to follow-up range between 1 and 9 months and 11 different criteria of restenosis have been applied by these investigators who in large majority used visual assessment of the coronary angiogram.

The variety of criteria in current use is tabulated in Table 5. Most are entirely arbitrary, some are based on doubtful logic and some, although of some relevance for visual estimation of percent diameter stenosis, are unrealistic when applied to the most accurate values obtained from quantitative angiography. Thus most of the discrepancies between these studies can be

Table 5. Criteria of restenosis in current use.

1. Loss of at least 50% of the initial gain (NHLBI IV)
2. A return to within 10% of the pre-PTCA diameter stenosis (NHLBI III)
3. An immediate post-PTCA < 50% diameter stenosis that increase to ⩾50% at follow-up
4. As for 3, but for a diameter stenosis ⩾70% at follow-up (NHLBI II)
5. Reduction ⩾20% in diameter stenosis
6. Reduction ⩾30% in diameter stenosis (NHLBI I)
7. A diameter stenosis ⩾50% at follow-up
8. A diameter stenosis ⩾70% at follow-up
9. Area stenosis ⩾85% [30]
10. Loss ⩾1 mm^2 in stenosis area [31]
11. Deterioration of ⩾0.72 mm in minimal luminal diameter from post-PTCA to follow-up [13]
12. Deterioration of ⩾0.5 mm in minimal luminal diameter from post-PTCA to follow-up [12]

attributed to three factors: 1) the selection of patients; 2) the method of analysis; and 3) the definition of restenosis used. In order to improve the situation these 3 factors need to be addressed [18].

1. The study population. This means a high angiographic follow-up rate (>80%) with a predetermined time for restudy; this will avoid a selection bias of symptomatic patient. Sample size of observational or randomized clinical trial should be adequately controlled to avoid a type II error commonly referred to as the power of the test.

2. A well validated system of analysis with known accuracy and variability should be employed. The use of a visual percent diameter stenosis measurement with its inherent variability precludes meaningful results and edge tracing by hand or other techniques that can produce values not physiologically possible are also unacceptable [24]. Videodensitometry may eventually provide the best measurement because the technique estimates the volume of the lumen independently of geometric assumption, but for technical reasons this theoretical method of choice has not (yet) proven practical [25].

3. The measured variables must be chosen so as to reflect the restenosis proliferative process and distinguish between the results of angioplasty (optimal or suboptimal) and this proliferative restenosis process. We believe that the conventional assessment of percent diameter stenosis is not sufficiently discriminating in doing this and that definitions based on percent diameter stenosis measurement fail to identify lesions undergoing significant deterioration [18, 26]. Percent diameter stenosis criteria are chosen to reflect the change in minimal luminal diameter in relation to the so-called normal diameter of the vessel in the immediate vicinity of the obstruction. In the first place, it is assumed that there is a normal diameter; diffuse intimal or subintimal thickening are not detectable on a coronary "shadowgram". Secondly, the choice of a socalled normal diameter, proximal or distal to the obstruction is arbitrary and will have major impact on the calculation of the percentage diameter stenosis. This is illustrated in Figure 4; in this particular

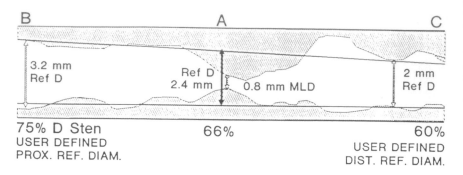

Figure 4. Graphical illustration of different percentage diameter stenosis values dependent on the arbitrary choice of the site of the reference diameter. With our quantitative analysis system it is possible to obtain an objective, independent value for the reference diameter and thus for the % diameter stenosis. This is called the 'interpolated reference diameter'. A computer derived reconstruction of the original arterial dimension at the site of obstruction (assuming there is no disease present) is used to define the interpolated reference diameter (tapering lines in figure).

example the percentage diameter stenosis is ranging from 75% to 60% according to the site of reference arbitrarily chosen. Thirdly, it is assumed that this normal diameter does not change as a result of angioplasty or during the immediate follow-up period when restenosis of the dilated lesion is a well recognized phenomenon. The socalled normal diameter might be diffusely affected by the barotrauma of the balloon which can induce a reactive hyperplasia in the area touched by the balloon [26]. This seriously questions the use of percent diameter stenosis as the only index of restenosis (Figure 5).

Restenosis definition, subject of debate

The restenosis definition of choice has been the subject of much debate and there is currently no satisfactory definition that takes into account both the functional and angiographic outcome after PTCA. The known discrepancy between these two parameter means that this objective will not be realized. A single "stenosis" measurement should not be confused with a measurement of "restenosis" which should represent the change in stenosis severity. The commonly used definition of 50% diameter stenosis at follow-up is historically based on the physiological concept of coronary flow reserve introduced by Lance Gould in 1974 and is taken because it represents the approximate value in animals with normal coronary arteries at which blunting of the hyperemic response occurs [27]. Although this value may be of some relevance in determining a significant stenosis in human atherosclerotic vessels, it tells us nothing about the way the lesion has behaved since the angioplasty procedure.

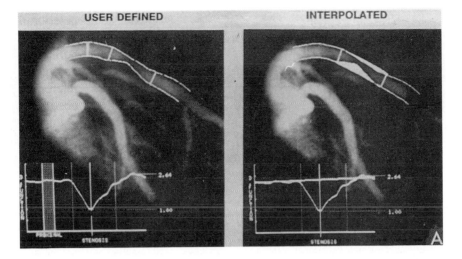

Figure 5(a).

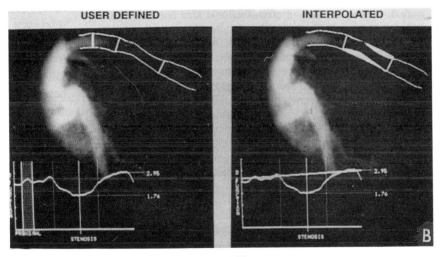

Figure 5.(b).

In 1988 2 different studies, performing follow-up angiography at different preselected follow-up intervals, gave remarkably similar results and showed more precisely how lesions behave after angioplasty [28, 29]. In a study carried out at the Thoraxcenter the minimal lumen diameter measured increased slightly from 2.06 mm to 2.11 mm at 30 days and then decreased steadily to 1.93, 1.77 mm and 1.69 mm at the subsequent follow-up times (2, 3, 4 months). Nobuyoshi and colleagues restudied 229 patients at 24 hours,

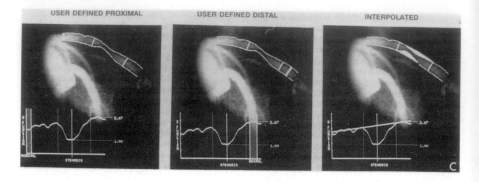

Figure 5(c).

Figures 5a–c. Single frame angiograms of a proximal left anterior descending artery stenosis. A. predilation (PRE-PTCA), B. postdilation (POST-PTCA), C. at follow-up. Quantitative coronary analysis was performed using a coronary angiography analysis system. The arterial boundaries detected by the system are shown on the angiogram and below the diameter function curve derived from these contours. The example illustrates the importance of the choice of reference diameter, the fact that the dilated but nonstenotic coronary artery may be involved in the restenosis process, and the value of the interpolated reference diameter for calculating the appropriate diameter stenosis. A. Before angioplasty, the lesion is relatively easy to analyze. The segments proximal and distal to the stenosis are of similar caliber and the lesion is relatively discrete, so that its length can easily be defined on the diameter function curve. B. After angioplasty, there is a satisfactory result, the diameter stenosis decreasing from 59% to 36% (area stenosis from 83% to 59%). C. At follow-up, the result is very dependent on the method of analysis. The artery proximal to the stenosis has already been involved in the restenosis process; if this is chosen as a reference diameter (left), a 42% diameter stenosis is obtained (no "restenosis"). The distal portion is of a larger caliber than the proximal portion; if it is chosen as a reference diameter (middle), the result is a 62% diameter stenosis ("restenosis"). If the interpolated technique is used (right), the reference diameter is similar to the postangioplasty value, and a 58% diameter stenosis is obtained that accurately reflects what is happening between the post-angioplasty result and the followup. Even with this high quality angiogram of a well visualized segment with a discrete stenosis, there are problems in obtaining accurate and realistic results.

and 1, 3, 6 and 12 months. Their findings were very similar to ours (Figure 6). In addition, it should be stressed that the individual changes in minimal luminal diameter of these lesions show that it is not just a limited number of lesions that "restenose", but rather almost all lesions deteriorate to some extent. This is a concept that is not well understood in the context of restenosis. A significant deterioration is also seen in the decreasing reference diameter which tends to minimize the change in the calculated percentage diameter stenosis. Furthermore, lesion progression after 6 months is unusual [28].

While accurate (quantitative) assessment suggests that the trend to restenosis applies to most dilated lesions, deciding which of these lesions should be defined as restenosis is less clear. Indeed, the factor that most influences

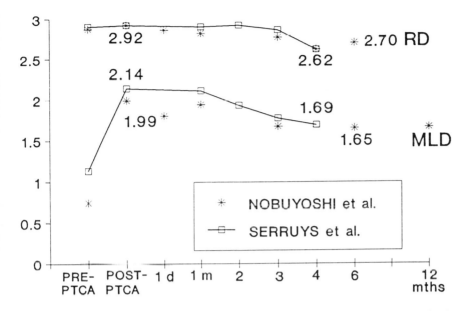

Figure 6. Minimal luminal diameter and reference diameter values found in the studies by Nobuyoshi ct al. [28] and Serruys et al. [29]. Results are remarkably similar. MLD=Minimal luminal diameter, RD=Reference diameter.

the restenosis rate is the definition of restenosis applied. Figure 7 shows the incidence of restenosis according to three criteria taken from a group of 490 lesions analyzed in the first 150 days after angioplasty [29]; the three criteria are the National Heart Lung Blood Institute criterion no IV, a loss of greater than half the gain, a diameter greater than 50% at follow-up and a change greater than 0.72 mm from postangioplasty to follow-up. From this figure two conclusions can be drawn: first, there is a variation in the incidence of restenosis according to the criterion applied; and second, the incidence of restenosis is progressive to at least the third month. At 5 months, the incidence of restenosis is not too dissimilar, ranging from 21% to 34%. However, it should be clear that even a similar incidence of restenosis using different criteria may be defining different patients. This is illustrated by Figure 8 which shows a Venn diagram of the number of lesions fulfilling three different restenosis criteria, taken from the same group of 490 lesions [29]. The 43 lesions that fulfill each criterions are enclosed by all three circles. Although the percentages of lesion, fulfilling the three criteria for restenosis were similar, it must be emphasized that each of the three criteria identified unique lesions that were not identified by the other two. This point has a particular relevance when determining the risk factors for restenosis: if restenosis cannot be reliably determined, then it is unlikely that the associated risk factors will be identified.

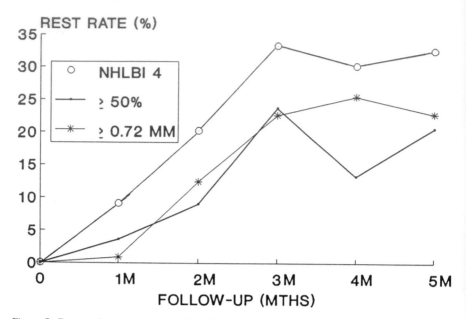

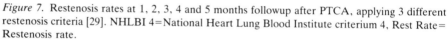

Figure 7. Restenosis rates at 1, 2, 3, 4 and 5 months followup after PTCA, applying 3 different restenosis criteria [29]. NHLBI 4=National Heart Lung Blood Institute criterium 4, Rest Rate= Restenosis rate.

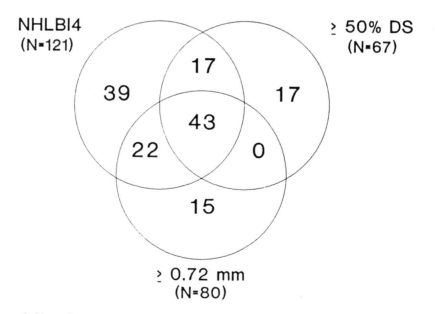

Figure 8. Venn diagram showing the number of lesions fulfilling 3 different restenosis criteria [28].

Restenosis definition, new concept

As a result of quantitative angiographic studies a new concept for defining restenosis criteria based on the change in minimal lumen diameter has been introduced. The changes in this value from post-PTCA to follow-up can be expected to give a good quantitative measurement of the degree of restenosis. The restenosis criterion or the cut-off point dividing the restenosis patients from the nonrestenosis patient is then derived by determining the variability of measurements (one standard deviation of the difference in means) of the same lesion from separate catheterization sessions. Twice the variability defines with reasonable certainty those lesions that have undergone significant deterioration from those that have not. We found this value to be 0.72 mm based on angiograms taken 90 days apart, whereas Nobuyoshi et al., using a different measurement system, found 0.5 mm based on angiograms taken 7–10 days apart. However, criteria based on the absolute change in minimal luminal diameter are nevertheless limited because they make no attempt to relate the extent of the restenosis process to the size of the vessel. Studies need to be undertaken to assess the variability of measurement on vessels with different diameters. "Sliding-scale" criteria should be created, which adjust for vessel size.

Restenosis definition, a categorical or continuous approach?

In studies evaluating the biology of restenosis, a continuous measure of the degree of luminal obstruction is preferable since any progression of the stenosis reflects the process of interest whether or not an arbitrarily defined threshold of obstruction is reached. However, when the main concern is clinical decision making, a binary or categorical measure of restenosis provides clinicians with more relevant information. Keeping in mind that an angiographic restenosis study assesses only the anatomical component of the restenosis problem, there is no threshold above which a loss of luminal diameter would have clinically significant functional or symptomatic consequences. Why then would one bother to try to define a threshold above which then would be "significant" quantitatively determined angiographic restenosis? To define the threshold on consideration of reproducibility of the measurement in individual patients is also questionable. The possible benefit of a treatment (pharmacological or interventional) can be measured with much greater precision by using the change in lumen diameter for the group. If treatment reduces the loss of luminal diameter from 0.4 mm under placebo [29] to 0.25 mm under active medication, 233 patients per treatment group are required in order to detect a significant difference with a power of 90%. The above reduction corresponds with restenosis rates (defined as a loss of minimal luminal diameter of $\geqslant 0.72$ mm) of 25% and 17.5%, respectively (Figure 9). This difference, however, can statistically be detected with a power of 90% with 620 patients per treatment group. Thus, statistically, the

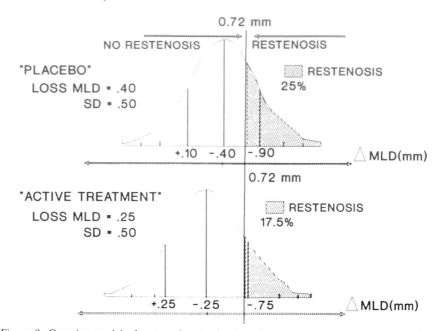

Figure 9. Gaussian model of restenosis rates in the reference group (upper panel) and in the treatment group (lower panel), considering a 30% reduction in minimal luminal diameter change in the second group. The upper panel denotes the change in minimal lumen diameter ($\triangle$ MLD) found in a prospective study of our institution [28]. A change of 0.72 mm was taken as the cutoff point for restenosis. This categorical model would mean 620 patients per group in order to have a power of 90%.

quantitative outcome determined from direct measurements of continuous variables can be evaluated with only one third of the number patients required for the categorical outcome. This is indeed logical because the categorical endpoints do not take full advantage of the available information.

Currently the results of 6 randomized trials, involving 76 cities and more than 2500 patients, are analyzed at the quantitative angiographic core laboratory in Rotterdam and at the data center in Givrins. In the future you might expect that the quantitative angiographic results will be presented according to a Gaussian model. Figure 10 shows the distribution of the change in minimal lumen diameter (MLD) from post angioplasty to 6 months follow-up angiography, excluding lesions that progressed to total occlusion. Superimposed is the theoretical Gaussian distribution curve, given the mean and standard deviation. It is clear that the change in MLD approximately follows this Gaussian distribution. Restenosis can thus be viewed as a the tail end of an approximately Gaussian distributed phenomenon with some lesions crossing a more or less arbitrary cut-off point. A cumulative distribution curve of change in MLD is an elegant way of showing results of restenosis

No of lesions

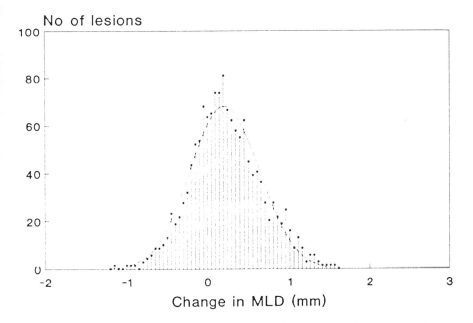

Figure 10. Distribution of the change in minimal lumen diameter (MLD) from post-angioplasty angiogram to 6 months followup angiography in 1375 lesions, excluding lesions that had progressed to total occlusion at followup. The curve superimposed on the distribution depicts the theoretical Gaussian distribution given the mean and standard deviation of the population. A change greater than 0 corresponds with a decrease in MLD.

trials. Figure 11 shows this for a restenosis prevention trial with a Thromboxane A2 receptor blocker [32].

In summary, with the advent of new technology of quantitative assessing coronary lesions, one should fully exploit the quantitative information (angiographic or ultrasonic) available (i.e. continuous approach). This is particularly important in view of the fact that the quantitatively measured anatomical changes do not specifically relate to functional endpoints.

Acknowledgements

We gratefully acknowledge the skillful secretarial assistance of Hanneke Roerade and technical assistance of Marie-Angèle Morel in the preparation of the manuscript.

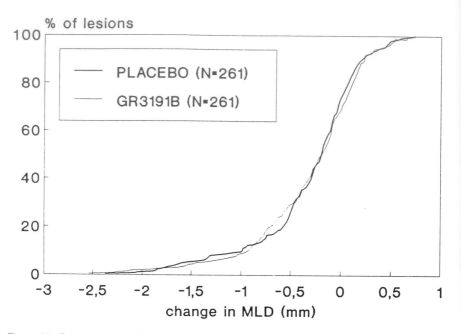

Figure 11. Cumulative distribution curve of the change in minimal lumen diameter (MLD) from post-angioplasty angiogram to follow-up angiography for the placebo and the treatment group in a restenosis prevention trial.

References

1. Waller BF. "Crackers, breakers, stretchers, drillers, scrapers, shavers, burners, welders and melters" – the future treatment of atherosclerotic coronary artery disease? A clinical-morphologic assessment. J Am Coll Cardiol 1989; **13**: 969–87.
2. McBride W, Lange RA, Hillis LD. Restenosis after successful coronary angioplasty. Pathophysiology and prevention. N Engl J Med 1988; **318**: 1734–7.
3. Serruys PW, Rensing BJ, Luijten HE, Hermans WM, Beatt KJ. Restenosis following coronary balloon angioplasty. In: Meier B (Ed.), Interventional cardiology. Toronto: Hogrefe & Huber: 79–115.
4. Schwartz RS, Murphy JG, Edwards WD, Camrud AR, Vlietstra RE, Holmes DR Jr. Restenosis after balloon angioplasty. A practical proliferative model in porcine coronary arteries. Circulation 1990; **82**: 2190–200.
5. Essed CE, Van den Brand M, Becker AE. Transluminal coronary angioplasty and early restenosis. Fibrocellular occlusion after wall laceration. Br Heart J 1983; **49**: 393–6.
6. Austin GE, Ratliff NB, Hollman J, Tabei S, Phillips DF. Intimal proliferation of smooth muscle cells as an explanation for recurrent coronary artery stenosis after percutaneous transluminal angioplasty. J Am Coll Cardiol 1985; **6**: 369–75.
7. Nobuyoshi M, Kimura T, Ohishi H, et al. Restenosis after percutaneous transluminal coronary angioplasty: pathologic observations in 20 patients. J Am Coll Cardiol 1991; 17: 433–9. Comment in: J Am Coll Cardiol 1991; **17**: 440–1.
8. Johnson DE, Hinohara T, Selmon MR, Braden LJ, Simpson JB. Primary peripheral arterial stenoses excised by transluminal atherectomy: a histopathologic study. J Am Coll Cardiol 1990; **15**: 419–25. Comment in: J Am Coll Cardiol 1990; **15**: 426–8.

9. Safian RD, Gelbfish JS, Erny RE, Schnitt SJ, Schmidt DA, Baim DS. Coronary atherectomy. Clinical, angiographic, and histological findings and observations regarding potential mechanisms. Circulation 1990; 82: 69–79. Comment in: Circulation 1990; **82**: 305–7.

10. Garratt KN, Holmes DR Jr, Bell MR, et al. Restenosis after directional coronary atherectomy: differences between primary atheromatous and restenosis lesions and influence of subintimal tissue resection. J Am Coll Cardiol 1990; **16**: 1665–71.

11. Stein, B, Fuster V, Israel DH, et al. Platelet inhibitor agents in cardiovascular disease: an update. J Am Coll Cardiol 1989; **14**: 813–36.

12. Coller BS. Platelets and thrombolytic therapy. N Engl J Med 1990; **322**: 33–42. Comment in: N Engl J Med 1990; **323**: 831.

13. Clowes AW, Schwartz SM. Significance of quiescent smooth muscle migration in the injured rat carotid artery. Circ Res 1985; **56**: 139–45.

14. Ross R. The pathogenesis of atherosclerosis – an update. N Engl J Med 1986; **314**: 488–500.

15. Liu MW, Roubin GS, King SB 3rd. Restenosis after coronary angioplasty. Potential biologic determinants and role of intimal hyperplasia. Circulation 1989; **79**: 1374–87.

16. Forrester JS, Fishbein M, Helfant R, Fagin J. A paradigm for restenosis based on cell biology: clues for the development of new preventive therapies. J Am Coll Cardiol 1991; **17**: 758–69.

17. Hermans WR, Rensing BJ, Strauss BH, Serruys PW. Prevention of restenosis after percutaneous transluminal coronary angioplasty: The search for a "magic bullet". Am Heart J 1991; **122**: 171–87.

18. Beatt KJ, Serruys PW, Hugenholtz PG. Restenosis after coronary angioplasty: new standards for clinical studies. J Am Coll Cardiol 1990; **15**: 491–8.

19. Block PC. Percutaneous transluminal coronary angioplasty: role in the treatment of coronary artery disease. Circulation 1985; **72**: V161–5.

20. Kent KM, Bonow RO, Rosing DR, et al. Improved myocardial function during exercise after successful percutaneous transluminal coronary angioplasty. N Engl J Med 1982; **306**: 441–6.

21. Joelson JM, Most AS, Williams DO. Angiographic findings when chest pain recurs after successful percutaneous transluminal coronary angioplasty. Am J Cardiol 1987; **60**: 792–5.

22. Califf RM, Ohman EM, Frid DJ, et al. Restenosis: the clinical issues. In: Topol EJ (Ed.), Textbook of interventional cardiology. Philadelphia: Saunders 1990: 363–94.

23. Lefkowitz CA, Ross BL, Schwartz L, et al. Superiority of tomographic thallium imaging for the detection of restenosis after percutaneous transluminal coronary angioplasty. J Am Coll Cardiol 1988; **13**(2 Suppl A): 161A (Abstract).

24. Reiber JH, Serruys PW. Quantitative coronary angiography. In: Marcus ML, Schelbert HR, Skorton DJ, Wolf GL (Eds.), Cardiac imaging: a companion to Braunwald's Heart Disease. Philadelphia: Saunders 1990: 211–80.

25. Reiber JH. Morphologic and densitometric quantitation of coronary stenoses: an overview of existing quantitation techniques. In: Reiber JHC, Serruys PW (Eds.), New developments in quantitative coronary angiography. Dordrecht: Kluwer 1988: 34–88.

26. Beatt KJ, Luijten HE, de Feyter PJ, van den Brand M, Reiber JH, Serruys PW. Change in diameter of coronary artery segments adjacent to stenosis after percutaneous transluminal coronary angioplasty: failure of percent diameter stenosis measurement to reflect morphologic changes induced by balloon dilation. J Am Coll Cardiol 1988; **12**: 315–23.

27. Gould KL, Lipscomb K, Hamilton GW. Physiologic basis for assessing critical stenosis: Instantaneous flow response and regional distribution during coronary hyperemia as measures of coronary flow reserve. Am J Cardiol 1974; **33**: 87–94.

28. Nobuyoshi M, Kimura T, Nosaka H, et al. Restenosis after successful percutaneous transluminal coronary angioplasty: serial angiographic follow-up of 299 patients. J Am Coll Cardiol 1988; **12**: 616–23.

29. Serruys PW, Luijten HE, Beatt KJ, et al. Incidence of restenosis after successful coronary

angioplasty: a time-related phenomenon. A quantitative angiographic study in 342 consecutive patients at 1, 2, 3 and 4 months. Circulation 1988; **77**: 361–71.
30. Meyer J, Schmitz HJ, Kiesslich T, et al. Percutaneous transluminal coronary angioplasty in patients with stable and unstable angina pectoris: analysis of early and late results. Am Heart J 1983; **106**: 973–80.
31. Fleck E, Dacian S, Dirschinger J, Hall D, Rudolph W. Quantitative changes in stenotic coronary artery lesions during follow up after PTC. Circulation 1984; **70** (4 Suppl II): II–176 (Abstract).
32. Serruys PW, Rutsch W, Heyndrickx G, et al. Effect of long term thromboxane A2 receptor blockade on angiographic restenosis and clinical events after coronary angioplasty. The Carport study. Circulation 1991; **84**: 1568–80.

20. CARPORT – Coronary artery restenosis prevention on repeated thromboxane antagonism. A multicenter randomized clinical trial

WOLFGANG RUTSCH, PATRICK W. SERRUYS, GUY R. HEYNDRICKX, NICOLAS DANCHIN, E. GIJS MAST, WILLIAM WIJNS, JEROEN VOS and J. STIBBE. On behalf of the CARPORT Study Group (Coronary Artery Restenosis Prevention On Repeated Thromboxane Antagonism).

Summary

GR32191B is a novel thromboxane A_2 receptor antagonist with potent antiaggregational and antivasoconstrictive properties. To study whether this compound is useful in restenosis prevention after coronary angioplasty, we have conducted a randomized, double blind, placebo controlled trial. Patients were randomized to receive either GR32191B, 80 mg intravenous before angioplasty and 40 mg orally for 6 months, or 250 mg intravenous aspirin before angioplasty and control for 6 months. Coronary angiograms before angioplasty, after angioplasty and at 6 months follow-up were quantitatively analyzed using an automated edge detection technique. Angioplasty was attempted in 697 patients. Failure of the procedure occurred in 47 patients (6.7%). Follow-up angiography was available in 88.5% (575 patients) of successfully treated patients. In 53 patients drug compliance was less then 80% or trial medication was discontinued for more then 3 consecutive days. Quantitative data from these patients were excluded from analysis in accordance with the protocol. Baseline clinical and angiographic parameters did not differ between the two treatment groups. Multiple matched view analysis was performed on 320 segments (261 patients) in the control group and on 316 segments (261 patients) in the active treatment group. The mean minimal luminal diameter after angioplasty was 1.77 ± 0.35 mm in the control group and 1.79 ± 0.33 mm in the treatment group. Minimal luminal diameter at follow-up angiography was 1.46 ± 0.59 mm in the control group and 1.49 ± 0.58 mm in the treatment group. The mean difference in coronary diameter between post angioplasty and follow-up angiogram was $- 0.31 \pm 0.54$ mm in the control group and $- 0.31 \pm 0.55$ mm in the treatment group. Clinical events during 6 months follow-up, analyzed on intention to treat basis, were ranked according to the highest category on a scale ranging from death, nonfatal myocardial infarction, bypass grafting, reangioplasty. No significant difference in ranking was detected between the

351

J.H.C. Reiber and P.W. Serruys (eds), Advances in Quantitative Coronary Arteriography, 351–364.
© 1993 Kluwer Academic Publishers. Printed in the Netherlands.

two treatment groups. Six months after angioplasty 75% of patients in the treatment group and 72% of patients in the control group were symptom free, 18% of the control group were in Canadian Heart Association class I/II versus 21% in the treated group and 8% of the control group was in Canadian Heart Association class III/IV versus 5% in the treated group. In conclusion: long term thromboxane A_2 receptor blockade with GR32191B does not prevent reactive intimal hyperplasia and does not favorably influence the long-term clinical course following angioplasty.

Introduction

Although major improvements in angioplasty techniques resulted in a high initial success rate, the late restenosis rate of 20–40% still limits the long term benefit of the procedure [1–5]. It is well known that restenosis after balloon angioplasty is a time related phenomenon, occuring in the first months after balloon angioplasty [5, 6].

Deendothelialisation and vascular disruption at the angioplasty site exposes vessel wall smooth muscle cells and collagen directly to blood. This causes platelet adhesion, platelet aggregation and activation of the clotting cascade. Adhesion and aggregation of platelets at the post-angioplasty plaque can lead to an early occlusion in the first 48 hours after angioplasty. Over the long term platelet and monocyte derived growth factors stimulate smooth muscle cell proliferation, leading to the fibroproliferative reaction of the vessel wall in the first months following balloon angioplasty [7–9]. Apart from the proliferation process, organization of mural thrombi may also be the cause of restenosis [10, 11]. Early platelet aggregation thus seems to play a pivotal role in the occurrence of post-angioplasty thrombotic occlusion and the restenosis process [12].

Thromboxane A_2 (TXA_2) is a potent platelet aggregational agent and vasoconstrictor released from activated platelets. A body of knowledge is now available, stressing the importance of the activated platelet and its production of TXA_2 in vascular disease states [13–17]. A promising approach towards inhibition of the detrimental effects of TXA_2 is the blockade of the receptor for thromboxane A_2 [18]. GR32191B has shown to be a potent and specific thromboxane A_2 receptor blocking drug that antagonizes the proaggregatory and vasoconstrictor actions of TXA_2, as well as those of agents that act indirectly via TXA_2, such as collagen and arachidonic acid, and agents that directly stimulate the receptor, such as PGH_2 and the TXA_2 mimetic U-46619 [18, 19]. While not affecting platelet adhesion, it potently inhibits the aggregation of platelets onto damaged blood vessels [18, 20]. This property, together with the ability of the compound to inhibit the platelet release reaction [18], indicates a potential clinical use of GR32191B in reducing early thrombotic events and late intimal hyperplasia and subsequent restenosis after angioplasty.

Coronary angiography has emerged as the most reliable method of judging in late results after coronary angioplasty. In the current trial quantitative angiography was performed with the extensively validated Cardiovascular Angiography Analysis System (CAAS) [23–26]. The conventional assessment of stenosis severity using percent diameter reduction measurements does not adequately reflect the changes occurring after angioplasty since the adjacent part of the dilated vessel segment may also be involved in the restenosis process [6, 29]. The comcomitant decrease in reference diameter can lead to a falsely low restenosis rate at follow-up. This observation lead us to select the minimal luminal diameter as a parameter for restenosis, which is independent of changes in an adjacent normal part of the dilated lesion.

The present multicenter, randomized, double-blind, aspirin-controlled trial was carried out to evaluate the role of GR32191B in the prevention of late restenosis and early thrombosis after angioplasty.

Methods

All patients with angiographically-proven coronary artery disease affecting single or multiple vessels, and with clinical symptoms of stable or unstable angina, who were scheduled for angioplasty, were considered candidates for the trial. In total 707 patients were enrolled in the study at six participating centers (see appendix).

Randomization and treatment protocol

One hour before angioplasty patients received either 80 mg of GR32191B orally and an intravenous injection of a physiological salt solution, or matching control tablets and 250 mg aspirin intravenously. Patients allocated to GR32191B continued to take 40 mg of the active drug twice daily, beginning the first evening after angioplasty and continuing for six months. Patients allocated to control tablets and aspirin intravenously received matching control tablets twice a day. The final dose of trial medication was taken one hour before the follow-up angiogram.

Angioplasty procedure and follow-up angiography

At the beginning of the angioplasty procedure all patients received 10.000 IU of intravenous heparin for the first two hours, afterwards 5.000 IU/hour for as long the procedure continued.

For the purpose of the study three coronary angiograms were obtained in each patient, one just before angioplasty, one immediately after and one angiogram at follow-up. The angiograms were recorded in such a way that they were suitable for quantitative analysis by the Cardiovascular Angiography Analysis System (CAAS), using fixed table systems and 35 mm cinefilm at a minimum speed of 25 frames per second. For calibration purposes the catheter tips were cut off and sent with the cinefilm to the angiographic core laboratory. To standardize the method of data acquisition and to ensure exact reproducibility, the following six measures were undertaken [21]. First, the angular settings of the X-ray system were recorded and repositioned to correspond exactly to the projections used during the previous angiographies. Second, cineframes to be analyzed were preferably selected at end-diastole to minimize possible foreshortening and blurring effect of motion. Third, the user defined beginning and end points of the analyzed segments were ident- ified according to the definitions of the Amercian Heart Association [22]. Fourth, to avoid the influence of vasomotion on vessel dimensions the same dose of intracoronary nitrates, either nitroglycerin or isosorbidedinitrate, was given before each angiographic study. Fifth, the same contrast medium was used for the angioplasty and follow-up angiograms at six months. Finally, photographs of the video image with the detected contours superimposed were taken to ensure that the analyses were performed on the same coronary segment in the consecutive angiograms.

Follow-up evaluation

After successful angioplasty, defined as at least one lesion successfully dilated (i.e. < 50% diameter stenosis on visual inspection after the procedure) as judged by the investigator, patients returned to the outpatient clinic after three weeks, three, six and seven months. Patients with an unsuccessful angioplasty were taken of the drug and received the standard medical care. At six months follow-up, 1 to 4 days prior to angiography a symptom limited exercise test was performed on a bicylce ergometer. The follow-up coronary angiogram was performed at the six month visit. If symptoms recurred within 6 months, coronary angiography was carried out earlier. If no definite re- stenosis was present and the follow-up time was less than 4 months, the patient was asked to undergo another coronary arteriogram at 6 months.

Quantitative angiography

All cineangiograms were analyzed using the CAAS-System [23–27]. Vessel contours were determined automatically based on the weighted sum of first and second derivative functions applied to the digitized brightness infor- mation along scanlines perpendicular to the local centerline directions of an arterial segment. A computer derived reconstruction of the original arterial dimension at the site of the obstruction was used to define the interpolated reference diameter. The absolute values of the stenosis diameter as well as the reference diameter were measured by the computer using the known contrast catheter diameter as a scaling device. All contour positions of the catheter and the arterial segment and the balloon were corrected for pin- cushion distortion.

Multiple matched view analysis was performed on each dilated lesion. This means that the mean change in minimal luminal diameter (MLD) from post angioplasty to follow-up angiography was derived from matched angiographic projections. In case of multivessel or multisite dilation, the change in MLD per patient was calculated as the average change of the different lesions.

End points

The primary end point of the study was the change in minimal luminal diameter between the post angioplasty angiogram and the follow-up angiogram. Only patients with a successful angioplasty continued with the trial medication. When discrete variables such as presence of angina or exercise test response were correlated with the outcome of quantitative angiography, categorical criteria of angiographic restenosis were applied to assess the positive and negative predictive value of these markers for restenosis. We have found a change in minimal luminal diameter of 0.72 mm or more to be a reliable indicator of angiographic lesion progression [5, 25]. This value takes into account the limitations of coronary angiographic measurements and represents twice the long-term variability for repeat measurements of a coronary obstruction using CAAS. The second criterion is an increase in diameter stenosis from less than 50% after angioplasty to greater than 50% at follow-up. This criterium was selected since common clinical practice continues to assess lesion severity by percentage stenosis. The secondary end points of the study refer to clinical events believed to be related to restenosis. The incidence of five different clinical events were compared between the two treatment groups. Each patient appears only once, placed within the highest category in the following priority: death, nonfatal myocardial infarction, CABG, repeat angioplasty at the original site and angina pectoris according to the Canadian Heart Association Classification I–IV. Only patients who received at least a single dose of trial medication, with at least one lesion that was reduced to a visually assessed diameter stenosis of less then 50% after angioplasty, who had a follow-up angiogram suitable for quantitative angiography and showed good compliance (i.e. taken at least 80% of the projected medication and did not stop taking medication for more than 3 consecutive days) were included in the analysis of the primary end point.

Statistical analysis

The minimal sample size was estimated at the outset of the study to be 233 patients in each group, on the assumption of a change of -0.40 mm in mean minimal luminal diameter between post angioplasty and follow up angiogram in the control group and -0.25 mm (i.e. a 30% difference) in the active drug group (two side test with an alpha error of 0.05 and a power of 0.90).

Table 1. Clinical baseline data of 697 patients included in analysis for clinical end points

	GR32191B n = 351	Control n = 346
Males	279 (80%)	276 (80%)
Ever smoked	280 (80%)	259 (75%)
Smoking at present	57 (16%)	40 (12%)
Hypertension	120 (34%)	111 (32%)
Diabetes	29 (8%)	28 (8%)
CCSI	42 (12%)	37 (11%)
CCS II	116 (33%)	111 (32%)
CCS III	140 (40%)	141 (41%)
CCS IV	52 (15%)	57 (16%)
Unstable Angina	48 (14%)	43 (12%)

Table 2. Flow chart

	GR32191B	Control
Randomized	353	354
No PTCA	2	8
Intention to treat	351	346
Failed PTCA	29 (8.3%)	19 (5.5%)
No QCA follow-up	35	39
Non compliance	26	27
Efficacy analysis	261	261

Results

In total 707 patients were randomized. Of these patients 353 were randomized to receive GR32191B and 354 to the control group. No baseline differences were observed between the two groups (Table 1). Angioplasty was successful in 322 of the patients in the treated group and 327 in the control group (Table 2). Quantitative angiographic follow-up was not available in 74 cases. Forty-six patients refused to undergo repeat catheterization, 2 patients died during follow-up. Eight cineangiograms were of insufficient quality to be quantitatively analyzed, and in 18 cases quantitative angiography could not be obtained for a variety of reasons.

Results of the angiographic efficacy analysis

At baseline, the minimal luminal diameter in the control and the treated group were 0.99 ± 0.35 mm and 1.06 ± 0.39 mm, respectively (Table 3). The increase in minimal luminal diameter were on average 0.78 ± 0.39 mm in the control group and 0.73 ± 0.39 mm in the treated group and did not differ

Table 3. Efficacy analysis of 636 lesions in 522 patients

	GR32191B $n = 261$	Control $n = 261$
MLD (mm)		
Pre-PTCA	1.06 ± 0.39	0.99 ± 0.35
Post-PTCA	1.79 ± 0.33	1.77 ± 0.35
Follow-up	1.49 ± 0.58	1.46 ± 0.59
Difference in MLD (mm)		
Post-pre PTCA	0.73 ± 0.38	0.78 ± 0.39
FUP-Post PTCA	−0.31 ± 0.55	−0.31 ± 0.54
Treatment effect:	0.0 (95%ci − 0.09, 0.09)	
Restenosis (0.72 mm)	21%	19%
Reference diameter (mm)		
Pre-PTCA	2.70 ± 0.50	2.64 ± 0.57
Post-PTCA	2.76 ± 0.48	2.71 ± 0.54
Follow-up	2.74 ± 0.52	2.72 ± 0.55
Difference in reference diameter (mm)		
Post-Pre-PTCA	0.06 ± 0.25	0.07 ± 0.24
FUP-post-PTCA	−0.02 ± 0.29	−0.01 ± 0.31
Percentage stenosis (%)		
Pre-PTCA	61 ± 12	62 ± 13
Post-PTCA	34 ± 9	34 ± 9
Follow-up	45 ± 19	46 ± 19
Difference in percentage stenosis (%)		
Post-pre-PTCA	−26 ± 14	−28 ± 14
FUP-post-PTCA	11 ± 19	12 ± 20

significantly. At follow-up the treatment effect was equal to 0 mm and the loss in minimal luminal diameter were identical in both groups, − 0.31 mm, so that the minimal luminal diameter at follow-up were 1.46 ± 0.59 mm in the control group and 1.49 ± 0.58 mm in the treated group. Figure 1 is a cumulative curve of the change in minimal luminal diameter observed in both groups. A loss of 0.72 mm corresponds to a restenosis rate of 19% in the control group and 21% in the treated group. The relative risk for restenosis in the treated group with respect to the control group is thus 1.15 (95% confidence intervals 0.82, 1.60). The reference diameters were comparable in both groups and did not change significantly post-angioplasty or at follow-up. Accordingly the percentage diameter stenosis decreased from 62 ± 13% pre-angioplasty in the control group and 61 ± 12% in the treated group to 34 ± 9% immediately post angioplasty for both groups with an increase in diameter stenosis at follow-up from 34 ± 9% to 46 ± 19% and 45 ± 19%, respectively.

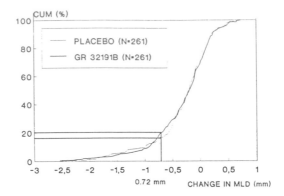

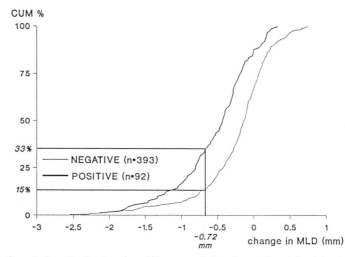

Figure 1. Cumulative distribution curve of the change in minimal luminal diameter pre-angioplasty, post-angioplasty and at 6 month follow-up.

Figure 2. Cumulative distribution (cum%) curve of the change in minimal luminal diameter (delta MLD (mm)). Patients with positive and negative exercise tests. Superimposed on the curve is the restenosis criterium of 0.72 mm. The corresponding restenosis rates can be read on the vertical axis.

Results of exercise testing

Out of 649 patients that had a successful angioplasty, 487 underwent exercise testing at follow-up. No significant difference in any parameter was observed at submaximal and maximal exercise. ST deviation of more than 0.1 mV associated with anginal symptoms was observed in 92 patients. Only 33% of these patients demonstrated angiographic restenosis with a decrease in the minimal luminal diameter of more than 0.72 mm; however, 15% of patients

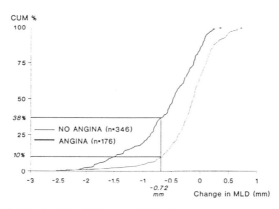

Figure 3. Cumulative distribution (cum%) curve of the change in minimal luminal diameter (delta MLD (mm)). Symptomatic versus asymptomatic patients. Superimposed on the curve is the restenosis criterium of 0.72 mm. The corresponding restenosis rates can be read on the vertical axis.

with a negative stress test had restenosis according to the -0.72 mm criterium (Figure 2). Thirty-eight% of patiens with angina pectoris demonstrated restenosis, while 10% of patients who were symptom free had clear evidence of restenosis (Figure 3).

Clinical follow-up

Clinical follow-up was done for all 697 patients randomized, who underwent angioplasty and received at least 1 dose of trial medication. During 6 months follow-up 10 patients died (Table 4). No death occurred in the first 24 hours. Procedural events included myocardial infarction in 10 patients. Myocardial infarction in the first 24 hours after guidewire removal occurred in 18 patients. During 6 months follow-up myocardial infarction was documented in 12 patients equally devided over the 2 groups. Procedural events included emergency bypass surgery in 10 patients, while early bypass surgery was performed in 7 patients. During 6 months follow-up 36 patients underwent bypass surgery with a total of 8% in each group for all time frames. Early repeat angioplasty in the first 24 hours was performed in 15 patients, and repeat angioplasty in 112 patients. At 6 months follow-up a comparable number of patients were either in Canadian Heart Association class III–IV or I–II. The total number of events during the 6 months follow-up are listed in Table 5.

Table 6 shows the ranking scale of clinical events. Finally 195 patients (56%) in the treated group and 197 (56%) in the control group were event- and symptom-free at 6 months follow-up. Adjusted chi square test revealed no difference in ranking between the two groups.

Table 4. Total number of events during 6 months follow-up

	GR32191B n = 351	Control n = 346
Death		
Late	4	6
All	4 (1%)	6 (2%)
Myocardial infarction		
Procedural	5	5
Early	7	11
Late	6	6
All	18 (5%)	22 (6%)
CABG		
Procedural	7	3
Early	2	5
Late	18	18
All	27 (8%)	26 (8%)
Repeat angioplasty		
Early	6	9
Late	53	59
All	59 (17%)	68 (20%)
Angina pectoris		
CCS IV	1 (0.3%)	5 (2%)
CCS III	18 (5%)	19 (6%)
CCS II	47 (14%)	36 (11%)
CCS I	32 (9%)	24 (7%)
None	248 (72%)	255 (75%)

Table 5. Total number of events during 6 months follow-up

	GR32191B n = 351	Control n = 346
Death	6 (2%)	4 (1%)
MI	22 (6%)	18 (5%)
CABG	26 (8%)	27 (8%)
Re-PTCA	68 (20%3	60 (17%)
CCS I–IV	86 (25%)	98 (28%)
No angina	254 (75%)	249 (72%)

Discussion

Although the subjective improvement of symptoms after angioplasty is probably the most desirable endpoint, it is also the least objective evaluation. The
reappearance of angina as a sole criterion of restenosis underestimates the
angiographic rate of restenosis. In the present trial repeat catheterization
with quantitative angiography was obtained in 88.5% of patients with a

Table 6. Ranking of clinical status 6 months after PTCA

	GR32191B n = 351	Control n = 346
Death	4 (1%)	6 (2%)
Myocardial infarction	18 (6%)	22 (6%)
CABG	22 (6%)	19 (6%)
Repeat angioplasty	48 (14%)	52 (15%)
CCS III–IV	12 (3%)	16 (5%)
I–II	49 (14%)	35 (10%)
None	197 (56%)	195 (56%)

successful angioplasty. The restenosis rate according to the 0.72 mm criterium was 33% in the symptomatic group versus 10% in the asymptomatic patients. The low positive predictive value found in this trial confirms the findings of many other studies and may be explained by the presence of other mechanisms for angina, such as incomplete revascularization or progression of disease in other vessels.

Several studies have examined the ability of the exercise treadmill test to detect restenosis after angioplasty [28]. These studies have generally found that the presence of exercise-induced angina or ST segment depression or both is not highly predictive of restenosis whether the test is performed early or late after angioplasty [11].

Continuous versus categorical approach

In studies evaluating the biology of restenosis, a continuous measure of the degree of luminal obstruction is preferable since any progression of the stenosis reflects the process of interest whether or not an arbitrarily defined threshold of obstruction is reached. Keeping in mind that an angiographic restenosis study assesses only the anatomical component of the restenosis problem, there is no threshold above which a loss of luminal diameter would have clinically significant functional or symptomatic consequences. Why then would one bother to try to define a threshold above which there would be significant quantiatively determined angiographic restenosis. The expected benefit of a treatment can be measured with much greater precision by using the change in lumen diameter.

In this trial thromboxane A_2 receptor blockade failed to demonstrate prevention of late restenosis following angioplasty. The question remains whether near complete inhibition of platelet aggregation can effectively prevent the intimal proliferative response to the barotrauma of balloon angioplasty. The restenosis process might be a multifactorial phenomenon. The injury due to stretching per se might trigger the change in phenotype of the smooth muscle cells from contractile to synthetic [30, 31], since in thrombopenic animals balloon angioplasty was followed by reactive intimal hyperplasia.

In conclusion, first, in the CARPORT study no difference was found in change in MLD between post-angioplasty angiogram and follow-up angiogram between the GR32191B treated group and the placebo group; second, no differences were detected in clinical events during the 6 months follow-up period between the GR32191B group and the placebo group.

Appendix

CARPORT Study Group

Study Chairman

Patrick W. Serruys, MD

Participating Clinics and Investigators
Thoraxcenter, Rotterdam, The Netherlands: P.W. Serruys, Principal Investigator; B.J. Rensing, MD
Universitätsklinikum Charlottenburg, Berlin, Germany: W. Rutsch, MD, Principal Investigator; M. Klose, MD
C.H.R.U. de Nancy – Hopitaux de Brabois, Nancy, France: N. Danchin, MD, Principal Investigator; Y. Juilliere, MD, A. Hueber, MD, F. Cherrier, MD
Onze Lieve Vrouw Ziekenhuis, Aalst, Belgium: G.R. Heyndrickx, MD, Principal Investigator; P. Nellens, MD, B. de Bruyne, MD, M. Goethals, MD, P. Goemare, RN
St. Antonius Ziekenhuis, Nieuwegein, The Netherlands: E.G. Mast, MD, Principal Investigator; F. Jonkman, MD, R. Tjon, MD
U.C.L. St. Luc University Hospital, Brussels, Belgium: W. Wijns MD, Principal Investigator; M. Delgadillo, MD, J. Renkin MD

Data Coordinating Center

SOCAR S.A., Nyon, Switzerland: M.Bokslag, J.Vos, MD, J.Lubsen, MD

Data Monitoring and Ethical Committee

University of Southampton, Southampton, UK: D.A. Wood, MD
Klinikum Bogenhausen, München, Germany: T. Ischinger, MD
Chest Hospital, London, UK: R. Balcon, MD

Critical Events Committee
University of Southampton, UK: D.A. Wood, MD
Onze Lieve Vrouw Ziekenhuis, Aalst, Belgium: G.R. Heyndricks, MD
C.H.R.U. de Nancy – Hopitaux de Brabois, Nancy, France: N.Danchin, MD

Quantitative Angiographic Core Laboratory

Rotterdam, The Netherlands: P.W. Serruys, MD, B.J. Rensing, MD, W.R.M. Hermans, MD, J. Pameyer

References

1. Holmes DR Jr, Vlietstra RE, Smith HC, et al. Restenosis after percutaneous transluminal coronary angioplasty (PTCA): a report from the PTCA Registry of the National Heart, Lung, and Blood Institute. Am J Cardiol 1984; **53**: 77C–81C.
2. Leimgruber PP, Roubin GS, Hollman J, et al. Restenosis after successful angioplasty in patients with single vessel disease. Circulation 1986; **73**: 710–7.
3. Kaltenbach M, Kober G, Scherer D, Vallbracht C. Recurrence rate after successful coronary angioplasty. Eur Heart J 1985; **6**: 276–81.
4. de Feyter PJ, Suryapranata H, Serruys PW, et al. Coronary angioplasty for unstable angina: immediate and late results in 200 consecutive patients with identification of risk factors for unfavorable early and late outcome. J Am Coll Cardiol 1988; **12**: 324–33.
5. Serruys PW, Luijten HE, Beatt KJ, et al. Incidence of restenosis after successful coronary angioplasty: a time related phenomenon. A quantitative angiographic study in 342 consecutive patients at 1, 2, 3, and 4 months. Circulation 1988; **77**: 361–71.
6. Nobuyoshi M, Kimura T, Nosaka H, et al. Restenosis after successful percutaneous transluminal coronary angioplasty: serial angiographic follow-up of 229 patients. J Am Coll Cardiol 1988; **12**: 616–23.
7. Stemerman MB. Vascular injury: platelets and smooth muscle cell response. Philos Trans R Soc Lond (Biol) 1981; **294**: 217–24.
8. Ross R. The pathogenesis of atherosclerosis – an update. N Engl J Med 1986; **314**: 488–500.
9. Faxon DP, Sanborn TA, Haudenschild CC, Ryan TJ. Effect of antiplatelet therapy on restenosis after experimental angioplasty. Am J Cardiol 1984; **53**: 72C–76C.
10. Steele PM, Chesebro JH, Stanson AW, et al. Balloon angioplasty. Natural history of the pathophysiological response to injury in the pig model. Circ Res 1985; **57**: 105–12.
11. Wilentz JR, Sanborn TA, Haudenschild CC, Valeri CR, Ryan TJ, Faxon DP. Platelet accumulation in experimental angioplasty: time course and relation to vascular injury. Circulation 1987; **75**: 636–42.
12. Chesebro JH, Lam JY, Fuster V. The pathogenesis and prevention of aorto-coronary vein bypass graft occlusion and restenosis after angioplasty: role of vascular injury and platelet thrombus deposition. J Am Coll Cardiol 1986; **8**(6 Suppl B): 57B–66B.
13. Davies MJ, Thomas A. Thrombosis and acute coronary-artery lesions in sudden cardiac ischemic death. N Engl J Med 1984; **310**: 1137–40.
14. Sherman DG, Hart RG. Thromboembolism and antithrombotic therapy in cerebrovascular disease. J Am Coll Cardiol 1986; **8**(6 Suppl B): 88B–97B.
15. Green K, Vesterqvist O. In vivo synthesis of thromboxane and prostacyclin in man in health and disease. Data from GC-MS measurements of major urinary metabolites. Adv Prostaglandin Thromboxane Leukotriene Res 1986; **16**: 309–24.
16. Catella F, Lawson JA, Fitzgerald DJ, Fitzgerald GA. Analysis of multiple thromboxane metabolites in plasma and urine. Adv Prostaglandin Thromboxane Leukotriene Res 1987; **17b**: 611–4.
17. Cairns JA, Gent M, Singer J, et al. Aspirin, sulfinpyrazone, or both in unstable angina. Results of a Canadian Multicenter Trial. N Engl J Med 1985; **313**: 1369–75.
18. Hornby EJ, Foster MR, McCabe PJ, Stratton LE. The inhibitory effect of GR32191, a thromboxane receptor blocking drug, on human platelet aggregation, adhesion and secretion. Thromb Haemost 1989; **61**: 429–36.
19. Lumley P, White BP, Humphrey PPA. GR32191, a highly potent and specific thromboxane A_2 receptor blocking drug on platelets and vascular and airway smooth muscle in vitro. Br J Pharmacol 1989; **97**: 783–94.
20. McCabe PJ, Stratton LE, Hornby EJ, Foster M. Inhibition of guinea-pig platelet function in vivo and ex vivo using the thromboxane A_2 receptor antagonist, AH23848 and GR32191. Thromb Haemost 1987; **58**: 182 (Abstract).

21. Reiber JHC, Serruys PW, Kooijman CJ, Slager CJ, Schuurbiers JCH, den Boer A. Approaches towards standardization in acquisition and quantitation of arterial dimensions from cineangiograms. In: Reiber JHC, Serruys PW (Eds.), State of the art in quantitative coronary arteriography. Dordrecht: Martinus Nijhoff Publishers 1986: 145–72.
22. Austen WG, Edwards JE, Frye RL, et al. A reporting system on patients evaluated for coronary artery disease. Report of the Ad Hoc Committee for Grading of Coronary Artery Disease, Council on Cardiovascular Surgery, American Heart Association. Circulation 1975; 51P Suppl: 5–40.
23. Reiber JHC, Kooijman CJ, Slager CJ et al. Coronary artery dimensions from cineangiograms: methodology and validation of a computer-assisted analysis procedure. IEEE Trans Med Imaging 1984; 3: 131–41.
24. Reiber JHC, Slager CJ, Schuurbiers JCH, et al. Transfer functions of the X-ray sine video chain applied to digital processing of coronary cineangiograms. In: Heintzen PH, Brennecke R (Eds.), Digital imaging in cardiovascular radiology. Stuttgart: Georg Thieme Verlag 1983: 89–104.
25. Reiber JHC, Serruys PW, Kooijman CJ, et al. Assessment of short-, medium-, and long-term variations in arterial dimensions from computer-assisted quantitation of coronary cineangiograms. Circulation 1985; 71: 280–8.
26. Serruys PW, Reiber JHC, Wijns W, et al. Assessment of percutaneous transluminal coronary angioplasty by quantitative coronary angiography: diameter versus densitometric area measurements. Am J Cardiol 1984; 54: 482–8.
27. Reiber JHC, Serruys PW, Slager CJ. Quantitative coronary and left ventricular cineangiography: methodology and clinical applications. Dordrecht: Martinus Nijhoff Publishers 1986: 162–89.
28. Califf RM, Ohman EM, Frid DJ, et al. Restenosis: the clinical issue. In: Topol EJ (Ed.), Textbook of interventional cardiology. Philadelphia: Saunders 1990: 363–94.
29. Beatt KJ, Luijten HE, de Feyter PJ, van den Brand M, Reiber JHC, Serruys PW. Change in diameter of coronary artery segments adjacent to stenosis after percutaneous transluminal coronary angioplasty: failure of percent diameter stenosis measurement to reflect morphologic changes induced by balloon dilation. J Am Coll Cardiol 1988; 12: 315–23.
30. Campbell GR, Campbell JH. Smooth muscle phenotypic changes in arterial wall homeostasis: implications for the pathogenesis of atherosclerosis. Exp Mol Pathol 1985; 42: 139–62.
31. Clowes AW, Reldy MA, Clowes MM. Kinetics of cellular proliferation after arterial injury. I. Smooth muscle growth in the absence of endothelium. Lab Invest 1983; 49: 327–33.

21. Angiotensin converting enzyme inhibition in the prevention of restenosis: the MERCATOR and MARCATOR trials

DAVID P. FAXON and RAPHAEL BALCON

Summary

Angiotensin II is recognized to result in hypertrophy, migration and proliferation of vascular smooth muscle cells. Recently it has been shown that the angiotensin converting enzyme inhibitor (ACE) cilazipril, inhibits myointimal proliferation following balloon injury in the rat. Confirmatory studies suggest that ACE inhibitors may prevent restenosis experimentally. Two large multicenter trials are now being conducted to evaluate the efficacy of cilazipril in the prevention of restenosis following angiography. The European study (the MERCATOR study) involves 27 centers. 736 patients have been randomized to placebo plus aspirin or cilazipril 5 mg bid. The primary endpoint is the change in minimal lumen diameter as assessed by quantitative angiography (CAAS system) at a core laboratory in Rotterdam. Other endpoints include death, non-fatal MI, function status, angina relief, and exercise stress testing. The final results will be presented in August 1991. The North American Study (MARCATOR) is a parallel study including 42 centers in the United States and Canada. It utilizes similar entry criteria and endpoints but differs in that patients are randomized into 4 groups (placebo, 1 mg, 5 mg or 10 mg of cilazipril bid plus aspirin). 1,428 patients have been enrolled and the study will conclude in December of 1991. Presentation of the results are expected in the spring of 1992. Together these studies will be the largest restenosis trial utilizing detailed angiographic endpoints.

Introduction

Restenosis remains the most troublesome complication of angioplasty. Solutions to the problem of restenosis following angioplasty have yet to be found despite efforts to reduce this problem with antiplatelet, anticoagulant and calcium antagonists [1]. It has become clear that the pathophysiology of this problem is complex. Recent studies would suggest that it involves the complex interaction of elastic recoil of the vessel, platelet deposition, thrombosis

J.H.C. Reiber and P.W. Serruys (eds), Advances in Quantitative Coronary Arteriography. 365–372.

and myointimal proliferation [2]. This latter process has been shown to be present in the majority of patients developing restenosis [3]. Balloon angioplasty initially results in denudation of the endothelium with creation of intimal and medial tears as a result of stretching of the vessel. These events are followed by a series of pathophysiological events that draw close analogy to wound healing [4]. Initially platelets adhere and aggregate. They release seratonin, ADP, Epinephrine as well as growth promoters such as platelet derived growth factor and platelet factor 4. Micro and often macro thrombi form with thrombin itself providing a stimulus for mitogenic activity [2]. Within 1 to 2 days an inflammatory response ensues and monocytes infiltrate into the damaged area. Mitogens from platelets and inflammatory cells as well as damaged smooth muscle cells themselves activate the quiescence smooth muscle cell to phenotypically change, migrate and proliferate in the intima [5]. These stimulated synthetic smooth muscle cells continue to divide and secrete large amounts of extracellular matrix. The final process is organization of this matrix with the laying down of collagen and elastin [4]. During this period of time the endothelium also regrows and by six months the smooth muscle cells have returned to a quiescence status and further progression of the lesion is unlikely. While many of the steps in the process are speculative and based upon basic in vitro and in vivo studies, histopathological examination of atherectomy specimens and of patients who have died following angioplasty emphasize the importance of neointimal proliferation as a central process in restenosis [3, 6]. Currently a great deal of attention is being focused on this aspect of restenosis and on the means of preventing excessive proliferation.

Antiproliferative effect of ace inhibitors

The rationale for angiotensin converting enzyme inhibition in the prevention of restenosis derives from the knowledge of the importance of angiotensin II's contribution to proliferation of endothelial and smooth muscle cells. It is recognized that endothelial and smooth muscle cells have converting enzyme and angiotensin II receptors [7]. Exogenous angiotensin II can result in hypertrophy, migration and proliferation of smooth muscle cells and culture [8]. It also induces PDGF A chain, c-myc, c-fos and c-june early oncogenes that signal the onset of DNA synthesis [9]. The most compelling evidence that angiotensin converting enzyme inhibitors may help in preventing restenosis comes from the work of Powell and Baumgartner [10]. In a rat carotid model of intimal proliferation these investigators demonstrated that a long acting converting enzyme inhibitor, cilazipril, was capable of reducing intimal hyperplasia 14 days after balloon injury. In a series of studies they demonstrated a dose response relationship between cilazipril and the development of intimal hyperplasia. At a dose of 10 mg/kg/day a 70% reduction was possible.

Approximately a 20% greater reduction was obtained when the treatment was started 6 days before injury. They also demonstrated that other ACE inhibitors including Captopril at a dose of 100 mg/kg was also capable of inducing a similar effect. Other antihypertensive agents including verapamil, minoxidil and hydralazine had no effect. The addition of heparin to cilazipril resulted in further inhibition of proliferation [11]. Recent cell culture studies would suggest that this effect is primarily due to angiotensin II rather than due to other potential mechanisms such as increasing tissue bradykinin or prostaglandin E1 (JS Powell, personal communication).

Another confirmatory study was recently reported by Bilazarian [12]. Using a hypercholesterolemic atherosclerotic rabbit model, animals were randomized to cilazipril 5 mg/kg/day or placebo one week before angioplasty. Angioplasty of focal > 50% stenoses in the iliac arteries were performed and the animals were then followed for four weeks in a high cholesterol diet. Repeat angiography demonstrated restenosis in all control animals but only 30% of the treatment group. Quantitative histology confirmed a smaller intima and media in the treatment group when compared to the control animals. In addition other studies have indicated that ACE inhibitors can retard the development of atherosclerosis. In the Wantanabe rabbit Choban- ian and colleagues showed a significant reduction in plaque area and arterial cholesterol content in the thoracic aorta after 26 weeks of treatment with 25–50 mg/kg/day of Captopril [13].

Recently two studies in a swine model has shown that cilazipril as well as another long-acting ACE inhibitor, trandolopril, were unable to reduce the proliferative response following balloon injury or placement of an intravascu- lar stent in the coronary artery [14, 15]. The discrepancy of this study with the previously mentioned studies is uncertain but may reflect differences in animal models and pathophysiological mechanisms.

In addition to the effect on smooth muscle cell proliferation, converting enzyme inhibitors may have been shown to have an effect on endothelial function that may also be important in the development of restenosis. Endo- thelium is critically important in regulating vascular constriction and relax- ation as well as regulating other arterial wall functions. Following de-endo- thelization and subsequent regrowth, the endothelium loses much of its normal function. Recent studies in the DOC salt rat model have demon- strated endothelial dysfunction that can be partially reversed by angiotensin converting enzyme inhibitor cilazipril [16].

These studies in a variety of different animal models with various angioten- sin converting enzyme inhibitors demonstrate that ACE inhibitors have im- portant inhibitory effects on neointimal proliferation and can restore normal endothelial function. On the basis of these studies, two large multicenter trials are currently being undertaken in Europe and the United States to evaluate the effect of cilazipril in the prevention of restenosis following angioplasty in man.

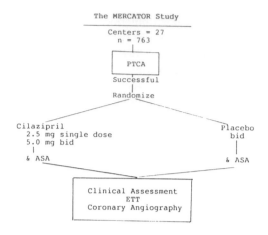

Figure 1. The study design for the MERCATOR study.

The MERCATOR study

The primary objective of the study was to determine whether cilazipril in a dose of 5 mg twice daily plus aspirin reduced the rate and/or extent of restenosis compared to placebo plus aspirin after successful PTCA as judged by repeat angiography 6 months after the procedure.

The secondary objectives were to assess the tolerability and safety of cilazipril and to assess the effect of cilazapril on the frequency of clinical events suggestive of re-occlusion; the incidence of myocardial ischemia on the 6 month exercise test; the frequency of repeat PTCA or by-pass surgery; and the progression of disease in the untreated vessels.

In addition to these objectives, clinical outcome was assessed. Survival free of symptoms or clinical sequelae of coronary artery disease was considered a favorable outcome. To assess this at 12 months each patient was assigned to the highest applicable category on the following six point scale:
– Death from any cause
– Myocardial infarction since randomization
– Repeat intervention for severe angina
– Severe LV dysfunction (NHYA III or IV)
– Need of increased anti-anginal therapy
– None of the above

The study was a multicenter, double-blind, parallel group trial. Quantitative angiograms were obtained on all patients on entry to the study and at 6 months (Figure 1). The angiograms were obtained after nitroglycerin using the same projections, x-ray settings and patient position. The quantitative angiograms were analyzed at the core laboratory in Rotterdam. Every center performed at least 2 "dummy runs" to ensure adequate angiographic technique and quality. The apparatus in each center was checked with a standard grid to assess the degree of pincushion distortion. Absolute measurements were obtained by calibration using the tip of the catheter used to take the angiogram. Restenosis was assessed by comparison of absolute measurements of minimal lumen diameter from the 2 angiograms.

Exercise testing was performed at follow-up using a bicycle ergometer according to the guidelines of the European Society of Cardiology.

The calculation of the sample size of three hundred evaluable patients per group was based on the assumption that the restenosis rate in the placebo group would be 30% and that this would be halved in the treatment group.

Baseline characteristics were compared using appropriate standard parametric and nonparametric statistical tests. The primary final analysis will be on an "Intention to treat" basis of those patients who had a successful angioplasty. The data were continuously monitored by an independent Critical Events Committee.

Patients aged 25 to 75 selected for PTCA were eligible for inclusion. The exclusion criteria were: childbearing potential; sustained hypertension; systolic BP = < 100 or diastolic BP < 65; Q wave myocardial infarction within 4 weeks; previous attempted PTCA at the same site.

Suitable patients who had signed informed consent were randomized, a quantitative angiogram performed followed by the PTCA. If successful, cilazapril 2.5 mg or placebo was given on the same day. The dose was increased to 5 mg the next day, and aspirin 100 mg added. This regime was continued for 6 months in all patients when an exercise test was performed and quantitative angiography repeated.

Recruitment

Twenty-seven centers in 8 European countries took part in the study, and undertook to recruit the necessary patients. A total of 763 patients were recruited in 5 months. All centers at least achieved their recruitment target and many exceeded it. Data collection was complete and angiographic standards were achieved. Data analysis is now being completed and the results will be available in the fall of 1991.

The MARCATOR study

The overall goal of the MARCATOR study is to evaluate the effect of incremental doses of cilazipril on prevention of restenosis following coronary angioplasty. The study is intended to complement the recently conducted European trial. It differs however in a number of important areas.

The study involves 41 centers in the United States and Canada. A core angiographic laboratory is located in Rotterdam under the direction of Patrick Serruys, M.D. and angiographic data is reviewed by an external angiographic committee. A Steering Committee oversees the conduct of the trial

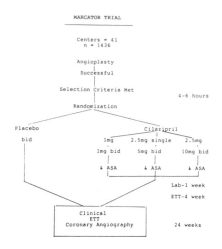

Figure 2. The study design for the MARCATOR study.

in concert with the study directors and sponsor. A safety data monitoring committee is responsible for reviewing the safety and efficacy endpoints of the trial.

The primary objective of the study is to assess relative to placebo the extent to which cilazipril in varying doses effects the angiographically measured absolute minimal lumen diameter at 24 weeks after initially successful PTCA. Other objectives include assessment of clinical benefit to the patient, assessment of the effect of treatment on exercise capacity at 24 weeks, a comparison of the exercise capacity between 4 and 24 weeks relative to the minimal lumen diameter and to assess angiographic restenosis rates using a variety of categorical definitions. Finally the safety and tolerability of cilazipril will also be evaluated.

The study is designed as a multicenter double-blind 4 parallel placebo controlled trial. After a successful PTCA and informed consent patients are randomly allocated to cilazipril 1 mg or 2.5 mg in a single initial dose and then 1.5 or 10 mg bid plus aspirin 325 mg once daily or to placebo bid plus aspirin (Figure 2). The first dose of medication is administered within 6 hours of a successful angioplasty and the patients are maintained in the hospital for 24 hours prior to discharge. Patients are then seen at 1 week at which time clinical status is assessed and renal function and blood pressure measured. The patient is again re-evaluated at four weeks at which time an exercise test is performed and a clinical status is assessed at 8 and 16 weeks. The patient returns for a repeat cardiac catheterization at 24 weeks at which time an exercise treadmill test is again repeated. The study medication is continued throughout the entire evaluation period.

Inclusion criteria for participation in the study include all patients between the age of 25 and 79 who undergo a successful angioplasty. Patients are excluded if they are known to be on maintenance therapy of diuretics or have severe essential hypertension. Patients who had a recent myocardial infarction or received thrombolytic therapy within seven days of the study entry are also excluded. Likewise patients with hemodynamically significant valve disease, left main disease or who have had prior bypass surgery and are undergoing dilation of a coronary bypass graft. Patients with previous angioplasty at the same site are likewise excluded. Other known severe cardiac or medical conditions are also not included in this study.

1,436 patients have been recruited into this study. This sample size was calculated by assuming that the restenosis rate of 30% in a placebo group and 20% in the cilazipril group with a significance level of 5% and a power of 80%. This will require a size of 293 available patients. 350 patients per group were estimated to be necessary accounting for 15% of the patients in whom the test drug would be discontinued.

As previously mentioned the primary endpoint of the study is angiographically determined minimal lumen diameter in the dilated vessel after 24 weeks of therapy. The analysis will use an intention to treat principle. However, subsequent analyses will also involve analysis of those who actually received therapy. For patients who do not obtain a final angiogram the minimal lumen diameter will be imputed as 0 for all patients who die or have an MI or coronary bypass surgery. All other patients will be assumed to be the same as the average for all patients. Clinical endpoints including death, severe symptomatic cardiac disease (New York Heart Association functional class III or IV), non fatal MI, repeat PTCA or bypass surgery, Canadian Cardiovascular Society anginal class II or greater or an increase in anginal medications will be determined for each patient on a clinical scale created and compared between treatment groups. The separate 5 and 10 mg doses of cilazipril will be compared independently to placebo. If these outcomes are similar then they will be combined and compared between the MERCATOR and MARCATOR studies. Again, if similar then the placebo group will be pooled and the 5 mg of the MERCATOR will be pooled with the 5 mg and 10 mg of MARCATOR and comparisons again made.

Conclusions

Based on experimental studies in a variety of animal models, it is evident that angiotensin converting enzyme inhibitors reduce intimal proliferation following vascular injury as well as the development of atherosclerosis. Two large multicenter trials are currently ongoing to examine whether cilazipril, a long-acting ACE inhibitor, prevents restenosis following successful angioplasty. The trials are appropriately sized to determine a 10% difference in restenosis and combined will be the largest clinical trial yet performed in the area of restenosis. It also should be a model for future studies in the prevention of restenosis and in addition to evaluating the efficacy of cilazipril will likely provide useful information about the angiographic patterns and clinical predictors of restenosis following angioplasty.

References

1. Califf RM, Ehman EM, Frid DJ, et al. Restenosis: the clinical issues. In: Topol EJ (Ed.), Textbook of interventional cardiology. Philadelphia: WB Saunders 1990: 363–94.
2. Ip JH, Fuster V, Israel D, Badimon L, Badimon J, Chesebro J. The role of platelets, thrombin and hyperplasia in restenosis after coronary angioplasty. J Am Coll Cardiol 1991; **17** (6 Suppl B): 77B–88B.
3. Nobuyoshi M, Kimura T, Ohishi H, et al. Restenosis after percutaneous transluminal coronary angioplasty: pathologic observations in 20 patients. J am Coll Cardiol 1991; 17: 433–9. Comment in: J Am Coll Cardiol 1991; **17**: 440–1.
4. Forrester JS, Fishbein M, Helfant R, Fagin J. A paradigm for restenosis based on cell biology: clues for the development of new preventive therapies. J Am Coll Cardiol 1991; **17**: 758–69.
5. Clowes AW, Schwartz SM. Significance of quiescent smooth muscle cell migration in the injured rat carotid artery. Circ Res 1985; **56**: 139–45.
6. Lui MW, Roubin GS, King SB III. Restenosis after coronary angioplasty. Potential biologic determinants and role of intimal hyperplasia. Circ 1989; **79**: 1374–87.
7. Dzau VJ. Circulating versus local renin-angiotensin system in cardiovascular hemostasis. Circ 1988; **77**: I4–13.
8. Campbell-Boswell M, Robertson AL Jr. Effects of angiotensin II and vasopressin on human smooth muscle cells in vitro. Exp Mol Pathol 1981; **35**: 265–76.
9. Naftilan AJ, Pratt RE, Dzau VJ. Induction of platelet-derived growth factor A-chain and c-myc gene expressions by angiotensin II in cultured rat vascular smooth muscle cells. J Clin Invest 1989; **83**: 1419–24.
10. Powell JS, Clozel JP, Muller RK, et al. Inhibitors of angiotensin-converting enzyme prevent myointimal proliferation after vascular injury. Science 1989; **245**: 186–8.
11. Powell JS, Muller RK, Baumgartner HR. Suppression of the vascular response to injury: the role of angiotensin converting enzyme inhibitors. J Am Coll Cardiol 1991; **17** (6 Suppl B): 137B–42B.
12. Bilazarian SD, Currier JW, Haudenschild CC, Heyman D, Powell J, Faxon DP. Angiotensin converting enzyme inhibition reduces restenosis in experimental angioplasty. J Am Coll Card 1991; **17** (2 Suppl A): 268A (Abstract).
13. Chobanian AV, Haudenschild CC, Nickerson C, Drago R. Antiatherogenic effects of Captopril in the Wantanabe heritable hyperlipidemic rabbit. Hypertension 1990; **15**: 327–31.
14. Lam JY, Bourassa MG, Lacoste L, Lachapelle C. Can Cilazipril reduce the development of atherosclerotic changes in the balloon injured porcine carotid arteries? Circulation 1990; **82** (4 Suppl III): III–429 (Abstract).
15. Schwartz R, Edwards W, Camrud A, Jorgenson, Murphy J, Holmes D. Effect of angiotensin converting enzyme inhibition or smooth muscle proliferation in a porcine coronary restenosis model: proceedings of the restenosis summit 1991. Sl.l.: S.N. 1991.
16. Clozel M, Kuhn H, Heft, F. Effects of angiotensin converting enzyme inhibitors and of hydralazine on endothelial function in hypertensive rats. Hypertension 1990; **16**: 532–40. Comment in: Hypertension 1990; 541–3.

22. Historic. A multicenter randomized clinical trial to evaluate feasibility and tolerability of recombinant congener of hirudin as an alternative to heparin during PTCA

GUY R. HEYNDRICKX on behalf of the Historic Study Group

Summary

Incidence of restenosis after conventional balloon dilatation has remained unchanged over the last decade despite major efforts to reduce its occurrence, underlining the lack of insight regarding trigger mechanisms and pathophysiological processes. In the course of elucidating the mechanisms of intimal proliferation after PTCA, it has become clear that thrombin formation plays a pivotal role in early and late reactive changes of the vessel wall. Hence a working hypothesis was proposed that blocking thrombin could favorably alter the course and sequence of events leading to restenosis. Hirudin, a potent thrombin inhibitor, was chosen to verify this hypothesis. Prior to a major restenosis trial, a pilot study was first designed to test the feasibility and safety of a 24 hour rec-hirudin infusion compared to heparin, during PTCA.

Introduction

Coronary angioplasty has been widely accepted as a valuable, safe and effective alternative to coronary bypass surgery by the medical community. Yet the incidence of late restenosis of 20–40% has remained much the same over the last decade, requiring often repeat interventions or coronary bypass surgery for lasting results [1, 2].

Sofar no procedural or technical act nor pharmacologic interventions have been shown to alter significantly the restenosis process.

Restenosis after PTCA seems to be more complex than first anticipated and numerous subtle theoretical considerations did not live up to the expectations in PTCA practice. Several pharmacological interventions along different lines of reasoning have failed to show any beneficial effects in large randomized clinical trials.

Thus research endeavour should be pursued and another step in this course is the Historic trial.

J.H.C. Reiber and P.W. Serruys (eds). Advances in Quantitative Coronary Arteriography, 373–376.
© 1993 *Kluwer Academic Publishers. Printed in the Netherlands.*

Aim of the trial

The primary objective of the Historic trial is to evaluate the feasibility for a much larger future trial i.e. the Helvetica trial (Hirudin in a European restenosis prevention trial versus heparin treatment in PTCA patients) designed to assess the efficacy of recombinant hirudin – in reference to standard heparin – in preventing restenosis in patients undergoing PTCA.

Hirudin is a potent selective, direct, and almost irreversible inhibitor of thrombin which was initially isolated from the salivary secretions of the medicinal leech. Its recombinant congener rec-hirudine (CGP 39393) is also a potent and selective thrombin inhibitor.

Rationale

The rationale for this trial stems from the knowledge that thrombin is generated at the time of arterial injury and through a potent amplifying effect on platelet adhesion and clotting cascade initiates early thrombus formation on the one hand and release of vasoactive and mitogenic substances on the other hand [3]. These effects may trigger early reocclusion after vessel wall injury as well as late smooth muscle cell proliferation and migration inducing late restenosis.

Hirudin is known to prevent thrombus induced platelet activation [4, 5]. Recent experimental evidence shows that r-hirudin not only prevents thrombosis after vessel wall injury but also reduces restenosis after balloon angioplasty of atherosclerotic arteries in rabbits [6]. Its seems thus that thrombin holds a pivotal role in the early and late adaptive changes of the vessel wall subjected to injury. Blocking these effects of thrombin is the next logical step to investigate.

Trial design

The trial was conducted in 5 hospitals in Belgium and the Netherlands. From January 1991 till May 1991 a total of 118 patients have been recruited, between 30 and 75 years with angiographically-proven atherosclerotic coronary artery disease affecting single or multiple vessel and with clinical symptoms of stable or unstable angina pectoris, who were scheduled for angioplasty.

After obtaining written informed consent patients were randomized between hirudin and heparin treatment. Two patients were allocated to hirudin for each patient allocated to heparin treatment.

Trial medication was started after puncture of the femoral artery and introduction of the sheaths. Hirudin was given 20 mg iv̇. followed by an infusion of 0.16 mg/kg/h.

Heparin was given 10.000 IU-iv̇. followed by infusion 12 IU/kg/h.

Intravenous infusions were ceased after repeat angiogram at 24 hrs.

The infusion rates were adjusted as to maintain APTT between 85 and 120 sec.

Experimental medication was packaged and supplied by Ciba-Geigy (Switzerland).

Angioplasty procedure and follow-up angioplasty

Coronary angioplasty was performed with a steerable, movable guide wire system via the femoral route. Standard available balloon catheters were used. Trial medication was started after puncturing the femoral artery. For study purposes three coronary angiograms were obtained in each patient, one just before PTCA, one immediately after angioplasty and one angiogram at 24 hours. The angiograms were recorded in such a way that they were suited for quantitative analysis by the Coronary Angiography Analysis System (CAAS) [7, 8].

End point

The end point assessment will include:
a) changes in cross-sectional area and area plaque at 24 hrs repeat angiography relative to baseline angiogram (post-PTCA);
b) changes in biological markers of early thrombosis. Laboratory test will include activated partial thromboplastin time, prothrombin time as well as platelet counts, thrombin induces aggregation, thrombin chromogenic assay, thrombin antithrombin complexes, anti-Xa, Di-dimer, tissue plasminogen activator antigen and plasminogen activator inhibitor antigen;
c) symptoms and signs of recurrent myocardial ischemia;
d) occurrence of silent myocardial ischemia during 24 hrs post PTCA using Holter-ECG;
e) bleeding complications;
f) occurrence of cardiac death, myocardial infarction, repeat angioplasty or CABG within one month after PTCA.

Conclusion

The Historic trial aims to compare the use of rec-hirudin (CGP 39393) and heparin in a randomized double blind fashion in order to test tolerability and safety of this new compound. Patient intake as well as data collection is now completed.

The final data analysis is expected for the end of this year (1991).

A decision regarding a larger trial will also be taken on the basis of the pilot study.

Appendix

Historic study Group.

Study Chairman: Patrick W Serruys, MD.

Participating Clinics:
- Thoraxcenter, Rotterdam, The Netherlands.
- Academisch Ziekenhuis, Leiden, The Netherlands.
- Cardiovascular Center, O.L.V.-Ziekenhuis, Aalst, Belgium.
- Onze-Lieve-Vrouwe Gasthuis, Amsterdam, The Netherlands.
- Ziekenhuis De Weezenlanden, Zwolle, The Netherlands.

References

1. Leimgruber PP, Roubin GS, Hollman J, et al. Restenosis after successful coronary angioplasty in patients with single-vessel disease. Circulation 1986; **73**: 710–7.
2. Serruys PW, Luijten HE, Beatt KJ, et al. Incidence of restenosis after successful coronary angioplasty: a time-related phenomenon. A quantitative angiographic study in 342 consecutive patients at 1, 2, 3, and 4 months. Circulation 1988; **77**: 361–71.
3. Harker LA. Role of platelets and thrombosis in mechanisms of acute occlusion and restenosis after angioplasty. Am J Cardiol 1987; **60**: 20B–28B.
4. Markwardt F. Pharmacology of hirudin: one hundred years after the first report of the anticoagulant agent in medicinal leeches. Biomed Biochim Acta 1985; **44**: 1007–13.
5. Kaiser B, Markwardt F. Antithrombotic and haemorrhagic effects of synthetic and naturally occurring thrombin inhibitors. Thromb Res 1986; **43**: 613–20.
6. Sarembock IJ, Gertz SD, Gimple LW, Owen RM, Powers ER, Roberts WC. Effectiveness of Recombinant Desulphatohirudin in Reducing Restenosis After Balloon Angioplasty of Atherosclerotic Femoral Arteries in Rabbits. Circulation 1991; **84**: 232–243.
7. Reiber JH, Kooyman CJ, Slager CJ, et al. Coronary artery dimensions from cineangiograms: methodology and validation of a computer-assisted analysis procedure. IEEE Trans Med Imaging 1984; **3**: 131–41.
8. Serruys PW, Reiber JH, Wijns W, et al. Assessment of percutaneous transluminal coronary angioplasty by quantitative coronary angiography: diameter versus densitometric area measurements. Am J Cardiol 1984; **54**: 482–8.

23. Angiopeptin in experimental models of restenosis

KENNETH M. KENT, MARIE L. FOEGH, MUN HONG and
PETER W. RAMWELL

Summary

Recurrent arterial obstructions, restenosis, after coronary angioplasty are
due to myointimal proliferation, probably due to the barotrauma of balloon
dilatation. This phenomenon has been studied extensively and although agents have been found to inhibit the response in experimental animal angioplasty, no agents have been proved to be useful in humans. The mitogenic
response which leads to proliferation is undoubtably controlled by growth
factors initiated by the initial arterial wall injury. Angiopeptin, a synthetic
octapeptide analogue of somatastatin, is effective in inhibiting myointimal
proliferation in a variety of animal models of vascular injury. Both in vitro
and in vivo models of injury have demonstrated decreased intimal proliferation by morphometric analyses and decreased thymidine incorporation as
an index of cellular proliferation. Physiologic amounts of these agents have
been used in these experiments, doses that are well tolerated in humans. A
controlled clinical trial is underway to assess the effectiveness of Angiopeptin
on the restenosis that occurs after coronary angioplasty in humans. The trial
will be completed in 1992.

Recurrent arterial stenoses which occur following balloon angioplasty in
human coronary artery disease limit the overall effectiveness of PTCA since
20–30% of patients require additional revascularization procedures in the
first year following PTCA. In addition to these clinical events, angiographic
restenosis occurs in up to 42% of patients [1]. No mechanical or pharmacologic strategy has been effective in limiting restenosis although many agents
are effective in experimental animal models. Frequently, the concentrations
of agents used in such models are toxic to humans, e.g. colchicine [2].

Biopsies of recurrent arterial obstructions with directional atherectomy
devices demonstrate that the composition is a myoproliferative response
similar to vascular responses to a variety of injuries [3]. The current hypothesis is that barotrauma induces arterial wall injury, which induces proliferation and migration of smooth muscle cells through the internal elastic lamina
and reduces the arterial lumen.

377

J.H.C. Reiber and P.W. Serruys (eds), Advances in Quantitative Coronary Arteriography, 377–383.
© 1993 *Kluwer Academic Publishers. Printed in the Netherlands.*

Smooth muscle cell proliferation is induced by circulating growth factors and a series of growth factors released at the time of the arterial injury. Platelet derived growth factor (PDGF) which is released during platelet aggregation at the site of arterial injury is now thought to be secondary to insulin-like growth factor (IGF-1). The activated IGF-1, epidermal growth factor, and PDGF increase tyrosine kinase activity which results in receptor autophosphorylation and induction of competence genes necessary for DNA replication. Stimulated smooth muscle cells release growth factors like IGF-1 and PDGF, which through self-stimulation leads to further replication. Furthermore, endothelial cells also release growth factors (IGF-1 and fibroblast growth factor). Somatostatin inhibits growth hormone release and reduces tissue concentrations of IGF-1. This may be one of the mechanisms related to its antiproliferative activity.

Angiopeptin, a synthetic octapeptide analogue of somatastatin has been examined in a variety of in vitro and in vivo models to determine its effectiveness in inhibiting myointimal proliferation following vascular injury. This phenomenon appears to be the pathophysiologic process leading to several important problems: transplantation atherosclerosis, vein graft stenosis after operative revascularization and restenosis after balloon angioplasty of coronary and peripheral arteries. To test the effectiveness of Angiopeptin on restenosis after balloon angioplasty in humans, a clinical trial is in progress. The purpose of this chapter is to summarize the effects of Angiopeptin in several animal models: rats, rabbits, pigs and non-human primates and to describe the experimental design of the current clinical trial.

Effects of Angiopeptin on the myoproliferative responses following vascular injury have been assessed by two different means, morphometric analyses and thymidine incorporation as an index of cellular proliferation.

Arterial injury by air drying was induced in one carotid artery using the contralateral artery as the control. The rats were sacrificed 15 days after the injury. At that time a myoproliferative response was evident in controls with an increase in the intima/media ratio to 1.6 ± 0.2 and a 12 fold increase in the 3H thymidine uptake compared to the sham operated contralateral carotid. Pretreatment with Angiopeptin 50 ug/kg/day continued for 5 days after injury decreased the intima/media ratio to 0.5 ± 0.1 ($p < 0.01$) [4]. Angiopeptin pretreatment 100ug/kg/day, but not 10 or 50 ug/kg/day, decreased cellular activity assessed by thymidine uptake [4].

In these experiments four other synthetic analogues of somatastatin were assessed. Only one, BIM20234 in one of the two doses, significantly inhibited the myoproliferative response although all inhibit growth hormone release (Figure 1) [4].

In rabbits, similar morphometric and physiologic responses have been documented after balloon injury of the aorta and iliac vessels. Angiopeptin 2,20 and 200 ug/kg/day in divided doses was effective in decreasing intimal thickness measured 3 weeks after balloon injury. There was no difference in the effect of the different doses, although the group treated with 2 ug/kg/day

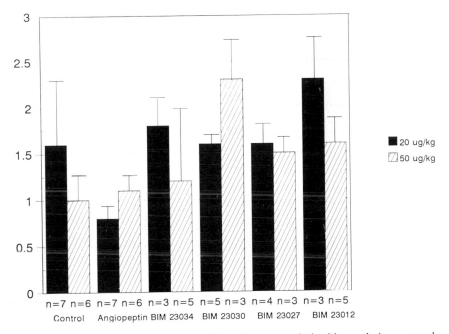

Figure 1. Effects of five different somatostatin analogs on myointimal hyperplasia expressed as the intimal/media ration in rat carotid arteries following air injury. Rats were treated from 2 days prior to endothelial injury to 5 days post injury, and sacrificed 14 days following injury. Only two of the analogs exert significant inhibition of myointimal hyperplasia. Reproduced with permission [4].

appeared to have less intimal hyperplasia (Figure 2) [5]. Rabbits were subjected to balloon injury from below the diaphragm to the femoral artery and the thoracic aorta was the control, untreated segment. Animals were pretreated with Angiopeptin 200 ug/kg/day in divided doses. The animals were sacrificed 3 days after balloon injury and 3H thymidine uptake of control, thoracic slices and injured, abdominal aortic slices were measured. There was a significant reduction of thymidine uptake in the abdominal aorta of the Angiopeptin treated animals (Figure 3) [6]. There was very little thymidine uptake of the aortic slices taken from the control, non-injured thoracic aorta and it was not different between saline and Angiopeptin treatment [6]. Thus, in two species of animals, anatomic and physiologic markers of myointimal proliferation following arterial injury are significantly reduced after Angiopeptin treatment (Figure 4.)

Intimal hyperplasia occurs in vein segments placed in the arterial system to revascularize obstructed arterial beds. Although this may initially be an adaptive response, as the intimal thickening progresses, it may result in failure of the graft. The effects of Angiopeptin on the proliferative response has been studied in rabbits. The jugular vein was reversed and interposed in

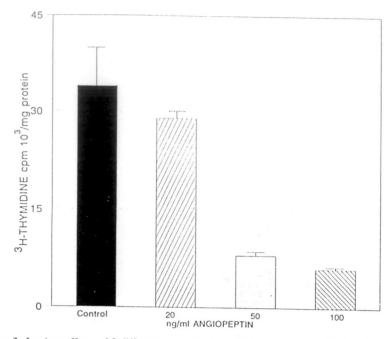

Figure 2. In vitro effects of 3 different concentrations of Angiopeptin on 3H-thymidine uptake in rat carotid arteries incubated for 24 hours with Angiopeptin. Mean ± SEM, $n = 3$. Reproduced with permission [5].

the carotid artery. Pretreatment with Angiopeptin 20 ug/kg/day in divided doses or saline was given prior to and continued until sacrifice 3 weeks later. Neointimal hyperplasia in control animals was $0.08 \pm 0.017 \, \text{mm}^2$ and was significantly less in Angiopeptin treated animals $0.022 \pm 0.006 \, \text{mm}^2$ ($p < 0.05$) [7].

Preliminary studies, in progress, have demonstrated similar inhibiting effects of angiopeptin in other species. Explanted coronary arteries from pigs were incubated in tissue culture media containing angiopeptin 48, 96 nM or forskolin, a known inhibitor of smooth muscle proliferation. Angiopeptin produced a dose dependant inhibition of thymidine uptake at 24 hours with inhibition by the largest concentration of Angiopeptin similar to that achieved with forskolin [8]. Smooth muscle proliferation in response to balloon injury was studied in cynomologous monkeys. Angiopeptin 25 ug/kg slow release over 3 weeks was effective in inhibiting this response. (Personal communication: Dr. Conor Lundergan.)

The time course of effective Angiopeptin treatment has been examined following arterial injury in rabbits. Angiopeptin was given to 4 groups of animals each, either at the time of injury or at 8, 18, 27 hours following injury. Only the group of animals in which angiopeptin was given at the time of injury had a significant reduction of the myoproliferative response [9].

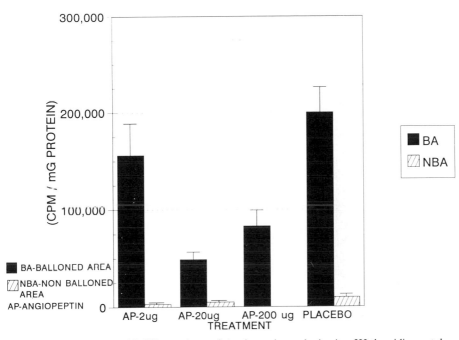

Figure 3. In vivo effects of 3 different doses of Angiopeptin on the in vitro 3H-thymidine uptake in rabbit aorta incubated with 3H-thymidine for 3 hours. Rabbits were sacrificed 72 hours following balloon injury of the aorta. Each experimental group consisted of five animals. Twenty and 200 ug/kg/day of Angiopeptin inhibited significantly ($p < 0.01$) thymidine uptake. Non-ballooned thoracic aorta was used as a control. Reproduced with permission [6].

    To determine the effects of localized delivery of Angiopeptin at the site of arterial injury, two experiments have been performed. I-125 Angiopeptin was infused in the abdominal aorta of rabbits through a Wolinsky (10) balloon. The animals were sacrificed 30 minutes later and radioactivity was found distributed in the cytoplasm and nuclei of smooth muscle cells. Next, 4 groups of animals were studied, saline control, 1, 10, 100 ug/ml Angiopeptin delivered locally through the Wolinsky balloon. Animals were sacrificed 3 weeks later and the aortas were fixed in situ. Neointimal hyperplasia was significantly reduced in the group, Angiopeptin 10 ug/ml, compared to control ($p = 0.05$) or other treatment groups.

    On the basis of these animal studies, a randomized, placebo controlled, double blind clinical trial was initiated in July, 1989. The primary endpoints include angiography at six months, exercise capacity, clinical events, and need for repeat revascularization procedures. The treated vessel is visualized before and after PTCA in orthogonal views after intracoronary nitroglycerin. Care is taken to visualize the contrast filled catheter in the cine run. Identical views are assured by recording imaging tube angles, table heights, etc. during the treatment studies so that they are repeated at the six month study.

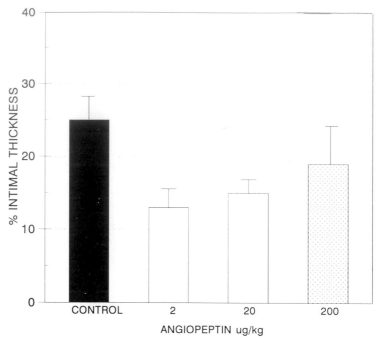

Figure 4. In vivo effects of three different doses of Angiopeptin on intimal hyperplasia of the rabbit common iliac artery following balloon injury. The animals were treated from the day prior to balloon injury and until sacrifice at day 21. The three doses inhibited significantly ($p < 0.05$) myointimal hyperplasia expressed as area of intimal thickening/total vessel area $\times$ 100. Reproduced with permission [5].

Quantitative angiography is being performed by The Angiographic laboratory, initially at the University of Michigan and now at the Washington Cardiology Center. The edge detection program is being run on the ImageCom system. Saline or Angiopeptin 20, 40 or 80 ug/kg/d in 2 divided doses are given subcutaneously before and for 10 days following PTCA. As of July 1992, all of the 1250 patients have been randomized. Initially successful PTCA with no complications was performed in 88%. No adverse responses to the drug have been seen in any of the four treatment groups. Angiographic follow-up has been obtained in > 90% of the eligible patients. Follow-up will be completed in 1992. A similar clinical trial is underway examining the effects of Angiopeptin 80 ug/kg/d on restenosis following directional atherectomy. Since the initial angiographic result is better defined after this technique, the effect of Angiopeptin on the proliferative response, alone, may be easier to delineate. Similar clinical studies are in progress examining other dose regimen, effects on endovascular stents, and others. It is hoped that this agent may have some impact on the enormous clinical problem of recurrent arterial obstructions after all forms of transcatheter therapeutics.

References

1. Klein LW, Rosenblum J. Restenosis after successful percutaneous transluminal coronary angioplasty. Prog Cardiovasc Dis 1990; **32**: 365–82.
2. Currier JW, Pow TK, Minihan AC, Haudenschild CC, Faxon DP, Ryan TJ. Colchicine inhibits restenosis after iliac angioplasty in the atherosclerotic rabbit. Circulation 1989; **80** (Suppl II): II–66 (Abstract).
3. Johnson DE, Hinohara T, Selmon MR, Braden LJ, Simpson JB. Primary peripheral arterial stenoses and restenoses excised by transluminal atherectomy: a histopathologic study. J Am Coll Cardiol 1990; **15**: 419–25. Comment in: J Am Coll Cardiol 1990; **15**: 426–8.
4. Lundergan C, Foegh ML, Vargas R, et al. Inhibition of myointimal proliferation of the rat carotid artery by the peptides, angiopeptin and BIM 23034. Atherosclerosis 1989; **80**: 49–55.
5. Conte JV, Foegh ML, Calcagno D, Wallace RB, Ramwell PW. Peptides inhibition of myointimal proliferation following angioplasty in rabbits. Transplant Proc 1989; **21**: 3686–8.
6. Asotra S, Foegh M, Conte JV, Cai BR, Ramwell PW. Inhibition of 3H-thymidine incorporation of angiopeptin in the aorta of rabbits after balloon angioplasty. Transplant Proc 1989; **21**: 3695–6.
7. Calcagno D, Conte JV, Howell MH, Foegh ML. Peptide inhibition of neointimal hyperplasia in vein grafts. J Vasc Surg 1991; **13**: 475–9.
8. Vargas R, Wroblewska B, Ramwell P. Angiopeptin inhibits myointimal proliferation in segments of porcine coronary artery. J Am Coll Cardiol 1991; **17** (Suppl A): 299A (Abstract).
9. Howell M, Trowbridge R, Foegh M. Effects of delayed Angiopeptin treatment on myointimal hyperplasia following angioplasty. J Am Coll Cardiol 1991; **17** (Suppl A): 181A (Abstract).
10. Wolinsky H, Thung SN. Use of a perforated balloon catheter to deliver concentrated heparin into the wall of the normal canine artery. J Am Coll Cardiol 1990; **15**: 475–81.

24. Cyclic flow alterations and neointimal proliferation following experimental coronary stenosis and endothelial injury

JAMES T. WILLERSON, SHENG-KUN YAO, JANICE McNATT, CLAUDE R. BENEDICT, H. VERNON ANDERSON, PAOLO GOLINO, SIDNEY S. MURPHREE and L. MAXIMILIAN BUJA

Summary

We evaluated the hypothesis that recurrent platelet aggregation as evidenced by the frequency and severity of cyclic coronary blood flow variations is an important pathophysiologic factor in the development of neointimal proliferation. In 24 chronically instrumented dogs, variable degrees of coronary artery neointimal proliferation were observed 3 weeks after mechanical injury of the arterial endothelium and the placement of an external coronary artery constrictor. The severity of neointimal proliferation at 21 days was closely related to the frequency and severity of cyclic coronary blood flow variations during the initial 7 days after instrumentation of the animals. Pharmacological therapy with a dual thromboxane A_2 synthetase inhibitor and receptor antagonist and a serotonin S_2 receptor antagonist frequently was successful in abolishing cyclic blood flow variations and appeared to attenuate neointimal proliferation.

Introduction

Acute coronary artery disease syndromes, including unstable angina pectoris and acute myocardial infarction may be caused by the accumulation of platelet aggregates at sites of coronary artery stenosis and endothelial injury [1–4]. Aggregating platelets release mediators that may promote further platelet aggregation, dynamic coronary artery vasoconstriction, and neointimal proliferation in the arterial wall [1, 5–11]. When coronary artery angioplasty is used as a treatment for focal atherosclerotic lesions, injury to the endothelium and media of the arterial wall occurs, and platelet aggregates form at these sites [12–16]. It has been postulated that platelet aggregates accumulating at angioplasty sites may release factors which mediate a fibroproliferative response [1, 3, 15–18]. A proliferative response of smooth muscle cells in the media and intima has been shown to cause the restenosis phenomenon after angioplasty [12–14, 18]. In this report, we show a strong association between

J.H.C. Reiber and P.W. Serruys (eds), Advances in Quantitative Coronary Arteriography, 385–393.
© 1993 Kluwer Academic Publishers. Printed in the Netherlands.

the frequency and severity of platelet aggregation, as detected by cyclic alterations in coronary blood flow, thrombosis, and neointimal proliferation following endothelial injury at sites of experimentally-created coronary artery stenoses in a canine model. Our data suggest that a potent antiplatelet regimen consisting of a combined thromboxane synthesis inhibitor and receptor antagonist and a serotonin receptor antagonist given continuously for 14 days usually markedly attenuates the neointimal proliferation in this experimental model.

Materials and methods

The experiments were performed in mongrel dogs. Anesthetized animals had a thoracotomy under sterile conditions. The left anterior descending (LAD) coronary artery was gently dissected free of surrounding tissues. A cylindrical pulsed-Doppler flow probe was placed around the exposed portion of the LAD and continuous recordings of LAD blood flow velocity were obtained. The arterial endothelium was injured by gently squeezing the external surface of the exposed artery with cushioned forceps. Next, a small plastic constrictor was placed around the artery at the site of endothelial injury. The chest was closed. Following surgery, all animals were monitored closely with continuous recordings of LAD blood flow velocities and aortic blood pressures.

A total of 24 dogs were followed for 21 days. Seven of the dogs did not receive any treatment and served as controls. Another 17 dogs received the antiplatelet agents, ridogrel (a dual thromboxane A_2 synthetase inhibitor and thromboxane A_2 receptor antagonist, Janssen Pharmaceuticals, Beerse, Belgium) [19] and either ketanserin (a serotonin S_2 receptor antagonist, Janssen Pharmaceuticals, Beerse, Belgium) [20] or LY53857 (another serotonin receptor antagonist, Eli Lilly, Indianapolis, IN) [21]. Of these antiplatelet agent-treated dogs, 7 received bolus doses of ridogrel at 5 mg/kg and either ketanserin at 0.5 mg/kg or LY53857 at 0.2 mg/kg every 8–12 hours for 7–14 days through catheters positioned in the left atrium. The remaining 10 dogs received ridogrel as 5–10 mg/kg bolus injections every eight hours and a 0.6 mg/kg/hour continuous infusion and ketanserin as 1–2 mg/kg bolus injections every eight hours and a 0.1–0.2 mg/kg/hour continuous infusion for 14 days. Ex vivo platelet aggregation was evaluated in these animals before applying the arterial constrictor and injuring the endothelium and every day during the period when the treatments were given using a modified Born's method and the agonists, ADP (at a final concentration of 10–20 micromolar), U46619 (a thromboxane mimetic, at 50–100 ng/ml), and serotonin (at 1–2 micromolar). The results of in vitro platelet aggregation studies were used to adjust in vivo dosages of the thromboxane A_2 and serotonin inhibitors given by sustained infusion so as to ensure complete or near complete abolition of in vitro responses to the platelet agonists as a result of the in vivo infusion of the combined antagonists.

After sacrifice, segments of the LAD and the circumflex coronary arteries were dissected from the hearts, fixed in phosphate-buffered formalin, and embedded into paraffin. Histological sections were prepared. On photographic prints of the sections, structures were drawn onto the prints while examining the original slides by light microscopy. These areas were the media, original lumen (outlined by the inner edge of the media and delineated by the circumferential projection of the internal elastic lamella), area of intimal proliferation, and residual lumen. These areas were measured using a computer-linked digitizing tablet. The percent stenosis was calculated as:

$$\frac{(1 - residual\ lumen\ area) \times 100}{residual\ lumen + intima\ area} \tag{1}$$

Results

Cyclic flow variations. Coronary artery cyclic flow variations (CFVs) (Figure 1) occur in dogs with coronary artery stenosis and endothelial injury, and they correlate with repetitive platelet aggregation and dislodgement and vasoconstriction at sites of coronary artery stenosis and endothelial injury [16, 22–29]. CFVs developed in 4 of the 7 non-treated dogs. CFVs also developed in 4 of the 17 dogs that received combined treatment with two antiplatelet agents, ridogrel and either ketanserin or LY53857, that have been shown to be effective in eliminating CFVs in anesthetized and awake dogs [22, 24–29]. During the initial coronary flow recordings after surgery, most dogs had CFVs that disappeared in the subsequent 12 hours. In the animals that developed CFVs later, they usually occurred during the second to fourth days following the surgical procedures.

Morphologic analyses. On the 21st day following surgery, animals were sacrificed with large doses of intravenous sodium pentobarbital. Coronary artery tissues were obtained for histological studies that revealed various degrees of neointimal proliferation with modified smooth muscle cells present in the thickened intima of the LAD at sites of endothelial injury and arterial constriction (Figure 1). Some vessels also showed evidence of organized thrombi.

Severity of neointimal proliferation. The severity of neointimal proliferation was related to the frequency and severity of CFVs (Figures 2 and 3). In the 6 dogs with severe CFVs defined as more than 9 flow reductions greater than 70% of baseline flow velocity values during the first week following surgery, the LAD lumens were narrowed 84 ± 5% (mean ± S.E.) by neointimal proliferation and/or organizing thrombi. In 2 dogs with mild to moderate CFVs, defined as more than 3 flow reductions that were 30–60% of baseline flow velocity levels, neointimal proliferation resulted in 40 ± 5% narrowing of the

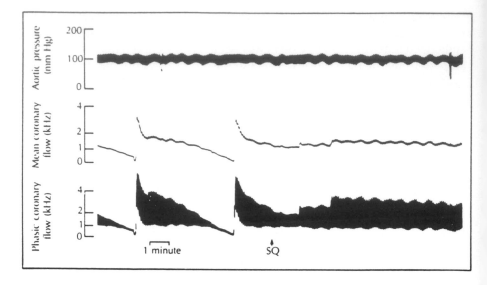

Figure 1. A representative tracing from a dog on the 4th day after surgery. The aortic pressure was recorded from a catheter placed in the aorta. Coronary artery blood flow velocity was recorded from a pulsed Doppler flow probe externally positioned on the left anterior descending coronary artery above a site of stenosis and endothelial injury. Coronary blood flow reductions are caused by in vivo platelet aggregation and dynamic vasoconstriction associated with the local accumulation of thromboxane A_2 and serotonin in this experimental model [1, 2]. SQ refers to the administration of a thromboxane A_2 receptor antagonist (Squibb, SQ29548) that abolished the cyclic flow variations as shown.

LAD lumen. In the remaining animals without CFVs, only $17 \pm 4\%$ narrowing of the LAD lumen by neointimal proliferation was observed. The correlation between the severity and frequency of CFVs and the severity of neointimal proliferation was significant (Pearson's $r = 0.90$, $p \leqslant 0.001$) (Figure 3).

Prevention of neointimal proliferation. Treatment with the combined thromboxane synthetase inhibitor and receptor antagonist, ridogrel, and the serotonin receptor antagonist, either ketanserin or LY53857, was started during surgery immediately following the appearance of the first 1–2 CFVs, and they eliminated CFVs within 5–10 minutes in all animals. Ex vivo platelet aggregations induced by U46619 and serotonin were also inhibited. Following surgery, 7 dogs received every eight hour injections of the two agents for 7–14 days. CFVs still developed in 4 of the 7 dogs receiving this regimen. The addition of continuous infusions of the two agents to the every eight hour injections prevented CFVs in 10 additional dogs. Coronary artery neointimal proliferation in the 4 dogs in whom CFVs were not prevented was similar to that found in untreated animals. In the dogs in whom ridogrel and ketan-

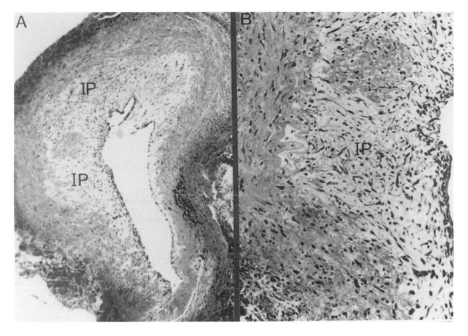

Figure 2. Histological sections of a coronary artery from a dog with endothelial injury and coronary artery stenosis of the proximal left anterior descending coronary artery. A, LAD constrictor site from a dog sacrificed 11 days after instrumentation and with frequent cyclic coronary blood flow variations during the first week following instrumentation and endothelial injury. This constrictor site shows extensive intimal proliferation (IP) × 62 (Panel A). In Panel B, the area of intimal proliferation (IP) is comprised of loose connective tissue containing numerous elongated cells shown to have features of modified smooth muscle cells by electron microscopy. There are also round monocytoid cells adjacent to the luminal surface (×150).

serin were effective in preventing CFVs, there was less neointimal proliferation (14 ± 6%) (Figures 2 and 3). Marked inhibition of the neointimal proliferation was observed in 8 of 10 dogs treated with bolus injections at 8 hour intervals and continuous infusions of ridogrel and ketanserin in whom ex vivo platelet aggregations induced by the thromboxane mimetic, U46619, and serotonin were also inhibited during the entire period of treatment (Figures 2 and 3). These data suggest that marked attenuation or inhibition of recurrent platelet aggregation at sites of endothelial injury and coronary artery stenosis may be necessary to markedly attenuate coronary artery neointimal proliferation in this experimental model. Two dogs developed mild-moderate neointimal proliferation (31 and 42 percent luminal diameter narrowings) after continuous infusions of ridogrel and ketanserin and prevention of CFVs as well as inhibition of ex vivo platelet aggregation (Figure

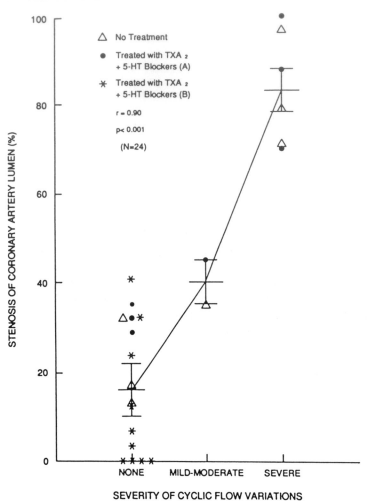

Figure 3. The correlation between the frequency and severity of cyclic coronary flow velocity variations and the severity of coronary artery neointimal proliferation is shown. Dogs (A) received ridogrel (a dual TXA_2 synthetase and receptor antagonist) at 5 mg/kg and ketanserin (a 5HT receptor antagonist) at 0.5 mg/kg or LY53857 (another 5HT receptor antagonist) at 0.2 mg/kg every eight hours bolus doses for 7 to 14 days. Dogs (B) received ridogrel 5–10 mg/kg every eight hours plus 0.6 mg/kg/hour continuous infusions and ketanserin at 1 to 2 mg/kg every eight hours plus 0.1–0.2 mg/kg/hour continuous infusions for 14 days. Reproduced from Proceedings of the National Academy of Sciences, 88: 10624–10628, 1991.

3). This suggests that factors in addition to recurrent platelet aggregation may contribute to the development of neointimal proliferation. Alternatively, these two animals may have had enough platelet deposition and growth factor activation to initiate moderate neointimal proliferation even though recurrent platelet attachment and dislodgement in the form of CFVs could not be identified.

Discussion

The processes which lead to neointimal proliferation after endothelial injury are incompletely understood. Platelet-derived growth factors (PDGF) as well as several other mitogens induce smooth muscle cell migration and proliferation [30–37]. PDGFs are released from alpha granules of platelets following their activation and adhesion. Inhibition of platelet aggregation would therefore be a logical step in attempting to prevent neointimal proliferation. Of course, growth factors may be released from other cells and tissues as well, including mononuclear cells and endothelium. Clinical use of antiplatelet agents, such as aspirin, has not prevented neointimal proliferation leading to restenosis after coronary angioplasty in patients with coronary artery disease [38]. Data from the present study stress the relatively "malignant" nature of recurrent platelet aggregation and dislodgement following mechanically induced endothelial injury and the need to give sustained antiplatelet therapy with combined inhibitors for thromboxane A_2 and serotonin in this experimental model. Therefore, insufficient inhibition of recurrent platelet aggregation when just aspirin is used might be at least one factor leading to the inability to markedly attenuate neointimal proliferation observed in previous studies [39, 40].

Recurrent platelet aggregation and thrombosis appear to play important roles in the development of coronary arterial neointimal proliferation following endothelial injury in this experimental model. Bolus administration and sustained infusions of a thromboxane synthesis inhibitor and receptor antagonist and a serotonin receptor antagonist prevent cyclic flow variations and usually markedly attenuate neointimal proliferation that occurs at sites of endothelial injury in this experimental model. However, complete prevention of neointimal proliferation may require large doses of specific inhibitors of platelet mediators, other antiplatelet strategies, direct inhibition of smooth muscle cell migration and/or proliferation, and/or antagonists of growth factor receptors or post receptor events to block several critical activation pathways simultaneously.

Acknowledgements

We thank Ms. Vanessa Smith for secretarial assistance, Dr. Fred DeClerck at Janssen Pharmaceuticals in Beerse, Belgium, for making ridogrel and ketanserin available for these studies, and Dr. Marlene Cohen at Eli Lilly Laboratories in Indianapolis, Indiana, for making LY53857 available for these studies.

This work was supported in part by NHLBI Ischemic SCOR HL17669, and this manuscript is a modification of a similar report from our group in Proc. Natl. Acad. Sci., 1991.

References

1. Willerson JT, Golino P, Eidt J, Campbell WB, Buja LM. Specific platelet mediators and unstable coronary artery lesions. Experimental evidence and potential clinical implications. Circulation 1989; **80**: 198–205.
2. Willerson JT, Campbell WB, Winniford MD, et al. Conversion from chronic to acute ischemic heart disease: speculation regarding mechanisms (editorial). Am J Cardiol 1984; **54**: 1349–57.
3. Ross R. The pathogenesis of atherosclerosis – an update. N Engl J Med 1986; **314**: 488–500.
4. Davies MJ, Woolf N, Rowles PM, Pepper J. Morphology of the endothelium over atherosclerotic plaques in human coronary arteries. Br Heart J 1988; **60**: 459–64.
5. Golino P, Ashton JH, Buja LM, et al. Local platelet activation causes vasoconstriction of large epicardial canine coronary arteries in vivo: Thromboxane A_2 and serotonin are possible mediators. Circulation 1989; **79**: 154–66.
6. Clowes AW, Reidy MA, Clowes MM. Mechanisms of stenosis after arterial injury. Lab Invest 1983; **49**: 208–15.
7. Harker LA, Harlan, JJ, Ross R. Effect of sulfinpyrazone on homocysteine-induced endothelial injury and arteriosclerosis in baboons. Circ Res 1983; **53**: 731–9.
8. Reidy MA. Endothelial regeneration. VIII. Interaction of smooth muscle cells with endothelial regrowth. Lab Invest 1988; **59**: 36–43.
9. Tada T, Reidy MA. Endothelial Regeneration. IX. Arterial injury followed by rapid endothelial repair induced smooth-muscle-cell proliferation but not intimal thickening. Am J Pathol 1987; **129**: 429–33.
10. Clowes AW, Reidy MA. Mechanisims of arterial graft failure: the role of cellular prolifation. Ann N Y Acad Sci 1987; **516**: 673–8.
11. Sprugel KH, McPherson JM, Clowes AW, Ross R. Effects of growth factors in vivo. I. Cell ingrowth into porous subcutaneous chambers. Am J Pathol 1987; **129**: 601–13.
12. Liu MW, Roubin GS, King SB. Restenosis after coronary angioplasty: potential biologic determinants and role of intimal hyperplasia. Circulation 1989; **79**: 1374–87.
13. Block PC, Myler PK, Stertzer S, Fallon JT. Morphology after transluminal angioplasty in human beings. N Engl J Med 1981; **305**: 382–5.
14. Uchida Y, Kawamura K, Shibuya I, Hasegawa K. Percutaneous angioscopy of the coronary luminal changes induced by PTCA Circulation 1988; **78** (4 Suppl II): II–84 (Abstract).
15. Faxon DP, Sanborn TA, Weber VJ, et al. Restenosis following transluminal angioplasty in experimental atherosclerosis. Arteriosclerosis 1984; **4**: 189–95.
16. Anderson HV, Yao S, Murphree SS, Buja LM, McNatt JM, Willerson JT. Cyclic coronary artery flow in dogs after coronary artery angioplasty. Coronary Artery Dis 1990; **1**: 717–23.
17. Essed CE, van den Brand M, Becker AE. Transluminal coronary angioplasty and early restenosis. Fibrocellular occulusion after wall laceration. Br Heart J 1983; **49**: 393–6.
18. Austin GE, Ratliff NB, Hollman J, Tabei S, Phillips DF. Intimal proliferation of smooth muscle cells as an explanation for recurrent coronary artery stenosis after percutaneous transluminal coronary angioplasty. J Am Coll Cardiol 1985; **6**: 369–75.
19. DeClerck F, Beetens J, de Chaffoy de Courcelles D, Freyne E, Janssen PAJ. Thromboxane A_2 synthetase inhibition and thromboxane A_2/prostaglandin endoperoxide receptor block-

ade combined in one molecule. I. Biochemical profile in vitro. Thromb Haemost 1989; **61**: 35–42.

20. DeClerck F, David J, Janssen PAJ. Inhibition of 5–hydroxytryptamine-induced and -amplified human platelet aggregation by ketanserin (R 41 468), a selective 5–HT_2-receptor antagonist. Agents Actions 1982; **12**: 388-97.

21. Cohen ML, Fuller RW, Kurz KD. LY53857, a selective and potent serotonergic (5–HT_2) receptor antagonist, does not lower blood pressure in the spontaneously hypertensive rat. J Pharmacol Exp Ther 1983; **227**: 327–32.

22. Bush L, Campbell WB, Buja LM, Tilton GD, Willerson JT. Effects of the selective thromboxane synthetase inhibitor dazoxiben on variations in cyclic blood flow in stenosed canine coronary arteries. Circulation 1984; **69**: 1161–70.

23. Folts JD, Crowell EB Jr, Rowe GG. Platelet aggregation in partially obstructed vessels and its elimination with aspirin. Circulation 1976; **54**: 365-70.

24. Ashton JH, Schmitz JM, Campbell WB, et al. Inhibition of cyclic flow variations in stenosed canine coronary arteries by thromboxane A_2/prostaglandin H_2 receptor antagonists. Circ Res 1986; **59**: 568–78.

25. Ashton JH, Ogletree ML, Michel IM, et al. Serotonin and thromboxane A_2/prostaglandin H_2 receptor activation cooperatively mediate cyclic flow variations in dogs with severe coronary artery stenoses. Circulation 1987; **76**: 952–9.

26. Golino P, Buja LM, Ashton JH, Kulkarni P, Taylor A, Willerson JT. Effect of thromboxane and serotonin receptor antagonists on intracoronary platelet deposition in dogs with experimentally stenosed coronary arteries. Circulation 1988; **78**: 701–11.

27. Eidt JF, Ashton J, Golino P, McNatt J, Buja LM, Willerson JT. Thromboxane A_2 and serotonin mediate coronary blood flow reductions in unsedated dogs. Am J Physiol 1989; **257**: H8 73–82.

28. Ashton JH, Benedict CR, Fitzgerald C et al. Serotonin is a mediator of cyclic flow variations in stenosed canine coronary arteries. Circulation 1986; **73**: 572–8.

29. Yao SK, Rosolowsky M, Anderson HV, et al. Combined thromboxane A_2 synthetase inhibition and receptor blockage are effective in preventing spontaneous and epinephrine-induced canine coronary cyclic flow variations. J Am Coll Cardiol 1990; **16**: 705–13.

30. Ross R, Raines EW, Bowen-Pope DF. The biology of platelet-derived growth factor. Cell 1986; **46**: 155-69.

31. Raines EW, Dower SK, Ross R. Interleukin-1 mitogenic activity for fibroblasts and smooth muscle cells is due to PDGF-AA. Science 1989; **243**: 393-6.

32. Geisterfer AA, Peach MJ, Owens GK. Angiotensin II induces hypertrophy, not hyperplasia, of cultured rat aortic smooth muscle cells. Circ Res 1988; **62**: 749–56.

33. Shuman MA. Thrombin-cellular interactions. Ann N Y Acad Sci 1986; **485**: 228-39.

34. Hansson GK, Jonasson L, Lojsthed B, Stemme S, Kocher O, Gabbiai G. Localization of T lymphocytes and macrophages in fibrous and commplicated human atherosclerotic plaques. Atherosclerosis 1988; **72**: 135–41.

34. Klagsbrun M, Edelman ER. Biological and biochemical properties of fibroblast growth factors. Arteriosclerosis 1989; **9**: 269–78.

36. Roberts AB, Sporn MB, Assoian RK, et al. Transforming growth factor type beta: rapid induction of fibrosis and angiogenesis in vivo and stimulation of collagen formation in vitro. Proc Natl Acad Sci USA 1986; **83**: 4167–71.

37. Wilcox JN, Smith KM, Williams LT, Schwartz SM, Gordon D. Platelet-derived growth factor mRNA detection in human atherosclerotic plaques by in situ hybridization. J Clin Invest 1988; **82**: 1134–43.

38. Percutaneous transluminal angioplasty. Council on Scientific Affairs. JAMA 1984; **251**: 764–8.

39. Fingerle J, Johnson R, Clowes AW, Majesky MW, Reidy MA. Role of platelets in smooth muscle cell proliferation and migration after vascular injury in rat carotid artery. Proc Natl Acad Sci U S A 1989; **86**: 8412–6.

40. Friedman RJ, Stemerman MB, Wenz B, et al. The effect of thrombocytopenia on experimental arteriosclerotic lesion formation in rabbits. Smooth muscle cell proliferation and re-endothelialization. J Clin Invest 1977; **60**: 1191–201.

PART SEVEN

QCA after recanalization techniques in coronary arteries

25. The use of quantitative coronary angiography (QCA) in interventional cardiology

BRADLEY H. STRAUSS*, MARIE-ANGELE M. MOREL,
ELINE J. MONTAUBEN VAN SWIJNDREGT, WALTER R.M.
HERMANS, VICTOR A.W. UMANS, BENNO J.W.M.
RENSING, PETER P. DE JAEGERE, PIM J. DE FEYTER,
JOHAN H.C. REIBER and PATRICK W. SERRUYS

Summary

Quantitative Coronary Angiography (QCA) has become the gold standard in the assessment of the immediate and long term results of various coronary interventions, both pharmacological and mechanical. In particular, the phenomenon of restenosis has been primarily described and researched on the basis of sequential QCA studies. Although initially intended as a system to assess the extent of disease within the coronary tree, the Cardiovascular Angiographic Analysis System (CAAS) has become the most utilized quantitative system for restenosis trials. At the Thoraxcenter, more than 1700 patients who have undergone PTCA, stenting, atherectomy or laser have had sequential angiographic studies analyzed by CAAS. Several new and unforseen problems have been encountered with this later application of the CAAS system, due to either the device or the effect of the intervention on the angiographic appearance of the treated coronary vessel. In this chapter, we review the capabilities of the CAAS system and outline some of the methodological problems and shortcomings of the system that have become evident from our experience with coronary devices. Specific examples include the immediate evaluation after a complicated dissection, the determination of the exact location of radioluscent stents within the coronary vessel and the difficulties of assessing reference diameters in segments that have been "overdilated" following stenting or atherectomy. Although our studies have relied almost exclusively on data based on a contour detection method, we have been interested in densitometry and discuss the use of information (and problems) of the data obtained by the densitometric method. Finally, we address the issue of how to use QCA-acquired data to compare the various coronary interventional devices with information currently available and for future randomized trials. We have evaluated the immediate results with the concept of the "expansion ratio". The late results have been compared by two methods: 1) historical angioplasty studies previously analyzed by CAAS;

*Dr. Strauss is a Research Fellow of the Heart and Stroke Foundation of Canada.

J.H.C. Reiber and P.W. Serruys (eds), Advances in Quantitative Coronary Arteriography. 397–441.

THORAXCENTER QCA INVENTORY

INTERVENTION	PATIENTS	LESIONS
PTCA	1234	1452
STENTS	393	446
WALLSTENT	283	335
WIKTOR	91	92
PALMAZ-SCHATZ	19	19
ATHERECTOMY	105	114
DIRECTIONAL	95	103
ROTATIONAL	10	11
EXCIMER LASER	20	20
TOTAL	1752	2032

Figure 1. Inventory of quantitative coronary angiographic (QCA) results following various coronary interventions at the Thoraxcenter in Rotterdam.

2) using the principles of the "dilating index", "restenosis index" and the "utility index" in patients that have been "matched" according to reference diameter and minimal luminal diameter. For future trials, the important angiographic endpoint should be the minimal luminal diameter at follow-up.

Introduction

Quantitative Coronary Angiography (QCA) has had a tremendous impact in the field of interventional cardiology. It has supplanted visual and hand-held caliper assessments of coronary arteriography due to its superior interobserver and intraobserver variability [1–3]. Currently it is the gold standard to assess the coronary tree for research purposes, although it has not gained widespread appeal for routine clinical use because of expense and time constraints. It has been particularly useful in interventional cardiology as the only reliable means to assess the short- and long- term effects of coronary interventions. In particular, the phenomenon of restenosis has been primarily described and researched most extensively on the basis of sequential QCA studies. At the Thoraxcenter in Rotterdam, we have been advocating the importance of QCA since the first publication by our group in 1978 [4]. The system developed at the Thoraxcenter by Johan Reiber and colleagues, the Cardiovascular Angiographic Analysis System (CAAS), has been extensively and rigorously validated [5–7]. In our database, we have now collected information from over 1700 patients who have undergone several different forms of nonoperative coronary revascularization (Figure 1). We have had to adapt the principles of QCA, which were initially designed for diagnostic studies to assess the extent of coronary artery disease, to more complicated

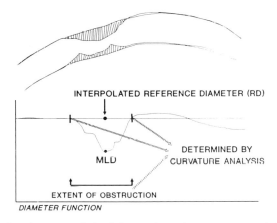

INTERPOLATED REFERENCE DIAMETER (RD)

MLD

DETERMINED BY
CURVATURE ANALYSIS

EXTENT OF OBSTRUCTION

DIAMETER FUNCTION

Figure 2. Diameter function curve derived from schematic coronary vessel. Minimal luminal diameter (MLD) and interpolated reference diameter are shown; the extent (or length) of the obstruction is determined by a curvature analysis.

and complex situations related to either the device or the effect of the intervention on the angiographic appearance of a damaged vessel. The introduction of several newer devices in the past 4 years, has presented several unique and unforseen problems in our interpretation of important quantitative data. The purpose of this chapter is to highlight the basic features and information that can be obtained by the CAAS system and to discuss some of the benefits and limitations of this important method in the analysis of results from the devices of interventional cardiology. At the conclusion of the chapter, it is hoped that QCA should be regarded as more than just setting up the cinefilm and returning 20–30 minutes later for the "perfect"

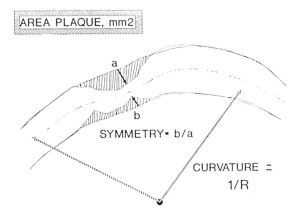

AREA PLAQUE, mm2

a

b

SYMMETRY= b/a

CURVATURE =
1/R

Figure 3. Determination of the area plaque, symmetry and curvature values. See text for details.

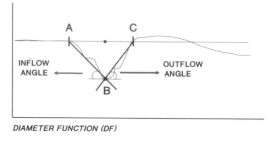

DIAMETER FUNCTION (DF)

INFLOW-ANGLE   : AVERAGE SLOPE OF THE DF
BETWEEN (B) AND (A)

OUTFLOW-ANGLE : AVERAGE SLOPE OF THE DF
BETWEEN (B) AND (C)

Figure 4. Determination of inflow and outflow angles from the diameter function. See text for details.

data. Only close scrutiny of the results combined with ongoing communication between the angiographer, the analyst and the programmer ensures that meaningful and useful data emerge from the use of QCA.

Part A: The CAAS system – what information can we learn?

The complexities of the algorithms essential for the operation of the CAAS system may intimidate the casual reader unfamiliar with image processing. In this chapter, we do not wish to explain the series of complicated steps that convert a cinefilm to a digitized image that is amenable to computer

OSTIAL LESION

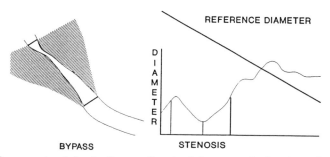

Figure 5. The computer-defined reference diameter is inaccurate in situations where there is no reliable proximal or distal boundary (e.g. ostial lesion or lesions located at the origin of a side branch). In this situation, the analyst must determine the reference diameter (user-defined).

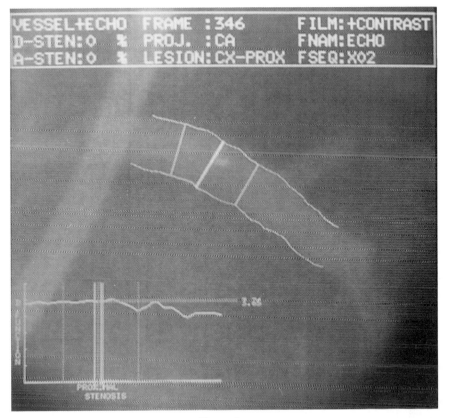

Figure 6a.

asssisted analysis. For the expert, this has been described in the literature [5–7]. Rather we would like to focus more on the clinician's ability to assess data generated by QCA. The prime aim of QCA is to provide precise and accurate measurements of coronary anatomy. The CAAS system can provide this information by two different methods: (1) detection of lumen borders (socalled edge detection), preferably in two orthogonal projections (to provide a three-dimensional approximation of the diseased segment) which can then be converted into absolute values after calibration with a known diameter object such as the shaft of the guiding catheter; and (2) densitometry, which is an approach that assesses the relative area stenosis by comparing the density of contrast in the diseased and "normal" segment. The method by which the relative area stenosis is converted to absolute area stenosis measurements will be explained later in the chapter. The advantage of the information acquired by the densitometric method is that meaningful data can be obtained by a single projection, even if the cross-sectional shape is highly irregular. In contrast, area measurements derived from edge detection

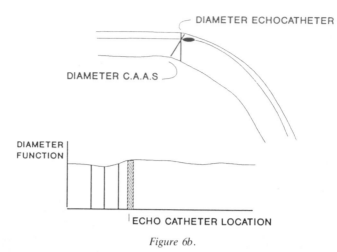

Figure 6b.

Figures 6a–b. The user-defined reference diameter is also useful when the exact diameter is required at a specific location in the coronary artery. (A) In the validation studies of intravascular echo catheters, the tip of the echo-catheter is visible and the diameter of the segment (3.26 mm) has been determined by the CAAS analysis. (B) It is also clear from the schematic diagram, that different diameters are measured by the two methods when the intravascular echo catheter is placed in a bend in the coronary artery.

data (and specifically from minimal luminal diameter values) by definition require an assumption of a circular cross-sectional shape in the diseased arterial segment, which is at odds with the observations of several pathologic studies [8, 9]. The limitations of both techniques will subsequently be discussed and discrepancies in the results of these two methods following coronary interventions will be presented later.

(1) *Edge detection*

The important parameters that can be obtained by edge detection are described below and in Figures 2–4.

Direct Measurements
1. minimal luminal diameter (MLD)
2. maximal luminal diameter
3. mean luminal diameter
4. extent of the obstruction
5. obstruction area (assumes circular model)
6. reference area (assumes circular model)

Interpolated Measurements
1. reference diameter (RD) (the assumed "normal" segment of the vessel)
2. symmetry
3. area plaque

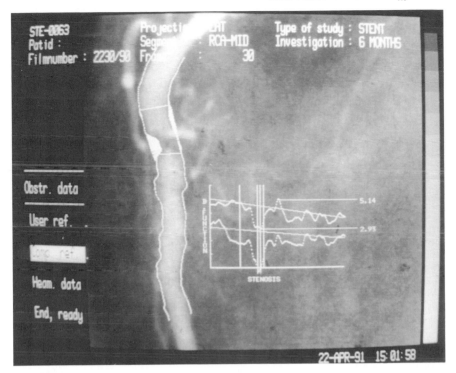

Figure 7. Densitometry measurements are affected and inaccurate in the presence of overlapping sidebranches. In this example, the upper curve (the diameter function) shows a minimal luminal diameter of 2.93 mm. However due to interference from side branches from the background subtraction, the densitometric determined minimal luminal cross-sectional area (MLCA) (lower curve) is a negative value.

MLD CHANGES POST PTCA

YEAR	N	PRE	POST	F\U
1988	88	1.13 ± .41	2.10 ± .40	1.69 ± .55
1990	309	0.99 ± .35	1.77 ± .34	1.46 ± .59
1991	261	0.98 ± .35	1.77 ± .34	1.49 ± .54

Figure 8. Minimal luminal diameter changes following PTCA. The reproducibility of QCA results by the CAAS system is seen in three different restenosis trials evaluated at the Thoraxcenter from 1988 [20], 1990 [21], and 1991 [22]. In the two latter trials, data is presented only for the control patients. PRE = Pre-PTCA, POST = Post-PTCA, F/U = Follow-up.

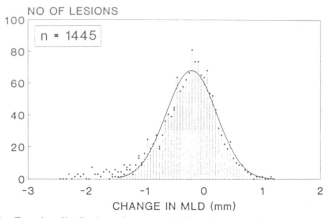

Figure 9. The Gaussian distribution of restenosis. The change in minimal luminal diameter (in mm) from post PTCA to follow-up is shown for 1445 patients from two restenosis trials approximately follows a normal distribution. Total occlusions at follow-up have been excluded. Reprinted with permission [23].

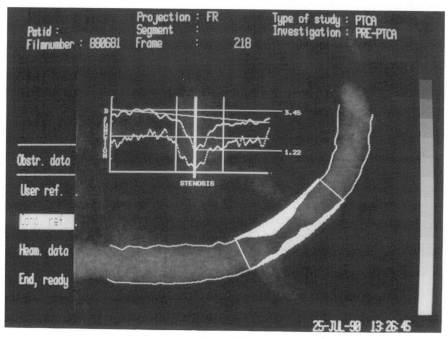

Figure 10a.

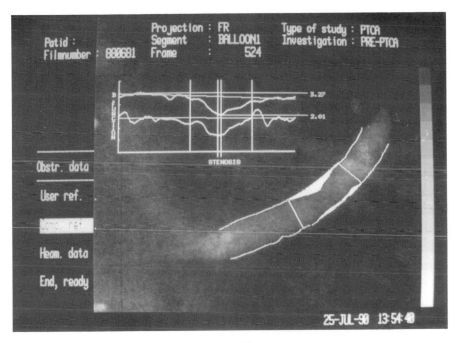

Figure 10b.

Derived Measurements
1. percent diameter stenosis (calculated from the MLD and RD)
2. percent area stenosis (assumes circular model)
3. curvature (calculated from the centerline of the vessel segment)
4. inflow angle/outflow angle (calculated from the diameter function)
5. roughness (calculated from the individual contour points, separately for the left and right-hand contours)

Hemodynamic Measurements
1. theoretical transstenotic pressure gradient
2. calculated Poisseuille resistance
3. calculated turbulent resistance

Contour detection is based on the use of first and second derivative functions applied to the brightness distributions along scanlines perpendicular to the centerline of the vessel segment and using minimal cost edge detection techniques [5]. The distances between corresponding left and right contour points in pixels can be converted into absolute values by using the catheter as a scaling device. The direct measurements are derived from the "diameter function" which represents the size of the analyzed vessel segment at intervals of approximately 0.1 mm as measured by the computed centerline (Figure 2). The diameter values are presented along the y-axis and the vessel length is represented along the x axis. The length of the lesion is specifically defined

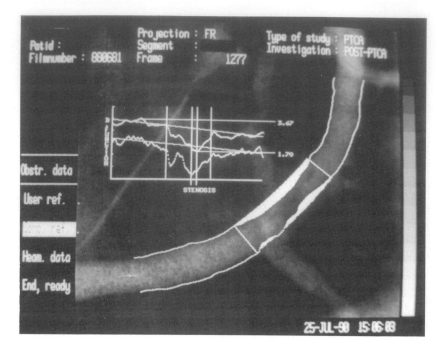

Figure 10c.

Figures 10a–c. Nonuniform balloon inflation during balloon angioplasty. Pre-PTCA minimal luminal diameter 1.22 mm (A). During balloon inflation with a 3.5 mm (manufacturer specification) balloon (B). The minimal balloon diameter is 2.01 mm and the maximal balloon diameter is 3.27 mm. Post-PTCA (C). Reprinted with permission [30].

by a curvature analysis of the diameter function curve. To estimate the original diameter values over the obstructive region, the reference diameter function is computed. To this end, a first degree least squares polynomial is determined through all the diameter values proximal and distal to the obstruction; this polynomial allows the vessels to taper. Next, the polynomial is translated upwards until 80% of the diameter values are below the polynomial. The resulting polynomial values are then assumed to be a measure for the normal size of the artery at the corresponding points; this polynomial function is denoted the reference diameter function and displayed in the diameter function by the straight line. Thus, the reference diameter is taken as the value of the reference diameter function at the minimum position of the obstruction.

On the basis of the proximal and distal centerline segments and the reference diameter function, the reference contours over the obstruction region are determined in the following way. Vessel midpoints for the proximal and distal portions are found by averaging the coordinates of the left and right contour positions. For the obstructive region, the vessel midpoints

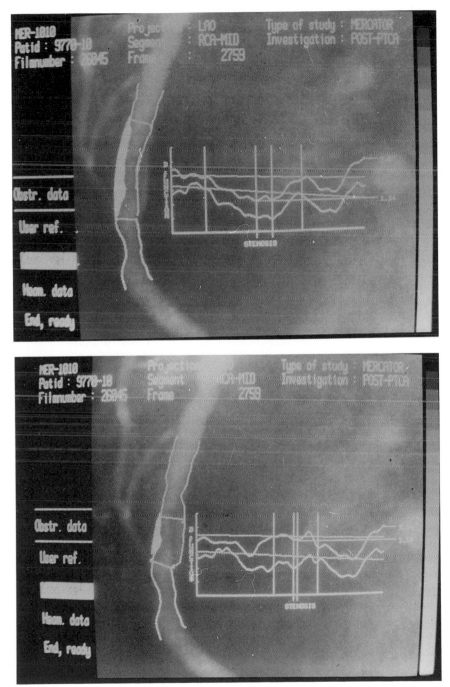

Figure 11. Edge detection of a lesion after PTCA has induced a large dissection. (A) Excluding dissection the minimal luminal dimater is 1.34 mm. (B) Including the dissection, the minimal luminal diameter is 2.53 mm.

INFLUENCE OF VASOMOTOR TONE ON QCA
MEASUREMENTS OF NON-DISEASED SEGMENTS

MEAN DIAMETER (MM)	WITHOUT NITRO POST-PTCA (N = 34)	WITH NITRO POST-PTCA (N= 168)
PRE-PTCA	3.12 ± 0.63	2.74 ± 0.63
POST-PTCA	3.01 ± 0.64	2.75 ± 0.59
F-UP	3.18 ± 0.55	2.82 ± 0.63
△POST-PRE	-0.11 ± 0.27 ⟷ +0.02 ± 0.21·)	
△F-UP↘PRE	+0.06 ± 0.22 ⟷ +0.07 ± 0.22··)	

·) P ‹ 0.001   ··) P = NS

Figure 12. Influence of vasomotor tone on QCA measurements of nondiseased segments. Thirty-four patients did not receive intracoronary nitroglycerin post-PTCA. In the nondiseased segments adjacent to the dilated site, these patients had a loss in the mean diameter of 0.11 mm compared with the pre-PTCA values (where nitro had been given). This change was not seen in the group who recieved nitro post-PTCA. The change in the mean diameter will affect the determination of percentage diameter stenosis.

AGREEMENT BETWEEN DENSITOMETRIC PERCENT
AREA STENOSIS AND THE CIRCULAR PERCENT-
AREA STENOSIS POST PTCA

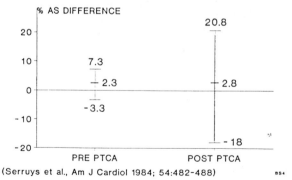

(Serruys et al., Am J Cardiol 1984; 54:482-488)

Figure 13. Agreement between densitometric percentage area stenosis and the circular (edge detection) percentage area stenosis pre- and post-PTCA. The mean difference (and standard deviation) for % area stenosis between the two methods was 2.3 ± 4.0% pre-PTCA and 2.8 ± 18% post-PTCA. Important discrepancies (i.e. large standard deviation) between the two methods after PTCA are likely related to the noncircular, asymmetric configuration of the lesion after angioplasty.

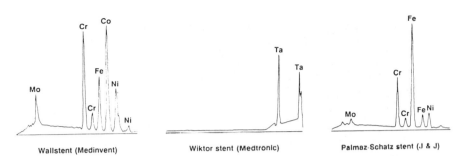

Figure 14. The metal composition according to X-ray energy dispersion spectrometry used in three currently investigated coronary stents. Ta = tantalum, Mo = molybdenum, Cr = chromium, Co = cobalt, Fe = iron, Ni = nickel. Reprinted with permission [40].

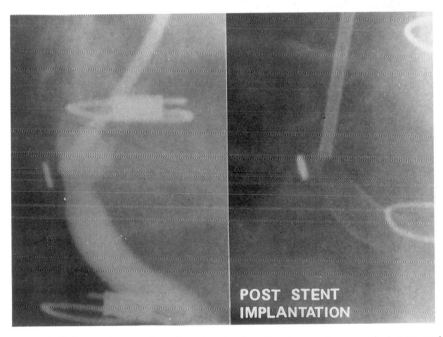

Figure 15. Wallstent (poor radiopacity) after implantation in a saphenous vein bypass graft. (A) in vessel without contrast. (B) in vessel filled with contrast.

are obtained by interpolation between the proximal and distal vessel mid-points with a second degree polynomial. The left and right reference contours are then obtained by centering the normal reference value for that position perpendicular to the local direction of the midline in each point. These computer-estimated predisease reference contours are superimposed in the image (Figure 3).

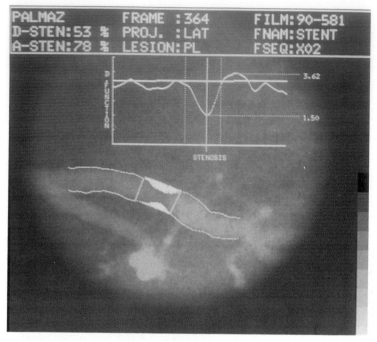

Figure 16a.

The area plaque is a measure of the atherosclerotic plaque in this angiographic view, expressed in mm^2 (Figure 3). This area is calculated as the sum of pixels between the computer-estimated predisease reference contours and the actual detected luminal contours of the obstructive lesion. Since measurement of area plaque is highly dependent on the length of the stenosis (which is subject to considerable variation) and the determination of the reference contours of the artery in the presumed prediseased state, the usefulness of this parameter is debatable.

The symmetry value is a measure of the eccentricity of a particular lesion. A symmetry measure of 1 denotes a concentric obstruction; the number decreases (down to 0) with increasing asymmetry or eccentricity of the obstruction. Unfortunately, this parameter has not yet been validated with pathologic studies and thus the pathologist and angiographer may not be talking about the same feature.

The curvature value is an attempt to assess the bend of the coronary segment analyzed (Figure 4). The view in which the vessel appears to be the least foreshortened (i.e. the lesion length is longest) is chosen for the curvature analysis. The inflow and outflow angles are derived from the slope of the diameter function at the descending and ascending limb of the diameter function curve at the defined site of the obstruction.

The CAAS system has also attempted to convert information on angiographic parameters into functional significance based on well-known fluid-

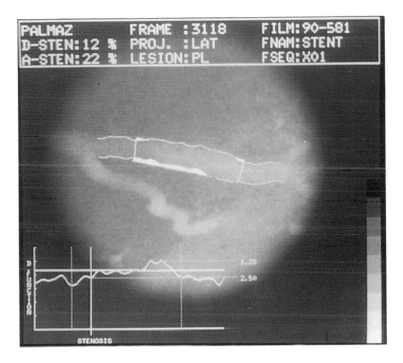

PALMAZ   FRAME :3118   FILM:90-581
D-STEN:12 %   PROJ. :LAT   FNAM:STENT
A-STEN:22 %   LESION:PL   FSEQ:X01

3.28
2.50

STENOSIS

Figure 16b.

Figure 16. (a) Pre-stent. (b) post-stent. Coronary segment overdilated by a Palmaz-Schatz stent. Although the minimal luminal diameter (MLD) in the stented segment should be greater than the reference diameter (which is determined by the smaller proximal and distal segments to the stented segment), the reference diameter remains larger than the MLD for unclear reasons and the diameter stenosis (8%) remains a positive value.

dynamic equations [6]. The calculated transstenotic pressure gradient over a particular stenosis derived from QCA describes the hemodynamic impact that a particular lesion would have under a range of flow conditions, within the range of "normal" aortic pressures. These calculations do not account for the effects of pulsatile flow or of curved and tapered vessels, more than one lesion in a vessel, the collateral circulation, or perfusion of areas of nonviable myocardium. The effects of the entrance and exit angle (along with the absolute lesion diameter, percent narrowing, length of stenosis, blood flow velocity, and inertial and frictional effects) are the important factors that determine the physiologic significance of a coronary stenosis [10]. The pressure gradient across a stenosis is determined by entrance effects, drag effects (frictional losses) and exit effects. Although the most important site of energy loss is at the exit of a stenosis where the separation of the fluid column occurs, neither the outflow nor inflow angle have yet been incorporated into the CAAS software package to calculate pressure gradients.

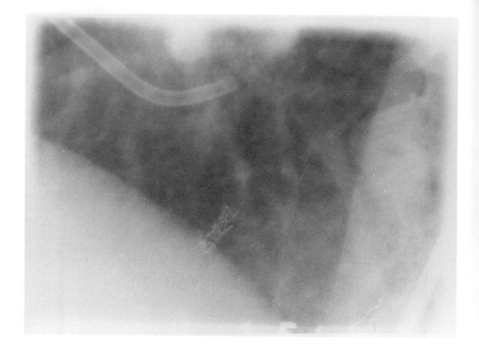

Figure 17a.

A word of caution in the interpretation of angiographic data

The limitations of angiographic information in the evaluation of the extent of coronary artery disease has been well recognized [11]. After all, coronary angiography is really just a two-dimensional shadowgram of an opacified vessel. It merely demonstrates the effect of arterial wall disease on the contour of the arterial lumen. Moreover, atherosclerotic changes of the arterial wall are not reflected precisely enough by changes in the lumen. Due to the diffuseness of the atherosclerotic process which can narrow the entire lumen of a segment of a vessel smoothly and evenly, angiography may not detect its existence. This is reflected in many studies that have shown that coronary angiography frequently underestimates the severity of coronary artery lesions or even misses significant narrowings regarding the underlying extent of coronary disease [12–14]. Furthermore, depending on the radiologic view, elliptical or D-shaped lumens may result in either under or overestimation of stenosis [15]. The interpolated measurements reconstruct the "normal" segment of the vessel at the site of the lesion. Accordingly, these measurements may be underestimations of the true diameter value in the disease-free segment.

It is also important in interpreting the results of angiographic studies to

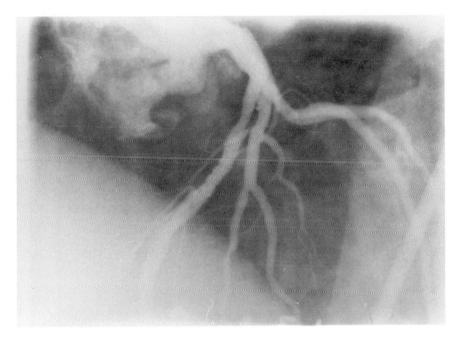

Figure 17b.

Figures 17a–b. Wiktor stent after implantation in left anterior descending artery. (A) in vessel without contrast. (B) in vessel filled with contrast, stent remains clearly visible.

know how the individual parameters were measured. Several angioplasty studies have identified multiple angiographic risk factors (e.g. lesion length (>10 mm), lesions on a coronary bend etc.) associated with a higher rate of restenosis [16–19]. However, measurement of lesion length and bend (curvature) may differ greatly depending on the type of system used.

Analyst-computer interaction

The entire analysis can be derived by the computer. However the analyst can interact at several steps, hence the term "computer-assisted" analysis. The contours of the vessel detected by the computer can be manually corrected by the analyst. This may be necessary when the angiogram is of poor technical quality, or in specific situations such as the presence of large side branches which interfere with the edge detection program or hazy vessel contours occasionally related to the presence of a dissection after an intervention. Excessive analyst interaction increases the risk of introducing bias and is discouraged. Thus, technically high quality angiograms are of paramount importance for reliable QCA. The second aspect of analyst-computer interaction is the definition of reference segment. Normally, the computer itself decides on the reference segment (i.e. computer-defined). Occasionally, the

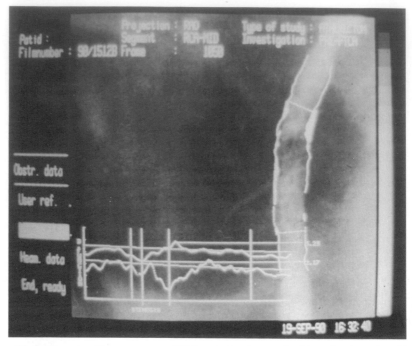

Figure 18. Restenosis within a coronary Wiktor stent not recognized by edge detection. Graph shows the diameter function (upper curve) and the densitometric area function (lower curve). Outside vertical lines on the graph and two horizontal lines in the angiographic image are lesion boundaries. The inner two vertical lines on the graph represent the minimal points on the diameter and densitometric graphs, respectively. The minimal luminal diameter by edge detection is 2.17 mm. A discrepancy between the two functions is present and most severe at the vertical line which denotes the minimal densitometric value (arrowhead). The edge detection algorithm followed the outline of the stent and was unable to recognize the stenosis within the stent. Reprinted with permission [40].

analyst may decide to choose a different part of the vessel as the reference diameter. This may be necessary in situations where there is no reliable proximal or distal obstruction boundary, such as lesions located at the ostia of a vessel or at the origin of side branches or in diffusely diseased vessels (Figure 5). A prerequisite to obtain reliable values for the reference diameter by the CAAS algorithm is comparable diameters proximal and distal to the lesion. The user-defined reference diameter may also be required when one wants to know the exact diameter at a specific location of the vessel segment. This has been useful in our validation studies of the intravascular echo (Figure 6).

(2) Densitometry

The important parameters that can be obtained by densitometry are:
1. % area stenosis

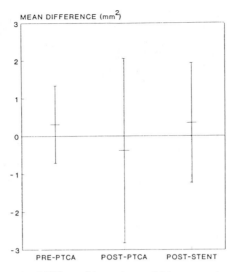

MEAN DIFFERENCE (mm^2)

PRE-PTCA   POST-PTCA   POST-STENT

Figure 19. Mean difference (and 95% confidence intervals) between edge detection and densitometry before and after percutaneous transluminal coronary angioplasty (PTCA) and after stenting. Mean differences were slightly positive (0.31, 0.35 mm^2) before PTCA and after stenting, respectively and slightly negative (-0.38 mm^2) after PTCA. The widest 95% confidence interval was in the analysis after PTCA, indicating the poorest association between the two methods, compared with the analysis before PTCA and stenting. Reprinted with permission [39].

2. minimal luminal cross-sectional area

It should be noted that these values are computed without making any assumption about the shape of the luminal cross-section of the obstruction.

As explained earlier, densitometry by itself can only provide relative measurements of area stenosis i.e. a ratio based on the relative differences in brightness (and thus density after appropriate transformations). For absolute measurements, the reference diameter must be determined from the edge detection data, and a circular cross section is assumed for this particular site.

The following steps are used by the computer in the calculation of the minimal luminal cross-sectional area measurements from densitometry and edge detection obtained data:
1. Edge Detection obtained: Reference Diameter. The Reference Area (RA) can then be calculated by assuming that the reference (or "normal") segment has a circular cross-sectional configuration.
2. Densitometry obtained: Ratio (R) =
  Integrated Density at Reference Segment

Integrated kDensity at Obstruction Segment

3. Minimal Luminal Cross-Sectional Area = RA/R
In this method, no assumption is made about the cross-sectional shape of the lesion in the most severely diseased segment of the vessel. Although densitometry is extremely attractive on a theoretical basis, numerous techni-

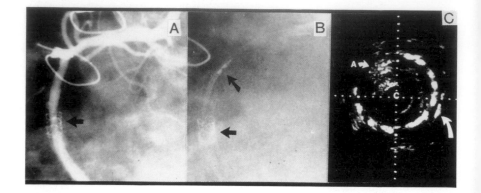

Figure 20. A) Right coronary angiogram showing a moderate restenosis (arrow) in a segment in which a Wiktor stent and a Wall-stent have been delivered as a bail-out procedure. B) The fluoroscopic image in the same projection (right oblique view) shows more clearly the highly radiopaque Wiktor stent while the underlying Wall-stent is radiographically hardly detectable. The curved arrow shows the mirror of the echographic catheter deflecting the ultrasound beam towards the vessel wall to create a cross-sectional image. The catheter was subsequently advanced up to the position marked with the straight arrow. C) Echographic cross-sectional image of the vascular segment in which the two stents are overimposed. The Wall-stent induces an almost continious circimferential series of intensely bright lines, *delimitating* inside a poorly echogenic area of intimal hyperplasia. The curved arrow shows the only imaged mesh of the Wiktor stent. A: artifact induced by the presence of the connection mirror-transducer and the guidewire. C: ultrasound catheter. Calibration: 0.5 mm.

cal problems have limited its use. The major limitation of this method is the strict requirement of a view that is perpendicular to the long axis of the vessel (i.e. to prevent oblique "cuts" which would lead to overestimate the luminal area) and absence of overlapping sidebranches in the segment or vessels running very closely to the analyzed segment (which would interfere with the density of the lesion due to background subtraction) (Figure 7). Densitometry is also more sensitive than edge detection to densitometric nonlinearities (X-ray scatter, veiling glare and beam hardening) and to inaccurate contrast filling of vessels.

QCA and coronary interventions

Prior to a discussion of the various devices used for coronary intervention, the utility of the information generated by QCA in general (and the CAAS system specifically) must be addressed. Anatomic information, such as minimal luminal diameter, reference diameter and percentage diameter stenosis, represent the most useful and reliable information obtained by this system. The physiologic and clinical significance of any individual value can not be

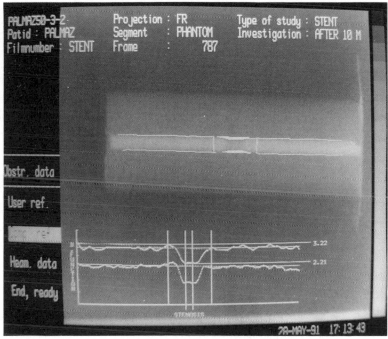

Figure 21a.

inferred although the CAAS system can generate theoretical measures of resistance based on the lesion characteristics and assumed coronary flow rates. Angiographic features of a particular lesion which may be important to the clinical outcome such as ulceration or complex, ragged morphology have not been a focus of our research in the natural history of large populations undergoing coronary interventions. The long-term variability of the CAAS system, under worst case or nonstandardized acquisition conditions has previously been validated [5]. Specifically, we have found that a change in minimal luminal diameter greater than 0.72 mm represents an angiographically detectable change. This does not infer physiologic significance but merely represents two times the standard deviation of measurements performed 3 months apart (i.e. the 95% confidence interval) under angiographic conditions in which no attempt was made to standardize on inspiratory level, volume and the rate of the contrast agent, nor on technical characteristics of the X-ray system. More importantly, the vasomotor tone in both conditions was unknown and neglected. If a more standardized acquisition protocol is followed, the medium term variability applies (2 s.d. = 0.44 mm). The physiologic significance will depend on the absolute minimal luminal diameter and other factors described earlier. For instance, if intervention A improves the MLD from 1.1 mm to 1.7 mm, and intervention B improves the MLD from 1.1 to 2.5 mm, a mean loss of 0.8 mm in the long term will be func-

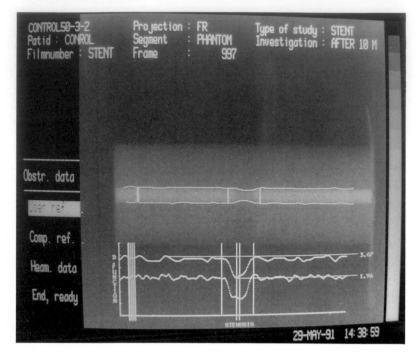

Figure 21b.

tionally more important to patients who have had intervention A. This lack of functional or physiologic significance in our definitions of restenosis of course applies to the other angiographic definitions (NHLBI 1–5) of restenosis. What QCA provides is an increased understanding of the natural history of lesions in populations of patients treated with a particular device, rather than aiding individual patient decisions.

Part B: QCA and specific coronary devices

A) Percutaneous Transluminal Coronary Angioplasty (PTCA)
The largest experience in the Thoraxcenter databank has been with serial studies following angioplasty. These studies have demonstrated several important advantages of QCA. The reproducibility of the CAAS system is extremely high (Figure 8). In several large trials, comparable values have been obtained in the determination of minimal luminal diameter pre PTCA, post PTCA and at 6 month follow-up [20–22]. Based on data obtained from these studies, we have learned that restenosis is not an all-or-nothing phenomenon as clinicians have been led to believe. Rather, the distributions of minimal lumen diameter pre angioplasty (1.03 ± 0.37 mm), post angioplasty (1.78 ± 0.36 mm), at 6 months follow-up (1.50 ± 0.57), as well as the

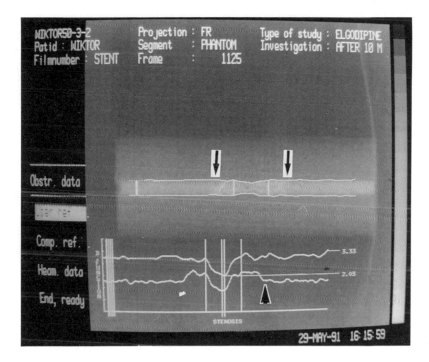

Figure 21c.

Figures 21a–c. Control (A), Palmaz-Schatz containing (B), and Wiktor containing (C) plexiglass phantom (4 × 3 mm) filled with 50 y% iopamidol contrast reagent. Graphs show the diameter function (upper curve) and the densitometric area function (lower curve). Outside vertical lines on the graph and rightward two vertical lines on the phantom are lesion boundaries. The inner two vertical lines represent the minimal points on the diameter and densitometric graphs, respectively. The multiple vertical lines in the left part of the graph and the leftward vertical line in the phantom represent the user-defined reference segment. The numbers in the graph represent the maximum and minimum diameter. The boundaries of the Wiktor stent are visible in the phantom (arrowheads) and as a step-up in the densitometry graph (arrows). As a result of the Wiktor stent contribution to the densitometry values, the minimal cross-sectional area determination is overestimated compared with the control and Palmaz-Schatz containing phantom. Reprinted with permission [40].

percentage diameter stenosis at 6 month follow-up approximately follow a normal distribution [23]. Therefore restenosis can be viewed as the tail end of an approximately Gaussian distributed phenomenon, with some lesions crossing a more or less arbitrary cut-off point, rather than a separate disease entity occurring in some lesions but not in others (i.e. a bimodal distribution) as suggested by the Emory group [24] (Figure 9). This has quite profound significance in the design of trials (pharmacologic or specific devices) to inhibit the restenotic process since a normal distribution is an underlying assumption for the use of parametric statistical tests (e.g. t-tail, analysis of variance).

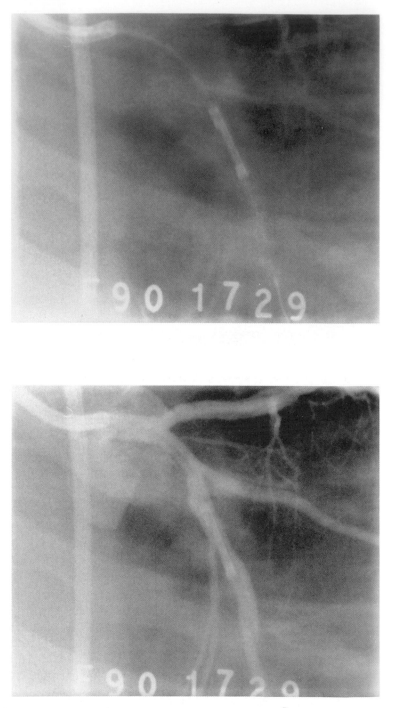

Figure 22. Radiopaque directional atherectomy device (atherocath^R). (A) in circumflex artery without contrast. (B) in circumflex artery containing contrast.

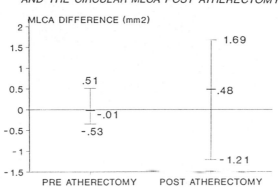

AGREEMENT BETWEEN DENSITOMETRIC MLCA
AND THE CIRCULAR MLCA POST ATHERECTOMY

Figure 23. Agreement between densitometric minimal luminal cross-sectional area (MLCA) and the circular (edge detection) MLCA pre- and post-directional atherectomy. Despite apparent smooth contours following atherectomy, similar discrepancy exists between analyses performed by edge detection or densitometry as occurs post-angioplasty. This may be due to preferential expansion of the bases of the atherectomy cuts creating a less circular configuration.

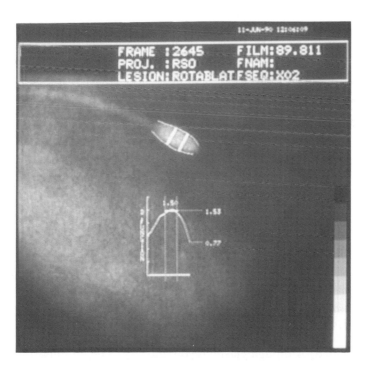

Figure 24a.

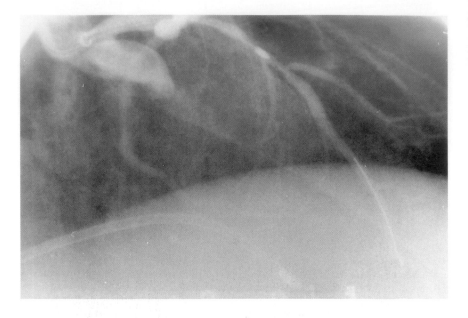

Figure 24b.

Figures 24a–b. Rotational abrasion (Rotablator™) in a coronary artery. (A) without contrast. Since the burr is nondeformable and of known diameter, calibration of the angiogram can occur at the site of the procedure in contrast to PTCA, stenting or directional atherectomy where we use the contrast-filled guiding catheter in one corner of the angiogram as the scaling device. In this case a 1.50 mm diameter burr was used. (B) in vessel containing contrast showing that the rotablator is clearly visible.

QCA has been useful to clarify conflicting data in the literature regarding angiographic risk factors associated with restenosis. In a recent report describing the restenosis rates in diverse segments of the coronary tree in 1445 patients, no differences were observed between coronary segments using a definition of either 50% diameter stenosis at follow-up or a continuous approach that compared absolute changes in minimal luminal diameter adjusted for the vessel size [25]. These results suggested that restenosis is an ubiquitous phenomenon without any predilection for a particular site in the coronary tree. In a second study, relative gain in minimal luminal diameter at angioplasty (post PTCA-pre PTCA) adjusted for vessel size, lesion length ⩾6.8 mm and total occlusions were independent predictors of restenosis [26]. Our interpretation of this data is that a too optimal result after PTCA, implying deeper arterial injury, adversely stimulates the fibroproliferative vessel reaction. Although elastic recoil appears to be an important aspect of the initial result, this study showed that no relationship between the extent of elastic recoil at the time of PTCA and late luminal narrowing.

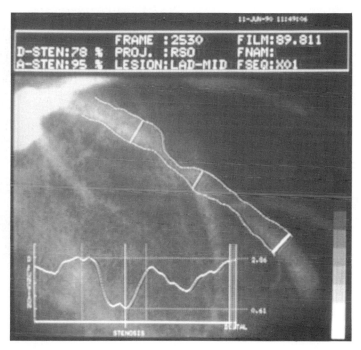

*Figure 25*a.

Insights into mechanisms of dilatation

The immediate result of percutaneous transluminal coronary angioplasty is influenced by both plastic (dissections, intimal tears) and elastic changes of the vessel wall. Experimental studies have shown that part of the angioplasty mechanism consists of stretching the vessel wall with a resulting fusiform dilation or localized aneurysm formation [27]. To evaluate elastic changes from our angiographic studies, we have defined elastic recoil as the difference between the minimal luminal diameter or area after angioplasty and the mean balloon diameter or cross-sectional area at the highest inflation pressure. We specifically have noted that elastic recoil after coronary angioplasty accounts for nearly 50% decrease in luminal cross-sectional area immediately after balloon deflation [28]. A follow-up study showed that asymmetric lesions, lesions located in less angulated parts of the artery and lesions with a low plaque content showed more elastic recoil [29]. Furthermore, lesions located in distal parts of the coronary tree were also associated with more elastic recoil, probably due to relative balloon oversizing in these distal lesions.

Although our initial work with balloon angioplasty was restricted to repeated measurements of at the lesion site, several concepts related to mechanisms of balloon dilatation required extension of our measurements to include the inflated balloon. These included *stretch* (theoretical maximal gain

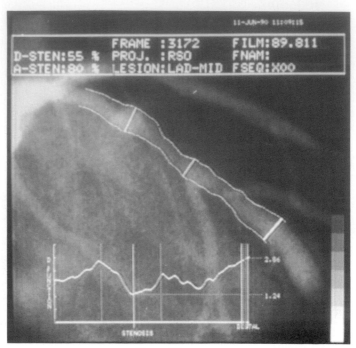

*Figure 25*b.

in diameter or area during the angioplasty procedure), *elastic recoil* (which appears to affect the immediate post-angioplasty result) and *relative balloon sizing* (which affects the incidence of dissection). Prior to these assessments, the inflated balloon was used as a scaling device and (incorrectly) assumed to be uniform along the entire balloon length at a diameter according to the manufacturer's specifications. However, we recently measured the balloon diameter over its entire length in 453 patients [30]. During an average inflation pressure of 8.3 ± 2.6 atm., we observed a difference of 0.59 ± 0.23 mm in diameter between the minimal and maximal balloon diameter (Figure 10). This difference results in large variations in the calculated stretch, elastic recoil and balloon-artery ratio depending on the site of the balloon chosen for the assessment.

Several technical considerations have emerged from these large studies. The analyst determines the length of the segment analyzed as the distance between two major side branches. This enables the analyst to be certain of the location during follow-up studies. Sidebranches crossing within the segment require manual correction and increase the risk of analyst bias. The major limitation of edge detection (aside from the technical quality of the cinefilm) is the analysis of the post angioplasty result. Dissections are a frequent

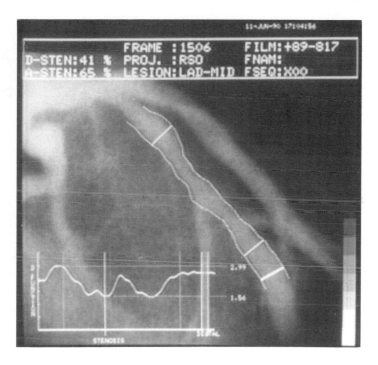

Figure 25c.

Figures 25a–c. Due to intense vasospasm following rotational abrasion, it may be necessary to repeat the study 24 hours later to assess the maximal benefit. (A) Pre-rotablator minimal luminal diameter (MLD) is 0.41 mm. (B) Immediately after the rotablator, MLD is 1.24 mm. (C) 24 hours later, MLD is 1.56 mm.

occurrence following PTCA and the resulting haziness, irregular borders or extravascular extravasation of contrast medium makes edge detection difficult (Figures 11A, B). There is no ideal solution to this problem. We usually rely on manual corrections while accepting this limitation. Secondly, as explained earlier, the computer generated interpolated measurements may be unreliable for ostial lesions or lesions located at sidebranches (see Figure 5). Manual contour correction may also be necessary when the angiogram is of poor technical quality. In our large scale restenosis trials, only 0.9% of films have been rejected for analysis due to poor technical quality [23].

An additional important technical point for all serial studies is the requirement of comparable vasodilator use for every study. In a recent study [31], the mean diameter of a normal segment of a nondilated vessel pre PTCA, post PTCA and at follow-up in 202 patients was analyzed (Figure 12). Thirty-four of these patients did not receive intracoronary nitrates prior to post-PTCA angiography. In the group that did not receive the nitrates post-procedure, there was a decrease in diameter of 0.11 mm versus the small

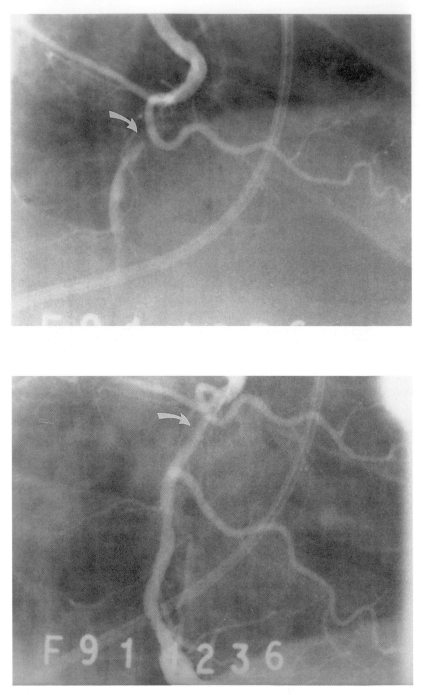

Figure 26a,b.

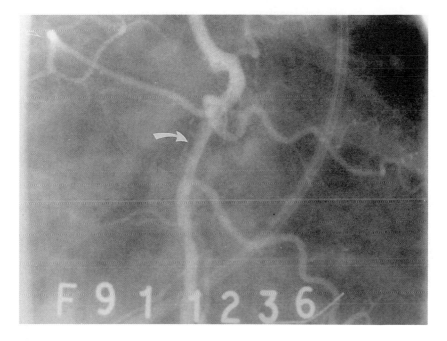

Figures 26c.

Figures 26a–c. Excimer laser. (A) narrowing in right coronary artery (arrow). (B) Post-laser, roughened hazy appearance (arrow). (C) Post balloon, haziness still present (arrow).

increase of 0.02 mm in the group that received nitrates post procedure. Lack of control of vasodilator therapy at follow-up angiograms may also partially explain an earlier observation from our group that there is significant deterioration in the mean reference diameter at four months post angioplasty since several subsequent studies that have controlled for this factor have not shown a loss of the reference diameter at follow-up [23, 32]. However, we still believe that in select patients, the reference segment is involved in the restenotic process and may contribute to the unreliability of an assessment of percent diameter stenosis at follow-up.

Densitometry may be more reliable than edge detection since it is theoretically independent of the projection chosen. In a study published in 1984, agreement between edge detection and densitometry was assessed by the standard deviation of the differrences of the% area stenosis, since absolute measurements of area by densitometry were not yet possible [33] (Figure 13). Prior to PTCA, reasonable agreement existed between the densitometric percent-area stenosis and the circular percent-area stenosis (standard deviation of the mean difference was 5%). However, important discrepancies between these two types of measurements were observed after PTCA (standard deviation 18%). This discrepancy suggested the creation of asymmetric

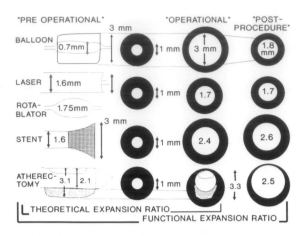

Figure 27. Comparison of various devices with the expansion ratio, which relates the final effect on the arterial diameter to the size of the catheter required to deliver this effect. (A) The far left column, pre-operational refers to the relationship between the profile of the various devices prior to the procedure and during the procedure. For example, balloon angioplasty catheter has a low profile (0.7 mm) but expands to a diameter of 3 mm in this case when it is fully dilated. The laser and the rotablator have the same profile prior to use and during use. The Wallstent is delivered on a 1.6 mm diameter catheter but can be expanded in this example to 3.0 mm (in fact it is possible to have a stent that expands to 6 mm). The directional altherectomy has a profile of 2.1 mm with balloon deflated and 3.1 mm with balloon inflated. The circles represent the diameter of the coronary artery pre-procedure (far left), during activation of the device (center circle) and post-procedure (far right). In this example, the pre-procedure diameter was 1 mm. During activation of the device, the vessel diameter is expanded from 1.7 mm to 3.3 mm depending on the device. The post-procedure results are based on the mean value of each procedure in the Thoraxcenter data bank. Elastic recoil is responsible for the immediate loss of 3 mm to 1.8 mm for balloon angioplasty and from 3.3 mm to 2.5 mm for directional atherectomy. The stent is an effective device against elastic recoil and due to the self-expanding property of the Wallstent, the vessel lumen continues to dilate (for at least the first 24 hours). Theoretical expansion ratio is the relation between the profile of the device and the maximal achievable diameter of the device. Functional (effective) expansion ratio represents the ratio between the post-procedure result and the profile of the device and thus indicates not only the initial effect of the device but also the effect of elastic recoil, which is primarily responsible for the deterioration in the diameter from the maximal achievable diameter to the postprocedure diameter. (B) the theoretical and effective expansion ratio for various interventional devices. The range for expansion ratios is due to ranges in the profiles of the device depending on the size of the balloon or stent mounted on the balloon catheter.

lesions after angioplasty, and an error in the circular assumption of cross-sectional area stenosis calculated from edge detection data.

B) *Stenting*

Three types of coronary stents have been implanted and followed with serial angiograms at the Thoraxcenter [34–38]. Two of these stents, the Wallstent and the Palmaz-Schatz stent are composed primarily of radioluscent stainless

INTER-VENTION	PTS	PRE	POST	FOLLOW-UP
PTCA	261	0.99 ±.35	1.77 ±.34	1.46 ± .59
WALLSTENT	166	1.17 ±.52	2.53 ±.53	*1.99 ± .81 **1.59 ±1.08
WIKTOR	62	1.09 ±.26	2.45 ±.35	1.71 ± .68
DCA	48	1.13 ±.40	2.52 ±.40	1.70 ± .58

* EXCLUDING IN HOSPITAL OCCLUSIONS
** INCLUDING IN HOSPITAL OCCLUSIONS

Figure 28. Results from the Thoraxcenter data bank for pre, immediately post and at follow-up in separate studies of angioplasty, stenting (Wallstent and Wiktor stent), and directional coronary atherectomy.

steel, whereas radiopaque tantalum is the principle constituent of the Wiktor stent (Figures 14A, B, C).

Stainless steel stents

The main problem with these stents is their poor angiographic visibility (Figures 15A, B). In particular, the Palmaz-Schatz stent which is the most difficult stent to visualize, can be dislodged from the balloon catheter and embolize distally without the stent operator's knowledge. Additionally, it can be quite difficult to ensure ideal placement of the stent across a lesion. For the analyst, this means that the stent boundaries may be uncertain at the time of implantation and the precise location of a late restenosis (within the stent or immediately adjacent) may be in some doubt. By carefully reviewing the angiograms done without contrast present, we usually can discern the position of the Wallstent for studies with contrast. In our follow-up reports of stenting, we have always included restenosis within and immediately adjacent to the stented segment to ensure restenosis is not underreported due to this problem [34].

A second problem with angiographic analysis of stented vessels is due to superior results immediately post stenting versus PTCA alone. Consequently, the "obstruction segment" may be completely corrected or in some cases overdilated in comparison to the reference diameter pre stenting. This causes problems specifically with the length of obstruction and the reference diameter. We arbitrarily define the length of the obstruction post stenting to be the actual length of the stent (which requires manual selection of the stent boundaries). Thus the extent of the stented segment is defined for future follow-up analyses. We perform each stent analysis either by stent and by vessel. In the former, the length of the lesion is the length of the stent as previously described. In the latter, there is no interaction with the choice of computer detected contours and the minimal luminal diameter may then be located outside the stent. In reporting our angiographic studies, we chose the pre and post PTCA frames to be analyzed by vessel, and the post stent and follow-up films according to the stent. This ensured that we could obtain the information related to the stent and its immediate adjacent segment rather than describing a more severe stenosis somewhere else in the coronary vessel.

Stenting has also taught us a limitation of the CAAS system in the measurement of the reference diameter in an overdilated segment. Theoretically, this should result in a negative value for diameter stenosis since the minimal luminal diameter (which we already mentioned was defined within the boundaries of the stent) was actually larger than the reference diameter which is determined according to the diameter of the proximal and distal segments (Figures 16A, B). However, for reasons still unclear to us, a negative diameter stenosis never occurred and the reference diameter always remained larger than the minimal luminal diameter. A further confounding factor in the determination of the reference diameter post stenting is the marked vasospasm occasionally seen immediately proximal and distal to the stent which persists despite nitrate administration.

Tantalum stents

The radiopacity of the Wiktor stent has greatly facilitated the implantation procedure (Figures 17A, B). The stent can easily be visualized in a vessel with and without contrast. However, this particular property of the Wiktor stent severely limits the assessment of follow-up studies by the CAAS system. Several cases have now been documented in which the radiopaque stent wires are traced by the contour detection program instead of the arterial borders of the narrowed intrastent hyperplasia (Figure 18). This invalidates the computer derived data and requires manual correction of the contours by the analyst, which is also difficult in a segment containing radiopaque wires.

Densitometry

In contrast to the situation after PTCA, there is excellent agreement between minimal luminal cross-sectional areas determined by edge detection and densitometry after stent implantation with the Wallstent [39]. In 19 patients, the standard deviation of the mean differences between edge detection and densitometric determination of minimal luminal cross-sectional area were 0.51 mm^2 pre PTCA, 1.22 mm^2 after angioplasty and 0.79 mm^2 after coronary stenting (Figure 19). This improvement is likely due to smoothing of the vessel contours by the stent and remodeling of the stented segment into a more circular configuration (Figure 20). Therefore we believe that both methods are appropriate to assess the immediate results post stenting. In a separate in-vitro study in which stents were placed in known stenoses within plexiglass phantoms, the Wallstent and Palmaz-Schatz stents had minor and likely clinically insignificant contributions to the densitometric determination of minimal luminal cross-sectional area within the known stenoses (Figures 21A, B) [40]. Conversely, the radiopacity of the tantalum Wiktor stent increased the MLCA in these same narrowings by 10–56% depending on the concentration of contrast and specific stenosis (Figure 21C). Therefore, the follow-up assessment of a lesion containing a Wiktor stent, is limited by both methods.

Directional atherectomy

Few problems have been encountered in the analysis of patients treated with directional atherectomy [41]. The radiopacity of the device, particularly when the support balloon is inflated, allows the operator excellent visualization of the position of the eccentric cutting apparatus (Figures 22A, B). The contours are typically smooth and much less ragged than after PTCA, facilitating the edge detection program. Despite the apparent smooth contours following atherectomy, similar discrepancy exist between analyses performed by edge detection or densitometry, as occurs post angioplasty (Figure 23) [42]. This suggest that the vessel wall assumes a less circular configuration as a result of atherectomy. As Baim's group has suggested, this may be due to preferential expansion of the bases of the atherectomy cuts [43]. Furthermore, QCA of atherectomy-treated lesions has provided some insight into the mechanisms of lesion improvement. Penny et al. have shown that approximately 28% of the effect of atherectomy can actually be attributed to tissue removal, although the individual values had a wide range (7–92%) [43]. The correlation between the volume of tissue retrieved and the change in luminal volume was poor ($r = 0.19$). The authors concluded that the major component of luminal improvement was due to "facilitated mechanical angioplasty" resulting from the high profile of the device and the low pressure balloon inflations. Data from our angiographic core laboratory seems to support this hypothesis. In 10 patients that had QCA performed pre atherectomy, after crossing the stenosis with the device and after directional atherectomy, it was shown that the dottering effect of the device accounted for 65% of the luminal improvement [44].

Rotational abrasion

The Thoraxcenter experience to date has been limited with this device (11 procedures) [45]. A unique feature of this particular device is its usefulness as a calibration unit. Usually we use the guiding catheter for this purpose.

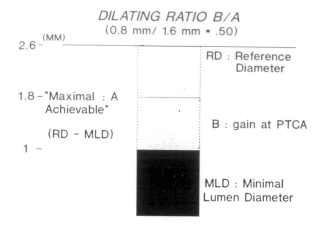

Figure 29a.

The tip (or shaft in the case of soft tip catheters) of the guiding catheter is measured by a micrometer and then the contrast-filled catheter in the angiogram is appropriately scaled. However, a limitation of this procedure is that the guiding catheter may be some distance away from the actual lesion (out-of-plane magnification) and thus introduce some error into the measurement. The rotablator™ contains a burr of known size and there is no question of completeness of expansion as with stents and PTCA catheters of specified sizes (Figures 24A, B). Precise measurement of the device at the site of lesion has been useful to assess the extent of elastic recoil which appears to be an important phenomenon since the effect immediately following rotational abrasion is always smaller than the diameter of the burr used. A unique feature of the Rotablator is that the optimal angiographic result is not realized until 24 hours later since the intense vasoconstriction induced by the burr is largely attenuated at that time (Figures 25A, B, C).

Excimer laser

Excimer lasers have seemed an attractive alternative to other forms of coronary interventions based on the experimental finding that a focused, pulsed, ultraviolet (UV) laser beam in air can ablate tissue with minimal adjacent tissue injury. However, in the clinical situation where the vessel is surrounded by a blood medium, contact is required to increase ablation efficiency which has actually resulted in considerable temperature accumulation and damage in the tissue due to expansion of gaseous debris trapped under the tip of the delivery system [46]. The angiographic correlate of this phenomenon appears to be haziness of the contours of lesions treated with the excimer laser, which can complicate the immediate post-procedure analysis (Figures 26A, B, C).

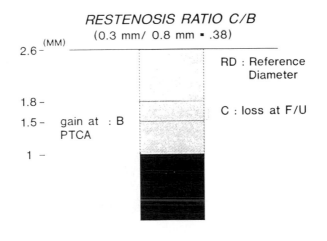

Figure 29b.

The lesion typically has a "roughened" appearance which may particularly be well suited to the detailed analysis of lesion morphology provided by the QCA system of Mancini et al. [47].

How should we use QCA data to compare interventional devices?

We have now reached the stage where the safety and favorable immediate results for the various devices have been demonstrated by ourselves and other groups. The logical next step is the comparison of the devices to determine what specific features of a device or clinical situation may favor the use of a particular device.

1) *Immediate results post procedure: The expansion ratio (Figures 27A, B)*

The expansion ratio is a useful concept to assess the immediate results of an intervention [37, 48]. It relates the final effect of the device on the arterial diameter to the size of the catheter required to deliver this effect. A favorable ratio is best exemplified by a small catheter delivery system that is able to pass severely narrowed segments and yet optimally dilate the stenosis. However, the maximum effect of the device may be partially lost due to the elastic recoil of the vessel. The current interventional devices may have differential effects in these two areas: the acute result, when the device is initially used and then the partial loss of the initial gain after the device has been removed. We have attemped to separate these two effects by subdividing the expansion ratio into the *theoretical* expansion ratio, which is a measure of the effect while the device is operational, and the *functional* expansion ratio, which takes into account vasoconstriction and the elastic recoil phe-

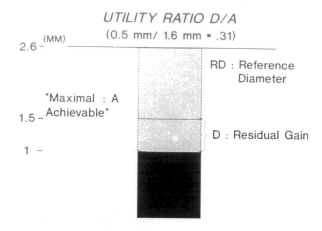

Figure 29c.

Figures 29a–c. Example of new indices to compare the effect of directional atherectomy versus balloon angioplasty. (A) The dilating index is the ratio between the gain in diameter during the intervention and the theoretically achievable gain i.e. the reference diameter. In this example, the minimal luminal diameter was 1 mm pre-procedure, the gain at PTCA (B) was 0.8 mm and the maximal achievable gain in diameter (A) was 1.6 (RD-MLD). The dilating ratio was then calculated as 0.50 (B/A). (B) The restenosis index is the ratio between the loss at follow-up (BC), which was 0.3 mm in this example, and the initial gain during the procedure (B), 0.8 mm. This gave an overall restenosis ratio of 0.38 (C/B). (C) The net result at long term is characterized by the utility index which is the ratio between the net gain in diameter at follow-up (D), i.e. the difference between the initial gain and then the late loss due to restenosis which is 0.5 mm in this example, and the maximal theoretically gain possible (A), i.e. the difference between the pre-procedure MLD and the reference diameter, which was 1.6 mm. The utility ratio is then calculated as 0.31 (D/A). (D) Comparison of directional coronary atherectomy (DCA) and balloon angioplasty (BA) for the three ratios in 30 matched patients with initially successfully treated lesions. Significantly higher dilating and restenosis ratios were seen with DCA in comparison to BA, suggesting that despite a superior immediate result with DCA, the late loss due to restenosis was much greater with DCA. As a result, there were no significant differences between the two procedures for the utility ratio which relates the immediate gain to the late loss.

nomenon. For example, a fully expanded 4 mm diameter balloon angioplasty catheter should achieve a vessel diameter of 4 mm at the time of balloon inflation but the lesion diameter may be considerably less after deflation, primarily due to the elastic recoil of the vessel. Balloon angioplasty and stenting give extremely favourable *theoretical* and *functional* expansion ratios since they may be delivered on low profile catheters. Although the directional atherectomy device is effective against elastic recoil, the bulky profile of the device limits introduction of the device and the theoretical expansion ratio. The dimensions of the rotational atherectomy device and the excimer laser do not change while in operation and therefore both exhibit lower theoretical expansion ratios. However, by physically removing or vaporizing tissue, the potential elastic recoil effect is diminished by atherectomy and excimer laser devices.

2) *Late results*

To date, no randomized trials have been reported that compare the various devices. In anticipation of this data, we have attempted to compare available data according to three methods. First, we have pre, immediately post and follow-up results in native vessels from separate angioplasty [21], directional atherectomy and stenting [51] studies (Figure 28).

Secondly, Kevin Beatt has devised 3 indices to assess the "utility" of each type of intervention [48]. This index can be subdivided into a dilating component and a restenosis component. The "dilating index" is the ratio between the gain in diameter during the intervention and the theoretically achievable gain i.e. the reference diameter. The "restenosis index" is the ratio between the loss at follow-up and the initial gain during the procedure. The net result at long term is characterized by the "utility index" which is the ratio between the final gain in diameter at follow-up and what theoretically could have been achieved. These indices are useful for studying the mean values for populations of patients who have undergone a particular intervention and have shown important differences between the initial effect of devices (atherectomy, stenting > PTCA) which are partially overcome by larger late losses in minimal luminal dimater. Recently, we have used these indices to compare the results of balloon angioplasty and directional atherectomy (Figure 29) [49]. The superior immediate results of atherectomy is shown in the dilating index, which is offset by the greater loss in MLD at late follow-up, resulting in a higher restenosis index. Thus the net effect at late follow-up is comparable i.e. utility ratio was not different.

Thirdly, we have used "matched" lesions to compare interventions [50] (Figures 30A–D). Matching is based on three principles: the angiographic dimensions of matched lesions are assumed to be "identical", the observed difference between the two "identical" lesions must be within the range of the CAAS analysis reproducibility of 0.1 mm (=1 s.d.), and finally that the reference diameter of the potentially "matched" vessels are selected within a range of ±0.3 mm (=3 s.d.; i.e. 99% confidence limits) (Figure 31 A, B). The appropriate lesions are selected by an independent observer who is unaware of the 6 month angiographic outcome.

3) *How should future trials be designed to compare devices using angiographic endpoints?*

In several large multicenter PTCA restenosis trials that have been analyzed by the CAAS system, we have used the mean difference in coronary diameter between post angioplasty and follow up angiograms as the primary angiographic endpoint. However, this would be inadequate to compare various devices since atherectomy and stenting both result in superior initial results

MATCHED PRE-PROCEDURAL STENOSIS CHARACTE-
RISTICS OF PTS WITH SUCCESSFUL DCA VS BA

	DCA	BA	P
REF–DIAM (mm)	3.03	3.07	NS
MLD (mm)	1.09	1.15	NS
D–Sten (%)	64	63	NS
A PLAQ (mm2)	9.5	8.4	NS
CURVATURE	15.9	22.2	< .02
SYMMETRY	0.6	0.5	NS
LENGTH (mm)	6.8	6.5	NS

QUANTITATIVE COMPARISON OF THE IMMEDIATE
AND LONG-TERM RESULTS OF DCA VS PBA
(MATCHED DATA)

	DCA	BA	P
RD (mm)			
PRE	3.03	3.07	NS
MLD (mm)			
PRE	1.08	1.15	NS
POST	2.61	1.92	10^{-5}
F–UP	1.69	1.57	NS
$\angle$ IN MLD (mm)			
POST–PRE	1.53	0.77	10^{-5}
POST–F\U	0.92	0.35	10^{-3}

Figure 30. Matching lesions to compare interventions. (A) Matched pre-procedural stenosis characteristics of patients. No significant differences exist between the two groups pre-procedure except for a lower curvature value for lesions treated by DCA. Ref diam = reference diameter, MLD = minimal luminal diameter, D-Sten = diameter stenosis, A PLAQ = area plaque, length = length of lesion, P = probability. (B) Quantitative comparison of the immediate and long-term results of directional coronary atherectomy (DCA), and percutaneous balloon angioplasty (PBA). Although there was a significant difference post-procedure with larger MLD with directional atherectomy, this superior initial result was not maintained at late follow-up due to a greater loss in MLD at follow-up in the DCA group. RD = reference diameter, F-UP = follow-up.

in addition to larger late losses than balloon angioplasty. We suggest that the important angiographic endpoint in these studies should be the minimal luminal diameter at follow-up provided that the lesions have comparable reference diameters and minimial luminal diameter prior to the initial intervention.

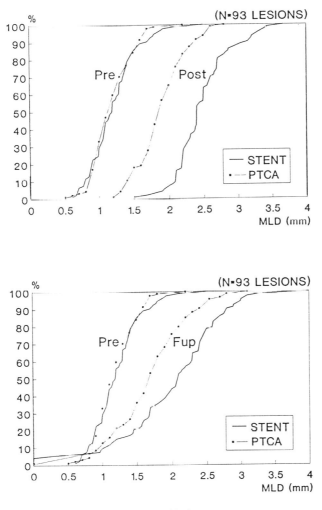

Figures 31a,b.

Conclusion

QCA remains the gold standard as the most objective and reproducible form of coronary artery disease. The Computer-Assisted Cardiovascular Angiography Analysis System (CAAS) has been the most extensively studied form of QCA. This system, which has provided important information about the natural history of coronary artery disease, now enables researchers in the field of interventional cardiology to accurately assess the immediate and late

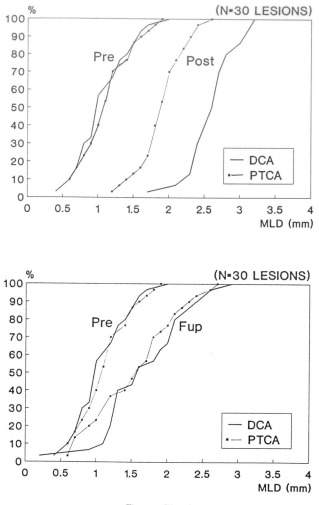

Figures 31c, d.

Figures 31a–d. Comparison of results in native vessels from matched studies of balloon angioplasty, stenting and directional atherectomy using a cumulative curve. On the x-axis is the minimal luminal diameter (MLD) and on the y-axis is the cumulative total. (A) Pre-procedure and immediately post-procedure results for PTCA and the Wallstent (93 lesions). (B) Pre-procedure and follow-up results for PTCA and the Wallstent. (C) Pre-procedure and immediately post-procedure for PTCA and directional atherectomy (30 lesions). (D) Pre-procedure and follow-up for PTCA and directional atherectomy.

results of devices utilized for nonoperative coronary revascularization. The introduction of new devices has exposed heretofore unknown limitations of this system in addition to the well known problems of cost and length of time required for analysis (approximately $\frac{1}{2}$ hour per lesion for 2 projections selected at any stage of the procedure). However, thanks to the rapid changes in computer technology over the years, second generation systems now appear on the market which are based on powerful personal computers (PC's) and workstations. These systems are characterized by improved contour detection with correction for the limited resolution of the x-ray imaging chain, automated pathline tracing, lower costs and significantly reduced processing time (complete analysis of coronary arterial segment can be done in less than 10–12 seconds).

References

1. Mancini GBJ. Quantitative coronary arteriographic methods in the interventional catheterization laboratory: an update and perspective. J Am Coll Cardiol 1991; **17** (6 Suppl B): 23B–33B.
2. Zir LM, Miller SW, Dinsmore RE, Gilbert JP, Harthorne JW. Interobserver variability in coronary angiography. Circulation 1976; **53**: 627–32.
3. Goldberg RK, Kleiman NS, Minor ST, Abukhalil J, Raizner AE. Comparison of quantitative coronary angiography to visual estimates of lesion severity pre and post PTCA. Am Heart J 1990; **119**: 178–84.
4. Reiber JHC, Booman F, Tan HS, et al. A cardiac image analysis system. Objective quantitative processing on angiocardiograms. Comput Cardiol 1978; 239–242.
5. Reiber JHC, Serruys PW, Kooijman CJ, et al. Assessment of short-, medium-, and long-term variations in arterial dimensions from computer-assisted quantitation of coronary cineangiograms. Circulation 1985; **71**: 280–8.
6. Reiber JHC, Serruys PW, Slager CJ. Quantitative coronary and left ventricular cineangiography: methodology and clinical applications. Boston: Martinus Nijhoff Publishers 1986.
7. Reiber JHC, Kooijman CJ, Slager CJ, et al. Coronary artery dimensions from cineangiograms: methodology and validation of a computer-assisted anaylsis procedure. IEEE Trans Med Imaging 1984; **3**: 131–41.
8. Vlodaver Z, Edwards JE. Pathology of coronary atherosclerosis. Prog Cardiovasc Dis 1971; **14**: 256–74.
9. Saner HE, Gobel FL, Salomonowitz E, Erlien DA, Edwards JE. The disease-free wall in coronary atherosclerosis: its relation to degree of obstruction. J Am Coll Cardiol 1985; **6**: 1096–9.
10. Marcus ML. Physiologic effects of a coronary stenosis. In: Marcus ML. The coronary circulation in health and disease. New York: McGraw-Hill 1983: 242–69.
11. de Feyter PJ, Serruys PW, Davies MJ, Richardson P, Lubsen J, Oliver MF. Quantitative coronary angiography to measure progression and regression of coronary atherosclerosis. Value, limitations and implications for clinical trials. Circulation 1991; **84**: 412–23.
12. Schwartz JN, Kong Y, Hackel DB, Bartel AG. Comparison of angiographic and postmortem findings in patients with coronary artery disease. Am J Cardiol 1975; **36**: 174–8.
13. Hutchins GM, Bulkley GH, Ridolf RL, Griffith LSC, Lohr FT, Piasio MA. Correlation of coronary arterigrams and left ventriculograms with postmortem studies. Circulation 1977; **56**: 32–7.
14. Arnett EN, Isner JM, Redwood DR, et al. Coronary artery narrowing in coronary heart disease: comparison of cineangiograms and necropsy findings. Ann Intern Med 1979; **91**: 350–6.
15. Thomas AC, Davies MJ, Dilly N, Franc F. Potential errors in the estimation of coronary arterial stenosis from clinical arteriography with reference to the shape of the coronary arterial lumen. Br Heart J 1986; **55**: 129–39.

16. Ellis SG, Roubin GS, King SB 3d, Douglas JS Jr, Cox WR. Importance of stenosis morphology in the estimation of restenosis risk after elective percutaneous transluminal coronary angioplasty. Am J Cardiol 1989; **63**: 30–4.
17. Leimgruber PP, Roubin GS, Hollman J, et al. Restenosis after succesful coronary angioplasty in patients with single-vessel disease. Circulation 1986; **73**: 710–7.
18. Myler RK, Topol EJ, Shaw RE, et al. Multiple vessel coronary angioplasty: classification, results, and patterns of restenosis in 494 consecutive patients. Cathet Cardiovasc Diagn 1987; **13**: 1–15.
19. Vandormael MG, Deligonul U, Kern MJ, et al. Multilesion coronary angioplasty: clinical and angiographic follow-up. J Am Coll Cardiol 1987; **10**: 246–52.
20. Serruys PW, Luijten HE, Beatt KJ, et al. Incidence of restenosis after successful coronary angioplasty: a time-related phenomenon. A quantitative angiographic study in 342 consecutive patients at 1, 2, 3, and 4 months. Circulation 1988; **77**: 361–71.
21. Serruys PW, Rutsch W, Heyndrickx GR, et al. Prevention of restenosis after percutaneous transluminal coronary angioplasty with Thromboxane A2 receptor blockade. A randomized, double-blind, placebo controlled trial. Circulation 1991; **84**: 1568–1580.
22. The MERCATOR study group. Does the new angiotensin converting enzyme inhibitor cilazapril prevent restenosis after percutaneous transluminal coronary angioplasty? Circulation 1992; **84**: 100–110.
23. Rensing BJ, Hermans WRM, Deckers JW, de Feyter PJ, Tijssen JGP, Serruys PW. Luminal narrowing after percutaneous transluminal coronary balloon angioplasty follows a near Gaussian distribution. A quantitative angiographic study in 1445 successfully dilated lesions. J Am Coll Cardiol 1992; **19**: 939–945.
24. King SB 3d, Weintraub WS, Xudong T, Hearn J, Douglas JS Jr. Bimodal distribution of diameter stenosis 4 to 12 months after angioplasty: implication for definitions and interpretation of restenosis. J Am Coll Cardiol 1991; **17** (2 Suppl A): 345A (Abstract).
25. Hermans WRM, Rensing BJ, Kelder JC, de Feyter PJ, Serruys PW. Postangioplasty restenosis rate between segments of the major coronary arteries. Am J Cardiol 1992; **69**: 194–200.
26. Rensing BJ, Hermans WRM, Vos J, et al. Angiographic risk factors of luminal narrowing after coronary balloon angioplasty using balloon measurements to reflect stretch and elastic recoil at the dilatation site. Am J Cardiol 1992; **69**: 584–591.
27. Sanborn TA, Faxon DP, Haudenschild CG, Gottsman SB, Ryan TJ. The mechanism of transluminal angioplasty: evidence for formation of aneurysms in experimental atherosclerosis. Circulation 1983; **68**: 1136–40.
28. Rensing BJ, Hermans WRM, Beatt KJ, et al. Quantitative angiographic assessment of elastic recoil after percutaneous transluminal coronary angioplasty. Am J Cardiol 1990; **66**: 1039–44
29. Rensing BJ, Hermans WRM, Strauss BH, Serruys PW. Regional differences in elastic recoil after percutaneous transluminal coronary angioplasty: a quantitative angiographic study. J Am Coll Cardiol 1991; **17** (6 Suppl B): 34B–38B.
30. Hermans WRM, Rensing BJ, Strauss BH, Serruys PW. Methodological problems related to the quantitative assessment of stretch, elastic recoil and balloon-artery ratio. Cathet Cardiovasc Diagn 1992; **25**: 174–185.
31. Hermans WRM, Rensing BJ, Paameyer J, Reiber JHC, Serruys PW. Experiences of a quantitative coronary angiographic core laboratory in restenosis prevention trials. In: Reiber JHC and Serruys PW (Eds.), Quantitative coronary arteriography 1992. Dordrecht: Kluwer Academic Publishers (in press).
32. Beatt KJ, Luijten HE, de Feyter PJ, van den Brand M, Reiber JHC, Serruys PW. Change in diameter of coronary artery segments adjacent to stenosis after percutaneous transluminal coronary angioplasty: failure of percent diameter stenosis measurement to reflect morphologic changes induced by balloon dilatation. J Am Coll Cardiol 1988; **12**: 315–23.
33. Serruys PW, Reiber JHC, Wijns W, et al. Assessment of percutaneous transluminal coronary

angioplasty by quantitative coronary angiography: diameter versus densitometric area measurements. Am J Cardiol 1984; **54**: 482–8.

34. Serruys PW, Strauss BH, Beatt KJ, et al. Angiographic follow-up after placement of a self-expanding coronary-artery stent. N Engl J Med 1991; **324**: 13–7.
35. Serruys PW, Juilliere Y, Bertrand ME, Puel J, Rickards AF, Sigwart U. Additional improvement of stenosis geometry in human coronary arteries by stenting after balloon dilatation. Am J Cardiol 1988; **61**: 71G–76G.
36. Puel J, Juilliere Y, Bertrand ME, Rickards AF, Sigwart U, Serruys PW. Early and late assessment of stenosis geometry after coronary arterial stenting. Am J Cardiol 1988; **61**: 546–53.
37. Serruys PW, Strauss BH, van Beusekom HM, van der Giessen WJ. Stenting of coronary arteries. has a modern Pandora's box been opened? J Am Coll Cardiol 1991; **17** (6 Suppl B): 143B–154B.
38. Serruys PW, de Jaegere P, Bertrand M, et al. Morphologic change of coronary artery stenosis with the Medtronic Wiktor™ stent. Initial results from the core laboratory for quantitative angiography. Cathet Cardiovasc Diagn 1991; **24**: 237–245.
39. Strauss BH, Julliere Y, Rensing BJ, Reiber JHC, Serruys PW. Edge detection versus densitometry for assessing coronary stenting quantitatively. Am J Cardiol 1991; **67**: 484–90.
40. Strauss BH, Rensing BJ, den Boer A, van der Giessen WJ, Reiber JHC, Serruys PW. Do stents interfere with the densitometric assessment of a coronary artery lesion? Cathet Cardiovasc Diagn 1991; **24**: 259–264.
41. Serruys PW, Umans VAWM, Strauss BH, van Suylen RJ, de Feyter PJ. Quantitative angiography after directional coronary atherectomy. Br Heart J 1991; **66**: 122–9.
42. Umans VA, Strauss BH, de Feyter PJ, Serruys PW. Edge detection versus videodensitometry for quantitative angiographic assessment of directional coronary atherectomy. Am J Cardiol 1991; **68**: 534–9.
43. Penny WF, Schmidt DA, Safian RD, Erny RE, Baim DS. Insights into the mechanism of luminal improvement after directional coronary atherectomy. Am J Cardiol 1991; **67**: 435–7.
44. Umans VA, Haine E, Renkin J, de Feyter PJ, Wijns W, Serruys PW. On the mechanism of directional coronary atherectomy (in press).
45. Laarman GJ, Serruys PW, de Feyter PJ. Percutaneous coronary rotational atherectomy (Rotablator). Neth J Cardiol 1990; **3**: 177–83.
46. Gijsbers GHM, Spranger RLH, Keijzer M, et al. Some laser-tissue interactions in 308 nm excimer laser coronary angioplasty. J Intervent Cardiol 1990; **3**: 231–41.
47. Kalbfleisch SJ, McGillem MJ, Simon SB, Deboe SF, Pinto IMF, Mancini GBJ. Automated quantitation of indexes of coronary lesion complexity. Comparison between patients with stable and unstable angina. Circulation 1990; **82**: 439–47.
48. Beatt KJ, Serruys PW, Strauss BH, Suryapranata H, de Feyter PJ, van den Brand M. Comparative index for assessing the results of interventional devices in coronary angioplasty. Eur Heart J 1991; **12** (Abstract Suppl): 395 (Abstract).
49. Umans VAWM, Strauss BH, Rensing BJWM, de Jaegere P, de Feyter PJ, Serruys PW. Comparative angiographic quantitative analysis of the immediate efficacy of coronary atherectomy with balloon angioplasty, stenting, and rotational ablation. Am Heart J 1991; **122**: 836–43.
50. Umans VAWM, Beatt KJ, Rensing BJWM, Hermans WRM, de Feyter PJ, Serruys PW. Comparative quantitative angiographic analysis of directional coronary atherectomy and balloon angioplasty: a new methodologic approach. Am J Cardiol 1991; **68**: 1556–63.
51. Strauss BH, Serruys PW, Bertrand ME, Puel J, Meier B, Goy J-J, Kappenberger L, Rickards AF, Sigwart U. Quantitative angiographic follow-up of the coronary Wallstent in native vessels and bypass grafts (European experience March 1986–March 1990). Am J Cardiol 1992; **69**: 475–481.
52. Reiber JHC, van der Zwet PMJ, von Land CD, et al. Quantitative coronary arteriography: equipment and technical requirements. In: Reiber JHC, Serruys PW (Eds), Advances in Quantitative Coronary Arteriography. Dordrecht: Kluwer Academic Publishers (in press).

26. Quantitative coronary arteriography in laser balloon angioplasty

H.W. THIJS PLOKKER, J. RICHARD SPEARS, E. GIJS MAST,
SJEF M.P.G. ERNST, EGBERT T. BAL and
MELVYN TJON JOE GIN

Summary

Percutaneous transluminal coronary angioplasty as developed by Grüntzig et al. has become an established therapeutic method to improve coronary blood flow in patients with obstructive coronary artery disease [1]. However, balloon angioplasty has three major limitations. First of all, there is the problem of restenosis within the first six months after a successful procedure, which has been reported to range between 17 and 40% [2–5]. Another limitation is the risk of abrupt closure during the procedure itself, which has been reported to be approximately 5%. Finally, balloon angioplasty can not predictably open chronic total coronary occlusions or very long diffusely atherosclerotic diseased segments.

Laser balloon angioplasty (LBA) as developed by Richard Spears and USCI primarily addressed the issue of improving on the initial balloon angioplasty result, which might lead to a lower restenosis rate. The hypotheses which had to be tested, were that the combination of laser-generated heat combined with pressure from the inflated balloon would:
1. leave a smoother endovascular surface;
2. improve luminal geometry;
3. prevent flow separation;
4. reduce elastic recoil;
5. weld intimal flaps; and
6. desiccate thrombus.
With the help of a quantitative coronary arteriography (QCA) system as developed by Spears et al. [6, 7], the LBA study group has been able to prove that points 2 and 4 are valid. QCA in general is unable to prove points such as 5 and 6, although the arteriografic results after LBA do suggest that these hypotheses are valid too.

Unfortunately, the QCA-system used does not incorporate a method to quantify the roughness (or smoothness) of the surface, to validate point 1. To prove the point of flow separation (point 3) other methods are required. However, we may conclude that LBA does improve on the results of ordinary

J.H.C. Reiber and P.W. Serruys (eds), Advances in Quantitative Coronary Arteriography, 443–458.

balloon angioplasty by improving luminal geometry, reducing elastic recoil, welding intimal flaps, and desiccating thrombus. Although the acute results of balloon angioplasty can be improved with LBA, restenosis rates have not been reduced, which severely limits the applicability of the LBA system.

Introduction

The neodymium-doped yttrium aluminum garnet (Nd: YAG) laser balloon angioplasty system as developed by Richard Spears and USCI was first used in the St Antonius Hospital in Nieuwegein on September 8, 1988. It was felt that the diffuse energy-scattering of Nd:YAG laser could be used to improve the results of conventional balloon angioplasty. The combination of heat (85–105°C) generated by laser, and the pressure from the inflated balloon would most likely yield the following results.
   It was expected to:
1. leave a smoother endovascular surface;
2. improve luminal geometry;
3. prevent flow separation;
4. reduce elastic recoil;
5. weld intimal flaps; and
6. desiccate thrombus.
   It is the purpose of this study to investigate with quantitative coronary arteriography whether these hypotheses can be supported or rejected.

Methods

LBA is always preceded by conventional coronary balloon angioplasty with a similar sized (3.0 mm) balloon. After an angiographically successful conventional balloon angioplasty procedure (defined as a reduction of the estimated diameter stenosis to less than 50%) the standard coronary guide wire (0.014 inch) is left across the dilated lesion to enable insertion of the LBA system.
   In the LBA-system a 15–40 Watt Nd:YAG air cooled laser delivery system from Quantronic Inc. (Smith Town, N.Y.) (Figure 1) is used to deliver laser radiation at 1064 nanometer into a fiber optic system. Standard fiber optic connectors allow rapid coupling of the catheter system to the laser source. The balloon catheter has a mechanical function which is similar to that of a conventional balloon catheter, in terms of balloon material (polyethylene terephthalate), shape and size (Figure 2). Within the balloon, a 100 micrometer optic fiber with a helical diffusing tip has been wrapped around the distal shaft. The balloon system, with a PVC-shaft of 4.3 French, is introduced via the standard 0.014 inch (exchange) guide wire. Prior to use, the LBA-balloon is filled with metrizamide and deuterium oxide which has a very low absorption of 1064 nm radiation. The pattern of radiation, provided

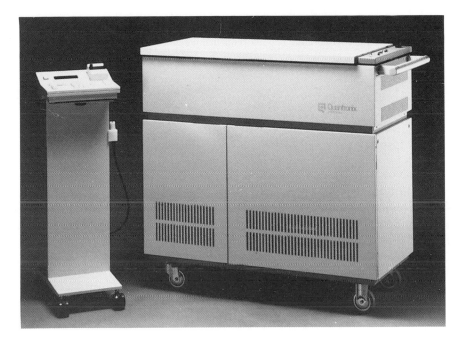

Figure 1. The Nd.YAG air cooled laser delivery system.

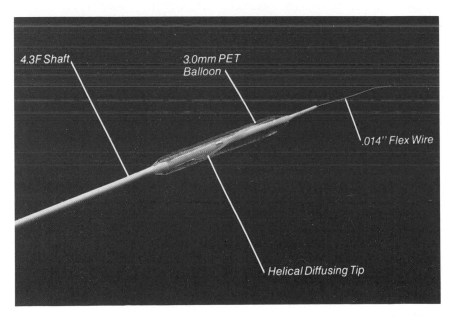

Figure 2. The laser balloon with a 100 micrometer optic fiber which ends with a helical diffusing tip wrapped around the shaft.

446   *H. Plokker et al.*

Table 1. Laser doses used during the LBA prospective randomized trial. The amount of laser energy was decreased stepwise, after 5, 10 and 20 seconds. This was followed by a 20 second cooling-down period. Therefore the balloon remained inflated during at least 40 seconds

	0–5 sec	5–10 sec	10–20 sec	20–40 sec
0 W group	0 W	0 W	0 W	0 W
15 W group	15 W	11 W	8 W	0 W
15 W group	15 W	11 W	8 W	0 W
20 W group	20 W	13 W	11 W	0 W
25 W group	25 W	15 W	12 W	0 W

by the diffusing tip can be visually assessed prior to insertion, with the use of a red helium-neon laser reference beam. Three different laser doses were used during the study (Table 1) to reach peak temperatures between 85°C and 105°C [8, 10].

Computerized image processing of digitized cineframes for quantitatation of absolute luminal diameters was used to evaluate both the relative immediate efficacy of laser balloon angioplasty compared with conventional balloon angioplasty, and the long-term efficacy of the procedure. In the initial patient group, coronary arteriography was repeated after 24 hours, to evaluate elastic recoil.

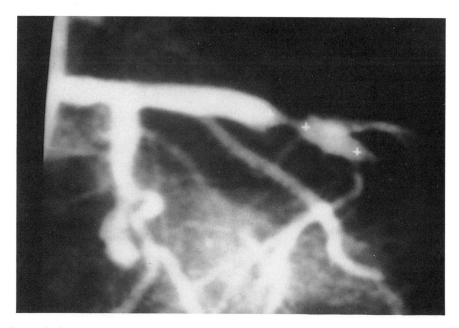

Figure 3. Computerized image processing of digitized cineframes. First step: manual marking of points along the centerline.

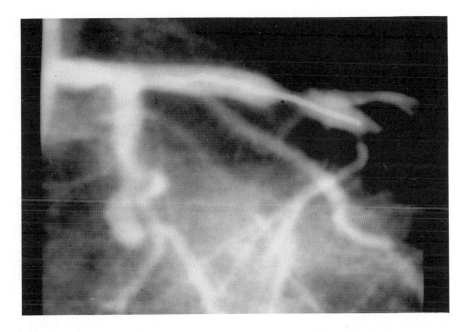

Figure 4. Computerized image processing of digitized cineframes: polynomial fit to centerline points.

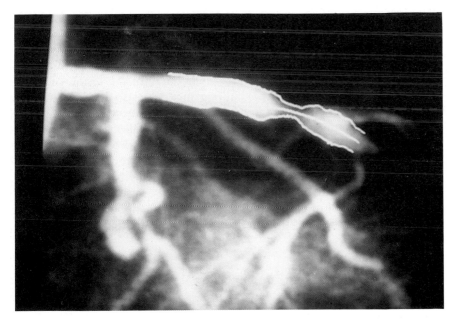

Figure 5. Computerized image processing of digitized cineframes: extraction of the vessel boundaries in first approximation and computation of improved centerline.

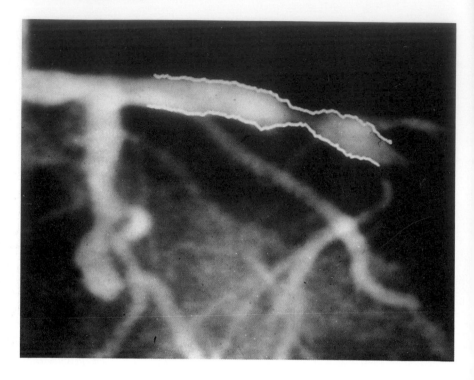

Figure 6. Computerized image processing of digitized cineframes: final edges found by scanning perpendicular to final centerline. Plotting of diameters versus axial location follows.

The rotation and angulation angles, and table and image intensifier height used for the initial optimal cineangiographic view of the lesion of interest were recorded before conventional balloon angioplasty so that identical views and magnification could be obtained for angiograms acquired after conventional balloon angioplasty, immediately after laser balloon angioplasty, and at 24 hours after the procedure. Computerized image processing of digitized cineframes (Figure 3–6) was performed in an unmasked manner at a core facility at Wayne State University. The accuracy of this system has been reported to be ≤ 100 μm and a reproducibility between sequential cineangiography studies ≤ 200 μm [6, 7]. Diameter measurements of the fully inflated 3 mm balloon were used as a reference to obtain absolute diameter measurements [8].

LBA-patients

After approval from the Medical Review Board of the St Antonius Hospital, all medically stable patients referred for elective PTCA with the anticipation

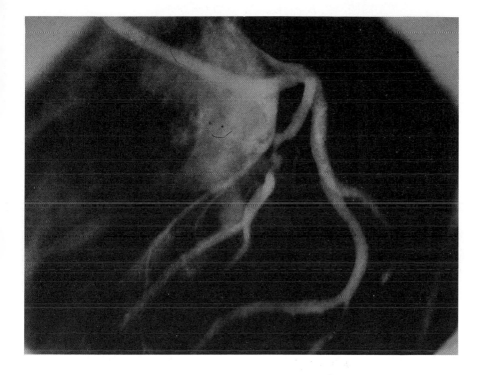

Figure 7. Eccentric lesion in the left anterior descending coronary artery (left anterior oblique cranial projection), prior to treatment.

of the need of a 3.0 mm diameter conventional balloon for treatment of a single lesion were considered to be candidates for LBA, with the following exclusion criteria: age >75 years, cholesterol >8.0 mmol/l, left main or mid vein graft lesions, presence of more than one lesion with >50% diameter stenosis, multivessel coronary artery disease and restenosis after prior PTCA. Informed consent was obtained in all patients. All patients were treated initially with a conventional 3.0 mm balloon, and were then randomized to the four treatment groups. In these groups three different laser doses (maximal energy 25,20 and 15 Watts, respectively) were compared with a 0 Watt (=PTCA only) group (Table 1). From January 19, 1989 to December 22, 1990, 48 patients from the St Antonius Hospital were entered into the study, following the first 7 patients in a pilot study. Another 14 patients have been treated in the St Antonius Hospital with the LBA-system for abrupt vessel reclosure after initially successful PTCA.

The following centers also contributed angiographic data to the core-lab in Detroit: Harper Hospital, Wayne State University, Detroit, Michigan; Sir Charles Gairdner Hospital, Perth, Australia; Toronto General Hospital,

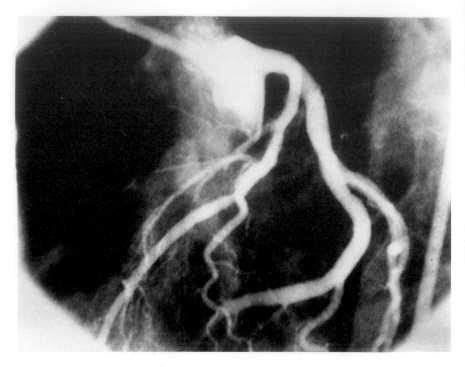

Figure 8. Left anterior descending coronary artery following conventional balloon angioplasty with a good result.

Toronto, Canada; St Antonius Ziekenhuis, Nieuwegein, The Netherlands; National Heart Hospital, London, England; Foothills Hospital, Calgary, Canada; Centre Hospitalier Universitair Vandois, Lausanne, Switzerland; Texas Heart Institute/St Lucs Episcopal Hospital, Houston, Texas; Beth Israel Hospital, Boston, Massachusetts; Emory University Hospital, Atlanta, Georgia.

In this way, the acute angiographic results of 200 patients, undergoing elective LBA could be analyzed.

Statistical analysis

Data are expressed as mean values ± 1 s.d. Minimal luminal diameter, reference segment diameter and percent diameter stenosis were analyzed using analysis of variance for repeated measures. When the result was statistically significant ($p < 0.05$) appropriate pairwise comparisons were made using Tukey's Studentized range test to control the experimentwise error rate. The unpaired Student's t-test was used to compare those patients who had a

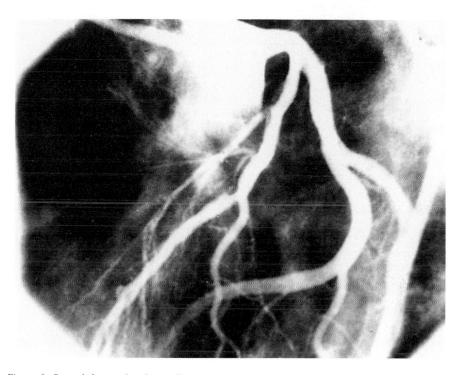

Figure 9. Same left anterior descending coronary artery as in Figures 7 and 8, following LBA. Note the smoother vessel contours.

postconventional balloon angioplasty minimal luminal diameter ⩽ 1.5 mm with those having postconventional balloon angioplasty minimum luminal diameter > 1.5 mm.

Results

There were few complications related to the laser balloon angioplasty procedure. In one of our 7 patients in the pilot phase a small thrombus was noted in a side branch distal to the laser site, without any apparent clinical consequence. In 11 of the 14 patients with abrupt vessel closure emergency coronary artery bypass surgery could be prevented by LBA.

The lesion of interest was succesfully crossed with a 0.014 High Torque Floppy guide wire (from ACS) followed by a conventional USCI Miniprofile 3.0 mm balloon in all patients. In some patients a smaller balloon was first used to cross and dilate the lesion. Quantitative coronary angiography later demonstrated (Table 2) that conventional balloon angioplasty had produced a successful angiographic result, defined as a minimal luminal diameter of

Table 2. Quantitative coronary arteriographic data of the LBA patients from the St Antonius Hospital

	Pre PTCA	Post PTCA	Post LBA	1 Day Post LBA	4–6 Months Post LBA
Minimal luminal diameter (mm)	0.59 ± 0.47	1.73 ± 0.63	2.15 ± 0.36	2.49 ± 1.14	1.4 ± 0.89
Percentage stenosis (%)	82.9 ± 11.9	42.6 ± 20.2	28.5 ± 11.3	9.7 ± 10.3	56.4 ± 25.7

Table 3. Quantitative coronary arteriographic data of the international LBA registry

	Pre PTCA	Post PTCA	Post LBA	1 Day Post LBA	1 Month Post LBA
Minimum diameter (mm)	0.67 ± 0.25	1.73 ± 0.57	2.27 ± 0.33	2.27 ± 0.39	2.39 ± 0.35
Reference diameter (mm)	3.00 ± 0.34	3.03 ± 0.32	3.05 ± 0.26	3.08 ± 0.40	3.10 ± 0.37
Percent stenosis (%)	77.7 ± 8.1	42.7 ± 18.1	26.6 ± 10.5	26.0 ± 10.7	22.5 ± 14.3

more than 1.5 mm in 42/48 patients (=87.5%) in our group. LBA succesfully increased the minimal luminal diameter to >1.5 mm in all 48 pts. The mean luminal diameter increased from 0.59 mm pre-angioplasty (± one standard deviation of 0.47 mm), to 1.73 mm (±0.63 mm) post-balloon angioplasty, with a significant further increase to 2.15 mm (±0.36 mm) after laser angioplasty. In the 9 patients from our hospital who underwent repeat angiography the following day, the lesion diameter had increased to 2.49 ± 1.14 mm. The percentage stenosis pre-angioplasty was 82.9 ± 11.9%, which decreased to 42.6 ± 20.2% following balloon angioplasty, and to 28.51 ± 11.3% after LBA. The day after the procedure the percentage stenosis had further diminished to 9.7 ± 10.3%. At follow-up angiography [9] (mean 4.6 months after the procedure) the mean luminal diameter had been reduced to 1.4 ± 0.89 mm, and the mean percentage stenosis had returned to 56.4% ± 25.7% (Table 2). In the internationally combined series results were quite similar. The mean luminal diameter of the vessel, immediately before the procedure was 0.67 ± 0.25 mm, after PTCA it had increased to 1.73 ± 0.57 mm and after LBA, the luminal diameter further increased to 2.27 ± 0.33 mm. The day following angioplasty, the vessel diameter had remained stable, at 2.27 ± 0.33 mm.

The mean stenosis percentage prior to the procedure was 77.7 ± 8.1%, which decreased to 42.7 ± 18.1% following balloon angioplasty and to 25.6 ± 10.5% after LBA. The day after LBA, the mean stenosis percentage had remained stable at 26.0 ± 10.7% (Table 3).

The reference luminal diameter did not change significantly over time (Table 3).

Of the 48 patients from our hospital who had been included in the prospec-

Elective LBA

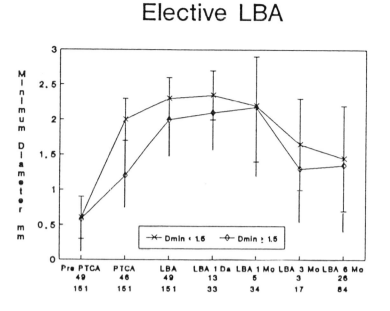

Figure 10. Minimal luminal diameters in elective patients of the international LBA registy. Note that in 49/200 patients (25%) the minimal luminal diameter failed to increase to over 1.5 mm after PTCA. After LBA, however, in these patients the minimal luminal diameter has improved to well over 1.5 mm.

tive randomized trial, 30 (=62%) remained free of angina pectoris. There were no myocardial infarctions during follow up. One patient died due to a ruptured abdominal aortic aneurysm; however, no postmortem examination was performed.

Discussion

The quantitative coronary angiography system as developed by Spears et al. docs not incorporate a method to quantify the roughness (or smoothness) of the endovascular surface [6, 7]. However, to the eye the vessel contours after LBA appear much smoother than after conventional balloon angioplasty (Figures 7–9). Quantitative coronary arteriography has been able to demonstrate that the luminal diameter increases significantly, both in the international registry and in the St Antonius patients group, if after standard balloon angioplasty with a 3 mm balloon, laser balloon angioplasty is performed with an otherwise similar 3.0 mm balloon. An increase in diameter from 1.73 mm to 2.25 mm corresponds with an increase by 30%. Which aspect contributes most to this significant increase in diameter is difficult to

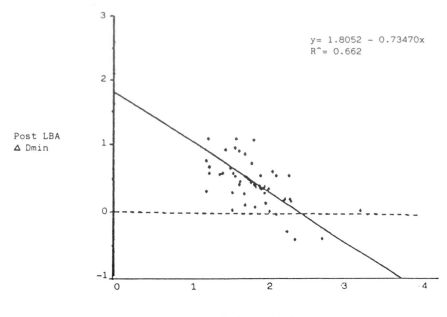

Figure 11. Inversely proportional relation between the degree of minimal luminal improvement by LBA (post LBA Δ Dmin) and the minimal luminal diameter after PTCA (post PTCA D min).

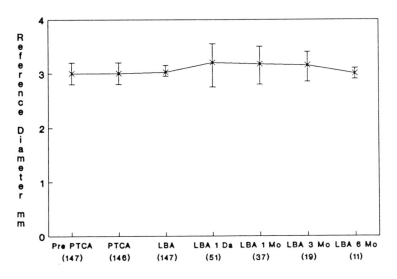

Figure 12. Reference luminal diameter measurements in 147 patients from the international registry.

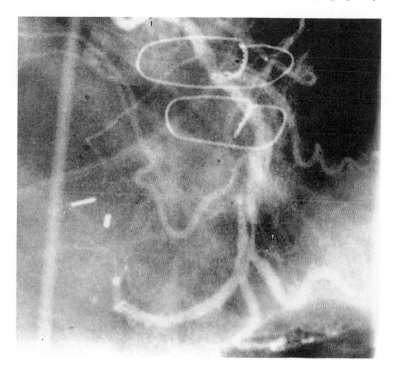

Figure 13. Example of a big dissection following balloon angioplasty of a stenosis in the left circumflex coronary artery.

establish. In the international registry in almost 25% of the patients the minimal luminal diameter failed to increase to more than 1.5 mm after conventional balloon angioplasty, despite multiple inflations (Figure 10). This means that only 75% of the balloon angioplasty procedures was successful if success is defined as a reduction of the percentage stenosis to less than 50%. After laser balloon angioplasty the minimal luminal diameter increased to >1.5 mm in all patients, making this a 100% successful procedure. In general, the degree of minimal luminal diameter improvement by LBA was inversely proportional to the minimal luminal diameter after conventional balloon angioplasty (Figure 11), which indicates that the poorer the PTCA results were, the bigger the benefit was from the LBA procedure. This improvement is not related to any change in reference luminal diameters, as measurements of the reference luminal diameters (Figure 12) revealed that these remained uninfluenced by the LBA procedure.

Part of the improvement might have been related to a reduction of the severity of dissections by LBA. An impressive example is given in Figures 13–14. However, because luminal diameters can hardly be quantified by any of the QCA systems in case of major dissections, most of these cases have

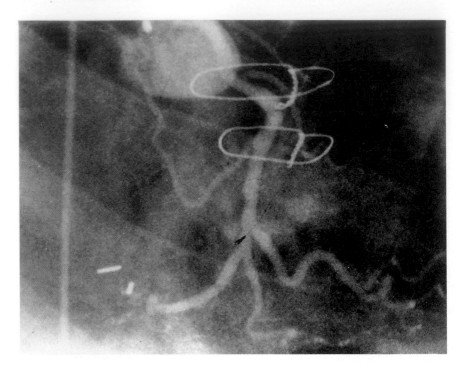

Figure 14. Same left circumflex coronary artery as in Figure 13 following laser balloon angioplasty: no more sign of dissection.

been considered to be unanalyzable. The true contribution of thermal fusion of separated tissue layers to the luminal diameter increase, therefore, could not be established, but the capacity of the LBA system to repair dissection has been impressive.

Reduction of arterial recoil also appeared to be contributive to the improvement of the minimal luminal diameter, especially since no reduction in luminal diameter after 24 hours post-LBA was observed. Although Nd:YAG laser energy itself can provoke arterial recoil, the pressure from the inflated balloon during laser energy application prevents this recoil mechanism and the remodeling of passive visco elastic properties by heat may prevent recoil later.

Another important LBA effect that cannot be quantified separately by any quantitative coronary anteriographic system is desiccation and remodeling of thrombus. A thin layer of thrombotic residue adherent to the LBA balloon surface in 4 patients (Figure 15) provided evidence of a thrombotic component in the lesions treated. Experimentally it has been observed that the 1060 mm Nd:YAG radiation is strongly absorbed by thrombus leading to

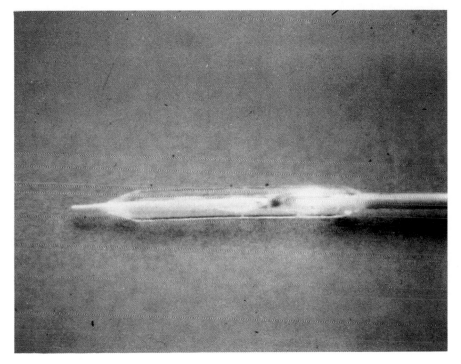

Figure 15. Thrombotic residue adhering to the balloon surface after removal of the LBA balloon (black dot).

selective, profound dehydration and associated volume reduction of the thrombus.

Conclusion

We conclude that laser balloon angioplasty is predictably effective in increasing minimal luminal diameters beyond what is achievable with conventional balloon angioplasty.

The hypotheses mentioned in the introduction were that laser balloon angioplasty would: 1) leave a smoother endovascular surface; 2) improve luminal geometry; 3) prevent flow separation; 4) reduce elastic recoil; 5) weld intimal flaps; and 6) desiccate thrombus.

With the help of quantitative coronary arteriography points 2 and 4 have been proven to be valid. Points 5 and 6 are valid too, but QCA in general remains unable to prove such points.

It is unfortunate that the laser balloon angioplasty system which provides such excellent acute results has such limited applicability sofar because of its high restenosis rate.

References

1. Gruentzig AR, Senning A, Siegenthaler WE. Nonoperative dilatation of coronary-artery stenosis: percutaneous transluminal coronary angioplasty. N Engl J Med 1979; **301**: 61–8.
2. Kaltenbach M, Kober G, Scherer D, Vallbracht C. Recurrence rate after successful coronary angioplasty. Eur Heart J 1985; **6**: 276–81.
3. Dangoisse V, Val PG, David PR, et al. Recurrence of stenosis after successful percutaneous transluminal coronary angioplasty (PTCA). Circulation 1982; **66** (4 Suppl II): II–331 (Abstract).
4. Jutzy KR, Berte LE, Alderman EL, Ratts J, Simpson JB. Coronary restenosis rates in a consecutive patient series one year post successful angioplasty. Circulation 1982; **66** (4 Suppl II): II–331 (Abstract).
5. Ernst SM, van der Feltz TA, Bal ET, et al. Long-term angiographic follow up, cardiac events, and survival in patients undergoing percutaneous transluminal coronary angioplasty. Br Heart J 1987; **57**: 220–5.
6. Spears JR, Sandor T, Als AV, et al. Computerized image analysis for quantitative measurement of vessel diameter from cineangiograms. Circulation 1983; **68**: 453–61.
7. Sandor T, D'Adamo A, Hanlon W, Spears JR. High precision quantitative angiography. IEEE Trans Med Imaging 1987; **6**: 258–65.
8. Spears JR, Reyes VP, Wynne J et al. Percutaneous coronary laser balloon angioplasty: initial results of a multicenter experience. J Am Coll Cardiol 1990; **16**: 293–303.
9. Plokker HW, Mast EG. Laser balloon angioplasty: European experience. In: Serruys PW, Strauss B, King SB (Eds.), Restenosis in the coronary arteries following interventions with new mechanical devices. Dordrecht: Kluwer 1991 (in press).
10. Spears JR. Sealing. In: Isner JM, Clarke RH (Eds.), Cardiovascular laser therapy. New York: Raven 1989: 177–99.

27. Quantitative coronary angiography after directional coronary atherectomy

DAVID R. HOLMES Jr., KIRK N. GARRATT,
STEPHEN G. ELLIS, and JEFFREY J. POPMA

Summary

Directional coronary atherectomy (DCA) has been developed to solve some of the shortcomings of conventional percutaneous transluminal coronary angioplasty (PTCA). By relying in part upon the excision of atheromatous tissue rather than solely on dilatation effect with remodeling, DCA may result in more favorable initial results of intervention and more favorably affect long-term results. DCA was performed in 378 patients with 400 lesions at six United States centers; quantitative angiography was performed in all patients. The left anterior descending was the most commonly treated segment (57%) followed by the right (25%), saphenous vein bypass grafts (13%), and the circumflex coronary artery. Of the 400 lesions, 44% were American Heart Association/American College of Cardiology class A, 37% class B1, and 18% class B2. Procedural success was achieved in 87.8% of lesions. The minimal lesion diameter at baseline was 1.2 ± 1.2 mm which increased to 2.9 ± 2.4 mm following DCA. The final minimal cross-sectional area was significantly larger for the circumflex compared to the other segments; this correlated with an increased incidence of postprocedural ectasia for this segment. Multivariate analysis was performed to assess associations with outcome. Of clinical factors, restenotic lesions were associated with a smaller final minimal cross-sectional area; of angiographic factors, a circumflex lesion was associated with a larger residual cross-sectional area while diffuse proximal disease and a long lesion were associated with a more severe residual stenosis. Of procedural factors, only one was significant, i.e. a larger device was associated with a smaller residual area of stenosis. Knowledge of these clinical, angiographic and procedural variables which are associated with improved outcome may help to optimize patient selection for this new evolving technology.

J.H.C. Reiber and P.W. Serruys (eds), Advances in Quantitative Coronary Arteriography, 459–472.

Introduction

Percutaneous transluminal coronary angioplasty (PTCA) has been widely used in the treatment of patients with coronary artery disease. Since its initial description in 1977, a wealth of data has accumulated on the mechanisms of angioplasty, the immediate and longer term results of the procedure, and risks and complications [1–6]. Our ideas and knowledge about the mechanisms of angioplasty have evolved from the initial thought that plaque compression was most important, to our understanding that successful dilatation involves stretching of the segment of adjacent arterial wall which is less involved with atheroma as well as fracturing of the plaque from the barotrauma induced by dilatation [7, 8]. Immediate and late events after PTCA include localized spasm, elastic recoil, arterial dissection, and restenosis [9–17]. Whether these events are as frequent with new interventional techniques remains unknown.

Directional coronary atherectomy has been developed in an attempt to solve some of the shortcomings of conventional PTCA [18–20]. Although this technique has now been approved for use by the Food and Drug Administration and has been clinically tested in more than 20,000 patients, there is limited information on specific mechanisms of action, angiographic findings, and complication patterns after atherectomy. Even such fundamental information as the relative importance of atheroma excision versus the "Dotter" effect of passing a 7 French device through the coronary artery versus balloon inflation when positioning the housing for cutting in producing the final angiographic result remains unclear [20, 21]. Quantitative coronary angiography may help to clarify the mechanism of directional atherectomy; in addition, it may be important for evaluating predictors of success or complications and for studying the long term outcome of directional coronary atherectomy [22,23].

Materials and methods

Over a 17 month period ending May 1990, directional coronary atherectomy was attempted in 378 patients at six centers (Appendix I) using the Simpson atherectomy device (AtheroCath, Devices for Vascular Intervention; Redwood City, California). These patients form the basis of this report. Quantitative coronary angiography was performed on these patients at the University of Michigan Angiographic Core Laboratory. Angiograms were reviewed by observers blinded to clinical characteristics and outcome. End diastolic cine frames were obtained at baseline immediately prior to and then after directional atherectomy. A computer-assisted edge detection algorithm was then applied to the digitized images [24]. The guiding catheter was used as the calibration standard. Reference diameters were determined from

Table 1. Quantitative morphologic analysis.

Vessel proximal to target lesion
  Diffuse proximal disease: ≥1/3 of the vessel proximal to the target lesion has luminal irregularities or stenoses
  Proximal vessel tortuosity: determined from a nonforeshortened end diastolic projection; tortuosity defined as present if there were two or more areas of vessel angulation ≥75°, or at least one angulation ≥90° proximal to the lesion
Stenosis characteristic
  Long lesion: ≥10 mm from the proximal to distal shoulder of the lesion in a nonforeshortened end diastolic projection
  Eccentric: lumen contained within outer one-quarter diameter of apparent normal lumen
  Irregularity: presence of an irregular "sawtooth" contour
  Calcification: patchy or nodular radio-opaque deposits within the wall of the stenotic segment
  Thrombus: discrete intraluminal filling defect anchored at least in part to the adjacent vessel wall with or without contrast staining
  Lesion bend: present when angle formed by centerline through the lumen proximal to the stenosis and the centerline through the lumen distal to the stenosis in a nonforeshortened view form an angle ≥45°
  Bifurcation lesion: the presence of a branch vessel of >1.5 mm originating at the target lesion
  Ostial lesion: a lesion which arises at the ostium of a major coronary arterial branch

orthogonal angiographic projections proximal and distal to the lesion in segments of the coronary artery which appeared to be unaffected or less affected by coronary disease. Minimal luminal diameters were also determined at the point of most severe stenosis.

The target lesions were assessed and analyzed according to the presence or absence of angiographic factors according to previously published criteria (Table 1) [25, 26]. In addition, lesions were classified using the modified American College of Cardiology/American Heart Association (ACC/AHA) lesion score of A, B1 (only one adverse B characteristic present), B2 (≥2 adverse characteristics present), and C. The device: artery ratio was measured by the ratio of the largest atherectomy device that crossed the stenosis and the normal adjacent coronary artery.

In a subset of patients undergoing atherectomy at Mayo Clinic, quantitative coronary angiography baseline, prior to, immediately following, and six months after atherectomy was available. In addition to luminal diameter and percent stenoses, in these patients plaque volume was assessed. For this assessment, magnified cine frames were digitized, the reference segment proximal to and downstream from the stenosis was identified, and a centerline determined. Diameters perpendicular to the center were determined and measured every 0.4 mm. Orthogonal views were used. With these orthogonal views, an eliptical formula was used to calculate volume. The hypothetical volume of the segment assuming no stenosis was calculated; then the actual luminal volume was calculated. The plaque volume was defined as the hypothetical lumen volume minus the measured lumen volume.

Statistical analysis

Chi square analysis was used to assess differences between dichotomous discrete variables. For differences between continuous variables, Student t test was used for two groups and analysis of variance for multiple groups. Multivariate analysis was performed using SYSTAT software (SYSTAT, Evanston, Illinois).

Atherectomy procedure

Atherectomy was carried out after informed consent with guidelines established by the individual centers' Institutional Review Boards. Patient selection was at the discretion of the individual cardiologist but included patients with symptomatic ischemia and anatomic stenoses amenable to atherectomy. In general, the lesions to be treated were located in the proximal portion of the coronary arteries or vein grafts; most arterial segments treated were ≥ 2.5 mm.

The procedure was carried out using a transfemoral retrograde arterial approach. Large guiding catheters of 9.5 to 11 French are required for atherectomy so that 10–11 French femoral sheaths were used. The guiding catheter (Devices for Vascular Intervention, Inc., Redwood City, California) was advanced under fluoroscopic guidance to the coronary ostium. Atherectomy devices of 5.5, 6 and 7 French were used; 7 French devices were selected in patients with arterial segments >3.5 mm, a 6 French device was used in segments of 3.0–3.5 mm, and a 5.5 French device was used for smaller segments. Predilatation of the lesion with conventional balloon angioplasty catheters was used in selected patients to facilitate passage of the atherectomy device across the stenosis.

As previously described, after coronary ostial intubation, a 0.014 guidewire was advanced across the lesion [18]. After crossing the lesion with the guidewire, the atherectomy device was then advanced into the coronary arterial tree. Gentle rotation of the device was often necessary to cross the lesion. If the device could not be positioned, it was withdrawn and preatherectomy dilatation was performed. After the housing was positioned across the stenosis, the balloon was inflated to push the atheroma into the open housing. The rotating cutter was retracted, the motor activated, and then the cutter readvanced thereby excising tissue protruding into the open housing. After excision, the balloon was deflated. The device was then rotated 30 to 90 degrees to position the cutter in a different portion of the atheroma. The procedure was then repeated.

The number of excisions per lesion varied. Usually following circumferential excisions, the atherectomy device was removed. Tissue specimens were flushed from the atherectomy device and the number of tissue fragments recorded. Repeat angiographic assessment after intracoronary nitrates was performed. If a significant stenosis remained, the procedure was repeated.

Successful atherectomy was defined by a residual percent stenosis of ≤50%, removal of tissue, and the absence of myocardial infarction, coronary bypass surgery, abrupt vessel closure (persistent or transient arterial segment occlusion with reduced blood flow), or death occurring during the hospital stay after atherectomy.

Results

There were 378 patients with 400 lesions which were treated. The mean age was 59 ± 11 years. Seventy-nine percent were male. Fifty-three percent had single vessel disease, the remainder had multivessel disease. Angina pectoris was unstable in 49.1%. In 47.9%, the lesion to be treated was a restenotic lesion; in the remaining 52.1%, the lesion treated was de novo without history of prior intervention.

The left anterior descending was the most commonly treated segment (57%, 226 lesions). The proximal left anterior descending segment was most commonly attempted (37%, 147/400) compared to the middle and distal segments (20%, 79/400). The right coronary artery was next most commonly treated (99 segments, 33 proximal and 63 in the mid or distal segment). Fifty-one saphenous vein grafts were treated. The proximal left circumflex was treated in 17 segments and the distal left circumflex in seven. Atherectomy of the left main coronary artery was attempted in three patients.

Of the 400 lesions, 44% were American Heart Association/American College of Cardiology classification A, 37% were B1, and 18% were B2. Only 1% of lesions were classified Type C [25, 26]. The majority (59.3%) of the lesions were eccentric. The next most common lesion feature was irregularity seen in 17%. The morphologic features of the lesions in each coronary artery can be seen in Table 2. As can be seen, right coronary artery lesions were characterized by more proximal disease and more proximal tortuosity compared to the remainder of the arterial segments. At baseline the mean minimal cross-sectional area was 1.2 ± 1.1 mm^2 with a percent area stenosis of 87 ± 10%.

At the time of atherectomy, a procedural success was achieved in 87.7% of lesions (351/400). In the remainder of lesions, atherectomy was unsuccessful. A major complication of death, myocardial infarction or emergency coronary bypass graft surgery occurred in 6.3% of patients.

Quantitative Analysis (Table 3)

The reference diameter and cross-sectional area remained relatively constant with the exception of the distal circumflex in which the reference diameter

Table 2. Lesion characteristics and morphology.

%	Lesion Location Overall	LAD	RCA	SVG	Circ
	N = 400	N = 229	N = 96	N = 51	N = 24
Proximal tortuosity	4.8	0.5	12.5	7.8	4.8
Proximal disease	12.2	4.9	29.1	14.0	12.2
Long lesion	10.8	9.3	15.6	11.8	4.2
Eccentricity	59.3	59.1	52.2	58.9	52.2
Irregularity	17.0	16.8	14.6	17.6	29.2
Calcification	12.0	20.0	7.3	0	4.2
Thrombus	6.4	3.7	9.4	11.7	8.3
Bend ≥45°	9.0	10.6	8.3	7.8	0
Bifurcation	10.0	15.7	1.0	0	16.7
Ostial	8.9	8.7	9.1	15.7	0

Abbreviations: LAD = left anterior descending; RCA = right coronary artery; SVG = saphenous vein graft; Circ = circumflex coronary artery.

increased from 3.2 ± 1.7 to 3.6 ± 2.3 mm. The minimal diameter and cross-sectional area for each group of arterial segments can be seen in Table 3. The minimal diameter for the entire group increased following atherectomy from 1.2 ± 1.2 mm to 2.9 ± 2.4 mm. Along with this, there was a reduction in percent area stenosis from $87 \pm 10\%$ to $31 \pm 42\%$ ($p < 0.001$). The final minimal diameter for the left anterior descending, right coronary artery and saphenous vein bypass grafts were similar at 2.8 ± 2.3, 2.8 ± 2.3., and 3.0 ± 2.5 mm. The final minimal cross-sectional area was significantly higher in the circumflex at 3.4 ± 2.6 mm^2. This increase in final minimal diameter in the circumflex was associated with an increased incidence of post-procedural ectasia (defined as a percent area stenosis <0%). This incidence of post-procedural ectasia was 30.4% for the circumflex compared to 8.3%, 5.5% and 20% for the left anterior descending, right coronary artery, and saphenous vein grafts respectively ($p < 0.05$).

Clinical angiographic and procedural variables were then tested to assess any relationship between these variables and the final minimal cross-sectional area (Table 4). With univariate analysis, the only clinical factor related to outcome was treatment of a restenotic lesion which had a negative correlation, that is, it was associated with a smaller final minimal cross-sectional area than treatment of primary atheromatous lesions ($p = 0.002$). Among angiographic factors, only three were significantly associated with final minimal cross-sectional area; treatment of the circumflex was associated with less severe residual cross-sectional area ($p = 0.004$); lesion calcification and lesion length ≥10 mm were negatively correlated and were associated with more severe residual cross-sectional areas. Finally, of procedural factors, only device size had a significant association with final minimal cross-sectional area.

Multivariate analysis of these factors was similar. Again, of clinical factors,

Table 3. Quantitative Angiography.

Segment		Reference Diameter (mm)	Reference Cross-sectional area (mm^2)	Area Stenosis (%)	Minimal Diameter (mm)	Minimal cross-sectional area (mm^2)
LAD						
Proximal	Pre	3.4 ± 2.0	9.2 ± 3.3	87 ± 9	1.2 ± 1.0	1.2 ± 0.9
($n = 147$)	Post	3.5 ± 2.1	9.7 ± 3.5	32 ± 39	2.9 ± 2.4	6.4 ± 4.4
Mid/distal	Pre	3.2 ± 2.0	8.2 ± 3.3	89 ± 8	1.1 ± 0.9	0.9 ± 0.7
($n = 79$)	Post	3.3 ± 2.0	8.6 ± 3.3	26 ± 56	2.8 ± 2.2	6.0 ± 3.7
RCA						
Proximal	Pre	3.8 ± 2.6	11.2 ± 5.3	88 ± 7	1.3 ± 1.1	1.3 ± 0.9
($n = 33$)	Post	3.7 ± 2.3	10.6 ± 4.0	37 ± 32	2.9 ± 2.2	6.6 ± 3.9
Mid/distal	Pre	3.6 ± 2.1	10.3 ± 3.5	85 ± 13	1.4 ± 1.4	1.6 ± 1.5
($n = 63$)	Post	3.5 ± 2.1	9.8 ± 3.4	39 ± 33	2.8 ± 2.3	6.1 ± 4.3
SVG						
($n = 51$)	Pre	3.6 ± 2.5	10.4 ± 4.8	86 ± 11	1.3 ± 1.3	1.3 ± 1.3
	Post	3.6 ± 2.5	10.1 ± 4.9	23 ± 43	3.0 ± 2.5	7.3 ± 5.0
Circ						
Proximal	Pre	3.7 ± 2.0	10.6 ± 33	91 ± 4	1.1 ± 0.9	1.0 ± 0.6
($n = 17$)	Post	3.8 ± 2.1	11.2 ± 3.6	20 ± 39	3.3 ± 2.4	8.7 ± 4.5
Mid/distal	Pre	3.2 ± 1.7	7.9 ± 2.4	88 ± 8	1.1 ± 0.8	0.9 ± 0.5
($n = 7$)	Post	3.6 ± 2.3	10.3 ± 4.3	2 ± 47	3.6 ± 2.9	10.4 ± 6.9

Table 4. Clinical, angiographic, and procedural correlates of final minimal cross-sectional area (mm^2) following directional atherectomy.

	Univariate Coefficient	p Value	Multivariate Coefficient	p Value
Constant			3.654	0.000
Clinical Factors				
Restenotic lesion	−1.409	0.002	−1.166	0.010
Angiographic Factors				
Circumflex artery	2.898	0.004	2.681	0.007
Calcification	−1.499	0.035	−1.615	0.081
ACC/AHA B2/C	−0.105	0.064	−1.531	NS
Diffuse proximal disease	−0.442	NS	−1.374	0.033
Lesion length ⩾10 mm	−1.778	0.018	−0.080	0.026
Procedural Factors				
Device size	2.139	0.001	1.386	0.003

a restenotic lesion was negatively correlated with outcome ($p = 0.010$). Of angiographic factors, only circumflex artery atherectomy had a positive correlation with outcome ($p = 0.007$) although the numbers of circumflex lesions treated were very small. The presence of diffuse proximal disease and a long lesion length of ⩾10 mm were negatively associated with final cross-sectional area, that is, a more severe final luminal cross-sectional area. Finally, of procedural factors, only device size had a positive correlation with smaller final minimal cross-sectional area. The remainder of the clinical, angiographic and procedural variables did not have a significant association. Even using multivariate analysis, however, correlation was suboptimal although statistically significant ($R = 0.436$, SEE $= 3.73$, $p < 0.001$).

Plaque volume

Data on minimal luminal diameter and plaque volume was available in a subset of 61 patients at baseline, immediately following atherectomy, and at the time of six month restudy. In this group, the mean preatherectomy minimal lesion diameter was 0.9 ± 0.6 mm; after atherectomy, the minimal luminal diameter had increased to 2.22 ± 0.6 mm while at the six month angiogram, the mean value had decreased to 1.47 mm. The mean baseline stenosis corresponding to this minimal luminal diameter was $70.6 \pm 12.9\%$, decreasing to $26.3 \pm 9.8\%$ but increasing at the time of follow-up to $47.1 \pm 18.6\%$.

Along with these changes in minimal luminal diameter and percent stenosis, plaque volume was determined. At baseline, plaque volume was 35.1 ± 28.9 mm^3. Immediately following atherectomy, the plaque volume had decreased significantly to 15.4 ± 12.5 mm^3 ($p = 0.0001$). At the time of follow-up angiography, the plaque volume had increased to $22.4 \pm 17.2 \, \text{mm}^2$ ($p = 0.0079$) but was still less than pre-atherectomy values ($p - 0.0002$).

Discussion

Conventional PTCA has been closely evaluated since its introduction in 1977. In the majority of patients, it results in improvement in luminal diameter stenosis and relief of symptoms. Although widely used, several limitations of PTCA have been well documented; these include the difficulty in treating diffuse disease and total occlusions, acute closure syndromes, and restenosis. Each of these areas limit application of the approach, result in increased complications, or increase socioeconomic costs. The new interventional procedures of atherectomy, lasers and stents have been developed in an attempt to solve these problems and thereby extend the application, safety and efficacy of PTCA.

Directional coronary atherectomy is the first new interventional device approved for marketing by the Food and Drug Administration. Preliminary data on acute results have been encouraging [19, 20, 22, 23, 27, 28]. As compared to PTCA, the technique involves atheroma excision and mechanical dilatation. Early reports have documented success rates of $\geqslant 85\%$ with a complication pattern at least as good as seen with conventional PTCA. In addition, atherectomy usually yields a stable angiographic result with a decreased incidence of dissection compared to conventional PTCA [30].

This current quantitative angiographic analysis underscores the early reported experience. In this group of 378 patients with 400 lesions, the procedure was successful in 87.7%. This success rate was seen despite the fact that this series involves early operator experience. In addition, many of the lesions had features which are usually associated with increased risk of complications with conventional PTCA. Thirty seven percent of the patients had B1 lesions and 18% had B2 lesions. Fifty-nine percent of the lesions were eccentric, while 17% had lesion irregularity. In eccentric or irregular lesions, atherectomy has potential advantages over conventional PTCA. A scientifically sound comparison of the two techniques with a randomized trial is currently underway.

In this group of patients, the initial angiographic results were excellent with a reduction in percent area stenosis from $87 \pm 10\%$ to $31 \pm 42\%$ ($p < 0.001$). The minimal diameter increased dramatically from $1.2 \pm 1.2 \, \text{mm}$ up to $2.9 \pm 2.4 \, \text{mm}$. The left anterior descending was the most commonly treated artery; the final minimal diameter for this artery was $2.8 \pm 2.3 \, \text{mm}$ and was similar to that seen for the right coronary artery and for saphenous vein bypass graft lesions. There was a significant difference in outcome with the circumflex coronary artery. The final area stenosis for this vessel was significantly smaller and the minimal cross-sectional area and diameter significantly larger than the other vessels which were treated. The final minimal diameter for the circumflex was 3.4 ± 2.6 mm. This increase in the arterial size in the circumflex is reflected in the increase in postprocedural ectasia compared to the other vessels (30.4% versus 8.3%, 5.5%, and 20% for the left anterior descending, right coronary artery and saphenous vein bypass graft respectively). Such aneurysmal dilatation has been previously reported for both PTCA and directional coronary atherectomy [9, 29]. In the former, it is very uncommon; with directional coronary atherectomy, the rates are probably increased. Bell et al., in a series of 86 consecutive patients undergoing atherectomy, found that 7 patients (11%) had had aneurysmal dilatation with a lesion/vessel diameter of >1. 2/1 [31].

The etiology of this aneurysmal dilatation is unclear. With the large size of the device, a "Dotter" effect may be partly responsible; the increase in reference vessel segment size lends some support to this concept [20, 21]. Alternatively, there may have been increased incidence of deep arterial resection of both media and adventitia with true luminal enlargement or over enlargement due to weakening of the support structure. Irrespective of the mechanisms, the immediate outcome of such lesions has been good without adverse effects [28]. If the mechanism of ectasia is increased incidence of deep arterial resection, restenosis rates may be increased. Garratt et al. found a definite increase in restenosis rates in vein grafts in which atherectomy resulted in deep arterial resection. In addition, they found a similar trend in native coronary arteries [32]. Not all investigators have found this. It is possible that the larger the residual lumen size, the better. With a very large lumen, although restenosis may occur, it may not be hemodynamically significant.

Comparison of the absolute dimensional changes between PTCA and directional coronary atherectomy is difficult because of the lack of well controlled trials comparing the two techniques in similar patients. The overall residual stenosis with directional atherectomy is usually less than with conventional PTCA [33]. This is probably the result of an improved acute outcome with decreased recoil; in addition, it may be the result of application of directional coronary atherectomy in larger vessels.

Lesion morphology has been important in assessment of the potential success rates as well as risks and complications of PTCA [25, 26]. As has been mentioned, specific lesion characteristics affect outcome. In the present study of atherectomy, specific arterial and lesion factors were assessed. With univariate analysis, two factors were found to be associated with a larger final cross-sectional area–circumflex target lesions and a larger atherectomy device. Characteristics associated with a less ideal final cross-sectional area were also identified and included longer lesion length and lesion calcification. The large size of the device and the limited cutting window could explain these correlations. Interestingly, a restenotic lesion was also associated with a less ideal result. The reasons for this are not clear; in general, these lesions are softer with less resistance to passage. There may be more residual tissue not removed however. With stepwise multivariate analysis, factoring in the reference cross-sectional area, atherectomy device size was most significant;

circumflex lesions were also associated with a larger final cross-sectional area. Four factors, a restenotic lesion, lesion length $\geqslant 10$ mm, diffuse proximal disease and lesion calcification, were associated with a smaller final minimal cross-sectional area.

A number of factors were not found to have a significant association with final minimal cross-sectional area. These included lesion characteristics of eccentricity, irregularity and thrombus. These characteristics have been associated with increased complication rates with conventional dilatation. The lack of adverse effect on outcome of directional coronary atherectomy reenforces the concept that atherectomy might be particularly suitable for these lesions [34–36].

There were also procedural details that did not have a significant association with outcome, including device:artery ratio, number of specimens excised, and number of atherectomy passes. This lack of association has some potential important implications as to the mechanism of atherectomy. Initially, atherectomy was felt to exert its effect by plaque excision. More recently, the relative importance of excision has been questioned. Safian et al. [14], using geometric calculation and an assumed plaque specific gravity of 1.0 concluded that complete atherectomy of an occluded vessel segment which was 3.0 mm in diameter and 10 mm in length should result in removal of approximately 70 mg of tissue. Despite this, in their series of 76 lesions, the average removed tissue weighed only 18.5 mg. In addition, in one patient there was clinical and angiographic success with removal of only 5.8 mg. The potential importance of passing the large device through the coronary artery and low pressure inflations to position the cutter by themselves may result in a substantial part of the improved lumen (Dotter effect). This has been demonstrated by other authors [21]. This is further supported by the results of intravascular ultrasound in which substantial luminal plaque remains after successful atherectomy [37].

Plaque volume was calculated in the present series of patients. Using an elliptical formula, baseline plaque volume was calculated at 35.0 mm^3. Although atherectomy resulted in a substantial improvement in plaque volume, a significant residual plaque volume of 15.36 ± 12.47 mm^3 remained. During follow-up in these patients, plaque volume increased along with an increase in stenosis severity but did not return to baseline levels.

Further studies are necessary to assess the relative importance of atheroma excision versus nonspecific Dotter effect on dilatation or dilatation on outcome. Serial angiographic studies at baseline, immediately after the procedure, and at 24 hours in addition to 3 to 6 months later would be helpful in separating these components. The addition of three dimensional ultrasound intravascular images will also be invaluable.

Conclusion

Directional coronary atherectomy has been demonstrated to be an effective means of coronary revascularization. In suitable patients, the technique results in excellent angiographic improvement with a low incidence of complication. Clinical, angiographic and procedural features can be identified which have substantial correlations with the final cross-sectional area, and are either associated with a better outcome (size of device, circumflex coronary artery) or are associated with a worse outcome (history of restenosis, diffuse proximal disease, a long lesion or calcification within the vessel). Knowledge of these factors can help to optimize patient selection.

Appendix

Angiographic Core Laboratory, Ann Arbor, Michigan.
  Jeffrey J. Popma MD, Nicoletta B. De Cesare MD, Stephen G. Ellis MD.
Christ Hospital, Cincinnati, Ohio.
  Dean J. Kereiakes MD, Charles Abbottsmith MD, Linda Martin RN.
Cleveland Clinic Foundation, Cleveland, Ohio.
  Patrick L. Whitlow MD, Jay Hollman MD, Sue DeLuca RN, Jennifer Malm RN, Michelle Webb RN.
Emory University Hospital, Atlanta, Georgia.
  Spencer B. King III MD, John S. Douglas Jr. MD, Nicholas Lembo MD, Ziyad Ghazzal MD, Susan Mead RN.
Mayo Clinic, Rochester, Minnesota.
  David R. Holmes Jr. MD, John F. Bresnahan MD, Kirk N. Garratt MD, Kris Menke RN.
St. Vincent's Hospital, Indianapolis, Indiana.
  Cass A. Pinkerton MD, Karen Wilson RN.
University of Michigan, Ann Arbor, Michigan.
  Eric J. Topol MD, Stephen G. Ellis MD, David W. Muller MBBS, Jeffrey J. Popma MD, Laura Gorman RN, Laura Quain RN.

References

1. Gruntzig AR, Senning A, Siegenthaler WE. Nonoperative dilatation of coronary-artery stenosis: percutaneous transluminal coronary angioplasty. N Engl J Med 1979; **301**: 61–8.
2. Detre K, Holubkov R, Kelsey S, et al. Percutaneous transluminal coronary angioplasty in 1985–1986 and 1977–1981. The National Heart, Lung, and Blood Institute Registry. N Engl J Med 1988; **318**: 265–70.
3. Holmes DR Jr., Holubkov R, Vlietstra RE, et al. Comparison of complications during percutaneous transluminal coronary angioplasty from 1977 to 1981 and from 1985 to 1986: the National Heart, Lung, and Blood Institute Percutaneous Transluminal Coronary Angioplasty Registry. J Am Coll Cardiol 1988; **12**: 1149–55.
4. Ellis SG, Roubin GS, King SB III, et al. Angiographic and clinical predictors of acute closure after native vessel coronary angioplasty. Circulation 1988; **77**: 372–9.
5. Detre KM, Holmes DR Jr., Holubkov R, et al. Incidence and consequences of periprocedural occlusion. The 1985–1986 National Heart, Lung, and Blood Institute Percutaneous Transluminal Coronary Angioplasty Registry. Circulation 1990; **82**: 739–50. Comment in: Circulation 1990; **82**: 1039–43.
6. Vlietstra RE, Holmes DR Jr. PTCA, percutaneous transluminal coronary angioplasty. Philadelphia: F.A. Davis Company 1987.
7. Castaneda-Zunega WR, Formanek A, Tadavarthy M, et al. The mechanism of balloon angioplasty. Radiology 1980; **135**: 565–71.

8. Waller BF. "Crackers, breakers, stretchers, drillers, scrapers, shavers, burners, welders and melters"–the future treatment of atherosclerotic coronary artery disease? A clinical-morphologic assessment. J Am Coll Cardiol 1989; **13**: 969–87.

9. Holmes DR Jr., Vlietstra RE, Mock MB, et al. Angiographic changes produced by percutaneous transluminal coronary angioplasty. Am J Cardiol 1983; **51**: 676–83.

10. Holmes DR Jr., Vlietstra RE, Smith HC, et al. Restenosis after percutaneous transluminal coronary angioplasty (PTCA): a report from the PTCA Registry of the National Heart, Lung, and Blood Institute. Am J Cardiol 1984; **53**: 77C-81C.

11. Austin GE, Ratliff NB, Hollman J, Tabei S, Phillips DF. Intimal proliferation of smooth muscle cells as an explanation for recurrent coronary artery stenosis after percutaneous transluminal coronary angioplasty. J Am Coll Cardiol 1985; **6**: 369–75.

12. Serruys PW, Luijten HE, Beatt KJ, et al. Incidence of restenosis after successful coronary angioplasty: a time-related phenomenon. A quantitative angiographic study of 342 consecutive patients at 1, 2, 3, and 4 months. Circulation 1988; **77**: 361–71.

13. Serruys PW, Reiber JII, Wijns W, et al. Assessment of percutaneous transluminal coronary angioplasty by quantitative coronary angiography: diameter versus densitometric area measurements. Am J Cardiol 1984; **54**: 482–8.

14. Muller DWM, Ellis SG, Debowey DL, Topol EJ. Quantitative angiographic comparison of the immediate success of coronary angioplasty, coronary atherectomy and endoluminal stenting. Am J Cardiol 1990; **66**: 938–42.

15. Fischell TA, Derby G, Tse TM, Stadius ML. Coronary artery vasoconstriction routinely occurs after percutaneous transluminal coronary angioplasty. A quantitative arteriographic analysis. Circulation 1988; **78**: 1323–34.

16. Sanz ML, Mancini GB, LeFree MT, et al. Variability of quantitative digital subtraction coronary angiography before and after percutaneous transluminal coronary angioplasty. Am J Cardiol 1987; **60**: 55–60.

17. Johnson MR, Brayden GP, Ericksen EE, et al. Changes in cross-sectional area of the coronary lumen in the six months after angioplasty: a quantitative analysis of the variable response to percutaneous transluminal angioplasty. Circulation 1986; **73**: 467–75.

18. Hinohara T, Robertson GC, Selmon MR, Simpson J. Directional coronary atherectomy. J Invasive Cardiol 1990; **2**: 217–26.

19. Kaufmann UP, Garratt KN, Vlietstra RE, Menke KK, Holmes DR Jr. Coronary atherectomy: first 50 patients at the Mayo Clinic. Mayo Clin Proc 1989; **64**: 747–52.

20. Safian RD, Gelbfish JS, Erny RE, Schnitt SJ, Schmidt DA, Baim DS. Coronary atherectomy. Clinical, angiographic, and histological findings and observations regarding potential mechanisms. Circulation 1990; **82**: 69–79. Comment in: Circulation 1990; **82**: 305–7.

21. Sharaf BL, Williams DO. "Dotter effect" contributes to angiographic improvement following directional coronary atherectomy. Circulation 1990; **82** (Suppl 3): III–310 (Abstract).

22. Popma JJ, DeCesare NB, Ellis SG, et al. Clinical, angiographic and procedural correlates of quantitative coronary dimensions following directional coronary atherectomy (in press).

23. Popma JJ, Topol EJ, Hinohara T, et al. Abrupt closure following directional coronary atherectomy: clinical, angiographic and procedural outcome (in press).

24. Mancini GB, Simon SB, McGillem MJ, LeFree MT, Friedman HZ, Vogel RA. Automated quantitative coronary arteriography: morphologic and physiologic validation in vivo of a rapid digital angiographic method (published erratum appears in Circulation 1987; **75**: 1199). Circulation 1987; **75**: 452–60.

25. Ellis SG, Vandormael MG, Cowley MJ, et al. Coronary morphologic and clinical determinants of procedural outcome with angioplasty for multivessel coronary disease. Implications for patient selection. Multivessel Angioplasty Prognosis Study Group. Circulation 1990; **82**: 1193–202. Comment in: Circulation 1990; **82**: 1516–8.

26. Guidelines for percutaneous transluminal coronary angioplasty. A report of the American College of Cardiology/American Heart Association Task Force on Assessment of Diagnostic and Therapeutic Cardiovascular Procedures (Subcommittee on Percutaneous Transluminal Coronary Angioplasty). J Am Coll Cardiol 1988; **12**: 529–45.

27. Ellis SG, Cowley MJ, Di Sciascio G, et al. Determinants of 2–year outcome after coronary angioplasty in patients with multivessel disease on the basis of comprehensive preprocedural evaluation-implications for patient selection. Circulation 1991; **83**: 1905–14.
28. Garratt KN, Kaufmann UP, Edwards WD, Vlietstra RE, Holmes DR Jr. Safety of percutaneous coronary atherectomy with deep arterial resection. Am J Cardiol 1989; **64**: 538–40.
29. Weston MW, Bowerman RE. Coronary artery aneurysm formation following PTCA. Cathet Cardiovasc Diagn 1987; **13**: 181–4.
30. Rowe MH, Hinohara T, White NW, Robertson GC, Selmon MR, Simpson JB. Comparison of dissection rates and angiographic results following directional coronary atherectomy and coronary angioplasty. Am J Cardiol 1990; **66**: 49–53.
31. Bell MR, Garratt KN, Bresnahan JF, Holmes DR Jr. Incidence of coronary artery aneurysmal dilatation following directional coronary atherectomy and the role of adventitial resection. (In press).
32. Garratt KN, Holmes DR Jr., Bell MR, et al. Restenosis following directional coronary atherectomy: differences between primary atheromatous and restenosis lesions and influence of subintimal tissue resection. J Am Coll Cardiol 1990; **16**: 1665–71.
33. Muller DW, Ellis SG, Debowey DL, Topol EJ. Quantitative angiographic comparison of the immediate success of coronary angioplasty, coronary atherectomy and endoluminal stenting. Am J Cardiol 1990; **66**: 938–42.
34. Hinohara T, Rowe M, Robertson G, Selmon M, Braden L, Simpson JB. Directional coronary atherectomy for the treatment of coronary lesions with abnormal contour. J Invasive Cardiol 1990; **2**: 257–63.
35. Dick RJ, Haudenschild CC, Popma JJ, Ellis SG, Muller DW, Topol EJ. Directional atherectomy for total coronary occlusions. Coronary Artery Dis 1991; **2**: 189–99.
36. Popma JJ, Dick RJ, Haudenschi 1 d CC, Topol EJ, El 1 i s SG. Atherectomy of right coronary ostial stenoses: initial and long-term results, technical features and histologic findings. Am J Cardiol 1991; **67**: 431–3.
37. Yock PG, Linder DT, White NW, et al. Clinical applications of intravascular ultrasound imaging in atherectomy. Int J Card Imaging 1989; **4**: 117–25.

28. Directional coronary atherectomy: evaluation by quantitative angiography

JEAN RENKIN, EMMANUEL HAINE, VICTOR UMANS, PIM
DE FEYTER, WILLIAM WIJNS and PATRICK W. SERRUYS

Summary

Directional Coronary Atherectomy has been introduced as an alternative to conventional balloon angioplasty for the treatment of selected coronary artery lesions characterized by a proximal localization in a large epicardial vessel and by a complex morphology at angiography.

To determine the immediate efficacy of coronary atherectomy we analyzed the first 113 attempts at atherectomy using quantitative angiography obtained in 105 consecutive patients from two centers. Procedural success, defined as a residual coronary diameter stenosis $\leq 50\%$ associated with effective tissue removal, was obtained in 90 (85.7%) of 105 patients. The primary angioplastic success rate combining atherectomy and balloon angioplasty in case of failed attempt at atherectomy was 94%. Assessed by quantitative angiography analysis, a mean residual minimal luminal diameter of $2.42 + 0.52$ mm and a mean diameter stenosis of $26 \pm 15\%$ were obtained immediately after successful directional coronary atherectomy in the 98 treated lesions. Major complications (death, emergency surgery and transmural infarction) were encountered in 5.7% of the patients.

In order to evaluate the results of these two interventional techniques we compared 51 atherectomy patients with 51 balloon angioplasty patients individually matched using quantitative angiography according to stenosis location and reference diameter. Atherectomy resulted in larger gains in luminal diameter as the minimal luminal diameter increased from 1.2 ± 0.4 to 2.6 ± 0.4 mm in the atherectomy group and from 1.2 ± 0.3 to 1.9 ± 0.4 mm in the angioplasty group ($p < 0.01$).

As the exact mechanism through which atherectomy enlarges the vessel lumen remains uncompletely understood, we evaluated a potential "Dotter" effect in 13 patients by performing quantitative angiography analysis before atherectomy, immediately after for- and backwards crossing the stenosis with the catheter but without inflation and cutting, and finally at the end of the successful procedure. The data suggest that simply crossing the stenosis with the atherectomy catheter contributes by more than 50% to the final luminal

J.H.C. Reiber and P.W. Serruys (eds), Advances in Quantitative Coronary Arteriography. 473–484.
© 1993 Kluwer Academic Publishers. Printed in the Netherlands.

improvement as the minimal luminal diameter increased from a mean of
0.96 ± 0.28 to 1.77 ± 0.37 mm, the final diameter reaching 2.39 ± 0.30 mm.

In conclusion, Directional Coronary Atherectomy (1) appears to be an
efficient technique for the treatment of complex coronary lesions with a
global success and complication rate similar to balloon angioplasty, (2)
achieves better immediate angiographic results than balloon angioplasty in
terms of minimal luminal diameter, and (3) is characterized by a complex
mechanism consisting of a mechanical or "Dotter" effect accounting for more
than 50% of the final obstruction improvement, and a functional effect
related to support balloon inflation and tissue removal.

Introduction

Balloon coronary angioplasty (PTCA) now plays a major role in the treatment of patients with coronary artery disease, as demonstrated by the large
number of procedures performed around the world. During the 15 years
following the performance of the princeps case by Gruentzig [1], a progressive but significant decrease in the immediate failure and complication rates
was achieved [2–3]. Nevertheless, two major limitations remain: firstly, the
occurrence of acute occlusion of the treated vessel during or early after
repeated inflations, which complication remains unpredictable and observed
in 2 to 5 per cent of the cases [4–5]; secondly, the high incidence of recurrent
angiographic restenosis reaching 30 to 40% within three to six months following an initially successful PTCA [6–8]. There is increasing evidence that both
limitations are inherent to the mechanism by which PTCA enlarges the
minimal diameter of the stenotic vessels. Indeed, the semiblinded balloon
inflations imply compressive disruption of both the atherosclerotic and normal vessel segments resulting in dissection in most cases [9]. The damage to
the vessel wall will eventually lead to acute occlusion or restenosis.

Various new techniques and devices [10] are under development to overcome these limitations of PTCA by a more controlled remodeling of the
coronary obstruction. In addition, data from the literature [11–12] suggest
that both the immediate and long term results of PTCA are related to the
level of vessel enlargement, i.e. the absolute minimal diameter obtained at
the end of the procedure, probably through improved lumen geometry and
blood rheology. Directional Coronary Atherectomy is such a new technique
that allows semi-selective removal of atheromatous or other deposits using
a special designed catheter including a rotating cutter [13]. Also, because
intracoronary material is being removed rather than just compressed or
splitted, atherectomy cuts should create a smoother surface and a wider
intraluminal opening as compared to PTCA. Theoretically, this should reduce the occurrence of highly irregular segments or dissections and improve
intracoronary hemodynamics.

Therefore, the present study reports on the clinical and angiographic
results obtained in the first 105 consecutive patients treated using Directional

Coronary Atherectomy at the Thoraxcenter, Rotterdam and the St-Luc University Hospital, Brussels. The clinical and angiographic indication for atherectomy and the procedural protocol were identical in both centers. More specifically, the aim of the study was (a) to evaluate the feasibility of coronary atherectomy in a series of consecutive patients, (b) to analyze the mechanisms of coronary obstruction improvement using quantitative angiography analysis and (c) to compare these results to the results obtained after conventional PTCA.

Methods

Patient and lesion selection

From September 1989 to March 1991, Directional Coronary Atherectomy was attempted in a total of 105 consecutive patients in the two participating centers (80 in Rotterdam and 25 in Brussels). In both centers, indication for atherectomy was essentially related to angiographic parameters not suitable for balloon PTCA. The technique was preferred in presence of at least two of the following criteria: (1) large vessel with a reference diameter >3 mm in absence of major bend or tortuosity, (2) excentric lesion, (3) large plaque area, (4) ostial or proximal lesion. In 10 patients, atherectomy was not performed because the device could not be placed within the coronary stenosis. Failures were related to the unability to selectively place the guiding catheter at the coronary ostium in 2 cases and to the unability to cross the lesion in 8 cases. Nine of these patients underwent a successful PTCA procedure while one patient was referred for elective bypass surgery.

The study group consisted of the remaining 95 patients including 81 men and 14 women (15%) with a mean age of 58 ± 11 years. Table 1 summarizes the baseline clinical and angiographic data. All procedures were performed in patients with significant coronary artery disease and stable ($n = 54$) or unstable angina ($n = 41$) despite medical therapy. Of the study group, 39 patients (41%) had a history of previous myocardial infarction, two patients had undergone a heart transplantation and 28 patients (24%) had a history of previous coronary revascularization: coronary balloon PTCA ($n = 15$), stenting ($n = 6$), atherectomy ($n = 2$) or bypass surgery ($n = 5$).

Coronary angiography showed multivessel disease in 29% of the patients and the 103 attempted stenoses were located in the left anterior descending artery in 61%, in the left circumflex artery in 12%, in the right coronary artery in 23% and in a saphenous graft in 4% of the cases.

Procedure

Before atherectomy was started, coronary angiograms in multiple views were performed using an 8 French guiding catheter after intracoronary infusion

Table 1. Baseline characteristics of the 95 patients

Age	58 ± 11	
Female	14	15%
History of previous:		
– infarction	39	41%
– balloon angioplasty	15	16%
– atherectomy	2	2%
– stenting	6	6%
– bypass surgery	5	5%
Angina:		
– stable	54	57%
– unstable	41	43%
Vessel Disease:		
– one	67	71%
– two	22	23%
– three	6	6%
Target vessel (n = 103)		
– left anterior descending	63	61%
– left circumflex	12	12%
– right coronary artery	24	23%
– bypass graft	4	4%

of 1–2 mg isosorbide dinitrate. Thereafter 10,000 IU heparin and 500 mg aspirin were administered as a bolus and the special 11 French guiding catheter (Devices for Vascular Interventions, California) placed at the coronary ostium. The atherectomy device was then advanced using the usual over-the-wire technique and the cutting chamber was positioned within the stenosis. When crossing with the atherectomy device was achieved without major difficulty ($n = 13$), we evaluated a potential "Dotter" effect by repeating angiograms immediately after for- and backwards crossing the target stenosis with the catheter but without inflation and cutting. Then, the standard atherectomy procedure was completed after recrossing, as explained hereunder. After low pressure (0.5 atm) inflation of the balloon, the cutter was retracted into the housing and the balloon pressure increased to 1 to 3 atm. After activation of the driving motor the rotating cutter was slowly advanced to cut and collect intracoronary material in the distal chamber of the device. After each pass, the balloon was deflated and the housing repositioned or removed into the guiding catheter. Atherectomy was considered successful in the presence of a visually estimated less than 50% residual diameter stenosis. The definition of success also implies removal of material from the collecting chamber. Repeat angiograms were performed at the end of the procedure, after repeat intracoronary infusion of 1–2 mg isosorbide dinitrate, using an 8 or 11 French guiding catheter. Clinical management after the procedure was similar to conventional balloon PTCA.

Clinical success was considered after technically successful procedure in the absence of major in-hospital complications including coronary reocclusion, myocardial infarction, bypass surgery or death.

Quantitative coronary angiography

Quantitative analysis of the treated vessels was performed using the computer based Coronary Angiography Analysis System (CAAS), as previously described [14]. In summary, boundaries of the selected coronary artery segment are automatically detected from optically magnified and video digitized regions of interest from a 35 mm cine-frame. The absolute diameter of the segment is determined using the catheter as scaling device. The percentage diameter and area stenosis and the minimal luminal diameter (mm) and cross sectional area (mm^2) are calculated, as well as some derived indexes (length, eccentricity and curvature).

Matching process

In absence of randomized data, we compared the quantitative angiography results obtained after atherectomy with the results obtained after conventional balloon PTCA using a matching process. To avoid selection bias, we selected primary lesions with comparable preprocedural characteristics. The lesions were individually matched according to stenosis location and reference diameter of the vessel. Only primary lesions (restenotic lesions were excluded) located on native coronary arteries were considered. Matching was considered adequate if the mean difference of the reference diameter between groups was identical. A total of 51 lesions analyzed after successful atherectomy were matched using the Thoraxcenter data base with twin lesions treated by balloon PTCA.

Statistical analysis

Paired and unpaired t test was used for statistical significance of difference for continuous variables shown as mean $\pm$ 1 s.d. A *p*-value of < 0.05 was considered as statistically significant.

Results

Procedural and clinical results

Considering the whole group, the procedural success rate for atherectomy was 85.7% (90 out of 105 patients), increasing to 94% (99 out of 105 patients) for atherectomy combined with balloon PTCA. Among the 95 patients in whom the device could be advanced in the stenosis, the primary success rate

Table 2. Quantitative angiography: Results in 98 lesions

	PRE-DCA		POST-DCA
Reference D (mm)	3.16 ± 0.63		3.26 ± 1.13
Min. luminal D (mm)	1.13 ± 0.38	*	2.42 ± 0.52
D. stenosis (%)	64 ± 11	*	26 ± 15
Reference area (mm²)	8.16 ± 3.28		8.55 ± 2.29
MLC area (mm²)	1.12 ± 0.75	*	4.84 ± 1.78
Area stenosis (%)	85 ± 8	*	43 ± 18

DCA: Directional Coronary Atherectomy.
D: Diameter; MLCA: Minimal Luminal Cross Sectional Area.
* $p < 0.001$.

was 95% (90 out of 95 patients). The procedure was unsuccessful in five patients. Two obstructive dissections at the atherectomy site were successfully treated by stent implantation in one case and by emergency surgery in the other. Two cases of total and irreversible occlusion of the vessel occurred during ($n = 1$) and one hour ($n = 1$) after the procedure despite emergency attempt at PTCA. These patients were referred for surgery (one urgent and one elective). Finally, one case of guiding-catheter induced dissection of the right coronary ostium was treated by emergency surgery.

Major complications, including death, emergency surgery and Q-wave myocardial infarction, were observed in 5.7% of the patients. One patient (0.9%) died from a delayed rupture of the atherectomized coronary vessel 3 days after an angiographically successful procedure, three patients (2.8%) underwent emergency surgery and 2 patients (2%) sustained a Q-wave myocardial infarction after an angiographically successful procedure. No patients required blood transfusions or vascular surgery because of arterial complications at the femoral puncture site.

Quantitative angiography

Quantitative angiography analysis was performed on all 98 successfully treated coronary lesions. Table 2 summarizes the mean values of the quantitative angiography measurements at baseline. The mean value for the area stenosis was 85 ± 8% and for the minimal cross-sectional area was 1.12 ± 0.75 mm².

The sequential changes in angiographic parameters immediately before and after atherectomy are shown in Figure 1. The reference diameter did not change significantly (3.17 ± 0.64 to 3.26 ± 1.13 mm) but, as expected, the minimal luminal diameter and cross-sectional area increased significantly (1.13 ± 0.38 to 2.42 ± 0.52 mm; $p < 0.01$ and 1.12 ± 0.75 to 4.84 ± 1.78 mm²; $p < 0.01$ respectively). Accordingly, the diameter stenosis and area stenosis decreased significantly from 64 ± 11% to 26 ± 15% ($p < 0.01$) and from 85 ± 8% to 43 ± 18% ($p < 0.01$), respectively.

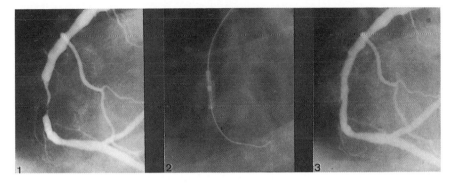

Figure 1. Angiographic example of a complex lesion located on a large right coronary artery: 1. Before atherectomy – MLD = 0.74 mm. 2. During atherectomy. 3. After atherectomy – MLD = 2.64 mm (MLD = Minimal Luminal Diameter).

The Dotter effect

According to the large profile of the atherectomy device, the hypothesis was tested in a subgroup of 13 patients that the mechanical effect of the catheter placement only, in absence of the functional effect related to balloon inflation or material retrieval, could partially explain for the improvement in coronary obstruction. The quantitative angiography data obtained in these patients are summarized in Table 3 and suggest that an immediate "Dotter" effect contributes by more than 50% to the improvement of the coronary stenosis as measured angiographically at the end of the procedure. Simply crossing the stenosis and withdrawing the atherectomy catheter resulted in an increase in minimal luminal diameter from a mean of 0.96 ± 0.28 to 1.77 ± 0.37 mm, which represents 57% of the final mean diameter reaching 2.39 ± 0.30 mm. The individual contribution of this effect ranged from 21 to 85%. In addition, the ratio of the catheter diameter/minimal stenosis diameter, an estimate of device oversize, ranged from 1.61 to 5.41 and was closely related to the observed Dotter effect ($r = 0.95$) as illustrated on Figure 2.

Table 3. Dotter Effect in 13 lesions

	PRE-DCA		DOTTER		POST-DCA
Reference D(mm)	3.45 ± 0.43		3.39 ± 0.48		3.67 ± 0.32
Min. luminal D (mm)	0.96 ± 0.28	*	1.77 ± 0.37	*	2.39 ± 0.30
D. stenosis (%)	72 ± 7	*	47 ± 9	*	34 ± 6

D: Diameter.
* $p < 0.001$.

DOTTER EFFECT

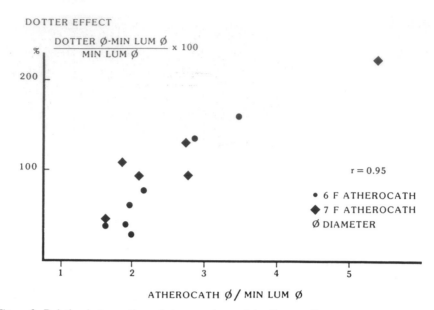

Figure 2. Relation between the catheter oversize and the Dotter effect.

Atherectomy versus balloon angioplasty

According to the matching process, no preprocedural differences were found between the atherectomy and the angioplasty group in reference diameter, minimal luminal diameter (Figure 3), diameter stenosis and area plaque. Table 4 summarizes the changes in minimal luminal diameter, diameter

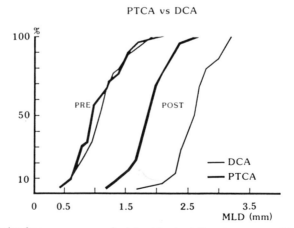

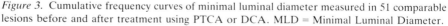

Figure 3. Cumulative frequency curves of minimal luminal diameter measured in 51 comparable lesions before and after treatment using PTCA or DCA. MLD = Minimal Luminal Diameter.

Table 4. Quantitative angiography: DCA vs Balloon PTCA[1]

	PRE		POST	
	DCA	PTCA	DCA	PTCA
Reference D (mm)	3.0 ± 0.6	3.0 ± 0.6	3.2 ± 0.4	3.1 ± 0.6
Min Luminal D (mm)	1.2 ± 0.4	1.2 ± 0.3	2.6 ± 0.4	* 1.9 ± 0.4
D. stenosis (%)	63 ± 11	62 ± 10	20 ± 11	* 36 ± 11

D: diameter; DCA: Directional Coronary Atherectomy; PTCA: Percutaneous Transluminal Coronary Angioplasty.
[1] Comparison performed using the matching technique in 51 lesions.
* $p < 0.01$.

stenosis and area plaque for the two groups of lesions. A significantly larger gain in mean luminal diameter was achieved by coronary atherectomy as compared to balloon PTCA (1.4 versus 0.7 mm; $p < 0.00001$).

Discussion

Since the initial application of Directional Coronary Atherectomy in peripheral artery disease in 1985 [13], the device has been improved in many ways as to allow successful application in coronary arteries. The procedural success rate in the present study was 86% of the attempted vessels. The success rate did not differ between the two centers and obviously included both learning curves. The vast majority of failures was observed during the initial experience and related mostly to our inability to cross the lesion with the atherectomy catheter. This again could suggest that an appropriate case selection in terms of vessel and stenosis morphology and dimensions largely determines the procedural success rate. Nevertheless, the final angiographic success rate of combined atherectomy and PTCA was 95%, which is not different from previously reported data on Directional Coronary Atherectomy [15–17] or conventional balloon PTCA [5].

Dilatation by intracoronary inflation of a balloon catheter has been shown to create a poorly controlled remodeling of the coronary obstruction leading to vessel wall damage and dissection [9]. In addition, many lesions are incompletely dilated because of elastic recoil of the vessel wall [18, 19] or incompressibility of complex atherosclerotic plaques. The advantage of atherectomy is to debulk the intracoronary plaque which should result in a greater "predictability" and improved immediate results in terms of vessel diameter. Since tissue removal is semi-selective, the incidence of dissections and abrupt closure is expected to be reduced, as compared with PTCA. This study using quantitative coronary angiography analysis confirms these theoretical advantages of atherectomy over PTCA. The incidence of acute or early occlusion (2%) compares favorably with recent studies reporting an incidence of such complication in 2 to 11% after conventional PTCA [4, 20,

21]. This becomes even more striking considering that many patients included in the present study were at particularly high risk of abrupt closure because of unstable angina (41%) or the presence of complex and eccentric lesions [4, 21]. We closely matched stenoses successfully treated by atherectomy with comparable lesions treated by balloon PTCA and found a significantly larger gain in minimal luminal diameter after atherectomy as compared to PTCA. This difference can be explained by the mechanism of action specific to each device. After balloon dilatation, the immediate luminal diameter increase obtained during inflations will be partially lost according to the recoil phenomenon [18, 19]. The mechanism of atherectomy appears more complex since the luminal diameter gain is due both to a "Dotter" effect and to physical removal of the plaque [22]. Our data demonstrate that the successful placement of the large atherectomy device across the stenosis accounted by itself for more than 50% of the final obstruction improvement. This pure mechanical or "Dotter" effect appears at least as important as the combined effects of tissue removal and dilatation by inflation of the support balloon.

Although Directional Coronary Atherectomy is technically feasible and yields high success rates in selected patients, some limitations remain related to the concept and to the characteristics of the presently available device. Firstly, although appealing, the idea of plaque excision carries potential risks whenever deep cuts are performed and atherectomy goes beyond the plaque. Recent studies [15, 23–25] reporting the presence of adventitial tissue in 30% of the resected specimen demonstrated the potential risk of removing normal vessel wall components. In the present study, major dissections were observed in 2 patients and a delayed vessel perforation occurred in one patient [26]. These complications suggest that the "predictability" of atherectomy is depending on the operator's aggressivity in terms of number of cuts and balloon inflation pressure. In addition, some data suggest [24] a direct relation between the depth of cut at histology and the restenosis rate. Enhanced operator experience and future technological improvements including intravascular imaging will hopefully avoid unnecessary removal of normal vessel wall components. The second limitation is related to the available guiding catheters and device. All our cases were performed using a guiding catheter which is significantly larger (11 French) and stiffer than conventional guidings used for balloon PTCA. These large guiding catheters have excellent torque control but their stiffness can induce coronary ostial damage during positioning and manipulations. Such complications were indeed reported, particularly on the right coronary ostium [16, 17]. The current coronary atherectomy catheter, which size ranging from 5 to 7 French, is also significantly larger as compared with balloon PTCA catheters and the metallic cutting and housing units give to its distal part an unusual rigidity. These technical characteristics currently limit the indications for the procedure to patients with easy peripheral vascular access and to proximal lesions located on large coronary vessels without tortuosity, usually the left anterior descending or the right coronary artery. The development of flexible housing on a lower profile device is likely to permit increasing application of Directional Coronary Atherectomy in the future.

Acknowledgements

William Wijns is supported by the C. and G. Damman Foundation. The authors express their gratitude to Mrs. R. Lauwers for careful secretarial assistance and Mrs. M. Lemaire for technical assistance.

References

1. Grüntzig A. Transluminal dilatation of coronary-artery stenosis [letter]. Lancet 1978; **1**: 263.
2. Holmes DR Jr, Holubkov R, Vlietstra RE, et al. Comparison of complications during percutaneous transluminal coronary angioplasty from 1977 to 1981 and from 1985 to 1986: the National Heart, Lung and Blood Institute Percutaneous Transluminal Coronary Angioplasty Registry. J Am Coll Cardiol 1988; **12**: 1149–55.
3. Ryan TJ, Faxon DP, Gunnar RM, et al. Guidelines for percutaneous transluminal coronary angioplasty. A report of the American College of Cardiology/American Heart Association Task Force on Assessment of Diagnostic and Therapeutic Cardiovascular Procedures. (Subcommittee on Percutaneous Transluminal Angioplasty). Circulation 1988; **78**: 486–502.
4. Ellis SG, Roubin GS, King SBIII, et al. Angiographic and clinical predictors of acute closure after native vessel coronary angioplasty. Circulation 1988; **77**: 372–9.
5. Savage MP, Goldberg S, Hirshfeld JW, et al. Clinical and angiographic determinants of primary coronary angioplasty success. M-Heart Investigators. J Am Coll Cardiol 1991; **17**: 22–8.
6. Serruys PW, Luijten HE, Beatt KJ, et al. Incidence of restenosis after successful coronary angioplasty: a time-related phenomenon. A quantitative angiographic study in 342 consecutive patients at 1, 2, 3 and 4 months. Circulation 1988; **77**: 361–71.
7. Nobuyoshi M, Kimura T, Nosaka H, et al. Restenosis after successful percutaneous transluminal coronary angioplasty: serial angiographic follow-up of 229 patients. J Am Coll Cardiol 1988; **12**: 616–23.
8. Leimgruber PP, Roubin GS, Hollman J, et al. Restenosis after successful coronary angioplasty in patients with single vessel disease. Circulation 1986; **73**: 710–7.
9. Block PC, Myler RK, Stertzer S, Fallon JT. Morphology after transluminal angioplasty in human beings. N Engl J Med 1981; **305**: 382–5.
10. Waller BF. "Crackers, breakers, stretchers, drillers, scrapers, shavers, burners, welders and melters" – the future treatment of atherosclerotic coronary artery disease? A clinical-morphologic assessment. J Am Coll Cardiol 1989; **13**: 969–87.
11. Hodgson JM, Reinert S, Most AS, Williams DO. Prediction of long-term clinical outcome with final translesional pressure gradient during coronary angioplasty. Circulation 1986; **74**: 563–6.
12. Renkin J, Melin J, Robert A, et al. Detection of restenosis after successful coronary angioplasty: improved clinical decision making with use of a logistic model combining procedural and follow-up variables. J Am Coll Cardiol 1990; **6**: 1333–40.
13. Simpson JB, Johnson DE, Thapliyal HV, Marks DS, Braden LJ. Transluminal atherectomy: a new approach to the treatment of atherosclerotic vascular disease. Circulation 1985; **72** Suppl. 3: III–146 (Abstract).

14. Serruys PW, Reiber JH, Wijns W, et al. Assessment of percutaneous transluminal coronary angioplasty by quantitative coronary angiography: diameter versus densitometric area measurements. Am J Cardiol 1984; **54**: 482–8.
15. Safian RD, Gelbfish JS, Erny RE, Schnitt SJ, Schmidt DA, Baim DS. Coronary atherectomy. Clinical, angiographic and histologic findings and observations regarding potential mechanisms. Circulation 1990; **82**: 69–79. Comment in: Circulation 1990; **82**: 305–7.
16. Hinohara T, Rowe MH, Robertson GC, et al. Effect of lesion characteristics on outcome of directional coronary atherectomy. J Am Coll Cardiol 1991; **17**: 1112–20.
17. Vlietstra RE, Abbotsmith CW, Douglas JC, et al. Complications with directional coronary atherectomy. Experience at eight centers. Circulation 1989; 80 Suppl. **2**: II–582 (Abstract).
18. Rensing BJ, Hermans WR, Beatt KJ, et al. Quantitative angiographic assessment of elastic recoil after percutaneous transluminal coronary angioplasty. Am J Cardiol 1990; **66**: 1039–44.
19. Hanet C, Wijns W, Michel X, Schroeder E. Influence of balloon size and stenosis morphology on immediate and delayed elastic recoil after percutaneous transluminal coronary angioplasty. J Am Coll Cardiol 1991; **18**: 506–11.
20. de Feyter PJ, van den Brand M, Laarman GJ, van Domburg R, Serruys PW, Suryapranata H. Acute coronary occlusion during and after percutaneous transluminal coronary angioplasty: frequency, prediction, clinical course, management and follow-up. Circulation 1991; **83**: 927–36.
21. Detre KM, Holmes DR Jr, Holubkov R, et al. Incidence and consequences of periprocedural occlusion. The 1985–1986 National Heart, Lung and Blood Institute Percutaneous Transluminal Coronary Angioplasty Registry. Circulation 1990; 82: 739–50. Comment in: Circulation 1990; **82**: 1039–43.
22. Penny WF, Schmidt DA, Safian ZD, Baim DS. Quantitation of tissue removal and luminal improvement following coronary atherectomy: the atherectomy index. Circulation 1990; **82** Suppl 3; II–623 (Abstract).
23. Johnson DE, Hinohara T, Selmon MR, Braden LJ, Simpson JB. Primary peripheral arterial stenoses and restenoses excised by transluminal atherectomy: a histopathologic study. J Am Coll Cardiol 1990; **15**: 419–25. Comment in: J Am Coll Cardiol 1990; **15**: 426–8.
24. Garratt KN, Holmes DR Jr, Bell MR, et al. Restenosis after directional coronary atherectomy: differences between primary atheromatous and restenosis lesions and influence of subintimal tissue resection. J Am Coll Cardiol 1990; **16**: 1665–71.
25. Garratt KN, Kaufmann UP, Edwards WD, Vlietstra RE, Holmes DR Jr. Safety of percutaneous coronary atherectomy with deep arterial resection. Am J Cardiol 1989; **64**: 538–40.
26. van Suylen RJ, Serruys PW, Simpson JB, de Feyter PJ, Strauss BH, Zondervan PE. Delayed rupture of right coronary artery after directional atherectomy for bail-out. Am Heart J 1991; **121**: 914–6.

29. Quantitative results and lesion morphology in coronary excimer laser angioplasty

ANDREAS BAUMBACH, KARL K. HAASE and
KARL R. KARSCH

Summary

The quantitative results and morphologic data of the first 147 patients treated with coronary excimer laser angioplasty at the University of Tübingen are presented. In regard of system parameters and catheter technology three subgroups are identified. The first 60 patients were treated with a prototype 1.4 mm catheter. In the second ($N = 40$) and third ($N = 47$, 48 target lesions) series an improved catheter system with improved and trusted energy transmission was used. The catheter diameters were 1.3 mm, 1.5 mm and 1.8 mm. In the third series of patients the pulse width could be increased from 60 ns to 115 ns, resulting in a further increase of the mean energy density at the catheter tip. The use of better catheters with higher flexibility and energy transmission lead to an increase in the primary success rate of stand-alone laser angioplasty. The lumen achieved with successful laser angioplasty corresponded to the catheter diameter and was independent of longer pulse duration and higher energy density. Morphologic analysis of all target lesions showed that failure of laser angioplasty was significantly increased in total occlusions and lesions with prestenotic vessel tortuosity. There was no morphologic parameter that correlated with the outcome as successful stand-alone laser angioplasty.

Introduction

Coronary excimer laser angioplasty has been introduced for experimental clinical trials two years ago [1–3]. Rapid technological progress and growing operator experience resulted in various changes of system parameters and patients selection. Since ablation of atheromatous tissue by pulsed laser energy is possible only by transmission of energy through waveguides from the light source to the target, catheter technology is a key issue in laser angioplasty. There are inherent technical limitations of the method. Pulsed excimer lasers are capable of ablating the tissue directly in front of the fibre

485

J.H.C. Reiber and P.W. Serruys (eds), Advances in Quantitative Coronary Arteriography, 485–495.
© 1993 Kluwer Academic Publishers. Printed in the Netherlands.

tip only. Furthermore, ablation of tissue is bound to a pulse energy exceeding the ablative threshold [4]. Thus, the quantitative effect of laser energy application in the coronary vessel is directly depending on sufficient energy transmission and the fibre area at the catheter tip. Insufficient energy transmission results in pure mechanical effects (Dotter effect). Small catheters are only capable of creating small channels. From these arguments it has to be suspected, that improvement of energy transmission and higher energy fluence together with larger catheter diameters might result in more efficacious stenosis reduction and may reduce the need for additional balloon angioplasty. A precise analysis of the quantitative results is neccessary to provide a basis for the ongoing discussion about ablation efficacy, interventional strategies and primary indications for the new technique [5–7].

This analysis represents the quantitative results of coronary excimer laser angioplasty with regard to different intervention parameters. It furthermore addresses the influence of morphologic parameters of the target lesion on the procedural outcome.

Patients

The data of 148 procedures of coronary excimer laser angioplasty in 147 consecutive patients (123 men, 24 women, mean age 57 ± 9 years) are presented. All patients had been previously selected for percutaneous transluminal coronary angioplasty on the basis of symptoms and angiographic findings. All patients had given informed consent to participate in the laser study protocol which had been approved by the local ethical committee. Medication consisted of a long-term treatment with acetylsalicylic acid (100–500 mg) in all patients and a combination of calcium antagonists, nitrates and β blockers according to the clinical course. The clinical state according to the Canadian Cardiovascular Society functional classification [8] was class I in 8, class II in 69, class III in 53 and class IV in 17 patients. In the first treatment series 11 patients had unstable angina pectoris. Since the major complications and adverse clinical outcome occurred in this subgroup, for the following series only patients with stable angina pectoris were included in the study. The patients baseline characteristics are listed in Table 1.

Laser system

Excimer laser angioplasty was performed using a commercially available xenon-chloride excimer laser (Max 10, Technolas Inc., Munich Germany) that emitted light at a wavelength of 308 nm at a repetition rate of 20 Hz. The differences in regard of catheter devices and energy transmission in the three treatment groups are listed in Table 2.

The first series of patients ($N = 60$) was treated with a prototype laser

Table 1. Patients baseline characteristics

	Series 1	Series 2	Series 3
Number of patients	60	40	47
Male/Female	49/11	31/9	43/4
Mean age (years)	59 ± 11	57 ± 9	56 ± 8
Extent of CAD			
1-vessel disease	41	24	27
1-vessel disease	13	12	12
3-vessel disease	6	4	8
Symptoms			
CCS 1	2	2	4
CCS 2	26	18	25
CCS 3	21	17	15
CCS 4	11	3	3
Target Vessel			
LAD	43	28	31
CX	7	3	3
RCA	10	9	14

CAD: Coronary artery disease; CCS: Canadian Cardiovascular Society Classification; LAD: Left anterior descending coronary artery; CX: Left circumflex coronary artery; RCA: Right coronary artery.

Table 2. Procedural parameters of coronary excimer laser angioplasty in the three consecutive treatment groups

	Series 1	Series 2	Series 3
	Xenon-chloride excimer laser Wavelength 308 nm Repetition rate 20 Hz		
Pulse width (ns)	60	60	115
Catheters (mm)	Prototype 1.4	1.3/1.5/1.8	1.3/1.5/1.8
No. of fibres (100 μ)	20	20/30/35	20/30/35
Energy fluence (mJ/mm^2)	30 ± 5	43 ± 14	67 ± 19
Time of laser energy delivery (sec)	123 ± 65	117 ± 72	51 ± 27
Mean loss of energy transmission	45%	30%	13%

catheter. This catheter had a diameter of 1.4 mm, consisting of 20 quartz fibres with a core diameter of 100 μm around a central lumen for the 0.014 inch guide wire. The pulse duration was 60 ns. The time intervals for laser energy delivery and intermission were operator dependent. The energy density, measured at the catheter tip pre procedural was 30 ± 5 mJ/mm^2. The total time of laser energy delivery was 123 ± 65s. Mean loss of transmission from before to after the laser procedure was 45% in this series. Fibre destruction and total loss of energy transmission was frequently observed.

In a second series of patients ($N = 40$) we employed a catheter system with variable diameters of 1.3, 1.5 and 1.8 mm consisting of 20, 30 and 35 quartz fibres with a core diameter of 100 μm each. The fibre quality had been improved, resulting in longer lifetime of the fibres and trusted energy transmission. The flexibility of the catheter devices was increased. Laser energy delivery was performed in trains of 3s with an intermission of at least 2s. Pulse duration was kept to 60 ns in this series. The mean energy density pre procedure was 43 ± 14 mJ/mm^2 with a mean loss of transmission of 30%. The total time of energy delivery was 117 ± 72 seconds. In the third series of patients the identical catheter system with further increased flexibility and improved coupling of the light into the fibres was used. The pulse duration was increased to 115 ns. Mean energy density before the procedure was 67 ± 19 mJ/mm^2 and mean loss of transmission was 13%. The total time of energy delivery was significantly reduced to 51 ± 27 seconds.

Laser angioplasty

Angioplasty was performed via the transfemoral approach. Heparine, 10000 U, was administered intraarterially. A 9Fr guiding catheter was placed in the ostium of the target vessel and the lesion was visualized after intracoronary application of 0.1 mg nitroglycerin. The laser catheter was advanced over a 0.014 inch flexible guide wire which had been placed in the distal vessel. After reaching the proximal edge of the stenosis laser energy application was started and the catheter was advanced, applying only moderate pressure on the device. Laser energy application was also performed during slow withdrawl of the catheter. The size of the improved catheters was selected according to the prestenotic vessel diameter and stenosis severity that was analysed in the previous diagnostic coronary angiogram. After each passage of the laser catheter control angiography was performed to examine the result of ablation. If the control angiography after laser passage revealed a residual stenosis of more than 50% on visual interpretation and the employment of a larger sized laser catheter was expected to be technically possible the laser catheters were changed. Criteria to stop laser angioplasty were: 1) a reduction of percent luminal diameter stenosis to less than 50%; 2) no further improvement of the result after the last laser irradiation cycle; 3) severe vasospasm (reduction in luminal diameter with vessel occlusion or reduced antegrade flow of contrast medium) or vessel occlusion due to dissection or thrombus formation. Additional balloon angioplasty was performed to improve an unsatisfactory result or to resolve vessel occlusion. After the final irradiation period or the last balloon inflation vessel patency was controlled by repeat angiograms for 20 minutes. The patients were monitored in the coronary care unit for 24 hours. An early follow-up angiog-

Table 3. Morphologic criteria

Target vessel
Involved vessel segment
Prestenotic lumen diameter
Minimal lumen diameter
Length of the lesion
AHA/ACC Task Force classification
Single discrete/complex lesion
Concentric/eccentric lesion
Tandem stenosis
Long segmental lesion
Total occlusion
Bifurcational lesion
Location in vessel curve
Prestenotic vessel tortuosity
Lasing direction in curved segments

ram of the target vessel was routinely performed within 24 hours after the intervention.

The outcome of the intervention was classified as "Failure" if no reduction in stenosis severity could be achieved and as "Successful stand-alone laser angioplasty" if the residual percent stenosis after laser treatment was < 50% and the vessel was documented to be patent at the early follow-up angiography.

Analysis

Quantitative coronary analysis was performed by a consensus of two experienced observers for the interventional and the follow-up angiographies. The angiograms were performed in identical projections and settings of the angiographic X-ray system (Poly Diagnost C, Philips). Only end-diastolic cine frames were used. All target vessels were traced on transparent paper and lumen diameter was measured with a milimeter ruler. The 9F guiding catheter was used for calibration of the measurement.

The prestenotic vessel diameter was measured as lumen diameter of the lesion-free vessel at the proximal edge of the stenosis. Minimal lumen diameter of the stenosis was measured in the projection that showed the highest degree of stenosis. Length of the lesion was defined as the distance between two points of the diseased segments, beginning and ending, where the lumen was reduced by 20% [9].

All target lesions were classified according to the morphological criteria that are listed in Table 3. Involved segments were defined to be in the proximal, mid or distal part of the vessel. The ACC/AHA Task Force classification [10] was used in the modification of Ellis et al. [11], therefore the lesions were classified as Type A, B1, B2 or C. Single discrete lesions were defined as lesions under 15 mm of length [12], they were additionally classified as concentric (symmetric luminal narrowing in two angiographic projections) or eccentric lesions (asymmetric luminal narrowing in at least 1 angiographic projection). Complex lesions were either longer lesions or tandem lesions (sequence of 2 significant stenoses), long segmental lesions (lesion involving a vessel segment with luminal narrowing on a length of ⩾20 mm), total occlusions (Thrombolysis in Myocardial Infarction (TIMI) trial flow grade 0 [13], at least one month old by clinical and angiographic findings) or bifurcational lesions (branch vessel of medium or large size originating within the lesion and being completely surrounded by significant stenotic portions of the lesion to be treated [12]). Criterion for the location in a curved vessel was the angle between 2 centerlines through the lumen from the middle of the lesion to points 5 cm proximal and distal to the stenosis, drawn and measured on the magnified copy. An angle of more than 45° indicated a curved vessel. Prestenotic vessel tortuosity was defined as >2 bends in the prestenotic vessel. The lasing direction in curves was assessed for eccentric lesions in curved vessels. It was classified directional if the laser catheter and laser beam headed the lesion and nondirectional if the laser catheter headed the opposite vessel wall.

All data were entered in the Statistical Analysis System (SAS Institute Inc., Cary, North Carolina). The frequency of morphologic parameters was compared for patients with failure of laser angioplasty, patients with successful stand-alone laser angioplasty and patients with laser and additional balloon angioplasty or not successful stand-alone laser angioplasty in an attempt to find predictors for failure and stand-alone success. Univariate (Chi-square and Fisher's exact test for qualitative parameters and U-test for quantitative parameters [14]) as well as multivariate (logistic regression) analysis was performed.

Results

Failure of the laser angioplasty attempt occurred in 5 patients of the first, 5 patients of the second and 7 patients of the third series. In 8 of these patients it was not possible to place the guide wire in the periphery of the target vessel, in 6 patients the target lesion could not be reached with the catheter and in three procedures the catheter failed to pass the lesion completely. Successful stand-alone laser angioplasty with a patent vessel at the 24 hours control angiography was performed in 23/55 patients of the first, 21/35 patients of the second and 24/41 procedures of the third group. Additional balloon dilatation was performed because of an insufficient result in 16 (29%), 6 (17%) and 5 (12%) patients of groups 1, 2 and 3, respectively. Balloon angioplasty was neccessary because of complications in 16, 5 and 12 patients. The acute quantitative results of coronary excimer laser angioplasty

Table 4. Procedural outcome

	Series 1	Series 2	Series 3
Number of procedures	60	40	48
Failure	5	5	7
%stenosis pre-intervention	81 ± 17	72 ± 12	70 ± 8
MLD pre-intervention (mm)	0.45 ± 0.36	0.76 ± 0.34	0.96 ± 0.31
Stand alone laser	23	24	24
Success	23	21	24
%stenosis post laser	27 ± 17	31 ± 14	35 ± 12
%stenosis at early follow-up	34 ± 15	35 ± 24	37 ± 9
MLD post laser (mm)	1.78 ± 0.45	1.88 ± 0.55	2.14 ± 0.45
MLD at early follow-up (mm)	1.77 ± 0.6	1.66 ± 0.55	1.94 ± 0.4
Laser and balloon	32	11	17
%stenosis post laser	44 ± 14	37 ± 15	42 ± 15
%stenosis post balloon	24 ± 15	20 ± 15	29 ± 14
%stenosis at early follow-up	32 ± 24	23 ± 18	31 ± 16
MLD post laser (mm)	1.53 ± 0.44	1.56 ± 0.38	1.86 ± 0.38
MLD post balloon (mm)	2.08 ± 0.46	2.35 ± 0.45	2.4 ± 0.5
MLD at early follow-up (mm)	1.79 ± 0.68	2.18 ± 0.59	2.0 ± 0.45
Procedural complications following laser angioplasty			
Death	1	1	–
MI	3	1	–
Occlusion	11	7	12
Perforation	–	1	1
Dissection	10	9	6
Reversible spasm	19	7	11

MI: Myocardial infarction; %stenosis: percentual luminal narrowing.
MLD: Minimal lumen diameter.

in the three patient series and the quantitative data of the early follow-up angiography are listed in Table 4. Figure 1 shows the luminal diameter achieved with the laser procedure alone with regard to the different catheter sizes.

Minor complications occurred in a high frequency in all three series. The onset of reversible vasospasm during and following laser energy delivery was constantly observed in 20 to 26% of the interventions. Membranes, indicating small dissection without reduction of antegrade flow were also frequently angiographically documented. Additional contrast reduction, suspective of thrombus formation, often affected the correct assessment of the angioplasty result immediately after the intervention, but in most of the cases was not present at the routinely performed early follow-up angiography. Vessel occlusion, probably as a result of dissections, thrombus formation and vasospasm was observed in 20 to 29% and is currently the main reason for additional balloon angioplasty. Vessel perforation with consecutive vessel

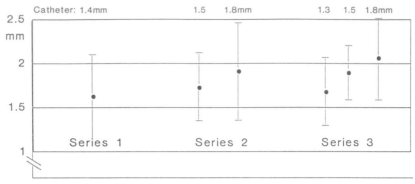

Figure 1. Minimal lumen diameter of the target lesion after laser angioplasty with different catheters. Mean ± standard deviation.

closure was observed in two patients, both complications were resolved with balloon angioplasty and had no further clinical sequelae [15]. Acute myocardial infarction occurred in 3 patients. One additional patient with unstable angina pectoris developed a cardiogenic shock and ventricular tachycardia and died three hours after laser and balloon angioplasty. In the second series one patient had abrupt vessel closure after laser treatment of an eccentric stenosis of the LAD, which could not be reopened by balloon dilatation. This patient developed a Q-wave infarction with an initially uncomplicated clinical course. 48 hours after discharge from the coronary care unit, this patient died suddenly. An autopsy was not performed. No fatal complication during the in-hospital period occurred in the third treatment series.

Analysis of the lesion morphology revealed 19, 26, 91 and 12 Type A, B1, B2 and C lesions consecutively. Complex lesions were found in 52 interventions. A total number of 15 occlusions, 15 long segmental lesions and 17 bifurcational lesions had been selected for laser angioplasty. Prestenotic vessel tortuosity was present in 10 patients. In the failure group a significantly higher frequency of complex lesions ($p < 0.001$), especially total occlusions ($p < 0.001$), and prestenotic vessel tortuosity ($p = 0.002$) was found.

In patients in whom stenosis reduction with the laser intervention could be achieved there was no morphologic parameter correlating with the outcome as successful stand-alone laser angioplasty.

Discussion

The presented data are the result of a single center experience using this new experimental technique. Due to the considerable changes of the laser system parameters, catheter quality, patients selection and operator experience, analysis is limited to subgroups with a reduced number of patients treated. As always in the development of new interventional methods data analysis was performed retrospectively. To exclude, however, additional operator bias, the quantitative data presented in this study were assessed by blinded review and quantitative coronary analysis (QCA) of independent observers.

In regard of the quantitative results in all three series of our patients population it is of interest that the luminal diameter of the target lesion achieved with laser irradiation corresponded to the diameter of the laser catheter used. In all three series, however, the increase of the luminal diameter was 0.2–0.3 mm higher than the diameter of the catheter. This is in contrast to the results of Torre et al. from the Mount Sinai group [16], who found the vessel diameter after treatment identical to the laser catheter diameter. The differences of the results are probably due to the different protocol of the interventions. Whereas all of the Mount Sinai patients were routinely dilated with conventional ballon angioplasty after a first pass with the laser catheter, we used in the majority of our patients multiple passes over the target lesion. With this strategy we had, at least in the two early series, considerably longer irradiation times. This procedural difference might reflect in the different luminal diameters achieved. Increase in energy fluence and the use of longer pulse durations resulted in a significantly shorter total time of irradiation (Series 1, 2 vs. series 3). The quantitative results, however, did not reveal any difference in the luminal diameter achieved in those patients with successful ablation using the same catheter system (Series 2 vs. series 3). The stand-alone success rate of excimer laser angioplasty improved considerably from series 1 to series 2 and 3. This is most probably the result of the increased catheter tip diameter. Furthermore, the qualtity of the quartz fibres was improved which resulted in a reduction of the mean loss of energy transmission during the intervention. Together with increased catheter flexibility, this may have resulted in a reduction of mechanical injury in the prestenotic vessel and at the lesion site. The quantitative results, combined with the clinical outcome indicate, that further improvement of catheter diameter and energy transmission may be an option for future trials.

Morphologic parameters for successful conventional balloon angioplasty have been previously analysed [11, 17–23]. Throughout the years, the major reason for failure of balloon dilatation was the inability to cross the lesion either with the guidewire in chronic total occlusions or to reach or pass the lesion due to severe vessel tortuosity. However, failed angioplasty attempts decreased from initially reported rates between 20 and 44% [17–19] to 3.7% [20] within a 10 years period of technical improvement and development of flexible, low profile balloon catheters.

In laser angioplasty fiberoptic catheter devices are used to transmit the energy from the light source to the target site in the coronary artery. Like in the early years of balloon angioplasty the catheters lack flexibility and steerability. Therefore the analysis of the failed laser attempts reveals similar problems as described for the early experience in balloon angioplasty. Individual predictors for failure were prestenotic vessel tortuosity and chronic total occlusion. These data suggest that failure of laser angioplasty is: 1) a problem of low flexibility of the catheter devices; and is 2) due to the requirement of guidewire support for save coaxial advancement in the treatment of totally occluded vessels. There was no morphologic parameter that correlated with a higher rate of successful stand-alone laser angioplasty. The stand-alone laser success, however, requires not only sufficient stenosis reduction but also the absence of complications. The considerable incidence of thrombus formation, vasospasm and vessel occlusion after laser angioplasty frequently neccessitated additional balloon treatment. This results in a considerable number of "not successful stand-alone interventions" despite initially successful plaque ablation. However, success rate of stand-alone laser angioplasty in complex lesions, such as long lesions and bifurcational lesions was comparable to single discrete lesions. Thus, once the catheter reaches the lesion and ablation of the plaque is possible, there is no morphologic parameter that goes along with reduced efficacy or increased risk of complications. This is in contrast to the experience in balloon angioplasty. The use of laser systems could therefore provide a viable alternative in the primary treatment of target lesions, that are associated with lower success rates and a higher incidence of complications using conventional balloon angioplasty [24–26].

References

1. Karsch KR, Haase KK, Voelker W, Baumbach A, Mauser M, Seipel L. Percutaneous coronary excimer laser angioplasty in patients with stable and unstable angina pectoris. Acute results and incidence of restenosis during 6–month follow-up. Circulation 1990; **81**: 1849–59. Comment in: Circulation 1990; **81**: 2018–21.
2. Litvack F, Eigler NL, Margolis JR, et al. Percutaneous excimer laser coronary angioplasty. Am J Cardiol 1990; **66**: 1027–32.
3. Sanborn TA, Torre SR, Sharma SK, et al. Percutaneous coronary excimer laser-assisted balloon angioplasty: initial clinical and quantitative angiographic results in 50 patients. J Am Coll Cardiol 1991; **17**: 94–9.
4. Litvack F, Grundfest WS, Goldenberg T, et al. Pulsed laser angioplasty: wavelength power and energy dependencies relevant to clinical application. Lasers Surg Med 1988; **8**: 60–5.
5. Forrester JS. Laser angioplasty. Now and in the future. Circulation 1988; **78**: 777–9.
6. Sanborn TA. Laser angioplasty. What has been learned from experimental studies and clinical trials? Circulation 1988; **78**: 769–74.
7. Isner JM, Rosenfield K, Losordo DW. Excimer laser atherectomy. The greening of Sisyphus. Circulation 1990; 81: 2018–21. Comment on: Circulation 1990; **81**: 1849–59. Comment in: Circulation 1990; **82**: 1076.
8. Campeau L. Grading of angina pectoris. Circulation 1976; **54**: 522–3 (Letter).
9. MacDonald RG, Barbieri E, Feldman RL, Pepine CJ. Angiographic morphology of restenosis after percutaneous transluminal coronary angioplasty. Am J Cardiol 1987; **60**: 50–4.

10. Ryan TJ, Faxon DP, Gunnar RM et al. Guidelines for percutaneous transluminal angioplasty. A report of the American College of Cardiology/American Heart Association Task Force on Assessment of Diagnostic and Therapeutic Cardiovascular Procedures (Subcommittee on Percutaneous Transluminal Coronary Angioplasty). J Am Coll Cardiol 1988; **12**: 529–45.

11. Ellis SG, Vandormael MG, Cowley MJ, et al. Coronary morphologic and clinical determinants of procedural outcome with angioplasty for multivessel coronary disease. Implications for patient selection. Multivessel Angioplasty Prognosis Study Group. Circulation 1990; **82**: 1193–202. Comment in: Circulation 1990; **82**: 1516–8.

12. Myler RK, Topol EJ, Shaw RE, et al. Multiple vessel coronary angioplasty: classification, results, and patterns of restenosis in 494 consecutive patients. Cathet Cardiovasc Diagn 1987; **13**: 1–15.

13. The Thrombolysis in Myocardial Infarction (TIMI) trial. Phase I findings. TIMI Study Group. N Engl J Med 1985; **312**: 932–6.

14. Sachs L. Angewandte Statistik: Anwendung statistischer Methoden. 6. Aufl. Berlin: Springer Verlag 1984.

15. Haase KK, Baumbach A, Voelker W, Kühlkamp V, Karsch KR. Gefäßwandperforation nach koronarer Excimer Laser Angioplastie. Z Kardiol 1991; **80**: 230–3.

16. Torre SR, Sanborn TA, Sharma SK, Cohen M, Ambrose JA. Percutaneous coronary excimer laser angioplasty: quantitative angiographic analysis demonstrates improved angioplasty results with larger laser catheters. Circulation 1990; **82** (4 suppl III): III–671 (Abstract).

17. Cowley MJ, Vetrovec GW, Wolfgang TC. Efficacy of percutaneous transluminal coronary angioplasty: technique, patient selection, salutary results, limitations and complications. Am Heart J 1981; **101**: 272–80.

18. Kent KM, Bentivoglio LG, Block PC, et al. Percutaneous transluminal coronary angioplasty: report from the Registry of the National Heart, Lung, and Blood Institute. Am J Cardiol 1982; **49**: 2011–20.

19. Meier B, Gruentzig AR, Hollman J, Ischinger T, Bradford JM. Does length or eccentricity of coronary stenoses influence the outcome of transluminal dilatation? Circulation 1983; **67**: 497–9.

20. Kahn JK, Hartzler GO. Frequency and causes of failure with contemporary balloon coronary angioplasty and implications for new technologies. Am J Cardiol 1990; **66**: 858–60.

21. Dorros G, Cowley MJ, Simpson J, et al. Percutaneous transluminal coronary angioplasty: report of complications from the National Heart, Lung, and Blood Institute PTCA Registry. Circulation 1983; **67**: 723–30.

22. Detre KM, Holmes DR Jr, Holubkov R, et al. Incidence and consequences of periprocedural occlusion. The 1985–1986 National Heart, Lung, and Blood Institute Percutaneous Transluminal Coronary Angioplasty Registry. Circulation 1990; **82**: 739–50. Comment in: Circulation 1990; **82**: 1039–43.

23. Ischinger T, Gruentzig AR, Meier B, Galan K. Coronary dissection and total coronary occlusion associated with percutaneous transluminal coronary angioplasty: significance of initial angiographic morphology of coronary stenoses. Circulation 1986; **74**: 1371–8.

24. Ghazzal ZM, Hearn JA, Goldenberg T, Eigler N, Kent KM, King SB 3d. Outcome predictors after excimer laser: detailed multicenter angiographic analysis. Circulation 1990; **82** (4 suppl III): III–670 (Abstract).

25. Cook SL, Eigler N, Goldenberg T, Forrester JS, Grundfest WS, Litvack F. Angiographic determinants of successful excimer laser coronary angioplasty. Circulation 1990; **82** (4 suppl III): III–671 (Abstract).

26. Baumbach A, Haase KK, Karsch KR. Usefulness of morphologic parameters in predicting the outcome of coronary excimer laser angioplasty. Am J Cardiol 1991; **68**: 1310–5.

30. Percutaneous transluminal coronary rotational ablation: early follow-up at 24 hours by quantitative angiography

KIRK L. PETERSON, ISABEL RIVERA, MARTIN McDANIEL, JOHN LONG, ALLAN BOND, VALMIK BHARGAVA and the Clinical Investigators* of the Multicenter Trial of the Rotablator™

Summary

Coronary rotational ablation with the Rotablator™ is manifesting significant promise for the treatment of atherosclerotic obstructions. Based upon careful serial measurements in 134 patients by quantitative coronary angiography, the device improved minimal luminal diameter from 0.69 ± 0.27 mm to 1.71 ± 0.33 mm 24 hours later. Lesions treated with the Rotablator™ do not show elastic recoil, but, by contrast, manifest even larger luminal diameters at 24 hours as compared to immediately post ablation. Although flow-mediated dilation or intrinsic metabolic factors may contribute to this phenomenon, the improvement in vessel lumen at 24 hours post-treatment appears to be related to relief of vasospasm. In some cases, balloon adjunctive dilation is used successfully when the initial minimal luminal diameter post-burr is in the range of 1.2 to 1.3 mm; however, the final result at 24 hours appears to be no different between those patients treated with burr alone as compared to burr ablation followed by balloon dilation. Further studies are necessary to determine if burrs of larger size can achieve a larger post-treatment luminal diameter and whether such use will be associated with higher complication and restenosis rates.

Introduction

A number of catheter devices for coronary plaque ablation have been developed in recent years to improve upon the clinical results of catheter balloon coronary angioplasty [1, 2]. Plaque ablation is aimed at increasing luminal patency, reducing dependence upon the reparative response to vessel

* Maurice Buchbinder, San Diego, Calif.; Gerald Dorros, Milwaukee, Wasconsin; Richard Podolin, San Diego, Calif.; Todd Sherman, Los Angeles, Calif; Simon Stertzer, San Francisco, Calif.; David Warth, Seattle Washington; Nadim Zacca, Houston, Texas

497

J.H.C. Reiber and P.W. Serruys (eds), Advances in Quantitative Coronary Arteriography, 497–513.
© 1993 *Kluwer Academic Publishers. Printed in the Netherlands.*

wall injury by balloon dilation, and expanding the use of percutaneous angioplasty techniques in more complex pathoanatomic lesions [3].

In addition to plaque ablation by excimer laser angioplasty and directional atherectomy [4–7], rotational ablation has been under intense investigation over the last three years [8–12]. One such promising device for rotational ablation (Rotablator™)is manufactured by Heart Technology, Inc. of Seattle, Washington, and has now been utilized in 17 centers in the United States and Europe in well over a thousand patients [9–12]. The device was first applied in animal models of coronary and peripheral atherosclerotic vascular disease [13, 14] and found to be safe and effective in improving luminal patency.

Shortly after the initiation of clinical trials, a core angiography laboratory for the coronary artery applications of the device was established. The goal was to assess by quantitative coronary angiography the effect of coronary rotational ablation on lesion geometry, immediate and long-term vessel patency, and coronary vasomotion. In this particular communication, we review the near-term (24 hour) effects of the Rotablator™ on 134 atherosclerotic lesions in 134 patients as assessed by quantitative mensuration of serial coronary artery cinefilms.

Device description

The Rotablator™ is a high-speed rotating catheter with a nickel burr tip impregnated with 5–10 micron diamond microchips over its distal one-half, creating an abrasive surface. An helical drive shaft, capable of rotating up to a speed of 200,000 revolutions per minute, energizes the burr. Saline is used to cool and lubricate the drive shaft system which is housed in a 4–French teflon catheter. The burr at the tip of the catheter is manufactured in sizes ranging in diameter from 1.25 to 2.50 mm. Any burr that is 2.15 mm or less in diameter is introduced via a 9 French guiding catheter; the 2.25 mm burr requires a 10 French catheter. For delivery of the device, a 0.009 inch stainless steel guidewire, with a 2 cm radio-opaque platinum spring tip, is threaded via a central lumen in the catheter, out the end of the burr, and through the lumen of the coronary artery lesion to be treated. The burr can then be advanced either manually or by forward rotation through the area of compromised vessel lumen.

Patient and film selection

Once the core angiography laboratory was established in March 1990, all active investigators were encouraged to contribute cinefilms to a central registry. A worksheet was devised which served to standardize the methods for cinefilm recording and to archive the geometric position of the radiographic imaging chain for each contrast injection before and subsequent to rotational ablation. All angiographers were encouraged to utilize projections which imaged optimally the treated lesion for purposes of edge recognition and quantitation, avoiding at the same time overlap of adjacent arteries and vessel foreshortening. Views recorded as part of the diagnostic cineangiogram were repeated 1) immediately after the burr ablation, 2) immediately after any adjunctive use of balloon dilation, 3) 24 hours later before the vascular sheaths were removed, and 4) at six-month's post-ablation unless recurrence or signs of myocardial ischemia mandated an earlier angiographic restudy. For this report, we have analyzed the serial films which were satisfactory for quantitation on the diagnostic study, immediately post-treatment, and then again at 24 hours.

Through May 1, 1991, 555 patients had undergone rotational ablation in the catheterization laboratories of the participating investigators of the Core Laboratory; 250 cinefilms of these 555 patients were submitted for analysis (a number of patients had been treated prior to the establishment of the Core Laboratory). Of the 250 patients for whom cinefilms were submitted, 173 were found suitable for quantitation on the diagnostic films. Rejection of films occurred for these reasons: 1) catheter positioning or imaging was not adequate for calibration of the coronary artery lesion, 2) cinefilm quality was insufficient (e.g., oversaturation or "blooming", excessive panning) for edge detection either by an automatic edge detection algorithm or with operator override, 3) problems with cine acquisitions including varying magnification or lesion projection at different times of filming (e.g., "diagnostic" versus "24 hours"), lesion obscured by diaphragm or other vessels, inadequate opacification of vessel, or choice of inappropriate view for quantitation.

In this communication, we report the serial measurements on 134 patients with suitable films for quantitation at the time of the diagnostic study, immediately post-rotational ablation, immediately post-balloon adjunctive dilation (if used, 59 patients), and at 24 hours of follow-up.

Hardware, procedures, and methods for cinefilm quantitation

All films are mounted on a CAP-35 (General Electric) cinefilm projector and magnified optically up to four times by an interposed lens. The iris, zoom, and mirrors are all remotely controlled and utilized to optimize the size and focus of any given coronary artery segment. The magnified images are recorded by a mounted, switchable videocamera (COHU), digitized as an interlaced television image (512 × 512 pixels, and 256 shades of gray) and stored in a Gould-DeAnza IP-8500 image processor interfaced to a Digital Equipment Corporation VAX 11/780 computer. The video camera can be rotated so as to align the lesion at any angle desired with respect to the raster lines of the television image. The operator can choose the proximal and distal ends of the segment of vessel to be analyzed, allowing for a significant length of reference vessel in order to compute percentage diameter and area stenosis.

The following general features are available as part of the coronary artery quantification program: 1) automatic edge detection with manual override, 2) correction for pincushion distortion based upon radial symmetric transformation and bilinear approximation to determine non-distorted from distorted intensity values, 3) three alternative methods for estimation of lesion cross-sectional area, including a) a geometric method based upon either single or biplane orthogonal views of the lesion, b) a videodensitometric method based upon background subtracted, log-transformed videointensities, and c) a combined geometric-videodensitometric method. For the patients undergoing rotational ablation with the Rotablator^{TM}, we have used the geometric approach because of its suitability for images archived on cinefilm.

Edge detection with the computer quantification program is accomplished using a two-dimensional search where, first, an edge likelihood matrix is created based upon two-dimensional gradients from Sobel operators (Figure 1, top panels). Thereafter, local edge correction is accomplished using first and second derivative thresholds and image weighted by the Laplacian; the image is then inverted so as to make the small values the likely edge points. Finally, each edge point is obtained as the least cost path through the modified gradient image (Figure 1, middle panels). The starting and ending points of the search along the vessel are provided by the operator. This heuristic makes the assumption that the slope of the edge will not change drastically at any given edge point, i.e., that successor points on the edge make an angle of no more than 90 degrees with the last path segment.

Once vessel edges have been established, a centerline is calculated based upon the shortest distance between successive points on either side of the vessel, as the computer interrogates down the path of the coronary artery segment chosen. Then, once a centerline has been determined, the algorithm recalculates perpendicular chords based upon intersections with the two edges on either side of the vessel. These perpendicular chords can then be plotted as a diameter function along the centerline; also, ten diameters from the proximal and distal reference segments, respectively, are averaged, and a linear fit of these two average values over the length of the coronary artery segment serves to estimate theoretic or expected diameters were there no luminal compromise present. The difference between the expected and actual diameters at each chord provides a measure of the plaque burden in that area. Moreover, filling in of that difference serves to graphically display the theoretic plaque area (Figure 1, bottom panels). Division of the average of a minimum of three successive diameters in the proximal reference segment by their theoretical (extrapolated) normal diameters provides a measure of the percent diameter and percent area obstruction of the atherosclerotic plaque. If only one projection is suitable for quantitation, minimal luminal cross-sectional area is derived from the minimal luminal diameter by assuming a circular model. If two views are available, the final vessel cross-

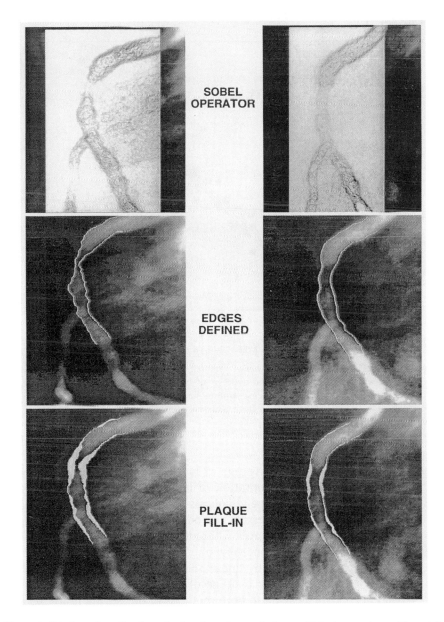

Figure 1. Display of application of edge detection and plaque fill-in in a patient with a right coronary artery lesion. Pre-treatment with rotational ablation is on the left; post-treatment at 24 hours is on the right. The top panels display the application of a Sobel operator to the region of interest around the treated stenosis. The middle panels display the ultimate determination of the vessel's edges (see text for details). The bottom panels display the theoretical plaque area fill-in based upon a linear interpolation between the proximal and distal reference segments (see text for details).

COMPARISON OF ONE VS. AVERAGE OF TWO DIAMETERS

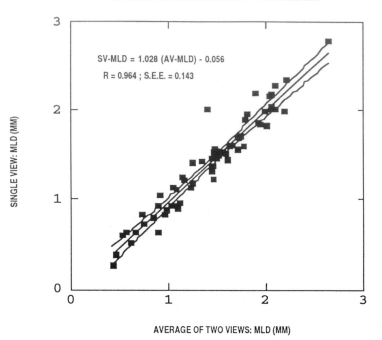

Figure 2. Plot of minimal luminal diameter obtained from a single view (SLV-MLD, vertical axis, in millimeters) as opposed to the average of two nearly orthogonal views (AV-MLD, horizontal axis, in millimeters). The least squares linear regression line, and associated 95% confidence intervals, are shown. Taken from Reference 15.

section is calculated from the average of two views. When one view only is utilized, it is accepted for quantitation of lesion severity when it meets the following criteria: a) near perpendicularity to the direction of imaging, b) lack of overlap of adjacent vessels, c) no seeming foreshortening of the vessel, due to tortuosity, in the area where the lesion is deemed most severe.

To evaluate the accuracy of one view only for assessment of lesion severity, we have previously compared by linear regression the single view minimal diameter (SV-MLD) versus the average of two relatively orthogonal views (AV-MLD) in 66 instances where both methods of measuring lesion severity were available (Figure 2) [15]. The correlation coefficient of this relation was 0.964 (standard error estimate = 0.143) with

$$SV\text{-}MLD = 1.028\,(AV\text{-}MLD) - 0.056 \qquad (1)$$

In those patients undergoing rotational ablation with the Rotablator™ the equivalency of SV-MLD and AV-MLD is promoted by the relatively tubular, concentric lumen which remains post-treatment. Balloon dilation, on the

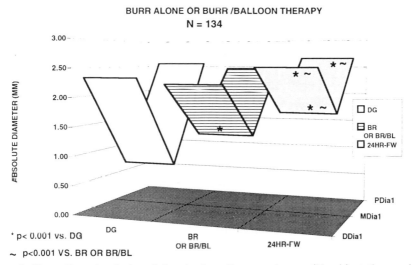

Figure 3. Three-dimensional plot of the absolute diameters in mm (Y axis) at the proximal reference segment (PDia1), at the minimum diameter (MDia1), and the distal reference segment (DDia1) (Z axis), taken from coronary arteriographic cinefilms recorded before rotational ablation (DG), immediately after either burr alone or burr/adjunctive balloon treatment (BR or BR/BL), and then again at 24 hours (24-HR FW) (X axis). Statistical symbols refer to average proximal, minimal and distal diameters of patient group. See Table 1 for other statistical parameters.

other hand, frequently give rise to a residual lumen which is quite complex in geometry and more difficult to model as a circle.

Quantitative results

For the 134 patients in whom quantitative coronary angiography was successfully accomplished upon diagnostic, immediate post-treatment, and at 24 hours post burr or burr/balloon, the average serial measurements (with relevant statistics, standard deviations, maximum and minimum values) are displayed in Table 1. All data were analyzed by analysis of variance for repeated measures, with the Tukey correction. Measurements are given for a proximal reference segment, at the minimum diameter, and for a distal reference segment. The calculated percentage diameter stenosis and percentage area stenosis are also given. The measurements for the absolute proximal, minimal, and distal diameters are graphed in Figure 3 for the pre-treatment diagnostic, immediately post-treatment, and 24 hour post-treatment studies. The proximal reference diameter did not change significantly between the diagnostic and immediately post-treatment films; however, at 24 hours this measure increased significantly to 2.64 ± 0.61 mm as compared to 2.50 ± 0.59 mm and 2.46 ± 0.64 mm on the diagnostic and immediate post-treatment film, respectively. Similarly, the distal segment increased to 2.50 ± 0.50 mm on the 24–hours study from 2.29 ± 0.49 and 2.23 ± 0.51 mm on the earlier films. At the same time, the minimal luminal diameter (MDia1) was 0.69 ± 0.27 mm on the diagnostic study, increased significantly to 1.33 ± 0.33 mm immediately post-treatment, and then increased significantly further to 1.71 ± 0.33 mm at 24 hours. The percentage stenosis, both by diameter and area, are also listed in Table 1; the percentage area stenosis was 90 ± 7% pre-treatment, declined to 64 + 17% immediately after burr or burr/balloon treatment, and then was found to be even further reduced to 51 ± 18% on the 24 hours follow-up film. Thus, some of the improvement in vessel lumen was ascribed to the effect of plaque ablation (followed in some cases by balloon adjunctive dilation); however, a further increment of improvement was attributable to dilation of the vessel as evidenced by the significant enlargement of the proximal and distal reference segments at 24 hours. The p-values for statistical significance are given in Table 1 and shown in the graph of Figure 3.

The total group of 134 patients were segregated into those where rotational ablation only was utilized (Figure 4, Table 2) and those where rotational ablation was followed by adjunctive balloon dilation (Figure 5, Table 3). In the 75 patients who had burr ablation alone, the minimal luminal diameter improved significantly from 0.73 ± 0.27 to 1.41 ± 0.33 mm immediately post-rotational ablation; then, at 24 hours later the average dimension had increased further to 1.70 ± 0.33 mm. As with the total group of patients, some of the improvement in the minimal luminal diameter between the time of diagnosis and 24 hours could be attributed to generalized enlargement of the vessel as evidenced by the significant increase in the size of the proximal and distal reference diameters.

In those 59 patients where balloon adjunctive dilation was utilized immediately following burr ablation, there was a progressive increase in the vessel dimensions. The average proximal and distal reference diameters did not change significantly between the diagnostic, post-burr, and post-balloon measurements; however, the distal reference segment was significantly increased at the time of the 24–hour follow-up study. The minimal luminal diameter in this subgroup averaged 0.65 ± 0.27 pre-treatment, increased significantly to 1.22 ± 0.30 mm post-burr plaque ablation, increased further to 1.51 ± 0.29 mm after balloon adjunctive balloon dilation, and then was found to be 1.73 ± 0.32 mm at the time of the 24 hour follow-up study.

In Figures 6, 7, and 8, cumulative histograms of the total population, burr only group, and burr/balloon groups are shown, respectively. The consistent improvement of luminal patency by rotational ablation is shown in both groups. In those patients where adjunctive balloon dilation was used, it appears that the operator was successful in effecting further improvement in the minimal luminal diameter which then improved even further at 24 hours.

Table 1.

	Diagnostic					Stat	Burr or Burr/Balloon					Stat	24-hour followup				Stat
	Mean	s.d.	Max	Min	N		Mean	s.d.	Max	Min	N		s.d.	Max	Min	N	
PDial	2.50	0.59	4.35	1.40	134		2.64	0.64	4.28	1.03	134		0.61	4.66	1.54	134	*-
MDial	0.69	0.27	1.54	0.01	134	*	1.71	0.33	2.93	0.55	134		0.33	2.79	0.97	134	*-
DDial	2.29	0.49	3.77	1.28	134		2.50	0.51	3.53	1.01	134	*	0.50	4.30	1.53	134	*-
%Dial	70.95	10.15	98.00	46.50	134		31.40	13.94	74.40	0.80	134		12.73	55.10	1.00	134	*-
%Arel	90.03	6.64	100.00	61.90	134		51.44	16.64	93.30	2.50	134		18.37	80.90	1.00	134	*-

Legend: PDial = Proximal Diameter, One View; MDial = Minimal Diameter, One View; DDial = Distal Diameter, One View; %Dial = percentage diameter stenosis, One View; %Arel = percentage area stenosis, One View; Max = Maximum value; Min = Minimum value; s.d. = Standard deviation; N = Number of lesions; Stat = Statistical significance by analysis of variance

Statistical Significance: * = p < .001 vs. DIAGNOSTIC; - = p < 0.001 vs BURR OR BURR/BALLOON.

N = 75

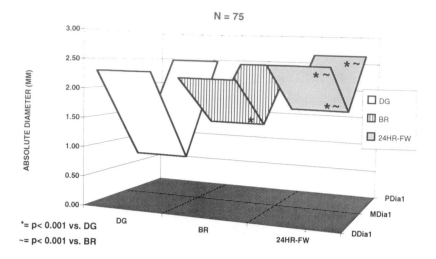

Figure 4. Three-dimensional plot of the absolute diameters in mm (Y axis) at the proximal reference segment (PDia1), at the minimum diameter (MDia1), and the distal reference segment (DDia1) (Z axis), taken from coronary arteriographic cinefilms recorded before rotational ablation (DG), immediately after burr alone (BR), and then again at 24 hours (24–HR FW) (X axis). Statistical symbols refer to average proximal, minimal and distal diameters of patient group. See Table 2 for other statistical parameters.

In no case of either population studied was there a worsening at 24 hours of the initially achieved lumen.

Conclusions

These initial studies, applying quantitative coronary angiography to patients undergoing rotational ablation of atherosclerotic plaque with the Rotablator, suggest that the device is remarkably and consistently successful in augmenting the minimal luminal diameter in an atherosclerotic coronary vessel. The quantitative analysis would also suggest that in some patients balloon adjunctive dilation is desirable to increase the minimal lumen further. Whichever approach is utilized, i.e. burr alone or burr with balloon adjunctive dilation, the ultimate luminal diameter at 24 hours follow-up ranges between 1.3 to 2.8 mm with an average of 1.71 mm. Initial clinical correlations indicate that this degree of luminal improvement is associated with relief of symptoms and signs of myocardial ischemia which is sustained out to at least six months. Some observations from this same core angiography registry in 69 patients also indicates that the loss of the initial gain at six months averages approximately 0.2 mm and is not higher than would be expected with balloon dilation angioplasty [15].

   In contrast to balloon dilation angioplasty, there does not appear to be

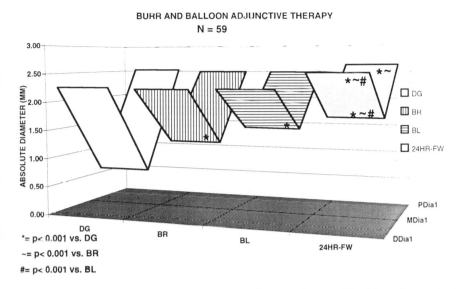

Figure 5. Three-dimensional plot of the absolute diameters in mm (Y axis) at the proximal reference segment (PDia1), at the minimum diameter (MDia1), and the distal reference segment (DDia1) (Z axis), taken from coronary arteriographic cinefilms recorded before rotational ablation (DG), immediately after burr (BR) treatment, after adjunctive balloon dilation (BL), and then again at 24 hours (24–HR FW) (X axis). Statistical symbols refer to average proximal, minimal and distal diameters of patient group. See Table 3 for other statistical parameters.

an immediate loss within the first 24 hours of the initial gain in luminal diameter, i.e. elastic recoil [16, 17]. In fact, the patients reported herein consistently demonstrated a further improvement in their luminal measurements, both the reference as well as the treated segments. This observation strongly indicates that there is an element of vasoconstriction associated with rotational ablation and which is relieved by 24 hours post-treatment. The improvement, however, may also be attributable to flow-mediated dilation brought about by enhancement of coronary blood flow after relief of the epicardial artery obstruction and clearance of particulate matter in the microvasculature. By protocol, all angiographic measurements were done during nitrate, and often calcium channel blocker, vasodilation; thus, the improvement at 24 hours cannot be accounted for by differences in pharmacologic vasodilation. It is of interest that improvement in the luminal diameter of all analyzed segments occurred also in the subgroup of patients treated with balloon adjunctive dilation. This would suggest that there is no prominent phenomenon of elastic recoil from balloon dilation once the plaque has been partially or totally ablated. Rather, the further improvement in the lumen would be attributable to compacting of the tissue underlying the area of rotational ablation.

It is also of interest that the luminal diameter achieved after burr therapy

Table 2.

	Diagnostic					Burr						24-hour followup				
	Mean	s.d.	Max	Min	N	Mean	Stat	s.d.	Max	Min	N	Mean	Stat	s.d.	Max	Min	N
PDia1	2.47	0.63	4.35	1.40	75	2.43		0.66	4.28	1.16	75	2.64	*-	0.65	4.66	1.54	75
MDia1	0.73	0.27	1.54	0.24	75	1.41	*	0.33	2.93	0.55	75	1.70	*-	0.33	2.79	0.97	75
DDia1	2.31	0.54	3.77	1.28	75	2.23		0.51	3.53	1.23	75	2.47	*-	0.50	3.49	1.53	75
%Dia1	69.42	9.62	89.60	46.50	75	37.59	*	11.77	61.60	10.90	75	31.31	*-	13.22	54.50	1.00	75
%Are1	89.26	6.44	98.90	68.80	75	59.71	*	14.60	84.30	21.00	75	51.05	*-	19.10	79.30	3.00	75

Legend: PDia1 = Proximal Diameter, One View; MDia1 = Minimal Diameter, One View; DDia1 = Distal Diameter, One View; %Dia1 = percentage diameter stenosis, One View; %Are1 = percentage area stenosis, One View; Max = Maximum value; Min = Minimum value; s.d. = Standard deviation; N = Number of lesions; Stat = Statistical significance by analysis of variance.
Statistical Significance: * = $p < 0.001$ vs. DIAGNOSTIC; - = $p < 0.001$ vs Burr or Balloon.

Table 3.

	Diagnostic					Burr						Balloon						24-Hour Followup					
	Mean	s.d.	Max	Min	N	Mean	Stat	s.d.	Max	Min	N	Mean	Stat	s.d.	Max	Min	N	Mean	Stat	s.d.	Max	Min	N
PDia1	2.52	0.54	4.03	1.52	59	2.49		0.61	3.87	1.03	59	2.49	*-	0.55	4.15	1.29	59	2.64	*-	0.57	3.95	1.58	59
MDia1	0.65	0.27	1.34	0.01	59	1.22	*	0.30	1.99	0.56	59	1.51	*-	0.29	2.09	0.95	59	1.73	*-#	0.32	2.50	1.14	59
DDia1	2.26	0.41	3.06	1.43	59	2.25		0.52	3.34	1.01	59	2.26		0.43	3.30	1.56	59	2.54	*-#	0.51	4.30	1.54	59
%Dia1	72.91	10.55	98.00	53.80	59	46.26	*	15.07	74.40	0.80	59	33.51	*-	15.25	61.90	1.00	59	31.53	*-	12.19	55.10	1.00	59
%Are1	90.96	6.80	100.00	61.90	59	69.14	*	17.54	93.30	2.50	59	53.62	*-	20.95	85.50	1.00	59	51.88	*-	17.64	80.90	1.00	55

Legend: PDia1 = Proximal Diameter, One View; MDia1 = Minimal Diameter, One View; %Dia1 = percentage diameter stenosis, One View; %Are1 = percentage area stenosis, One View; Max = Maximum value Min = Minimum value; s.d. = Standard deviation; N = Number of lesions; Stat = Statistical significance by analysis of variance.
Statistical Significance: * = $p < 0.001$ vs. DIAGNOSTIC; - = $p < 0.001$ vs BURR; # = $p < 0.001$ vs Balloon.

CUMULATIVE HISTOGRAMS: MINIMAL LUMINAL DIAMETER

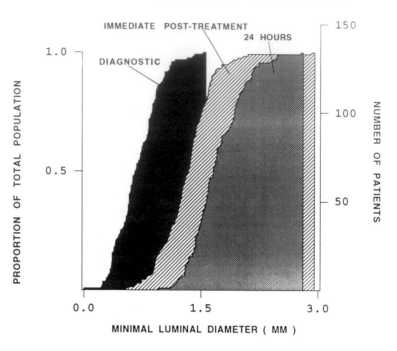

Figure 6. Cumulative histogram of the minimal luminal diameter in 134 patients undergoing burr treatment alone or burr treatment followed by adjunctive balloon dilation. Population statistics are accumulated at the time of the diagnostic study, immediately after treatment, and again at 24 hours post-treatment.

alone averaged 1.41 ± 0.33 mm in the burr alone group and 1.22 ± 0.30 mm in those patients treated with subsequent balloon adjunctive dilation. These dimensions are less than the diameter of the burr itself which ranges between 1.5 to 2.25 mm; in most cases reported herein a final burr size of 1.75 mm or greater was utilized. This suggests that there is some degree of "watermelon seed" slippage as it traverses through an area of narrowing. Alternatively, there may yet be some element of vasospasm, even at 24 hours, which mitigates the size of luminal opening achieved by the rotating burr. Whether use of larger burrs will lead to larger luminal results in the area of ablation is yet to be proven. Moreover, it is yet uncertain as to whether larger burrs will incite greater injury to the medial layer of the vessel wall and a more prominent neointimal and proliferative response.

CUMULATIVE HISTOGRAMS: MINIMAL LUMINAL DIAMETER
BURR THERAPY ONLY

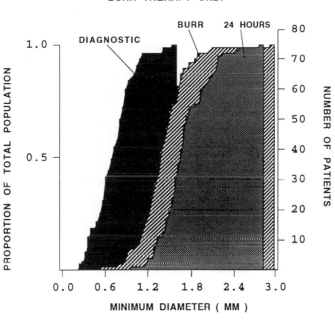

Figure 7. Cumulative histogram of the minimal luminal diameter in 75 patients undergoing burr treatment alone. Population statistics are accumulated at the time of the diagnostic study, immediately after treatment, and again at 24 hours post-treatment.

In conclusion, rotational ablation with the Rotablator™ manifests significant promise for the treatment of coronary atherosclerotic obstructions. Based upon careful serial measurements by quantitative coronary angiography, the device improves the minimal luminal diameter by approximately 100 percent or greater. In contrast with balloon angioplasty, it does not appear to be associated with elastic recoil, but, rather, is noted to produce even larger luminal diameters at 24 hours post-ablation. This latter phenomenon can be attributable to relief of vasospasm, although flow-mediated improvement in luminal dimensions or intrinsic metabolic factors related to intimal abrasion also may be playing a role. Only further studies will reveal if larger lumens can be attained by using burrs of greater size,and, secondly, whether such use will be associated with higher vascular complications and restenosis rates.

CUMULATIVE HISTOGRAMS: MINIMAL LUMINAL DIAMETER
BOTH BURR AND ADJUNCTIVE BALLOON THERAPY

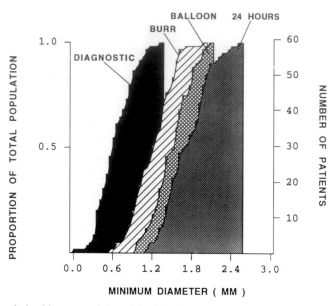

Figure 8. Cumulative histogram of the minimal luminal diameter in 59 patients undergoing burr treatment followed by adjunctive balloon dilation. Population statistics are accumulated at the time of the diagnostic study, immediately after burr treatment, again after balloon dilation, and finally at 24 hours post-treatment.

References

1. Evaluation of emerging technologies for coronary revascularization. Circulation 1992; **85**: 357–61 (Editorial).
2. King SB 3rd. Role of new technology in balloon angioplasty. Circulation 1991; **84**: 2574–9.
3. Guidelines for percutaneous transluminal coronary angioplasty. A report of the American College of Cardiology/American Heart Association Task Force on Assessment of Diagnostic and Therapeutic Cardiovascular Procedures (Subcommittee on Percutaneous Transluminal Coronary Angioplasty). J Am Coll Cardiol 1988; **12**: 529–45.
4. Litvack F, Eigler NL, Margolis JR, et al. Percutaneous excimer laser coronary angioplasty. Am J Cardiol 1990; **66**: 1027–32.
5. Spears JR, Reyes VP, Wynne J, et al. Percutaneous coronary laser balloon angioplasty: initial results of a multicenter experience. J Am Coll Cardiol 1990; **16**: 293–303.
6. Safian RD, Gelbfish JS, Erny RE, Schnitt SJ, Schmidt DA, Baim DS. Coronary atherectomy. Clinical, angiographic, and histological findings and observations regarding potential mechanisms. Circulation 1990; **82**: 69–79.
7. Hinohara T, Selmon MR, Robertson GC, Braden L, Simpson JS. Directional atherectomy. New approaches for treatment of obstructive coronary and peripheral vascular disease. Circulation 1990; **81** (3 Suppl): IV 79–91.

8. Sketch MH Jr, O'Neill WW, Galichia JP, et al. The Duke multicenter coronary transluminal extraction-endarterectomy registry: acute and chronic results. J Am Coll Cardiol 1991; **17** (2 Suppl A): 31A (Abstract).

9. Fourrier JL, Bertrand ME, Auth DC, LaBlanche JM, Gommeaux A, Brunetaud JM. Percutaneous coronary rotational angioplasty in humans: preliminary report. J Am Coll Cardiol 1989; **14**: 1278–82.

10. Buchbinder M, O'Neill W, Warth D, et al. Percutaneous coronary rotational ablation using the rotablator: results of a multicenter study. Circulation 1990; **82** (4 Suppl III): III–309 (Abstract).

11. Warth D, Buchbinder M, O'Neill W, et al. Rotational ablation using the rotablator for angiographically unfavorable lesions. J Am Coll Cardiol 1991; **17** (2 Suppl A): 125A (Abstract).

12. Buchbinder M, Warth D, O'Neill W, et al. Multi-center registry of percutaneous coronary rotational ablation using the rotablator. J Am Coll Cardiol 1991; **17** (2 Suppl A): 31A (Abstract).

13. Hansen DD, Auth DC, Vracko R, Ritchie JL. Rotational atherectomy in atherosclerotic rabbit iliac arteries. Am Heart J 1988; **115**: 160–5.

14. Hansen DD, Auth DC, Hall M, Ritchie JL. Rotational endarterectomy in normal canine coronary arteries: preliminary report. J Am Coll Cardiol 1988; **11**: 1073–77.

15. Peterson KL, Rivera I, McDaniel M, Long J, Bond A, Bhargava M. Serial follow-up by quantitative angiography. In: Serruys PW, Strauss BH, King SB 3rd (Eds.), Restenosis after intervention with new mechanical devices. Dordrecht: Kluwer Academic Publishers. In press.

16. Fischell TA, Nellessen U, Johnson DE, Ginsburg R. Endothelium-dependent arterial vasoconstriction after balloon angioplasty. Circulation 1989; **79**: 899–910.

17. Fischell TA, Derby G, Tse TM, Stadius ML. Coronary artery vasoconstriction routinely occurs after percutaneous transluminal coronary angioplasty. A quantitative arteriographic analysis. Circulation 1988; **78**: 1323–34.

31. Quantitative assessment of the residual stenosis after percutaneous transluminal cororonary rotary ablation: European Experience

MICHEL E. BERTRAND, FABRICE LEROY,
JEAN M. LABLANCHE, EUGENE McFADDEN,
CHRISTOPHE BAUTERS and GAETEN J. KARILLON

Summary

Quantitative assessment of the residual stenosis after percutaneous transluminal coronary rotary ablation was performed in a population of 77 patients who underwent Rotary ablation in 3 European Centers.

This study showed that the minimal luminal diameter obtained with Rotary ablation is relatively small: 1.44 mm on average. In 30 cases, the residual stenosis was still significant and the procedure was completed by adjunctive coronary balloon angioplasty. The residual lumen after treatment reaches only 75% of the expected result taking into account the size of the burr. Quantitative coronary angiography performed 24 hours after the procedure, showed that the residual stenosis remained unchanged and this suggests the absence of recoil after treatment with Rotablator.

Introduction

Percutaneous transluminal coronary angioplasty [1–2] is now recognized as a very effective method of myocardial revascularization. Nevertheless coronary angioplasty has still several limitations. Therefore, engineers and interventional cardiologists, have sought to develop new methods of recanalization trying to remove atherosclerotic material. There are several atherectomy devices including the atherocath described by J. Simpson [3], the Transluminal extracting catheter of R. Stack [4] and the Rotablator[TM] (Heart Technology, Seattle) designed by D. Auth to grind obstructive atheroma into fine particles [5–16]. In this chapter we analyze with quantitative coronary angiography the modifications of the coronary vessels treated by Rotary ablation.

J.H.C. Reiber and P.W. Serruys (eds), Advances in Quantitative Coronary Arteriography, 515–523.

Methodology

Patient group

The study population included 77 patients (60 males,17 females) mean age 56 years, who underwent Rotary ablation with the Rotablator. These patients can be subdivided into two groups. Forty-seven patients (Group A) were treated by Rotablator alone. In thirty patients the procedure was completed by an adjunctive balloon angioplasty owing unsatisfactory results or abrupt closure which was recrossed by the guidewire and dilated by a balloon.

In 17 of the 77 patients the coronary angiography was repeated the day after the procedure. In all cases the coronary angiograms were obtained after intracoronary injection of 2 mg of isosorbide dinitrate.

Rotary ablation procedure

The Rotablator™ consists of a rotative abrasive burr welded to a long flexible drive shaft tracking along a central flexible guide wire. The abrasive tip is an elliptically shaped burr of various sizes (1.0, 1.25, 1.5, 1.75, 2 mm diameter) The burr is coated with diamond chips of 30 to 40 um embedded into the metal. The drive shaft is housed in a 4F teflon sheath and connected to a turbine driven by compressed air. The shaft and the turbine spins at up to 190,000 rpm. The burr and the drive shaft track along a central coaxial guide wire (0.009 inch) of which the last 2 centimeters is radioopaque platinum. The central guide wire can be controlled and moved with a pin vise. The wire and abrasive tip can be advanced independently; thus, the wire could be placed in the selected artery, thereby directing the burr safely through the diseased artery. The steerable guide wire does not rotate with the burr during abrasion.

After local anesthesia, a 9F sheath was inserted into the femoral artery. A standard 9F guiding catheter was placed into the ostium of the coronary artery to perform an initial angiogram made in 3 different projections after i.c injection of 2 mg of isosorbide dinitrate. Ten thousand units of heparin were then intravenously injected. The atherectomy device was introduced into the guiding catheter and positioned just before the distal tip of the 9F guiding catheter. Under fluoroscopy, the steerable guide wire was advanced through the narrowing and directed into the distal part of the coronary artery. The abrasive tip was then advanced along the guide wire, placed in contact with the stenosis and rotation was started. When the adequate speed of rotation was reached (175,000 rpm) the abrasive tip was advanced gently over the guidewire. If a resistance was encountered, the tip was successively pulled back and advanced to maintain a high speed rotation. Once the abrasive tip crossed the lesion, it was withdrawn and several passages were performed until the impression of mechanical resistance completely disappeared. On the average, after 6 to 8 passages, the rotation was stopped and the abrasive tip was pulled back into the guiding catheter while the guidewire remained in the distal part of the vessel. Dye injection verified the quality and the success of the procedure; then the rotational device and guidewire were completely withdrawn.

Quantitative coronary angiography

The quantitative analysis of the treated vessel was carried out with the Caesar system (Computerized angiographic evaluation of stenosis and restenosis). The 35 mm films were mounted on a 35AX Tagarno projector. Cineframes were selected in most cases at the end-diastole to minimize any possibly blurring effect. The selected image was projected onto a high-resolution (1024 × 1024) CCD video camera. A zoom allowed to select the appropriate optical magnification ranging from 1 to 5. The resulting video signal was then digitized in matrix size of 1024 × 768 pixels with 9 bits (512 levels) brightness resolution and displayed on a video monitor. In the analysis procedure, user-interaction was possible by means of a writing tablet.

The three following steps were performed to analyze the dimensions of the vessel:

1) *Computation of the calibration factor.* To compute absolute sizes of the arterial segment analyzed, a calibration factor was determined by detection of the boundaries of the guiding catheter. The comparison of the computed mean diameter in pixels with the known size in millimeters resulted in the calibration factor expressed in mm/pixel. The delineation of the catheter boundaries was carried out with the technique applied for measurement of the different coronary segments.

2) *Contour analysis.* With the help of the writing tablet, two regions of interest were delineated on the vessel: (1) The "normal" or "reference" segment, proximal to the narrowing; and (2) the narrowed segment.

In these two matrices, a center line was manually traced from three points along the vessel. Then the contours of the arterial segment were automatically detected on the basis of the weighted sum of first and second derivative functions applied to the digitized brightness information.

3) *Calculations.* The diameter data of the vessels in absolute values were calculated in mm by using the guiding catheter as a scaling device.

The following parameters were obtained: the mean reference ("normal" proximal) (N) segment, the minimal luminal diameter (MLD) and the percentage of reduction of luminal diameter was calculated as follows: Percentage of stenosis = ((N-MLD)/N)* 100.

4) *Accuracy, precision, reproducibility of the CAESAR system.* The accuracy and precision of the edge detection technique were determined according to the recommendations by Herrington and Walford [17]. The parameters were calculated from measurements performed with a perspex phantom (Dr Do-

Table 1. Accuracy & Precision of the CAESAR system

	Load (kV)	Accuracy (mm)	Precision (mm)
Mode			
7"	70	0.05	0.15
7"	90	0.10	0.15
5"	70	0.12	0.11
5"	90	0.07	0.12
Contrast Concentration			
100%	80	0.02	0.16
50%	80	0.04	0.15
25%	80	0.04	0.17
Overall results		0.07	0.15

Table 2. Variability Inter & Intra Observer

	Standard deviation (mm)
Inter Observer	
Observer 1	0.12
Observer 2	0.11
Intra Observer	0.10

riot, Geneva) consisting of a number of tubes of known diameters (1.0 mm, 2.0 mm, 3.0 mm, 4.15 mm, 5.15 mm and 5.95 mm). The phantom was filled with different concentrations of contrast medium (100%, 50%, 25%) and filmed with the different modes of the image intensifier (7"; 5"). The accuracy was defined as the average signed difference between the measured and true diameter values;the precision was defined as the standard deviation of these differences.

The reproducibility of the system was determined with two consecutive measurements made by two different observers. These data are summarized in Tables 1 and 2 which allow to conclude that the CAESAR system performance was satisfactory for evaluation of coronary arterial dimensions.

Results

Group A: Rotablator as a stand alone procedure

The results for this group are reported in Table 3.

The reference diameter was measured at 2.84 ± 0.61 mm before Rotablator and decreased slightly but unsignificantly to 2.70 ± 0.62 mm after treatment.

Table 3. Measurements of the coronary arteries before and after the procedure

	Before RA	After RA	After RA + Ball
Group A			
Reference Diameter (mm)	2.84 ± 0.61	2.70 ± 0.62*	
MLD (mm)	0.75 ± 0.28	1.54 ± 0.41*	
Stenose (%)	72 ± 10	40 ± 13*	
Group B			
Reference Diameter (mm)	2.74 ± 0.36	2.64 ± 0.36	2.69 ± 0.42
MLD (mm)	0.60 ± 0.25	1.19 ± 0.42*	2.04 ± 0.49*
Stenose (%)	74 ± 9.2	57 + 15*	30 ± 9.8*

MLD = Minimal luminal diameter; RA = Rotary ablation.
* $p < 0.001$.

The size of the burr used in this group of patients was slightly smaller than the reference diameter of the vessel: the ratio burr/reference diameter was calculated at 0.70 ± 0.17.

The minimal luminal diameter increased significantly ($p < 0.0001$) from 0.75 ± 0.28 to 1.54 ± 0.41 mm ($p < 0.001$).

As a result, the percentage of reduction of luminal diameter significantly decreased from 72 ± 10% to 40 ± 13%.

Group B: *Rotary ablation completed by adjunctive balloon angioplasty* ($N =$ 30) Before Rotablator the reference vessel diameter measured 2.74 ± 0.54 mm and the minimal luminal diameter reached 0.60 ± 0.25 mm. Thus, the treated narrowing was 74 ± 9.2%.

The ratio burr/reference diameter was 0.69 ± 0.16.

After Rotary ablation the reference diameter was unchanged (2.74 ± 0.36 before vs 2.64 ± 0.36 mm after n.s.). The minimal luminal diameter significantly increased from 0.60 ± 0.25 to 1.19 ± 0.42 mm. However, the residual stenosis (calculated at 57 ± 15%) was most often still significant (>50%). Due to this unsatisfactory result, the procedure was completed by a balloon angioplasty. Then, the minimal luminal diameter increased to 2.04 ± 0.49 mm and the residual stenosis was considered as acceptable (30 ± 10%).

Quantitative coronary angiography 24 hours after the procedure

These results are reported in Table 4.

In patients treated by Rotablator alone there were no significant changes in the vessel sizes the day after the procedure: the reference diameter was unchanged. The most important observation is the absence of change in the minimal luminal diameter: 1.76 ± 0.48 mm after Rotablator vs

Table 4. Measurements of the treated segments before, immediately after treatment and the following day

	Before RX	After RX	Day after
Group A			
Reference	3.00 ± 0.46	3.04 ± 0.38	2.99 ± 0.62
Diameter (mm)			
MLD (mm)	0.87 ± 0.32	1.76 ± 48*	1.77 ± 0.46
Stenose (%)	69.8 ± 11	40 ± 16*	38 ± 15
Group B			
Reference	2.68 ± 0.42	2.81 ± 0.38	2.78 ± 0.23
Diameter			
MLD (mm)	0.67 ± 0.30	1.56 ± 0.53*	1.89 ± 0.31
Stenose (%)	74 ± 13	41 ± 20*	31 ± 10

MLD: Minimal luminal diameter; RX: treatment.
* $p < 0.001$.

1.77 ± 0.46 mm n.s. the day after. As a result, the residual stenosis remained unchanged (40 ± 16 vs $38 \pm 15\%$ n.s.).

This observation can also be applied to the group of patients treated by Rotablator and an adjunctive PTCA.

Relationship between the burr size and the residual luminal diameter

We compared the size of the residual luminal diameter to the size of the burr.

Figure 1 shows that in most of the cases the residual luminal diameter is under the identity line. The ratio minimal residual luminal diameter/ burr was on average 0.75 ± 0.19. This clearly demonstrates that the burr was unable to completely remove the atherosclerotic material.

Discussion

These results suggest two different comments: 1) The minimal luminal diameter obtained with Rotary ablation is relatively small: For the whole group the minimal luminal diameter increased from 0.73 ± 0.28 to 1.44 ± 0.44 mm ($p < 0.001$). In 30 cases the residual stenosis was still significant and the procedure was completed by adjunctive coronary balloon angioplasty. It is obvious that the size of the burr is limited by the internal diameter of the guiding catheter: even with large lumen guiding catheters (11F) the largest burr which can be used is 2.5 mm. In our study the ratio burr size/diameter of the proximal reference segment was only 0.70 ± 0.16 and the treatment of stenosis located in large vessels (>3.5 mm) should be avoided since it is very likely that rotary ablation will leave a significant residual stenosis. Thus,

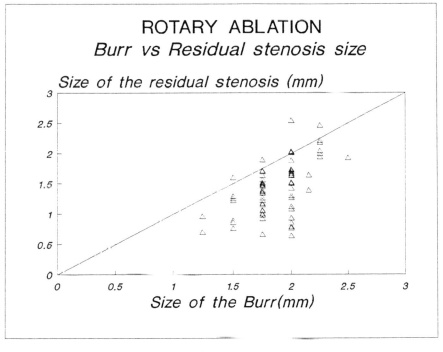

Figure 1.

at a first glance, this technique should be applied to relatively small (2 or 2.5 mm) distal vessels. However, a different strategy has been proposed for large vessels. This implies to start with an undersized burr to "debulk" the atherosclerotic material and then to complete the procedure with an adequately sized balloon in order to obtain a larger lumen. Obviously, this strategy increases the length and the cost of the procedure. Whether or not this strategy is able to decrease the rate of restenosis requires further informations and even randomized studies comparing Rotary ablation as a stand alone procedure versus rotary ablation completed by adjunctive PTCA.

2) The concept of the expansion ratio applied to this technique, as presented by Schatz [18] and applied to different devices by Umans [19] is relatively simple. These authors consider that the procedures of interventional cardiology include three stages. The first or prefunctional stage is characterized by the evaluation of the intrinsic dimensions of the device in order to determine its introduction into the coronary vessel. In the particular case of Rotablator it consists of measuring the reference proximal diameter and comparing it with the internal luminal diameter of the guiding catheter.

As soon the size of the burr has been chosen, the second stage or operational phase starts during which the tool is producing its specific mode of action i.e. to grind the atherosclerotic material into millions of tiny particles.

With the Rotablator, the diameter of the device is constant as opposed to the expansion of the balloon or other devices, directional atherectomy or stent. Theoretically, the removal of atherosclerotic material with the Rotablator should lead to a minimal luminal diameter equal to the size of the burr. Our study demonstrates that in most of the cases the residual luminal diameter is smaller than the diameter of the burr.

The residual lumen after treatment reaches only 75% of the expected result taking into account the size of the burr. This may be due to the location of the abrasive part at the front part of the burr. One can imagine that when the new channel reaches a certain diameter, the push exerted via the flexible shaft is able to distend the elastic wall and allows the device to reach into the distal part of the vessel beyond the narrowing. Thus, possible improvements could be obtained by a modification of the shape of the burr: better results could perhaps be obtained with a cylindric shape rather than an elliptical shape.

The last stage is depending on the recoil phenomenon and vascular reactivity. This latter phenomenon can be evaluated with the Rotablator. It is very likely that the abrasion of the endothelium of the normal segments adjacent to the narrowing induces spasm. This has been observed in the preliminary experience with the Rotablator. Therefore, most of the procedures are now conducted under continuous infusion of nitrates. Moreover, in this particular study with quantitative coronary angiography, all the measurements were done after intracoronary injection of isosorbide dinitrate. Thus, the real influence of the vascular reactivity could not be assessed accurately in this particular study. Nonetheless the results obtained the day after the procedure are interesting, since they clearly show the absence of the recoil phenomenon within the following 24 hours. Moreover, this was observed not only after stand alone rotary ablation, but also when the treatment with Rotablator was completed with adjunctive balloon angioplasty.

In conclusion, this study conducted with quantitative coronary angiography demonstrates that the results obtained with the Rotablator are very similar to those of coronary balloon angioplasty. The absence of recoil phenomenon is a very important issue but the device still requires further modifications: improvement of the guide wire, and modifications of the shape of the burr which could be cylindrical or even expandable.

References

1. Gruntzig AR, Senning A, Siegenthaler WE. Nonoperative dilatation of coronary artery stenosis: percutaneous transluminal coronary angioplasty. N Engl J Med 1979; 301: 61–8.
2. Kent KM, Bentivoglio LG, Block PC, et al. Long term efficacy of percutaneous transluminal coronary angioplasty (PTCA): report from the National Heart Lung and Blood Institute PTCA Registry. Am J Cardiol 1984; 53: 27C–31C.

3. Simpson JB, Robertson GC, Selmon MR. Percutaneous coronary atherectomy. J Am Coll Cardiol 1988; **11** (2 Suppl A): 110 A (Abstract).
4. Stack RS, Quigley PJ, Sketch MH Jr, Walker C.Hoffman PU, Phillips HR. Treatment of coronary artery disease with the transluminal extraction-endarterectomy catheter: initial results of a multicenter study. Circulation 1989; **80** (4 Suppl II): II–583 (Abstract).
5. Hansen DD, Auth DC, Vrocko R, Ritchie JL. Rotational atherectomy in atherosclerotic rabbit iliac arteries. Am Heart J 1988; **115**: 160–5.
6. Ahn SS, Auth DC, Marcus DR, Moore WS. Removal of focal atheromatous lesions by angioscopically guided high speed rotary atherectomy. Preliminary experimental observations. J Vasc Surg 1988; **7**: 292–300.
7. Fourrier JL, Stankowiak C, Lablanche JM, Prat A, Brunetaud JM, Bertrand ME. Histopathology after rotational angioplasty of peripheral arteries in human beings. J Am Coll Cardiol 1988; **11** (2 Suppl A): 109A (Abstract).
8. Zacca NM, Raizner AE, Noon GP, et al. Short term follow up of patients treated with a recently developed rotational atherectomy device and in vivo assessment of the particules generated. J Am Coll Card 1988; **11** (2 Suppl A): 109A (Abstract).
9. Hansen DD, Auth DC, Hall M, Ritchie JL. Rotational endarterectomy in normal canine coronary arteries. Preliminary report. J Am Coll Card 1988; **11**: 1073–7.
10. Fourrier JL, Auth D, Lablanche JM, Brunetaud JM, Gommeaux A, Bertrand ME. Human percutaneous coronary rotational atherectomy: preliminary results. Circulation 1988; **78** (4 Suppl II): II–82 (Abstract).
11. Fourrier JL, Bertrand ME, Auth DC, Lablanche JM, Gommeaux A, Brunetaud JM. Percutaneous coronary rotational angioplasty in humans: preliminary report. J Am Coll. Cardiol 1989; **14**: 1278–82.
12. Ginsburg R, Teirstein PS, Warth DC, Haq N, Jenkins NS, McCowan LC. Percutaneous transluminal coronary rotational atheroblation: clinical experience in 40 patients. Circulation 1989; **80** (4 Suppl II): II–584 (Abstract).
13. Teirstein PS, Ginsburg R, Warth DC, Haq N, Jenkins NS, McCowan LC. Complications of human coronary rotablation. J Am Coll cardiol 1990, **15** (2 Suppl A): 57A (Abstract).
14. Bertrand ME, Lablanche JM, Fourrier JL, Bauters C, Leroy F. Percutaneous rotary ablation. Herz 1990; **15**: 285–91.
15. Buchbinder M, O'Neill W, Warth D, et al. Percutaneous coronary rotational ablation using the Rotablator: results of a multicenter study. Circulation 1990, **82** (4 Suppl III): III–309 (Abstract).
16. Bertrand ME, Fourrier JL, Dietz U, De Jaegere P. European experience with percutaneous transluminal coronary rotational ablation. Circulation 1990, **82** (4 Suppl III): III–310 (Abstract).
17. Herrington DM, Walford GA, Pearson TA. Issues of validation in quantitative coronary angiography. In: Reiber JHC, Serruys PW (Eds.), New developments in quantitative coronary arterioography. Dordrecht: Kluwer Academic Publishers 1988: 153–66.
18. Schatz RA. A view of vascular stents. Circulation 1989; **79**: 445–57.
19. Umans VA, Strauss BH, Rensing BJ, de Jaegere P, de Feyter PJ, Serruys PW. Comparative angiographic quantitative analysis of the immediate efficacy of coronary atherectomy with balloon angioplasty, stenting and rotational ablation. Am Heart J 1991; **122**: 836–43.

32. Quantitative coronary angiography after revascularization with the transluminal extraction-endarterectomy catheter (TEC™)

DONALD F. FORTIN, MICHAEL H. SKETCH, Jr.,
HARRY R. PHILLIPS III and RICHARD S. STACK

Summary

Despite a seemingly exponential rise in the number of coronary angioplasty procedures since the introduction of the procedure in 1977, several major limitations to more widespread use still remain. These include difficulty traversing chronic total occlusions, the development of major dissection with an attendant increase in the risk of abrupt closure and the continuing problem of restenosis in a significant minority of patients. This has resulted in the development of a number of new technologies to address some facet of each of the above limitations. One promising new device is the Transluminal Extraction-endarterectomy Catheter (TEC). The device is introduced percutaneously and consists of a flexible torque tube that tracks over a flexible guidewire under standard fluoroscopic guidance. A unique feature of the TEC is the simultaneous application of suction while the conical cutter rotates and removes atheromatous plaque. This reservoir allows for the collection of the excised fragments for later analysis.

Preliminary data suggest that while the TEC can be used for lesions able to be treated with conventional balloon angioplasty devices, it may have special utility in two situations that are not particularly well suited for balloon angioplasty – long diffuse disease and bypass grafts. As a result of the need to compare this new technology to established devices, the TEC Multicenter Registry was formed with the goal of enrolling 317 patients. Core lab evaluation includes determination of absolute dimensions, i.e. lesion length, minimal lumen diameter and average reference diameter as well as conventional parameters such as percent diameter and area stenosis. A particular emphasis of our laboratory has been on the methodology for calibration of images in order to calculate absolute dimensions, as well as determining the role of lesion morphology in choosing new devices. The TEC is a promising new technology which may have special utility in treating long, diffuse disease and bypass grafts, further expanding the realm of interventional cardiology.

J.H.C. Reiber and P.W. Serruys (eds), Advances in Quantitative Coronary Arteriography, 525–533.
© 1993 *Kluwer Academic Publishers. Printed in the Netherlands.*

Introduction

Recent data document a nearly exponential increase in the number of angioplasty (PTCA) procedures being performed from approximately 100,000 in 1985 to 220,000 in 1987 and approximately 300,000 in 1989 in the United States alone. Assuming a conservative 30% restenosis rate, this translates to 30,000 restenosis events occurring in 1985 with an increase to 90,000 restenosis events occurring in 1989. As yet no single approach to this problem has been shown to be effective in preventing its occurrence. While this represents one of the major limitations of PTCA and garners much of the attention of the interventional cardiology world, other problems related to the basic mechanism of balloon dilation limit its usefulness. As a result of the tremendous improvement in dilation catheter technology, crossing of the attempted lesion occurs in excess of 99%. The mechanism of balloon inflation after traversing the lesion and subsequent procedural details remain essentially unchanged since the introduction of the procedure by Gruentzig in 1977 [1]. The mechanism of action involves stretching of the intima and media with an unpredictable degree of plaque fracture. A number of adverse sequelae result from plaque fracture in a significant minority of lesions undergoing PTCA. These include the development of major occlusive events such as abrupt closure in 2–12% of patients, as well as elastic recoil and intimal hyperplasia [2, 3], each of which may also contribute to the multifactorial problem of restenosis. In addition, difficulty in traversing total occlusions remains a major obstacle to the more widespread use of PTCA.

These limitations have resulted in the development of a number of new technologies each designed to address some facet of each of the above problems. The new technologies include intraluminal splints or stents made of a variety of metallic compounds in a number of geometric configurations, and the application of laser energy in a number of ingenious ways including via a hot tip catheter, as well as a balloon dilation catheter that radially directs energy to remodel the intima and media. Atraumatic excision and removal of plaque was hypothesized by John B. Simpson to result in a smoother intraluminal surface with a reduction in the risk of occlusive events and neointimal hyperplasia leading to restenosis [4]. In addition to the Transluminal Extraction-endarterectomy Catheter (TEC^{TM}), 2 other atherectomy catheters are in clinical use – the Simpson Atherocath, a directional coronary atherectomy through which fragments of atheromatous plaque are excised via a cutting edge directed laterally – the Rotablator^{TM}, an oblong metal burr with fine diamond abrasive particles on the distal half of the burr. The burr rotates at approximately 180,000 revolutions per minute over a central guide wire. In contrast to the other atherectomy devices, it emulsifies the plaque material rather than extracting it.

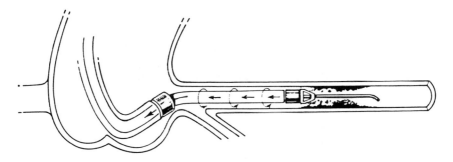

Figure 1. Diagrammatic representation of the transluminal extraction-endarterectomy catheter that has been advanced across an atherosclerotic lesion over a steerable 0.014-inch guide wire. (Reproduced with permission from Am J Cardiol 1988; 62: 3F–24F.)

TEC device: design and procedure

The TEC is an atherectomy device designed by Interventional Technologies, Inc. (San Diego, CA) and developed at Duke University Medical Center. The TEC was designed to take advantage of the many technical improvements made since the introduction of the PTCA technique. The TEC is a wire-based, motor-driven rotating steerable torque tube (1.8 to 2.5 mm in diameter) designed to excise and extract atherosclerotic plaque (Figure 1).

The device is introduced percutaneously via a #10.5 French (F) arterial sheath and is delivered to the coronary artery through a specially designed #10.0 F guide catheter [5, 6]. The catheter tracks over a flexible guidewire (0.014-inch) under standard fluoroscopic guidance. Once radiographic position has been confirmed, a two-stage trigger is activated on the catheter drive unit (Figure 2). The catheter drive unit contains the motor and trigger with attachment sites for a remote battery power source as well as a glass reservoir to capture excised fragments of plaque. The trigger activates the conical cutter head containing two stainless steel blades which rotate at 750 rpm (Figure 3). A unique feature of the TEC is the simultaneous application of vacuum suction and cutter blade rotation.

The device is available in a variety of cutter sizes (#5.5F (1.8 mm), #6F (2.0 mm), #6.5F (2.2 mm), #7F (2.3 mm) and #7.5F (2.5 mm)). This enables the operator to select a smaller cutter size initially to traverse severely stenotic lesions. The use of progressively larger cutter sizes results in maximal increases in luminal diameter. If the procedural result remains unsatisfactory after TEC alone, adjuvant PTCA may be performed. In addition, since the TEC device traverses the lesion for approximately 15 seconds at a time, only minimal interruption of blood flow occurs during therapy, minimizing ischemic injury.

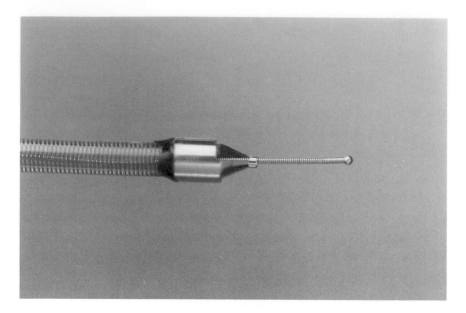

Figure 2. A close-up view of the torque tube and cutter head advanced over a 0.014–inch guide wire. (Reproduced with permission from Health Management Publications, Inc. (J Invas Cardiol 1991; 3: 15.))

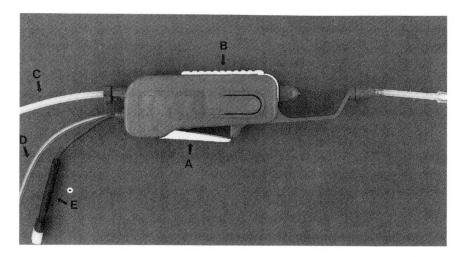

Figure 3. The TEC™ drive unit: (A) trigger, (B) advancement control lever, (C) rear extension tubing, (D) suction tubing, and (E) power connector. (Reproduced with permission from Health Management Publications, Inc. (J Invas Cardiol 1991; 3: 15.))

Historical development

The safety and efficacy of the TEC was tested in both normal arterial segments (human cadaveric and in vivo canine) and atherosclerotic human cadaveric segments. These experimental studies documented that the catheter could easily be maneuvered percutaneously in canine coronary arteries [6]. Histological examination of the normal arterial segments revealed focal intimal disruption limited to 25% of the medial thickness. In atheromatous vessels, TEC atherectomy successfully excised plaque leaving a smooth intraluminal surface with the depth of excision typically limited to the media [5], although occasional disruption of the internal elastic lamina has been noted.

In July, 1988, clinical investigation of the coronary TEC was begun at Duke University Medical Center. After the initial 50 clinical cases, a pilot multicenter study to evaluate the feasibility of using the TEC device was initiated. During this pilot phase, it became apparent that the device may have special utility in two situations that are not particularly well suited for balloon angioplasty – long diffuse disease and bypass grafts.

Procedural outcome after TEC

At the present time, use of the TEC to treat coronary lesions is underway at 19 sites (Duke Medical Center and 18 additional sites) in the United States, with over 900 coronary TEC procedures having been performed to date. As a result of the need to compare this new technology to established devices, the Duke Multicenter Coronary TEC Registry was formed [7] and to date has enrolled 317 patients. Catheter performance is to be evaluated by an angiographic core lab using commercially available hardware and software previously validated at our institution (ADAC Laboratories, Milpitas, CA) [8]. The evaluation process includes determination of absolute dimensions, i.e. lesion length, minimal lumen diameter and average reference diameter as well as conventional parameters such as percent diameter and area stenosis.

Preliminary results from this multicenter registry revealed that TEC was performed on 223 lesions (76 TEC alone and 147 TEC plus adjuvant PTCA) in 201 patients at 5 centers [7] (Table 1). Primary success (< 50% diameter stenosis by quantitative coronary arteriography) was achieved in 94% (130 of 139) native coronary lesions and 98% (82 of 84) vein graft lesions. The mean percent diameter stenosis of 76 ± 12% pre-procedure was reduced to 36 ± 17% in this series, while the minimal luminal diameter increased from 0.7 ± 0.4 mm pre-procedure to 2.0 ± 0.5 mm post-procedure (Table 2).

Follow-up angiography at 6 months post-procedure is an integral part of the Registry protocol. Angiographic follow-up at 6 months was obtained in 95 of 102 eligible patients (93%). Restenosis as defined by the presence of

Table 1. Lesion Distribution in the Duke Multicenter Coronary TEC Registry

Native Coronary Arteries	n	%
Protected Left Main	8	4
Left Anterior Descending Artery	53	24
Circumflex Artery	23	10
Right Coronary Artery	55	25
Procedural Success	130/139	94%
Bypass Grafts	n	%
Saphenous vein Graft	84	38
Procedural Success	82/84	98%

Table 2. Procedural Results Based on the Initial 223 Lesions in the Duke Multicenter Coronary TEC Registry

	Pre-Procedure	Post-Procedure
Diameter Stenosis (%)	76 ± 12	36 ± 17
Minimal Luminal Diameter (mm)	0.7 ± 0.4	2.0 ± 0.5
Restenosis Rate	44%	

>50% diameter stenosis by quantitative coronary arteriography at follow-up was present in 42 of 95 lesions (44%).

In a separate analysis, the preliminary results of the safety and efficacy of TEC in treating saphenous vein graft stenoses was evaluated. TEC was used to treat 98 patients with 125 vein graft lesions. Fully 30% of lesions in this series were considered unsuitable for PTCA secondary to diffuse disease or the presence of intraluminal thrombus [9]. Graft age ranged from 1 to 18 years, with a mean age of 8.8 years. Despite these complicating factors, procedural success remained high at 96% (120 of 125 lesions attempted).

Importance of lesion morphology

The continual evolution of the selection criteria for lesions to undergo TEC has been inexorably tied to a thorough evaluation of lesion morphology. Initially, lesion selection was similar to the original PTCA criteria – proximal, discrete concentric lesions in a nontortuous segment. The present criteria have evolved as a result of considerable operator experience (Table 3). As a result, the majority of lesions treated with the TEC device today would be considered to be unfavorable for conventional PTCA and include many Type C lesions (venous bypass grafts with friable thrombus or long, diffuse (>2 cm) lesions) [10]. The AHA/ACC Committee placed special emphasis on these two descriptors of lesion morphology suggesting that a lower success rate

Table 3. Lesion Exclusion Criteria

Tortuous anatomy proximal to lesion
Major side branch (>2 mm) involvement at target lesion
Severe eccentricity or angulation* of target lesion
Heavily calcified lesion
Total occlusion unable to be recanalized with guidewire
Coronary ectasia
Major dissection**
Severe peripheral disease
Aspirin allergy
Bleeding diathesis, including theombolytic therapy

* Lesions with marked angulation (>45 degrees) should be considered as a contraindication because of the risk of vessel perforation.
** Atherectomy of lesions with major dissections should be avoided secondary to the increased risk of vessel perforation due to pre-existing poor integrity of the vessel wall.

and freedom from adverse events, both acutely and during follow-up might be encountered. While this classification system has been tested for acute outcomes after PTCA [11], no data are available to determine the usefulness of this approach to predict restenosis. A review of available literature suggests that at least for bypass grafts the classification is accurate. In addition, data from the M-HEART Study suggested that increasing lesion length was an important independent predictor of restenosis [12]. This compares favorably with historical controls for both types of lesions, where restenosis rates in excess of 60% have been reported [13]. Many of the lesions attempted with TEC would be considered unsuitable for PTCA based on excessive lesion length rendering comparison of restenosis rates difficult, at best.

An adequate comparison of new technologies cannot occur until stratification of lesions into risk groups (low, medium, high) for adverse events – both short (abrupt closure, major dissection and thrombus formation, fatal and non-fatal myocardial infarction) and long-term (restenosis, need for subsequent revascularization, fatal and non-fatal MI and death). Reporting restenosis results based solely on changes in either absolute dimensions or changes in percent diameter stenosis tell only part of the story. Until data become available detailing outcomes after PTCA or other interventional techniques based on an integrated approach including detailed lesion morphology pre- and post-procedure as well as information regarding the hemodynamic significance of the lesion (minimal luminal diameter, percent stenosis, stenosis flow reserve), adequate comparisons of new interventional techniques and their proper role in therapy cannot be accomplished.

To address these needs, we have developed an integrated approach for the evaluation of all new technologies at our institution involving both quantitative and qualitative descriptors of lesion morphology [14]. The data acquisition system has been called DUQUES – Duke University Quantitative/ Qualitative Evaluation System. The data is entered and manipulated via a graphical user interface with integrated lesion location, detailed lesion morphology and quantitative coronary arteriography. All data entered is stored in a relational database server that is linked to the Duke Databank for Cardiovascular Diseases where extensive clinical, laboratory and procedural data is also stored for subsequent analysis and statistical modeling. It is hoped that analysis of data acquired in this format will lend insights to aid in evaluating the effect of new technologies on post-procedure outcomes.

Conclusion

The experience to date with transluminal extraction-endarterectomy reveals that the device can safely excise atheromatous plaque in a percutaneous fashion with improvement in luminal diameter in the vast majority of patients. At the present time the restenosis rate appears similar to an unstratified group of patients undergoing conventional PTCA. Procedural success remains high despite the inclusion of at least 30% of lesions that would be considered unsuitable for PTCA. At the present time, the maximum cutter size is #7.5 Fr (2.5 mm), necessitating adjuvant PTCA in a number of patients to achieve maximal results in patients with large coronary vessels or in saphenous vein grafts. Current development strategy for the more widespread use of the TEC involves fashioning an expandable cutter as well as an eccentric cutter, to achieve further increases in luminal diameter.

The Transluminal Extraction-Endarterectomy Catheter or TEC is a promising new technology which may have special utility in treating long, diffuse disease and bypass grafts, further expanding the realm of interventional cardiology. At the present time the device is still in its infancy with continually evolving lesion selection criteria. Preliminary data suggest that the device has safety and efficacy rates similar to conventional PTCA.

Acknowledgments

Supported in part by a research grant from the Andrew W. Mellon Foundation, New York, NY

References

1. Gruntzig AR, Senning A, Siegenthaler WE. Nonoperative dilatation of coronary artery stenosis: percutaneous transluminal coronary angioplasty. N Engl J Med 1979; **301**: 61–8.
2. Simpfendorfer C, Belardi J, Bellamy G, Galan K, Franco I, Hollman J. Frequency, management and follow-up of patients with acute coronary occlusions after percutaneous transluminal angioplasty. Am J Cardiol 1987; **59**: 267–9.
3. Califf RM, Ohman EM, Frid D, et al. Restenosis: the clinical issues. In: Topol EJ (Ed.),

Textbook of interventional cardiology. Philadelphia: W. B. Saunders Company 1990: 363–94.

4. Simpson JB. Future interventional techniques. In: Califf RM, Mark DB, Wagner GS (Eds.), Acute coronary care in the thrombolytic era. Chicago: Year Book Medical Publishers 1988: 392–404.

5. Perez JA, Hinohara T, Quigley PJ, et al. In-vitro and in-vivo experimental results using a new wire guided concentric atherectomy device. J Am Coll Cardiol 1988; **11** (Suppl A): 109A (Abstract).

6. Stack RS, Califf RM, Phillips HR, et al. Interventional cardiac catheterization at Duke Medical Center. Am J Cardiol 1988; **62**: 3F–24F.

7. Sketch MH Jr, O'Neill WW, Galichia JP, et al. The Duke Multicenter Coronary Transluminal Extraction-Endarterectomy Registry: acute and chronic results. J Am Coll Cardiol 1991: **17** (Suppl A): 31A (Abstract).

8. Skelton TN, Kisslo KB, Mikat EM, Bashore TM. Accuracy of digital angiography for quantitation of normal coronary luminal segments in excised, perfused hearts. Am J Cardiol 1987; **59**: 1261–5.

9. O'Neill WW, Meany TB, Kramer B, et al. The role of atherectomy in the management of saphenous vein grafts disease. J Am Coll Cardiol 1991; **17** (Suppl A): 384A (Abstract).

10. Guidelines for percutaneous transluminal coronary angioplasty. A report of the American College of Cardiology/American Heart Association Task Force on Assessment of Diagnostic and Therapeutic Cardiovascular Procedures (Subcommittee on Percutaneous Transluminal Coronary Angioplasty). J Am Coll Cardiol 1988; **12**: 529–45.

11. Ellis SG, Vandormael MG, Cowley MJ, et al. Coronary morphologic and clinical determinants of procedural outcome with angioplasty for multivessel coronary disease: Implications for patient selection. Multivessel Prognosis Study Group. Circulation 1990; **82**: 1193–1202. Comment in: Circulation 1990; **82**: 1516–8.

12. Pepine CJ, Hirshfeld JW, Macdonald RG, et al. A controlled trial of corticosteroids to prevent restenosis after coronary angioplasty. M-Heart Group. Circulation 1990; **81**: 1753–61.

13. Douglas JS Jr. Angioplasty of saphenous vein and internal mammary artery bypass grafts. In: Topol EJ (Ed.), Textbook of interventional cardiology. Philadelphia: W. B. Saunders Company 1990: 327–43.

14. Spero LA, Hanemann JD, Cusma JT, Fortin DF, Bashore TM. A multiuser networked system for the large scale study of coronary restenosis using quantitative and qualitative coronary angiography. Comput Cardiol 1991: 195–8.

PART EIGHT

QCA and intracoronary prostheses

33. An experimental cardiologist's view on coronary stents

WILLEM J. VAN DER GIESSEN, HELEEN M.M. VAN
BEUSEKOM, CORNELIS J. SLAGER, JOHAN C.H.
SCHUURBIERS and PIETER D. VERDOUW

Summary

Currently four metallic coronary stent devices are undergoing clinical investigation. At least three other permanent and two temporary stent devices are under experimental evaluation. Results from experimental studies with the Wallstent™, the Palmaz-Schatz Coronary Stent™, the Gianturco-Roubin Coronary Flex-Stent™, and the Wiktor™ Coronary Stent, and preliminary clinical results indicate that neither of them fulfills all requirements for an ideal intravascular support device. All have not only been proven to be thrombogenic, but also show significant neointimal hyperplasia, eventually resulting in angiographically or clinically demonstrable restenosis in 15 to 35% of the lesions treated with these devices.

We conclude that this first generation of metallic coronary stents will most likely be replaced by devices which are more resistant to thrombosis, and are at least as tissue compatible as stainless steel stents. Devices constructed of non-metal materials, such as synthetic polymers, may offer an attractive alternative.

Introduction

One of the first reports in the literature describing an endovascular splinting device was published in 1912 [1]. The author Alexis Carrel, a French surgeon, sociologist and biologist, described the implantation of aluminium endoluminal tubes in the thoracic aorta of dogs. In the year of publication Carrel received the Nobel prize for Physiology or Medicine for developing a method of suturing blood vessels, but this did not result in an increased interest in endoluminal prostheses, since it was not until 1969 that Charles Dotter reported his experiments with a stainless steel spiral tube graft [2]. The valiant work by the groups in Lausanne, Switzerland, and Toulouse, France, resulted in 1987 in the publication by Sigwart, Puel and co-workers, who described the first stent implantations in human coronary arteries [3]. Since

J.H.C. Reiber and P.W. Serruys (eds), Advances in Quantitative Coronary Arteriography, 537–552.
© 1993 *Kluwer Academic Publishers. Printed in the Netherlands.*

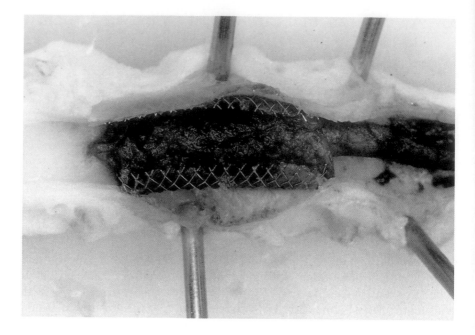

Figure 1. Macroscopic specimen showing a massive, white platelet-rich thrombus, which occludes a stainless steel Wallstent within 24 hours after implantation.

then, several metallic stent devices have entered the stage of clinical evaluation [4–7].

These first clinical reports describing the multicenter experience with stents, unfortunately show that these metallic stents are thrombogenic, resulting in acute or subacute thrombotic occlusion (Figure 1), or serious bleeding complications due to the requirement of an extensive anticoagulant and antithrombotic regimen. Subsequently, experience in hundreds of patients has taught the investigators to optimize the anticoagulant treatment. This learning curve, combined with the proper use of haemostasis parameters [8, 9], substantially decreased the number of thrombotic occlusions. On the other hand, using stents for bale-out indications, like acute occlusion after PTCA, will increase the demands for blood compatibility already made on these devices. A randomized trial studying the value of the Gianturco-Roubin stent for the bale-out indication has recently started.

Controlled clinical studies evaluating restenosis rates after stenting and those after balloon angioplasty alone are not yet available. At this moment we can only relate the restenosis rates after stent implantation with historic controls or angiographically matched clinical cases. Preliminary results indicate that restenosis rates in patients with stents are some 10 to 15 percent lower than in patients who underwent only PTCA. More reliable data ob-

Table 1. Biomaterial surface modification techniques*

I. Physicochemical
    a. physical deposition of coating (*polyurethane*)
    b. chemical modification (*PEO, -OH blocking*)
    c. graft copolymerization (*hydrogels*)
    d. plasma gas discharge (*silanes, fluorocarbons*)

II. Biological
    a. presorption of proteins (*albumin, fibronectin*)
    b. drug-, enzyme immobilization (*heparin, hirudin*)
    c. cell seeding (*endothelial cells*)
    d. preclotting (*fresh whole blood*)

* Modified from Hoffman, 1987 [10].

tained by randomized trials, as initiated for the Palmaz-Schatz stent, have to be awaited.

A third, potential application of vascular endoprostheses is using stents as vehicles for local drug delivery.

Towards less thrombogenic stents

Most manufacturers of coronary stents have been attempting to produce less thrombogenic stents by applying an active or passive coating to the stent filaments. Generally, any biomaterial surface can be modified using either physicochemical or biological techniques (Table 1). Physicochemical techniques deposit a passive polymer coating [11, 12], or change the composition of a thin layer at the surface of the biomaterial by binding biocompatible chemical groups. Biological techniques aim to interfere with the initial biomaterial-blood interaction. This can be done in a passive way, by presorption of bland biopolymers like albumin or preclotting grafts with whole blood. Biologically active techniques use drug or enzyme immobilization, either directly on the biomaterial surface [13] or incorporated in a thin polymer layer. Seeding unaltered or genetically engineered endothelial cells on the biomaterial surface provides an alternative approach [14, 15]. The full potential of these biological techniques has not yet been reached. For instance, it is very likely that a considerable number of the covering cells detach from a cell-seeded stent during placement or in the first seconds of contact with flowing blood. Furthermore, probably only that side of the balloon-expandable stent which is in contact with the vessel wall, and not the luminal side can be seeded.

The most promising approach appears to be the construction of pure polymer stents. At least for the bale-out indication where intimal flaps and/or mural thrombus are involved, stents have to be structurally stable for hours to days. Polymers are an inexhaustible source of materials combining blood

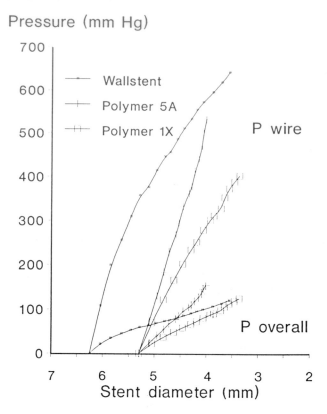

Figure 2. Pressure-diameter relation of stainless steel (Wallstent) and two polymer (polyethenet-erephthalate) stents. Note the steep buildup of pressure during only minor changes in the diameter of all three stents. P overall: actually measured overall pressure buildup; P wire: calculated values derived from correcting the P overall for actual wire-open space relation.

compatibility and high stiffness. Figure 2 illustrates that by reducing the diameter of the unconstrained Wallstent from 6.2 to 5 mm, a global pressure of about 75 mmHg is exerted. Expressing this pressure after correction for the actual surface area of a single wire, because of the open weave structure of the stent, this yields a local pressure of more than 400 mmHg. The curves for both polymers in this figure show that polymer stents can be constructed with at least the same radial force as stainless steel stents. Subtle changes in the mechanical behavior of polymer stents can be introduced by modifications in the heat setting process. Preliminary results of implanted polyester stents in porcine peripheral arteries in our institution, show that these polymer stents combine good blood compatibility with favorable mechanical properties (Figure 3).

Specifically for the treatment or prevention of acute complications during balloon angioplasty permanent metallic or polymer or biodegradable polymer

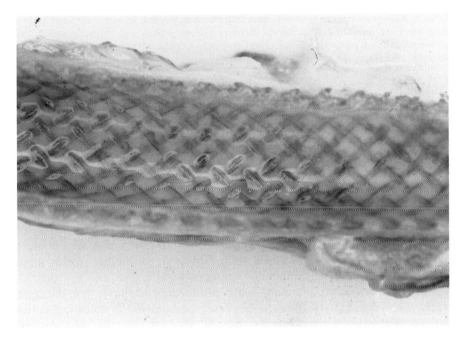

Figure 3. Macroscopic specimen of a polymeric (PETP) stent four weeks after implantation in a normal femoral artery of the pig.

stents have to compete with either the perfusion balloon or temporary stents [16–18]. Temporary stent catheters may allow better perfusion when placed in the coronary artery as compared to autoperfusion balloons [17]. On the other hand first generation temporary stents proved to be thrombogenic, especially in smaller sized (< 2 mm) arteries. Recently designed temporary stent catheters with a more open structure, exerted insufficient radial force to overcome focal vasoconstriction. However, the attractive idea behind temporary stenting warrants further evaluation.

Stents for the prevention of restenosis

Although studies evaluating new devices for coronary recanalization are uncontrolled, they suggest that restenosis rates after stent implantation are lower than with all other devices (Table 2). Although randomized clinical trials comparing the several techniques in the same patient population have to be awaited, it is tempting to speculate about the causes of the observed differences. A likely explanation is that some devices result in more damage to the arterial wall than others. This hypothesis has been tested in an experimental model [19], in which the amount of neointimal hyperplasia post-

Table 2. Restenosis rates at 6 months after different interventions in native coronary arteries. Data are from uncontrolled studies in different patient groups and originate mainly from presentations at international meetings (1991 American College of Cardiology Annual Scientific Sessions, 1991 European Congress of Cardiology)

Balloon angioplasty	27.5% (recent 48–52%)
Excimer laser	51% (N = 1400)
Directional atherectomy	36% (N = 721)
Rotational ablation	32% (N = 316)
Transluminal extraction	46% (N = 293)
Stent (Palmaz-Schatz)	19% (N = 191)
Stent (Wallstent)	19% (N = 265)
Stent (Wiktor)	20% (N = 95)
Laser balloon (Spears)	64% (N = 243)

stenting correlated with a scoring system describing the cumulated injury to the individual layers of the vessel wall. However, variability in this model was large when histological damage was considerable.

If damage is the predominant factor producing restenosis, less damaging methods of angioplasty have to be developed. Using a so-called cutting balloon, Forrester and colleagues recently showed that the reparative response after balloon angioplasty can be favorably influenced in normal peripheral arteries of pigs [20]. However, local vessel wall or intralesion characteristics have also to be taken into account, but this may prove to be extremely difficult, as even the histological features of normal coronary arteries are considerably different at their proximal and distal parts. For instance, the main stem is an elastic artery (Figure 4a), while a few tenth of a millimeter downstream in the proximal LAD, the amount of elastic tissue diminishes sharply. The arterial media contains only 5–10 layers of elastin at its origen from the mainstem (Figure 4b), while before the septal branch, this artery has become muscular in type, containing only three elastin layers (Figure 4c). So within the length of an angioplasty balloon or a stent device, an essentially elastic artery changes gradually into a muscular artery. In diseased human vessels intralesion morphology may vary considerably more. Figure 5a demonstrates this within a section of a human atherosclerotic coronary artery: a thinned media, and opposite to that an eccentric lesion containing calcified areas, and soft lipid-rich areas all covered with a fibrotic cap of variable thickness. If we apply considerable radial force within this segment by inflating a balloon or deploying a stent, the impact of the trauma will be very different for those several regions. The same phenomenon can also be found at the anastomosis sites of aortocoronary bypass grafts (Figure 5b). The different compliance of arteries and veins, and the firm fibrous tissue which has replaced normal vessel wall structures, will inevitably result in an uneven distribution of wall stress after applying radial force.

The employment of polymer stents may form a means to reduce acute vessel wall damage, because of a slower buildup of radial force. At variance

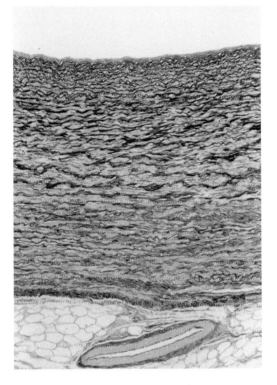

Figure 4(a).

Figure 4. Photomicrograph showing an elastin stain of a normal main stem of Göttingen minipig. Note the abundance of elastic lamellae in black (magnification 100×). b) Left anterior descending coronary artery (LAD) a few micrometers distal to the bifurcation from the main stem (magnification 200×). c) Proximal LAD approximately 1 mm distal to picture 4b (magnification 200×).

with stainless steel stents, self-expanding polymer stents will not immediately return to their unconstrained diameters after release from their delivery catheter (Figure 6). Considerable variation in this hysteresis-like behavior exists between a polyester stent and a polyester/polyether copolymer device. Although the ultimate radial force of polyester stents is in the same range as of metal stents (Figure 2), the slower buildup of radial force may allow a softer settling of the polymer stent with less acute trauma (Figure 7a vs 7b).

A potential problem when using biodegradable polymer stents may be the bioabsorption process itself, as most polymers will be hydrolysed and subsequently removed by macrophages. The latter may also convert into foam cells and create new atherosclerotic lesions. A foreign body reaction per se will not be an objection to the introduction of bioabsorbable material

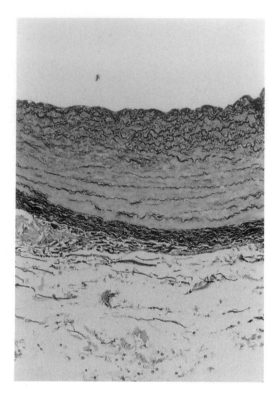

Figure 4(b).

in the coronary arteries, as signs of the former have also been observed after placement of metal and non-absorbable polymer stents (Figure 8a, b).

Stents as vehicle for local drug delivery

One of the most exciting, applications of coronary stents is their potential to act as a carrier of pharmacological agents, normal endothelial cells or genetically engineered cells [14, 15]. Stents constructed from a variety of materials, including stainless steel, can be used for the transmission of specific cells to the site of a lesion in a coronary artery (Figure 9). The practical problem remains that balloon expandable stents can only be seeded on their abluminal side and cell-seeding of this type of stents to enhance endothelialization will therefore be limited. It is also not known whether seeded/cells remain viable after stent implantation. Especially by using genetically engineered cells a variety of endogenous peptides interfering with the process of restenosis can be administered locally at any selected site.

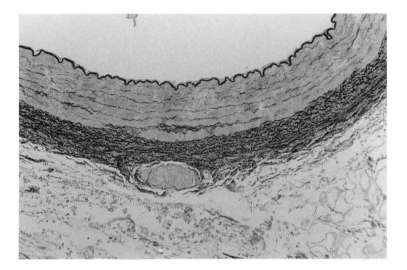

Figure 4(c).

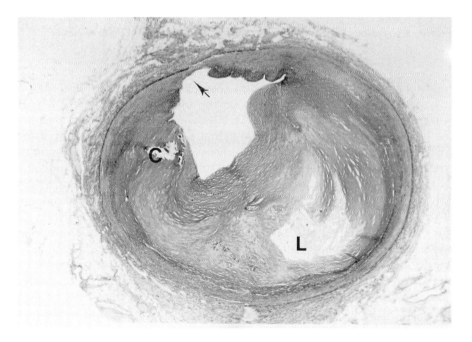

Figure 5a. Photomicrograph showing an elastin stain of human coronary artery. The very thin media (arrowhead) is probably the remnant of an ulceration. Within the eccentric atherosclerotic lesion a distinct calcification (c) and a large lipid core (l) can be seen (magnification 20×).

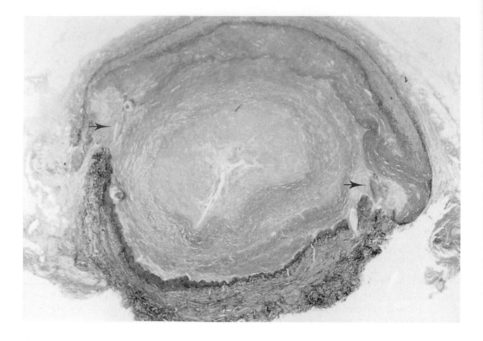

Figure 5b. Photomicrograph (magnification 20×), showing an elastin stain of an anastomosis site of a human saphenous vein aortacoronary bypass graft with the left anterior descending coronary artery. Note the lack of normal vessel wall architecture at the suture sites (arrows).

Metal stents are probably not attractive for the local delivery of drugs or enzymes, although favorable results on the blood compatibility of heparin bonded stents have been reported [13]. However, it is very difficult to control the release of the heparin from its binding sites. Drug binding of polymer coated stents appears to be a more attractive alternative. Depending on the type of polymer the drug can be diluted, absorbed, adsorbed or bonded to its inner or outer surface [21]. One of the theoretical objections against polymer-coated stents as drug vehicle is that only relatively small amounts of drug can be carried. Potentially, stents consisting of merely polymer can carry not only a larger amount of a drug, but even several different drugs, which can be released locally at different rates and with different time intervals. The polymer technology to realize this rather futuristic outlook is already available. However, implementation of this technology in invasive cardiology may take some time. If this can be achieved, stents may prove to be ideal carriers for not only spatial but also temporal drug delivery in potentially all the tubular systems of the body.

Candidate drugs for local delivery can already be selected and tested in animal models of restenosis using microporous balloon catheters [22]. We believe that stents may prove superior carriers compared to microporous

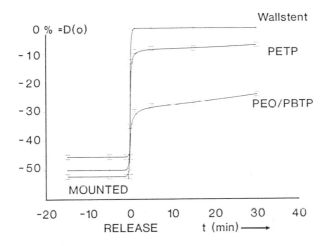

Figure 6. Percentage change in stent diameter from unconstrained diameter (D0) of three different stents. Mounting these stents on a delivery system reduces their diameter to about 50%. Subsequent release causes the Wallstent to regain its original diameter immediately. The polyester stent looses 10% of its original diameter immediately and 8% after 30 minutes. The biodegradable copolymer looses an immediate 35% at release to end up with 25% reduction in diameter after 30 minutes.

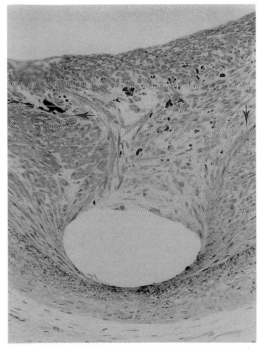

Figure 7a. Photomicrograph showing a toluidine blue stain of a porcine LAD four weeks after implantation of a tantalum Wiktor stent. Note that the stent has ruptured the internal elastic lamina (arrow) and virtually rests on the external elastic lamina (magnification 200×).

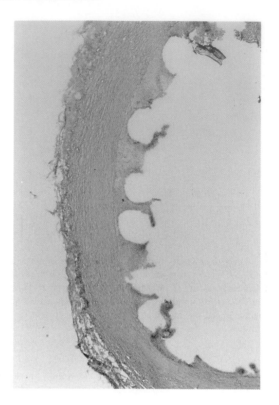

Figure 7b. Photomicrograph of a porcine femoral artery four weeks after implantation of a polyester stent. Note that there are no signs of medial compression (magnification 40×, haematoxylin azafloxine stain).

balloons or permeable balloons, as microporous balloons are yet not suitable for temporal drug delivery, exact dosing is still unreliable, and, especially at high inflation pressures, are potentially damaging to the arterial wall (unpublished observations).

Several other alternative local treatment modalities are now under investigation. For instance, the local application of drugs contained within albumin microspheres [23], or bioactive capsules such as liposomes [24], permeabilised and resealed platelets [25] or red cell ghosts [26] have been reported. Another exciting development is the local transduction of endothelial and vascular smooth muscle cells, achieved by direct retroviral infection or liposome-mediated recombinant DNA transfection, resulting in site-specific gene expression [27].

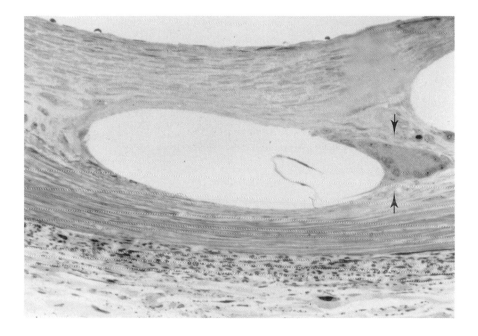

Figure 8a. Photomicrograph of a porcine coronary artery three months after implantation of a stainless steel Wallstent. Note the multinucleated giant cell (between arrows) next to the void formerly occupied by the stent filaments (magnification 400×, stain toluidine blue).

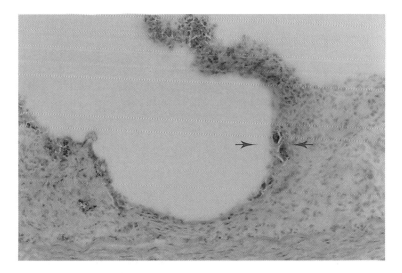

Figure 8b. Photomicrograph of a porcine femoral artery four weeks after implantation of a polyester stent. Note the two giant cells (arrow) next to one of the stent wire voids (magnification 320×, stain haematoxylin azafloxine).

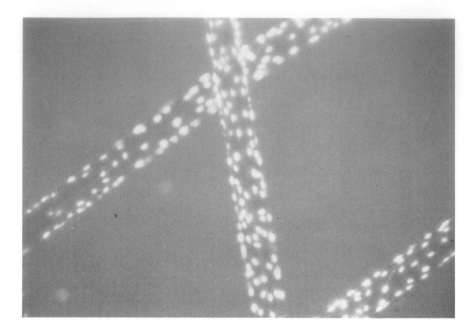

Figure 9. Detail of Wallstent showing wires covered with seeded endothelial cells obtained from human umbilical cord vein. The nuclei of the endothelial cells (white dots) are marked by a vital DNA stain.

Conclusion

Results from experimental studies with the Wallstent™, the Palmaz-Schatz Coronary Stent™, the Gianturco-Roubin Coronary Flex-Stent™, and the Wiktor™ Coronary Stent, and preliminary clinical results indicate that neither of them fulfills all requirements for an ideal intravascular support device. This first generation of metallic coronary stents will most likely be replaced by devices which are better resistant to thrombosis, and are at least as tissue compatible as stainless steel stents. Devices constructed of non-metal materials, such as synthetic polymers, may offer an attractive alternative.

Acknowledgments

Supported in part by grant nr. 88–077 from The Netherlands Heart Foundation

References

1. Carrel A. Results of the permanent intubation of the thoracic aorta. Surg Gynecol Obstet 1912; **15**: 245–8.
2. Dotter CT. Transluminally-placed coilspring endarterial tube grafts. Long-term patency in the canine popliteal artery. Invest Radiol 1969; **4**: 329–32.
3. Sigwart U, Puel J, Mirkovitch V, Joffre F, Kappenberger L. Intravascular stents to prevent occlusion and restenosis after transluminal angioplasty. N Engl J Med 1987; **316**: 701–6.
4. Serruys PW, Strauss BH, Beatt KJ, et al. Angiographic follow-up after placement of a self-expanding coronary-artery stent. N Engl J Med 1991; **324**: 13–7. Comment in: N Eng J Med 1991; **324**: 52–3.
5. Schatz RA, Baim DS, Leon M, et al. Clinical experience with the Palmaz-Schatz coronary stent. Initial results of a multicenter study. Circulation 1991; **83**: 148–61.
6. De Jaegere PP, Serruys PW, Bertrand ME, et al. Wiktor stent implantation in patients with restenosis following balloon angioplasty of a native coronary artery lesion. Am J Cardiol. 1992; **69**: 598–602.
7. Roubin GS, Hearn JA, Carlin SF, Lembo NJ, Douglas JS Jr, King SB 3rd. Angiographic and clinical follow-up in patients receiving a balloon expandable, stainless steel, stent (Cook, Inc.) for prevention or treatment of acute closure after PTCA. Circulation 1990; **82** (4 Suppl III): III–191 (Abstract).
8. Haude M, Erbel R, Straub U, Steffen W, Swars H, Meyer J. Subacute thrombotic occlusions after intracoronary implantation of Palmaz-Schatz stents: acute management and long-term outcome. Eur Heart J 1991; **12** (Abstract Suppl): 166 (Abstract).
9. Swars H, Hafner G, Erbel R, Ehrenthal W, Prellwitz W, Meyer J. Prothrombin fragment F1 + 2: early sign of subacute thrombotic occlusion after coronary stent implantation. Eur Heart J 1991; **12** (Abstract Suppl): 166 (Abstract).
10. Hoffman AS. Modification of material surfaces to affect how they interact with blood. Ann N Y Acad Sci 1987; **516**: 96–101.
11. Van der Giessen WJ, Strauss BH, Van Beusekom HM, Van Loon H, Van Woerkens LJ. Self-expandable mesh stents: an experimental study comparing polymer coated and un-coated Wallstent stents in the coronary circulation of pigs. Circulation 1990; **82** (4 Suppl III): III–542 (Abstract).
12. Bailey SR, Guy DM, Garcia OJ, Paige S, Palmaz JC, Miller DD. Polymer coating of Palmaz-Schatz stent attenuates vascular spasm after stent placement. Circulation 1990; **82** (4 Suppl III): III–541 (Abstract).
13. Cavender JB, Anderson P, Roubin GS. The effects of heparin bonded tantalum stents on thrombosis and neointimal proliferation. Circulation 1990; **82** (4 Suppl III): III–541 (Abstract).
14. Van der Giessen WJ, Serruys PW, Visser WJ, Verdouw PD, Schalkwijk WP, Jongkind JF. Endothelialization of intravascular stents. J Intervent Cardiol 1988; **1**: 109–20.
15. Dichek DA, Neville RF, Zwiebel JA, Freeman SM, Leon MB, Anderson WF. Seeding of intravascular stents with genetically engineered endothelial cells. Circulation 1989; **80**: 1347–53. Comment in: Circulation 1989; **80**: 1495–6.
16. Gaspard P, Didier B, Delsanti G, Gallice G, Frieh JP. Temporary stenting: a new method for treatment of coronary artery dissection during coronary angioplasty. Eur Heart J 1989; **10** (Abstract Suppl): 409 (Abstract).
17. Muller DW, White CJ, Friedman HZ, Willard L, Topol EJ. Temporary coronary "splinting" for abrupt closure post-PTCA: initial in vivo studies. J Am Coll Cardiol 1991; **17** (2 Suppl A): 235A (Abstract).
18. Didier BP, Gaspard PE, Lienhart YA, Frieh JP. Emergency temporary stenting for acute occlusion during PTCA: immediate and mid term results. J Am Coll Cardiol 1991; **17** (2 Suppl A): 302A (Abstract).
19. Schwartz RS, Murphy JG, Edwards WD, Camrud AR, Vlietstra RE, Holmes DR. Re-

stenosis after balloon angioplasty: a practical proliferative model in porcine coronary arteries. Circulation 1990; **82**: 2190–200.

20. Barath P, Fishbein M, Vari S, Yao F, Forrester J. Endovascular incisions with a novel device: a new approach to angioplasty. J Am Coll Cardiol 1991; **17** (2 Suppl A): 235A (Abstract).

21. Hrushesky WJ, Langer R, Theeuwes F (Eds.), Temporal control of drug delivery. New York: New York Academy of Sciences 1991.

22. Wolinsky H, Thung SN. Use of a perforated balloon catheter to deliver concentrated heparin into the wall of the normal canine artery. J Am Coll Cardiol 1990; **15**: 475–81.

23. Spears JR, Kundu SK, McMath LP. Laser balloon angioplasty: potential for reduction of the thrombogenicity of the injured arterial wall and for local application of bioprotective materials. J Am Coll Cardiol 1991; **17** (6 Suppl B): 179B–88B.

24. Allen TM, Hansen C, Rutledge J. Liposomes with prolonged circulation times: factors affecting uptake by reticuloendothelial and other tissues. Biochim Biophys Acta 1989; **981**: 27–35.

25. Hughes K, Crawford N. Reversible electropermeabilisation of human and rat blood platelets: evaluation of morphological and functional integrity "in vitro" and "in vivo". Biochim Biophys Acta 1989; **981**: 277–87.

26. Zimmermann U, Riemann F, Pilwat G. Enzyme loading of electronically homogeneous human red blood cell ghosts prepared by dielectric breakdown. Biochim Biophys Acta 1976; **436**: 460–74.

27. Nabel EG, Plautz G, Nabel GJ. Site-specific gene expression in vivo by direct gene transfer into the arterial wall. Science 1990; **249**: 1285–8.

34. The Palmaz-Schatz™ stent

DAVID L. FISCHMAN, MICHAEL P. SAVAGE, STEPHEN ELLIS,
DONALD S. BAIM, RICHARD A. SCHATZ, MARTIN B. LEON and
SHELDON GOLDBERG

Summary

Our experience indicates that stenting provides an intravascular scaffold which is effective in resolving intimal dissection, which may develop after standard PTCA. If the subacute thrombosis rate can be controlled, the stent may prove beneficial in the management of patients with suboptimal PTCA results.

Concerning restenosis, the data indicate there may be a reduction in certain patient subgroups, i.e. when a single stent is placed for a de novo lesion. However, analysis of the results of our prospective randomized trial will be necessary to assess the true efficacy of stenting in the prevention of restenosis.

Introduction

The concept of intravascular stenting was put forth even before Gruentzig's description of nonsurgical balloon recanalization of obstructed coronary arteries. Charles Dotter, in 1964, advocated the use of intravascular splints to preserve luminal patency of peripheral arteries [1]. He later developed a coil spring prosthesis, and described the results of canine experiments with the use of the coil stent in popliteal arteries [2]. Although there was reasonable long-term patency, the idea of stenting did not progress in an important way in the clinical setting. This was due to the bulky design of the early devices, along with problems of unpredictable expansion, stent migration due to stent-vessel mismatch, and stent thrombosis. After more than a decade of experience with the benefits and limitations of standard balloon angioplasty, there has been a resurgence of interest in the concept of placing a permanent intravascular "scaffold" to both optimize and improve on the initial results of standard percutaneous coronary angioplasty and also to ameliorate the stubborn problem of coronary restenosis [3].

The purpose of this report is to review preliminary data generated from

J.H.C. Reiber and P.W. Serruys (eds), Advances in Quantitative Coronary Arteriography, 553–566.

a central core angiographic facility of the results with the use of one type of permanent intravascular implant, the Palmaz-Schatz™ balloon expandable stent in the coronary circulation.

Description of core laboratory

The stent investigators agreed to establish a core angiographic laboratory at the Thomas Jefferson University Hospital in Philadelphia, PA. A list of the participating investigators along with their institutional affiliation is shown in the appendix. All cineangiograms from patients undergoing stent implantation are sent to the core facility for both qualitative and quantitative assessment. An angiographic manual has been developed for the individual investigators to assist in optimizing the quality of the studies so that accurate determinations of outcome can be made. A panel of two to three experienced observers review the baseline, post-PTCA, post-stent, and six- and twelve-month follow-up films. Detailed morphologic analysis of the cineangiograms includes assessment of lesion and vessel related variables known to affect the outcome of PTCA. These include lesion eccentricity, calcification, plaque ulceration and complexity, location on a bend $\geq 45°$, presence of thrombus, vessel tortuosity, and diffuse disease.

Appropriate cineframes are selected for quantitative coronary angiographic analyses. Frames from paired orthogonal views where available are acquired via a television camera mounted on a 35 mm cineviewer (GE, Caps 35 projector). The video signal is then digitized at $512 \times 512 \times 8$ bit resolution onto a digital angiographic computer (ADAC Laboratories, Model DPS-4100). The images are magnified fourfold using bilinear interpolation. After the region of interest is identified by the operator, an automatic edge detection algorithm is used to determine the arterial contour by assessing the brightness along scan lines which are perpendicular to the centerline of the artery [4, 5] (Figure 1). Absolute measurements are determined by using the coronary catheter as a scaling device. To obtain an accurate scaling factor, the catheter is filmed as close to the center of the magnified image field as possible so that pincushion distortion is minimized. Large lumen catheters ≥ 7 French are used to assure adequate vessel opacification. Adequate contrast injection to opacify the vessel for at least one cycle allows for analysis of the coronary segment at end diastole. This reduces artefact due to cardiac motion and eliminates variation in arterial diameter secondary to change in arterial pressure. Angiographic angles are selected so that the stented vessel is optimally visualized. These angles are precisely duplicated for the follow-up films. The quantitative measurements include stenosis length and diameter. Proximal and distal segments considered to be free of coronary disease and outside the stented segment are selected and averaged; the average value is considered to represent the "normal reference" diameter which is used to calculate the percent diameter stenosis. The validity of this quantitative technique has been confirmed by the use of phantom models and patient

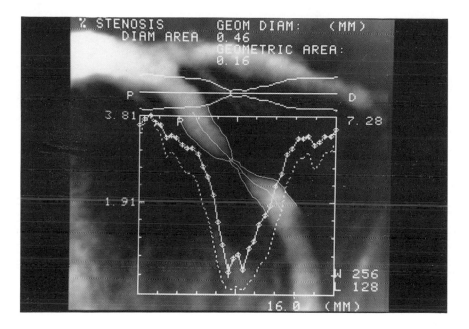

Figure 1. Illustration of automatic edge detection method used by core laboratory. The arterial contour is determined by assessing brightness along scan lines perpendicular to the centerline of the artery.

studies. Accordingly, a series of precision-drilled plexiglass models of vessel stenosis along with contrast-filled coronary catheters were filmed at 30 fps over the left thorax. There was excellent correlation between quantitative angiography and actual measurements ($r = 0.98$) (Figure 2). We have established that the intraobserver variability for repeated measurements of patient cineangiograms is 0.16 mm for absolute diameter and $<5\%$ for percent diameter stenosis.

Description of Palmaz-Schatz™ stent

The Palmaz-Schatz™ stent is constructed of stainless steel and consists of two 7.0 mm rigid, slotted tubes which are joined by a central bridging strut [6] (Figure 3). The stent is balloon expandable; it has a diameter of 1.6 mm in the unexpanded state and is 15 mm in length; when the appropriately-sized balloon is inflated, the stent struts take on a diamond-shaped configuration which is associated with a high free space to metal mass ratio, a factor which is believed to be responsible in part for the relatively low thrombosis rate. The articulation point of the stent gives the device longitudinal flexibility so that the balloon-stent assembly can negotiate bends in the coronary ves-

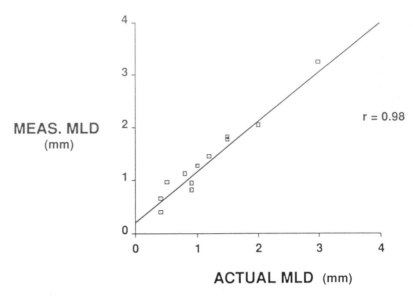

Figure 2. Correlation of measured minimal lumen diameter (MLD) and actual MLD using contrast-filled phantom models of arterial stenoses.

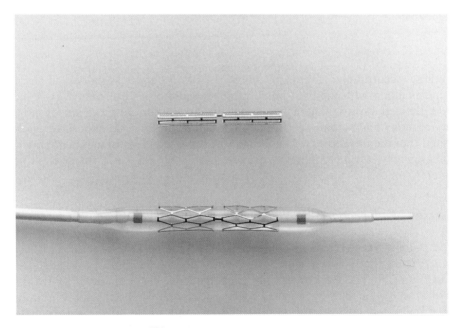

Figure 3. The Palmaz-Schatz^TM balloon expandable stent. The stent consists of two stainless steel slotted tubes connected by a central bridging strut. The stent is 15 mm in length and the unexpanded diameter is 1.6 mm. In the expanded state, the struts take on a diamond configuration with a high free space to metal ratio.

Table 1. Inclusion and Exclusion Criteria

Inclusions
Objective evidence of myocardial ischemia
Critical stenoses ⩾70%
Left ventricular ejection fraction ⩾40%
Suitability for coronary artery bypass graft surgery

Exclusions
Presence of bleeding diathesis
Recent acute myocardial infarction ⩽7 days
Diffuse distal disease – poor stent outflow
Ostial stenoses
Large, diseased side branches
Preexistent intracoronary thrombi
Lesion length greater than length of stent (15 mm)
Unprotected left main coronary artery stenoses
Extreme vessel tortuosity

sels. The stent is delivered by means of a sheath system which is designed to aid in delivery and prevent proximal deployment and stent embolization.

Patient selection criteria

The current criteria for patient selection and exclusion are shown in Table 1. These criteria represent an evolution in thinking as the clinical results of the study became available. At present, patients with objective evidence of myocardial ischemia who have discrete, critical stenoses, preserved left ventricular function and are suitable for coronary artery bypass graft surgery are candidates for stenting. Conversely, we exclude patients with bleeding diatheses, because of the required anticoagulation regimen. Importantly, patients with recent acute myocardial infarction and those with unstable angina with a significant amount of intracoronary thrombus are not offered this device. In addition, patients with diffuse distal disease which would result in reduced stent outflow, and those patients with ostial stenoses, large diseased side branches, long lesions (>15 mm), unprotected left main stenoses and extreme vessel tortuosity are also excluded.

Medication protocol

A very intense pharmacologic protocol is necessary in order to minimize the risks of stent thrombosis. Accordingly, ASA 325 mg and dipyridamole 75 mg tid, as well as a calcium antagonist are started 24–48 hours prior to the procedure; low molecular weight dextran 40 is given at 50–100 cc/hr beginning 3 hours prior to stenting and continued intraprocedurally and afterwards for a total dose of 1 liter. Heparin 10,000 units is given as a bolus after the sheaths are placed; additional heparin is administered as necessary and

Table 2. Pharmacologic Protocol

A.	Prior to procedure	
	aspirin 325 mg per day	
	dipyridamole 75 mg tid	
	calcium antagonist	
	low molecular weight dextran 40; 100 ml/hr	
B.	During procedure:	
	heparin 10,000 units intravenously + infusion	
	low molecular weight dextran	
C.	After procedure:	
	heparin	until PT $\geq$ 16 seconds
	warfarin	1 month
	aspirin	indefinite
	dipyridamole	3 months
	calcium antagonist	3 months

monitored by frequent checks of the activated clotting time (ACT); we aim for an ACT > 300 s during the procedure. We allow the heparin to wear off after the procedure, and remove the vascular sheaths when the ACT has dropped below 180 seconds. This is done while the LMW Dextran 40 is still being infused. Warfarin is begun on the day of the procedure; heparin is restarted several hours after sheath removal and continued until the warfarin has caused the prothrombin time to be stable in the 16–18 second range. Warfarin is continued for 1 month and dipyridamole for 3 months. Aspirin is continued indefinitely. The medication protocol is summarized in Table 2.

Clinical results with the Palmaz-Schatz™ stent

Efficacy of stenting in reducing intimal dissection

The investigators were interested in the effect of the stent on intimal dissection following balloon angioplasty and accordingly qualitative and quantitative analyses were performed on 87 lesions in 75 patients [7]. The baseline arteriograms, the immediate post-PTCA angiograms and the film after stent implantation were analyzed. The degree of intimal disruption was graded by the following definitions: grade 0– no dissection; grade 1– a simple dissection which consisted of a linear defect or extraluminal dye extravasation forming a "cap;" grade 2– a complex dissection, which was a nonlinear spiral tear or a luminal defect with multiple irregular borders. Quantitative analysis of the digitized cineangiograms was performed as described above. A total of 99 stents were placed for 87 lesions with a range of 1–6 stents per patient. The mean reference vessel diameter was 3.2 ± 0.5 mm with a range of 2.3 to 4.4 mm. The mean lesion length was 8.6 ± 5.0 mm with a range of 1.9 to

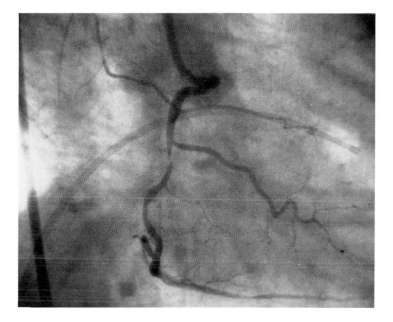

Figure 4(a).

32.7 mm. The distribution of vessels stented was the right coronary artery in 48, the left anterior descending in 31, and the left circumflex in eight. Intimal dissection occurred in 32 of 87 lesions (37%) following conventional balloon angioplasty. Of the 32 dissections, 20 (63%) were simple and 12 (37%) were complex. An example of the efficacy of the Palmaz-Schatz™ stent on resolving intimal tears is shown in Figure 4. Eighteen of 20 simple dissections (90%) were completely reduced to grade 0. Eleven of 12 complex dissections were reduced to grade 0, while one improved to grade 1. Therefore, intimal dissection improved by at least one grade in 30 of 32 lesions (94%). In no case was a complex dissection present at the completion of the stenting procedure (Figure 5). The results of quantitative analysis showed that at baseline the mean percent diameter stenosis was $74 \pm 17\%$; after balloon angioplasty, it was $47 \pm 17\%$; this result improved substantially to $15 \pm 10\%$ after stent placement (Figure 6).

Of note, there was one instance of thrombotic occlusion in a patient in whom the stent was placed for intimal dissection.

Based on these results, we concluded that stenting was extremely effective in improving the angiographic appearance of intimal dissection after standard balloon angioplasty; this reduction in dissection grade was accompanied by a marked improvement in percent diameter stenosis. Since the development of an intimal tear is the most important predictor of a major ischemic compli-

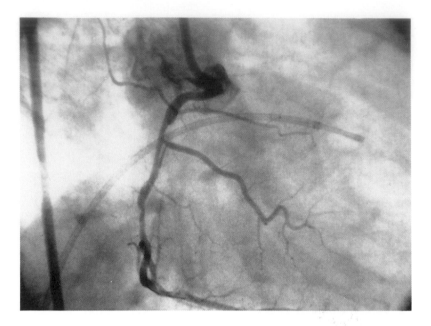

Figure 4(b).

cation in the early hours after standard balloon angioplasty [8–10], the stent may become a powerful tool in resolving this problem if the rate of subacute thrombosis proves to be reliably low.

Effect on restenosis

In the first phase of our trial, 226 patients underwent attempted stent place-ment [6]. Successful implantation was achieved in 213 patients (94%) and subacute thrombosis occurred in eight patients (3.8%). As a result, 205 patients remained eligible for follow-up angiography, which was done 5.5 ± 1.7 months in 165 patients (Figure 7); this represents an angiographic follow-up rate of 80% [11]. The lumen dimensions and percent diameter stenoses for this group of patients are presented in Table 3.

For this study, we used the following definition of restenosis: an immediate post procedure percent stenosis <50% that increased to ⩾50% at the time of follow-up angiography. Based on this definition, restenosis occurred in 56 out of 165 patients, yielding an overall restenosis rate of 34%. The restenosis rates for single and multiple stents for de novo and repeat procedures is shown in Figure 8. We also attempted to define restenosis rates in a clinically relevant subgroup.

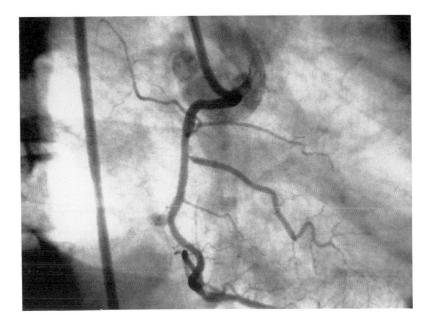

Figure 4. Efficacy of the stent in sealing an intimal tear. A. The baseline angiogram shows a severe mid right coronary artery stenosis. B. Result after PTCA shows significant intimal dissection. C. Resolution of dissection after stent placement.

DISSECTION GRADE

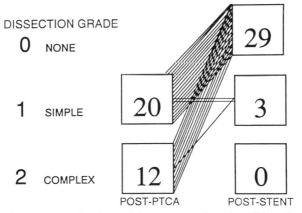

Figure 5. Results of coronary stenting in resolving coronary dissections. Dissections were graded as described in text. In no instance did the patient leave the catheterization suite with a complex (grade 2) dissection.

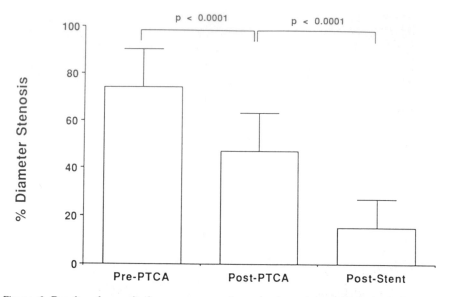

Figure 6. Results of quantitative coronary angiography in patients with intimal dissections following standard balloon angioplasty. There is marked improvement in percent diameter stenosis after stenting.

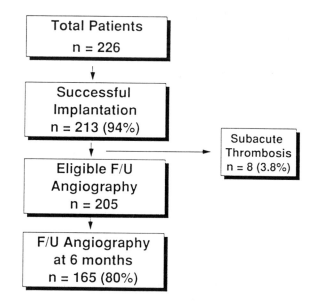

Figure 7. Flow chart of initial 226 patients who underwent stent placement.

Table 3. Quantitative Coronary Arteriography Measurement in Patients Undergoing Stent Implantation

	Pre-PTCA	Post-PTCA	Post-Stent	F/U
Reference Vessel	3.16 ± 0.49	3.17 ± 0.47	3.12 ± 0.47	2.92 ± 0.44
Minimum Lumen Dia	0.85 ± 0.48	1.85 ± 0.56	1.85 ± 0.56	1.71 ± 0.71
% Dia. Stenosis	72 ± 16	42 ± 16	42 ± 16	41 ± 23
Lesion Length (mm)	9.2 ± 6.6			

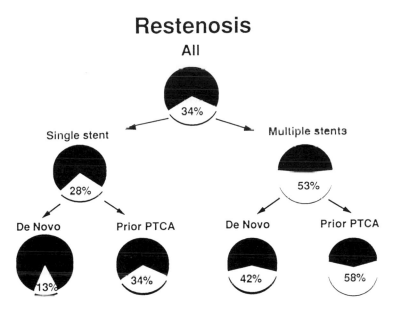

Figure 8. Restenosis rate for single vs. multiple stents for both de novo lesions and repeat PTCA attempts.

Single vs. multiple stents

A single stent was placed in 125 patients and 35 patients or 28% developed restenosis. This compared favorably to the restenosis rate in the multiple stent group: recurrence developed in 21 of 40 patients (53%) with multiple stents ($p = 0.007$) (Figure 8).

Effect of de novo lesions vs. prior PTCA

There was an important influence of prior PTCA in patients who received a single Palmaz-Schatz™ stent. For de novo lesions, in which a single stent was placed, the restenosis rate was 13%, which was significantly less than the 34% restenosis rate noted in the patients that had undergone prior PTCA procedures.

Acute angiographic result

We analyzed whether the final percent stenosis after stenting was a predictor of restenosis. Patients were divided by an arbitrary cutoff of ⩽5% and >5% stenosis after stent placement. Based on this, there was a clear trend for a lower restenosis rate when an optimal post stent angiographic result was obtained.

Effect of vessel diameter

We also assessed the effect of reference vessel diameter on occurrence of restenosis. The average reference vessel diameter was 3.2 mm. Of the 43% of patients with reference vessel diameter >3.2 mm, the restenosis rate was 21%; in contrast, there was a trend towards a higher restenosis rate in the patients with smaller vessels (37% restenosis), $p = 0.09$.

LAD vs. non-LAD location

Because of the well-known high restenosis rate for lesions located in the LAD, we analyzed the restenosis rate according to lesion location. Interestingly, there was no significant difference in restenosis rates for LAD vs. other location (33% vs. 34%). Therefore, the stimulus responsible for restenosis seems to occur irrespective of lesion location in the stented vessels.

Longer term follow-up

We sought to determine whether stenting might delay the temporal progression of the restenosis process [12]. Therefore, follow-up coronary angiography was carried out in a cohort of 37 patients (39 lesions), who reached the one-year follow-up after placement. A comparison of the six- and 12-month angiograms revealed no change in minimum lumen diameter (1.92 ± 0.57 vs 1.93 ± 0.56) or percent stenosis (36 ± 17 vs 35 ± 17). We concluded that stent placement does not delay the time course of the restenosis process.

Future goals

Based on the results of these findings, the stent investigators have organized a prospective randomized trial in order to compare the restenosis rates in patients who receive a single stent versus patients who undergo standard balloon angioplasty. We plan to enroll 600 patients whose de novo lesions can be treated with a single stent.

The major end point of the trial will be restenosis defined as ⩾50% narrowing on the 6-month angiogram. In addition, complication rates including the incidence of vessel closure, non-fatal infarction, death, emergency surgery and clinically significant bleeding will be analyzed for the two groups.

Appendix

Johnson and Johnson Interventional Systems Intracoronary Stent Study Group

Clinical Sites and Investigators
Scripps Clinic & Research Foundation – LaJolla, CA. Richard A. Schatz, MD; Paul Teirstein, MD.
Washington Hospital Center – Washington, DC. Martin B. Leon, MD.
Beth Israel Hospital – Boston, MA. Donald S. Baim, MD.
University of Michigan Medical Center – Ann Arbor, MI. Stephen G. Ellis, MD; Eric J. Topol, MD.
Thomas Jefferson University Hospital – Philadelphia, PA. Sheldon Goldberg, MD; Michael P. Savage, MD.
Yale University Medical School – New Haven, CT. Michael W. Cleman, MD; Henry S. Cabin, MD.
Cardiovascular Institute of the South – Houma, LA. Craig M. Walker, MD; Jody Stagg, MD.
University of California – San Diego, CA. Maurice Buchbinder, MD.
Hospital of the University of Pennsylvania – Philadelphia, PA. John W. Hirshfeld, MD.
Arizona Heart Institute, Phoenix, AZ. Richard Heuser, MD.
The University of Texas Health Science Center at San Antonio – San Antonio, TX. Julio A. Perez, MD; Steven Bailey, MD.
Florida Hospital – Orlando, FL. R. Charles Curry, MD; Hall B. Whitworth, MD.

Core angiographic laboratory
Thomas Jefferson University Hospital. David L. Fischman, MD; Glenn Morales, RCPT; Michael P. Savage, MD; Sheldon Goldberg, MD.

References

1. Dotter CT, Judkins MP. Transluminal treatment of arteriosclerotic obstruction. Description of a new technique and a preliminary report of its application. Circulation 1964; **30**: 654–70.
2. Dotter CT. Transluminally-placed coilspring endarterial tube grafts. Long-term patency in canine popliteal artery. Invest Radiol 1969; **4**: 329–32.
3. Goldberg S. Coronary angioplasty in the 1990's – new tools for old troubles. J Invasive Cardiol 1990; **2**: 211–6.
4. LeFree MT, Simon SB, Mancini GBJ, Vogel RA. Digital radiographic assessment of coronary arterial geometric diameter and videodensitometric cross-sectional area. Proc SPIE 1986; **626**: 334–41.
5. Mancini GB, Simon SB, McGillem MJ LeFree MT, Friedman HZ, Vogel RA. Automated quantitative coronary arteriography: morphologic and physiologic validation in vivo of a rapid digital angiographic method. Circulation 1987; **75**: 452–60 (published erratum appears in Circulation 1987; **75**: 1199).
6. Schatz RA, Baim DS, Leon M, et al. Clinical experience with the Palmaz-Schatz coronary stent. Initial results of a multicenter study. Circulation 1991; **83**: 148–61.
7. Fischman DL, Savage MP, Leon MB, et al. Effect of intracoronary stenting on intimal dissection following balloon angioplasty: results of quantitative and qualitative coronary analysis. J Am Coll Cardiol. In Press.
8. Bredlau CE, Roubin GS, Leimgruber PP, Douglas JS Jr, King SB 3d, Gruentzig AR. In-hospital morbidity and mortality in patients undergoing elective coronary angioplasty. Circulation 1985; **72**: 1044–52.

9. Ellis SG, Roubin GS, King SB 3d, et al. Angiographic and clinical predictors of acute closure after native vessel coronary angioplasty. Circulation 1988; **77**: 372–9.
10. Detre KM, Holmes DR Jr, Holubkov R, et al. Incidence and consequences of periprocedural occlusion. The 1985–1986 National Heart, Lung, and Blood Institute Percutaneous Transluminal Coronary Angioplasty Registry. Circulation 1990; **82**: 739–50. Comment in: Circulation 1990; **82**: 1039–43.
11. Fischman DL, Savage MP, Ellis S, et al. Restenosis after Palmaz-Schatz™ stent implantation. In: Serruys P, Strauss B, King S (Eds.), Restenosis after intervention with new mechanical devices. Dordrecht: Kluwer Academic Publishers. In press.
12. Savage M, Fischman D, Ellis S, et al. Does late progression of restenosis occur beyond six months following coronary artery stenting? Circulation. 1990; **82** Suppl 3: III–540 (Abstract).

35. The Wallstent experience: 1986–1990

PATRICK W. SERRUYS and BRADLEY H. STRAUSS* on behalf
of MICHEL E. BERTRAND, JACQUES PUEL, BERNHARD
MEIER, URS KAUFMANN, JEAN-CHRISTOPHER STAUFFER,
ANTHONY F. RICKARDS, LUCAS KAPPENBERGER and
ULRICH SIGWART

Summary

Coronary stenting has been investigated as an adjunct to percutaneous transluminal coronary angioplasty (PTCA) to obviate the problems of early occlusion and late restenosis. From March 1986–March 1990, 265 patients (308
lesions) were implanted with the coronary Wallstent™ in six European
centers. For this study, the patients were analyzed according to date of
implantation (Group 1: March 1986–January 1988; Group 2: February 1988–
March 1990) and vessel type (native arteries versus bypass grafts). Quantitative angiographic follow-up was performed in 82% of the study patients.

The early in-hospital occlusion rate in the overall group was 15%. Group
1 patients had a 20% rate in contrast to 12% rate in Group 2 (p = n.s.).
The early occlusion rate in native vessels and bypass grafts was 19% and
8%, respectively (p = 0.019). Restenosis was determined by two criteria
(Criterion 1: $\geq$0.72 mm loss in minimal luminal diameter (MLD) from post
stent to follow-up; Criterion 2: $\geq$50% diameter stenosis at follow-up) within
the stent and in the segments immediately proximal and distal to the stent.
The restenosis rate with Criterion 1 was 43% in the overall group of patients;
35% in Group 1 versus 49% in Group 2 (p = n.s.); 34% in native vessels
versus 54% in bypass grafts (p = 0.016). The second criterion was met by
27% of patients in the overall group; 21% in Group 1 versus 32% in Group
2 (p = n.s.); 18% in native vessel patients versus 39% in bypass grafts (p =
0.005).

The association between 16 variables and restenosis was determined by a
relative risk ratio assessment. Variables with significant risk ratios for restenosis with Criterion 1 were use of multiple stents/lesion (relative risk 1.56,
95% confidence interval (CI) 1.08–2.25) and oversized (unconstrained stent
diameter exceeding reference diameter >0.7 mm) stents (relative risk 1.64,
95% CI 1.10–2.45); and for Criterion 2, oversizing by >0.70 mm (RR 1.93,
95% CI 1.13–3.31), bypass grafts (relative risk 1.62, 95% CI 0.98–2.66), use

* Dr. Strauss is a Research Fellow of the Heart and Stroke Foundation of Canada.

J.H.C. Reiber and P.W. Serruys (eds), Advances in Quantitative Coronary Arteriography, 567–591.
© 1993 *Kluwer Academic Publishers. Printed in the Netherlands.*

of multiple stents/lesion (relative risk 1.61, 95% CI 0.97–2.67) and residual diameter stenosis >20% post stenting (relative risk 1.51, 95% CI 0.91–2.50).

The overall mortality during the study period was 6.6% in native vessel patients and 8.9% in patients with bypass grafts (6% and 7.9% at 1 year, respectively). The actuarial event-free survival (freedom from death, myocardial infarction, bypass surgery or PTCA) for native artery patients was 46% at 40 months and for bypass graft patients was 37% at 20 months.

It is concluded that early in-hospital occlusions remain a major problem with this device despite improvement in the later experience. Although bypass grafts had a significantly lower early occlusion rate than native vessels, a significantly higher rate of late restenosis limited the early benefits of stenting. Restenosis occurs in a significant number of patients, particularly in bypass grafts. The indications for stenting remain unknown and require results of randomized clinical studies.

Introduction

In 1986, the first coronary Wallstent implantation ushered in a new era in interventional cardiology with the purpose of circumventing the two major limitations of coronary angioplasty, early acute occlusion and late restenosis [1]. As with all new procedures, operators of the device had to struggle with their own learning curves at the same time that anticoagulation regimens and clinical indications and contraindications evolved from their clinical experience.

Since March 1986, the coronary Wallstent[R] has been the most intensively studied endovascular prosthesis in Europe. As a result of cooperation among the six participating European centers, a central core laboratory was set up in Rotterdam to objectively assess the follow-up of stents with quantitative coronary angiography.

In a previous publication from our group, the late angiographic and clinical follow-up of the inital 105 patients implanted between 1986–1988 was reported [2].

In the period from January 1989 until March 1990, a further 160 patients underwent stent implantation in the coronary circulation.

In this chapter, we compare the late quantitative angiographic and clinical follow-up of this second group of patients with the initial group, and, to further characterize the factors associated with angiographic restenosis within the stented segment, we retrospectively studied the predictive ability of several angiographic variables.

Table 1. Stent implantations according to date of implantation.

	Group 1 (March 1986-Dec 1988)	Group 2 (Jan 1989-March 1990)
Vessels	107	175
Bypass	18%	60%
Native	82%	40%
LAD	54%	15%
CX	7%	5%
RCA	21%	20%
Stent/Lesions	117/114	266/194

Table 2. Stent implantations according to vessel type.

	Natives	Bypass Grafts
Patients	166	101
Vessels	171	110
Stent/Lesion	193/173	192/135
LAD	55%	
CX	10%	
RCA	35%	

Methods

Study patients

Two hundred and sixty-five patients (308 lesions) were enrolled after obtaining informed consent between March 1986 and March 1990 at the participating centers.

The study patients were grouped according to the date of implantation (prior to or after January 1, 1988; Groups 1 and 2, respectively) and the vessel type stented (native vessel versus bypass graft) (Tables 1, 2).

In Group 1, 117 stents were implanted in 114 lesions, of which 82% were in native vessels (and in particular the left anterior descending artery). In group 2, 266 stents were implanted in 194 lesions, predominantly in bypass grafts (60% of cases). In this group, the right coronary artery was the most common vessel stented in the native circulation.

The indications for stenting also differed between the two vessel types (Figure 1). Native vessels were primarily stented to prevent a second restenosis or as a bail-out procedure for angioplasties complicated by abrupt closure or large dissections that interrupted anterograde flow and were associated with clinical and electrocardiographic signs of ischemia. However, in bypass grafts, the principle indication was for primary lesions in bypass grafts that had not been previously treated with angioplasty.

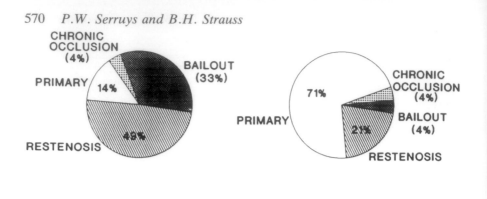

NATIVE   BYPASS

Figure 1. The indications for stenting in native arteries and bypass grafts. (Primary = Primary atherosclerotic lesion that has not been previously treated by PTCA or stenting.)

In the overall group, angiographic follow up was obtained in 218 patients (82%). However, in-hospital occlusions occurred in 40 patients (41 lesions).

Follow-up angiograms were quantitatively analyzed in 176 patients (78%) of the 225 patients who were discharged from hospital without known occlusion (Figures 2 and 3).

They had a total of 259 stents implanted in 214 lesions. The mean length of angiographic follow-up in the study group was 6.6 ± 4.8 months.

The anticoagulation for the first period of implantation has previously been described [2]. Based on this initial clinical experience, a uniform anticoagulation schedule was followed at the centers. Acetylsalicylic acid 1 gram orally was started 1 day before the procedure. At the beginning of the

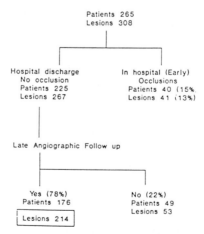

Figure 2. Flow diagram showing the angiographic follow-up in 265 stented lesions. In hospital (early) occlusions occurred in 40 patients (15%). In the remaining 225 patients that were discharged from hospital without known stent occlusion, 176 patients (78%) with 214 stented lesions had quantitative angiographic follow-up.

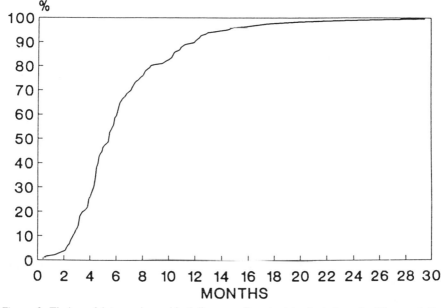

Figure 3. Timing of late angiographic follow-up after stent implantation. In this cumulative curve, the interval (in months) between date of implantation and final angiographic follow-up is shown for the study group.

procedure, patients recieved heparin 10,000 international units intravenously and in some cases, dextran infusions (500 mg/ 4 hours) were also given. Additional heparin (10,000 international units) and urokinase 100,000 units intracoronary were administered during the procedure. Following the procedure, the heparin infusion was adjusted according tho the activated partial thromboplastin time (APTT 80–120 seconds) in addition to initiating oral Vitamin K antagonist therapy. Heparin was discontinued after the therapeutic oral anticoagulation level was stabilized (International Normalized Ratio of 2.3 or more). Acetylsalicylic acid 100 mg daily, dipyridamole (300 to 450 mg/day) and in some patients sulfinpyrazone 400 mg daily were also administered.

In this trial, the endovascular prosthesis, Wallstent[R], was provided by Medinvent SA, Lausanne. The method of implantation and description of this stent has previously been reported [1, 2]. This stent is a self-expandable stainless steel woven mesh prosthesis that can be positioned in the coronary artery using standard over-the-wire technique through a 8F or 9F guiding catheter. The device is constructed of 16 wire filaments, each 0.08 mm wide. It is constrained in an elongated configuration on a 1.57 mm diameter delivery catheter with the distal end covered by a removable plastic sleeve. As the sleeve is withdrawn, the constrained device returns to its original unconstrained larger diameter and becomes anchored against the vessel wall. Unconstrained stent diameter ranged from 2.5–6 mm and was selected to be 0.50 mm larger than the stented vessel based on a visual estimate of the pre stent angiogram by the investigator. In an effort to alleviate the problem of acute thrombosis, the stent design was changed in April 1989 with the introduction of a polymer coated stent (Biogold^R) for certain stent sizes. By August 1989, all manufactured stents contained this particular polymer coating.

Quantitative coronary arteriography

All cineangiograms were analyzed at the core laboratory in Rotterdam using the computer assisted cardiovascular angiography analysis system (CAAS) which has previously been discussed in detail [3, 4]. The important steps will be briefly described. Selected areas of the cineframe encompassing the desired arterial segment (from side branch to side branch) are optically magnified, displayed in a video format and then digitally converted. Vessel contour is determined automatically based on the weighted sum of the first and second derivative functions applied to the digitized brightness information. A computer-derived estimation of the original arterial dimension at the site of the obstruction is used to define the interpolated reference diameter and area. The absolute diameter of the stenosis as well as the reference diameter are measured by the computer which uses the known guiding catheter diameter as a calibration factor, after correction for pincushion distortion. The percentage diameter of the narrowed segment is derived by comparing the observed stenosis dimensions to the reference values. *The length* of the lesion (mm) is determined from the diameter function on the basis of a curvature analysis. Using the reconstructed borders of the vessel, the computer can calculate a symmetry coefficient for the stenosis. Differences in distance between the actual and reconstructed vessel contours on both sides of the lesion are measured. *Symmetry* is determined by the ratio of these two differences with the largest distance between actual and reconstructed contours becoming the denominator. Values for symmetry range from 0 for extreme eccentricity to 1 for maximal symmetry (that is, equal distance on both sides between reconstructed and actual contours). The angiographic analysis was done pre- and post-angioplasty, immediately post-stent implantation and at long term follow-up in all patients using the average of multiple matched views with orthogonal projections wherever possible.

Restenosis

Two different set of criteria were applied to determine the restenosis rate. We have found a change in minimal luminal diameter (MLD) of 0.72 mm or more to be a reliable indicator of angiographic progression of vessel narrowing and by no means implies functional or clinical significance [3, 4]. This value takes into account the limitations of coronary angiographic

Table 3. Angiographic follow-up

Implantations (Lesions/Pts)	308/265	
Early Occlusions	41/40	
Late Follow Up	214/176	
Total	255/216	(82%)
No Angiographic Follow-up	53/49	(18%)
Death	10	(4%)
Early CABG	11	(4%)
Refusal	25	(9%)
Technical	3	(1%)
Time to Angiographic Follow Up		
Excluding Early Occlusions	6.6 ± 4.8	
Including Early Occlusions	5.7 ± 5.0	

measurements and represents two times the long term variability (i.e. the 95% confidence intervals) for repeat measurements of a coronary obstruction using CAAS. The other criterion for restenosis chosen was an increase of the diameter stenosis from less than 50% after stent implantation to greater than or equal to 50% at follow-up. This criterion was selected since common clinical practice continues to assess lesion severity by a percentage stenosis. The two criteria were assessed within the stent and in the segment immediately adjacent (proximal and distal) to the stent.

Late (i.e. documented after the initial discharge from hospital) occlusion ($n = 10$ patients, 16 lesions) were regarded as restenoses.

Angiographic variables

Based on the quantitative angiographic data, multiple variables were identified and recorded for each lesion. These variables, either discrete (two or three distinct responses) or continuous (a range of responses), were grouped according to lesion, stent or procedural factors (Tables 3, 4). These particular variables were of a priori clinical interest on the basis of previously published PTCA and stent reports [5–11].

Statistical methods

The data obtained by quantitative angiographic analysis are given as mean ± s.d. The mean of each angiographic variable pre-PTCA, post-stent and at follow-up were compared using analysis of variance. If significant differences were found, two tailed T-tests were applied to pairs of data. The occlusion and restenosis rates were compared using a chi square test. A statistical probability of less than 0.05 was considered significant.

A relative risk analysis was performed for the aforementioned discrete and continuous variables [12]. The continuous variables were dichotomized for the risk ratio analysis. To avoid arbitrary subdivision of data in continuous

Table 4. Angiographic results: Early occlusions

	Total	Group 1	Group 2	Native Vessels	Bypass Grafts
Lesions	308/265	114/105	194/160	173/166	135/101
Early Occlusions	40(13%)/39(15%)	21(18%)/21(20%)	20(10%)/19(12%)	32(18%)/32(19%)	9(7%)/8(8%)

Table 5. Late angiographic follow up: Restenosis within and immediately adjacent to the Stent

	Total	Group 1	Group 2	Native vessels	Bypass grafts
Lesions/Patients	214/176	85/75	129/101	111/104	103/74
0.72 mm Criterion					
Within Stent	75/61	25/21	50/40	34/30	40/31
Adjacent to Stent	14/14	5/5	9/9	5/5	9/9
Total	89/75	30/26	59/49	40/35	49/40
	(42%/43%)	(37%/35%)	(46%/49%)	(36%/34%)	(48%/54%)
50% DS Criterion					
Within Stent	51/42	17/15	34/27	21/18	30/24
Adjacent to Stent	6/6	1/1	5/5	1/1	5/5
Total	57/48	18/16	39/32	22/19	35/29
	(27%/27%)	(22%/21%)	(30%/32%)	(20%/18%)	(34%/39%)

variables, cutpoints were derived by dividing the data into two groups, each containing roughly 50% of the total population. This method of subdivision has the advantage of being consistent for all variables and thus avoids any bias in selection of subgroups which might be undertaken to emphasize a particular point. The incidence of restenosis in the two groups was compared using a relative risk analysis. A relative risk of 1 for a particular variable implies that the presence of that variable poses no additional risk for restenosis; relative risks greater than 1 or less than 1 imply additional or a reduction in risk, respectively. For example a relative risk of 2 for a particular parameter implies that the presence of that factor increases the likelihood of restenosis by a factor of two. The 95% confidence intervals were calculated to describe the statistical certainty. Statistical significance was defined as $p < 0.05$ and was determined using the Pearson Chisquare (BMDP statistical software, University of California, Berkeley, California, 1990).

The late clinical follow-up was determined according to a life table format using the Kaplan-Meier method [13].

The following events were considered clinical endpoints: death, myocardial infarction, bypass surgery or nonsurgical revascularization (PTCA or atherectomy). The life table was constructed according to the initial clinical event.

Results

A: Occlusion and restenosis rate

The angiographic follow-up for the entire study population was 82% (Table 3). This includes patients with documented early occlusions during hospital admission ($n = 40$) in addition to patients who had late (after the initial hospital discharge) angiographic controls. The reasons why follow-up angiography could not be performed are listed in Table 3. The time to angiographic follow-up was 6.6 ± 4.8 months if early occlusions are excluded and 5.7 ± 5.0 months with the early occlusions.

The angiographic data for individual lesions in bypass grafts and native vessels is presented in Figures 4A and B. In native vessels, there was a mean increase in minimal luminal diameter from 1.17 ± .52 mm to 2.53 ± .53 mm immediately post stenting but a late deterioration to 1.99 ± .81 mm if early occlusions are excluded and 1.59 ± 1.08 mm with the inclusion of the early occlusions ($p = < 0.0001$) (Figure 5). Similarly, the minimal luminal diameter increased in bypass lesions from 1.39 ± .64 mm to 2.81 ± .69 mm post stenting with a late reduction to 2.21 ± 1.16 mm and 2.03 ± 1.27 mm with the exclusion and inclusion of early occlusions, respectively ($p = < 0.0001$). Diameter stenosis was reduced from immediately post stenting in bypass grafts from 60 ± 14% to 23 ± 10%, but increased at late follow-up to 43 ± 31% and to 38 ± 27% with and without the early occlusions respectively

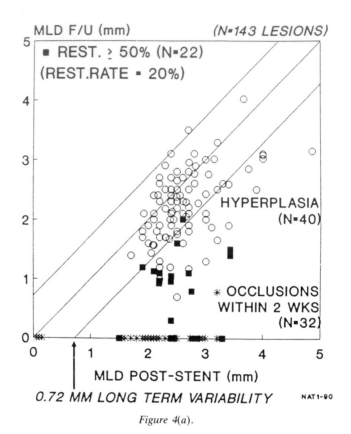

ANGIOGRAPHIC F/U OF NATIVE
ARTERIES (MARCH 86 - MARCH 90)

Figure 4(a).

($p = < 0.0001$). Similar changes were observed in native vessels (data not shown).

In the overall group, the incidence of early in-hospital occlusion was 15% by patient and 13% by lesion (Table 4). In bypass grafts, early occlusions were documented in 7% of lesions (8% of patients) versus 18% of lesions (19% of patients) in native vessels (by lesion $p = 0.005$; by patient $p = 0.016$). Three of these native vessel occlusions occurred during the procedure and could not be recanalized. The remaining occlusions presented clinically as acute ischemic syndromes following a successful stenting procedure. Early occlusions were less frequent in Group 2 patients (12%) than in Group 1 (20%) but not statistically significant. Detectable angiographic narrowing (0.72 mm loss in MLD) in the overall group was 42% by lesion and 43% by patient (Table 5). Using the 50% diameter stenosis criterion, restenosis occurred in 27% of lesions (27% of patients).

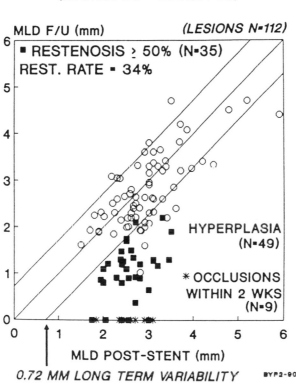

ANGIOGRAPHIC F/U OF BYPASSES
(MARCH 86 - MARCH 90)

Figure 4(b)

Figures 4(a–b). Change in the minimal luminal diameter (MLD) for individual lesions in native vessels (Figure 4A) and in bypass grafts (Figure 4B) between stent implantation and angiographic follow-up (F/U). The diameter of each segment immediately after implantation is plotted against the diameter at follow-up. The lines on each side of the identity line (diagonal) represent the limits of long-term variability of repeat measurements (a change of $\geqslant 0.72$ mm [arrow]). All symbols below the right-hand line represent stents with involvement of angiographic detectable hyperplasia. The filled squares represent lesions with follow-up diameter stenosis $\geqslant 50\%$. Occlusions are located along the x axis and those lesions that occurred within the first two weeks are marked by an asterisk.

Restenosis according to either definition was significantly higher in bypass grafts (MLD criterion: 54% by patient; DS criterion:39% by patient) than in native vessels (34% and 18% respectively) (MLD: $p = 0.016$; DS: $p = 0.001$). Group 2 patients (MLD criterion:49% by patient; DS criterion: 32% by patient) did not have significantly greater restenosis than Group 1 patients (MLD criterion: 35%; DS criterion: 21%).

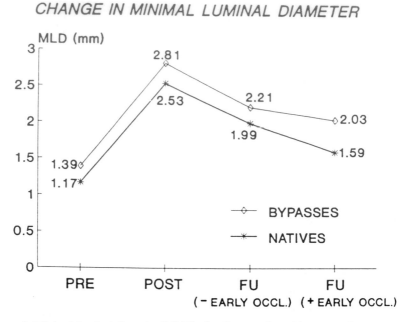

Figure 5. Minimal luminal diameter (MLD) of native vessels and bypass grafts pre procedure, post stenting, and at follow-up. The mean values at follow-up have been calculated with and without the inclusion of the early in-hospital occlusions.

B: *Relative risk analysis*

The relative risk and 95% confidence intervals for each variable using either of the two criteria for restenosis are shown in Figure 6. The variables with statistically significant associations with restenosis using the 0.72 mm criterion were multiple stents and oversizing the stent (unconstrained diameter) with respect to the reference diameter by more than 0.70 mm which had relative risk ratios (RR) (and 95% confidence intervals (CI)) of 1.56 (1.08–2.25) and 1.64 (1.10–2.45), respectively. The second criterion, $\geq$ 50% diameter stenosis at follow up, was associated with oversizing by > 0.70 mm (RR 1.93, 95% CI 1.13–3.31), bypass grafts (RR 1.62, 95% CI 0.98–2.66), multiple stents/lesion (RR 1.61, 95% CI 0.97–2.67) and residual diameter stenosis > 20% post stenting (RR 1.51, 95% CI 0.91–2.50). The actual restenosis rates for these variables are included in Tables 6 and 7.

C: *Long term follow-up*

The overall mortality during the study period was 8.9% for bypass grafts and 6.6% for native vessels (7.9% and 6% at 1 year, respectively). In the

RELATIVE RISK WITH 95% CI

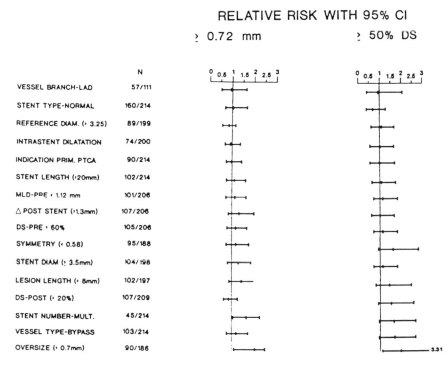

Figure 6. Relative risk ratios (with 95% confidence intervals) for the angiographic variables using the two restenosis criteria (≥0.72 mm loss in minimal luminal diameter from immediately post stenting to follow-up and diameter stenosis ≥50% at follow-up). The relative risk is indicated by the thick vertical line in the center and the outside vertical lines represent the 95% confidence limits. The hatched vertical line signifies a relative risk of 1 (no additional risk for restenosis). Variables with values greater than or less than 1 imply additional or a reduction in risk respectively (see text for details). The variables are listed in the left hand column. N represents the number of lesions analyzed for each particular variable. Although 214 lesions were analyzed in total, some lesions could not be analyzed for certain variables. The denominator for vessel branch (111) represents the total number of lesions that were stented in native vessels. (CI, confidence interval; DS, diameter stenosis; LAD, left anterior descending artery; DIAM., diameter; PRIM., primary; PTCA, percutaneous transluminal coronary angioplasty; MLD, minimal luminal diameter; /, absolute change; MULT, multiple.)

Table 6. Restenosis rates according to Criterion 1. (≥0.72 mm loss in minimal luminal diameter)

		n	Restenosis Rate
Stent Number	Multiple	22/44	50%
	Single	53/165	32%
Stent Oversize	>0.7 mm	40/90	44%
	≤0.7 mm	26/96	27%

Table 7. Restenosis Rates according to Criterion 2. (>50% Diameter Stenosis at Follow Up)

Parameter		n	Restenosis Rate
Vessel Type	Bypass	30/103	30%
	Native	20/111	19%
Stent Oversize	>0.7 mm	29/90	32%
	≤0.7 mm	16/96	17%
Diameter Stenosis Post Stent	>20%	30/107	28%
	≤20%	19/102	19%

bypass group, four of the nine deaths occurred during the initial hospitaliz-ation. Two of these deaths resulted from intracerebral hematomas related to the anticoagulation and two were from myocardial infarctions due to stent occlusion. Two of the 5 late deaths were sudden (at 2 and 18 months), two were clearly unrelated to the stent (chronic congestive heart failure, chronic renal failure) and the other death occurred after bypass surgery. In the group with native vessels, 7 of the 11 deaths were in-hospital. These were all due to myocardial infarctions resulting from stent occlusion with the exception of one intracerebral bleed and one patient who was stented 24 hours after an extensive myocardial infarction with cardiogenic shock. Two of the four late deaths were sudden (at 1.5 and 19 months), one was noncardiac (pneu-monia) and the other resulted from complications post bypass surgery.

The actuarial event-free survival (freedom from death, myocardial infarc-tion, bypass surgery or PTCA) for native artery patients was 46% at 40 months and for bypass graft patients was 37% at 20 months (Figure 7).

Discussion

Despite progress in techniques and equipment, the rate of late angiographic narrowing following PTCA, a process popularly termed "restenosis", has not been altered since its clinical introduction 13 years ago. This failure has provided the impetus for the development of newer alternative forms of coronary revascularization such as stenting, atherectomy and laser. However the effectiveness of all forms of nonoperative coronary interventions remains limited by the restenosis process(es).

A: Early occlusion, late restenosis

The coronary Wallstent was initially introduced as an endovascular device to prevent the late restenosis process that limits percutaneous transluminal coronary angioplasty. The indications for and management of patients im-planted with this particular prosthesis have evolved as experience and knowl-edge have increased. In this study, an attempt has been made to separate

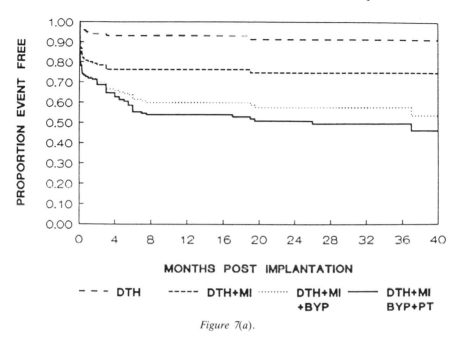

Figure 7(a).

two important factors in the late outcome of patients with stent implantations. The first division, according to date of implantation, provides the clearest picture of the changes in stent applications based on the early experience. Investigators originally believed that the stent could be safely implanted in native vessels and that the benefit of stents would be most apparent in lesions that had already restenosed on at least one occasion. However, a high in-hospital occlusion rate was noted, particularly in patients with unstable syndromes, evolving myocardial infarction or angiographic evidence of thrombus. These occlusions, often with disastrous clinical sequelae, convinced most of the investigators that native vessels in general and particularly in the left anterior descending artery (due to the large territory at risk), should only be stented in bail-out situations. Group 2 mainly consisted of patients with bypass grafts who were stented for primary lesions and native vessels who stented as part of a bail-out strategy following complicated balloon angioplasty. Bypass grafts in particular were selected for stent implantations due to an extremely high rate of restenosis after PTCA alone and the larger diameter of these grafts seemed less likely to thrombose than smaller calibre native arterial vessels [14–17].

Bypass lesions, which were the majority of lesions stented in Group 2, were more complex in general than Group 1 lesions due to the advanced age and diffuse nature of the disease in the bypass grafts. As a result, more stents per lesion (1.4 versus 1.1 in native vessels) were required to cover these lesions. Therefore, the significantly lower rate of in-hospital occlusion

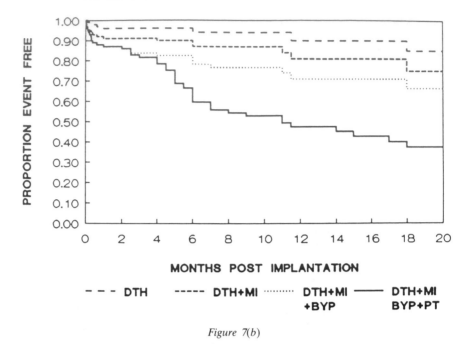

Figure 7(b)

Figures 7(a–b). Clinical follow-up in native vessels up to 40 months (Figure 7A) and bypass grafts up to 20 months (Figure 7B). Death, myocardial infarction, bypass surgery, and PTCA or atherectomy were considered clinical endpoints.

in bypass graft patients versus patients with native vessels (8% versus 19%) and trend in Group 2 versus Group 1 (12% versus 20%) is indicative of several possible factors including improvements in anticoagulation regimens, operator experience and/or larger calibre vessels despite more complex case selection.

Recently, the initial clinical experience with the Palmaz-Schatz stent has been reported [18]. Using a similar anticoagulation schedule in 174 patients, a 0.6% in hospital occlusion rate was demonstrated. The discrepancy between a substantially higher occlusion rate in our series with the Wallstent and the Schatz study can not be entirely explained. The stent itself does not appear to be more thrombogenic. In a model of stents placed inside a polytetrafluoethylene graft in exteriorized arteriovenous shunts in baboons, no difference in acute platelet deposition and thrombus formation was noted between the two types of stents [19]. Differences in study design such as patient selection (collateralized vessels, predominantly right coronary arteries and exclusion of patients with recent myocardial infarction and abrupt closure following PTCA in the Schatz study) may account for some of the differences.

Higher restenosis rates by both criteria were demonstrated in bypass grafts compared with native vessels and in Group 2 than in Group 1. There are two possible explanations for this increase. First, bypass grafts, which are overrepresented in Group 2, are known to have higher restenosis rates than native vessels [14, 15, 16]. Secondly, higher restenosis rates may be the "price" for lower occlusion rates. Organization of thrombus at the site of intimal damage may be an important cause of late restenosis after stenting. Although it is often difficult to histologically differentiate thrombus organization from intimal hyperplasia, we have observed an extremely disorganized pattern of intimal thickening in the stented segments of several bypass grafts that have been surgically retrieved or obtained by atherectomy 1–5 months following stent implantation [20]. By diminishing the formation of early occlusive thrombus with more effective anticoagulation, the residual nonocclusive thrombus could form the substrate for late restenosis. Although the second group had a higher proportion of bail-out cases, we did not identify increased relative risk for restenosis from bail-out, cases in comparison to stent implantations performed in primary or restenosed lesions [21].

B: *Relative risk analysis*

Restenosis is a complex process that is only partially understood. Pathological studies of patients who have died more than 1 month following angioplasty have demonstrated the presence of intimal hyperplasia, presumably due to proliferation and migration of medial smooth muscle cells into the intima, and associated production of extracellular matrix collagen and proteoaminoglycans [22, 23]. It has been suggested by Liu et al. that the two major factors that determine the absolute amount of intimal hyperplasia are (1) the depth of injury and (2) the regional flow characteristics (which are determined by the geometry of the dilated lumen of the lesion and blood flow velocity patterns across that lumen) [24]. Two separate PTCA follow-up reports support the concept that the greater the diameter change post-PTCA (implying a greater degree of disruption to the vessel wall), the more extensive is the absolute amount of reactive hyperplasia [25, 26]. On the basis of several angiographic studies from the Thoraxcenter, immediate results following stent implantation are superior to angioplasty alone (mean minimal luminal diameter of 2.5 mm versus 2.0–2.1 mm) and thus favor a more aggressive proliferative response post procedure [2, 4, 27]. The second factor is illustrated by the inverse relationship between the level of wall shear stress and subsequent intimal thickening. In the presence of a significant residual stenosis, the post-stenotic region is a site of flow separation and low wall shear stress. This may retard endothelial recovery and prolong the period of smooth muscle cell proliferation which is partially dependent on restoration of regenerated endothelial barrier [28]. Stenting appears to diminish the effect of post-stenotic wall shear stress by significantly improving the hemodynamic effects of the stenosis (based on the calculated reductions in Poiseuille and turbulent contributions to flow resistance [29]).

It is extremely difficult, if not impossible, to predict restenosis in the individual patient following PTCA [30]. This problem can be partially under-stood when one considers that the two factors (i.e. depth of injury and regional flow characteristics) affecting the extent of intimal proliferation act in opposition to the other and thus make it hazardous to predict outcome of this interaction in a particular patient. In large population of patients, relative risk analyses following PTCA have identified several patient, lesion, and procedural variables that predict late restenosis. However, the situation fol-lowing stenting may be different where the mean loss of minimal luminal diameter at late follow-up is twice that of PTCA alone (0.62 mm versus 0.31 mm) [2, 27]. Therefore, this study was designed to identify factors that were associated with an increased risk of restenosis following stenting.

Lesion factors
Stented bypass grafts had a greater risk of restenosis than native vessels (30% versus 19%) but this finding was restricted to the DS criterion. The increased susceptibility of bypass grafts to the restenosis process has pre-viously been documented following PTCA [9, 14–16, 31, 32]. Although left anterior descending (LAD) lesions have been shown to be a risk factor in several PTCA studies [5], this was not evident in our study. The reference diameter of the vessel also had no relationship to restenosis. Forty-three percent of the vessels had a reference diameter between 3–4 mm and 43% were 3 mm or less. Lesion length and the severity of the lesion, in absolute minimal luminal diameter or diameter stenosis, prior to the procedure have been cited by several authors as important risk factors for restenosis following angioplasty although our data did not show this association [5–7]. Lesion length is probably not an important factor for restenosis if lesions can be covered by a single stent (see below). We believe that this is due to a more uniform and optimal dilatation with stenting. Long lesions treated with angioplasty are frequently less successfully dilated along the entire length of the lesion and the ragged irregular surface of the vessel may predispose to rheological factors critically involved in restenosis. Total occlusions have been reported as an important predictor of restenosis in angioplasty studies. However, this accounted for only 4.5% of the lesions in our study which was too few for this analysis. Although there was a trend for higher restenosis in more eccentric lesions, this was not statistically significant.

Stent factors
Multiple stents (RR: MLD 1.56 (1.08–2.25); DS 1.61 (0.97–2.67)) and un-constrained stent diameter exceeding reference diameter by > 0.7 mm (RR: MLD 1.64 (1.10–2.45); DS 1.93 (1.13–3.31)) significantly predicted re-stenosis with both criteria. Preliminary reports from four separate groups working with the Palmaz-Schatz stent have shown a similar relationship between multiple stents/lesion and restenosis [33–36]. In our study, multiple stents placed in tandem were overlapped at the extremities (so called "tele-scoping") which may be the reason for the observed increase in restenosis

rates. The segment of the vessel that was covered by the overlapping stents was subjected to the dilating force of two separate stents as well as an increased density of metal. We have observed that restenosis commonly occurred at these sites of overlapping between extremities of stents. Since the length of the lesion and the absolute length of the stent required to cover a lesion were not significant predictors, it seems prudent to implant longer stents rather than two or more shorter stents in tandem.

Selecting an oversized stent (unconstrained diameter >0.7 mm larger than the reference diameter) was a particularly important stimulus for hyperplasia with the self-expanding Wallstent. Schwartz et al. have described an aggressive proliferative response in a porcine model as a result of severe stent oversizing (0.5 to 1.5 mm) [37]. This effect, which they attributed to penetration of the internal elastic lamina by the stent wires and subsequent deep medial injury, was much less pronounced when the stent diameter was matched more closely to the vessel diameter. Furthermore, due to its self expanding property, the Wallstent (and particularly when it is oversized) continues to expand the vessel wall for at least 24 hours post implantation [38]. The vessel is subjected to increasingly higher wall stress than after implantation of a balloon expandable stent (which is maximally expanded at the time of implantation), a factor which may adversely stimulate the proliferative process. It may seem paradoxical that oversizing the stent by >0.7 mm would result in a higher restenosis rate with the 50% DS criterion. However, the diameter stenosis post stent was not different in the two groups despite the oversizing. The main effect of oversizing then was not particularly a superior immediate result but rather a more aggressive "hyperplastic" reaction and a smaller MLD at follow-up than if less oversized stents were implanted. The absolute value of the unconstrained stent diameter and the addition of the polymer coating (Biogold^R) had no significant relationship to late restenosis.

Procedural factors
No significant relative risk could be attributed to a particular indication for the procedure. Restenosis rates for primary cases were not significantly different than for bail-out or restenosis cases (MLD Criterion: 37%, 42%, 33%; DS Criterion: 24%, 27%, 24%) although an increased rate of restenosis has been described with the Palmaz-Schatz stent in patients with previous restenosis [36]. The absolute change in diameter from the pre- to the post-stent result and dilatation within the stent after implantation (the so-called "Swiss Kiss") did not appear to affect the late restenosis. This post-stent dilatation was performed to dissipate clot within the stent and to accelerate early expansion of the stent. A post-stent diameter stenosis >20% tended to be predictive of a follow-up diameter stenosis >50% (RR 1.51, 95% CI 0.91–2.50) although not for the MLD criterion. The larger the residual stenosis following stenting (i.e. less optimal result), the less hyperplasia is

required to reach a particular diameter stenosis at follow-up such as the 50% diameter stenosis criterion.

Limitations of study

Several important limitations of this study must be mentioned. Although this study suggest several factors that may be predictive of restenosis following stenting, it does not address the actual mechanisms of restenosis in the stented vessel. By comparing the predictors of restenosis following stenting to angioplasty, we have assumed that the underlying mechanism(s) responsible for late angiographic narrowing are similar (i.e. primarily intimal hyperplasia). Although almost every stenting procedure was accompanied by balloon dilatation at some particular time during the procedure, several other mechanisms may be important. Elastic recoil, which in the first few days following the procedure may be a significant factor in causing renarrowing, may be less important in stented vessels than angioplasty alone due to the scaffolding function of the stent. Although organization of thrombus at the site of intimal damage following PTCA has been recognized as a cause for late restenosis, it has not been particularly regarded as an important factor based on late pathological studies following PTCA. However, this may be an extremely important cause of late restenosis after stenting. Although it is difficult to histologically discriminate thrombus organization from intimal hyperplasia, we have observed a disorganized layer of intimal thickening directly above the stent wire associated with remnants of thrombus in segments of several bypass grafts that have been surgically retrieved up to 10 months following stent implantation [20, 39] (Figure 8). Therefore we consider organization of residual thrombus to be a potentially important cause of late angiographic narrowing in addition to the major occlusion problems early after stenting. This may partially explain why commonly regarded determinants of restenosis following PTCA (e.g. lesion length, Left Anterior Descending Artery) do not appear to be significant in this analysis since, a different pathological process may predominate. This also has important clinical implications since therapy to limit smooth muscle proliferation may be quite different than therapy to minimize thrombus formation.

There are two statistical limitations to this study. Due to the relatively small sample size, we can not rule out a significant beta error. Secondly, in performing multiple statistical comparisons, there is a risk that some of them may be significant by chance alone. Therefore, this data requires confirmation by other studies.

In conclusion, the European coronary Wallstent experience has demonstrated that restenosis following stenting is increased in bypass grafts and in the presence of multiple stents and excessive oversizing of the stent (>0.7 mm) and less optimal results immediately post stenting (>20% diameter stenosis). Since some of these factors can be modified, we recommend against

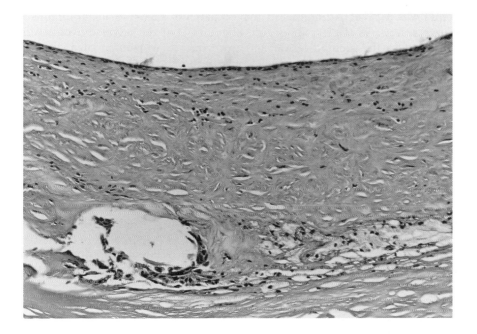

Figure 8. Light micrograph of stented bypass graft removed 10 months after stent implantation. The void (*) represents a 70 micron diameter stent wire. Immediately adjacent to the stent wire are cellular debris and foam cells (arrowhead). Directly above the stent wire is a layer of disorganized fibrointimal hyperplasia. (courtesy of HMM van Beusekom)

the use of multiple stents and excessive oversizing to reduce the probability of late restenosis.

C: *Short and long term follow-up: clinical events*

The problems of prolonged anticoagulation are an additional consideration. Increased morbidity (increased femoral hematomas, gastrointestinal and genito-urinary tract bleeding) and mortality (3 patients died from intracerebral hemorrhage) are directly attributable to the intensive anticoagulation regimen. The duration of hospitalization is also lengthened to ensure therapeutic levels of anticoagulation.

The high incidence of late adverse clinical events in stented patients is a cause for concern. A mortality rate of 8.9% in bypass grafts and 6.6% in native vessels is higher than in reported PTCA studies [40, 41, 42]. However, it must be stressed that a large number of stents in native vessels were implanted for abrupt closure following PTCA which dramatically increases the risk of the procedure [42]. Actuarial event free survival (freedom from death, myocardial infarction, bypass surgery or repeat PTCA or atherectomy) was 37% at 20 months in bypass patients and 46% at 40 months in native vessels. In the bypass group, about 30% of the adverse events were unrelated to the stented lesion and were due to worsening of a different lesion or to development of new lesions. In the native vessel group, 12% of the adverse events were unrelated to the stented lesion. In addition, 9 of the 30 bypass operations in stented native vessel patients were performed as part of a protocol for patients stented for the bail-out indication [43]. Although there are no comparable series of native vessel patients in the literature because of the unique set of indications in our study, three recent reports have been published of late clinical follow-up (Kaplan-Meier analysis) after PTCA in bypass grafts. The Thoraxcenter reported that only 41% of patients were alive and event-free (myocardial infarction, repeat CABG, repeat PTCA) at a median follow-up of 2.1 years [44]. A review of the overall Dutch experience also showed limited late beneficial results with a two year and five year event free survival of 52% and 26%, respectively in 454 bypass patients [45]. Webb et al. have described a 71% freedom from death, infarction and surgery at 5 years in bypass patients who underwent PTCA at their institution, but did not include the 27% incidence of second angioplasty procedures also required in their patient group [14]. However, it must be stressed that our study was not a randomized trial designed to compare stenting with PTCA but rather an observational study with a first generation coronary stent. Nevertheless, all of these late follow-up studies of nonoperative coronary revascularization clearly show that these are palliative procedures and not long-term solutions to the underlying problems of progression of underlying coronary disease and iatrogenically induced restenosis. Several important points emerge from this study. First, although in hospital occlusion rates improved in the later experience, Wallstent[R] coronary thrombosis continues to limit its use. Restenosis rates with the 50% DS criterion do not seem to be significantly improved when compared with historical post angioplasty results, although definitive statements must await randomized trials. Bypass grafts in particular have a high incidence of late restenosis rate although early occlusion occurred less significantly than in patients with native vessels. Based on our experience, there is insufficient evidence at this time to suggest implantation of this particular stent outside of a randomized trial with the following exceptions: (1) bail-out for abrupt occlusion, (2) suboptimal (inadequate dilalatation) results following PTCA, and (3) bypass grafts at high risk for distal embolization with PTCA (friable lesions that may benefit from the scaffolding property of the Wallstent[R]). If the low occlusion rate with the Palmaz-Schatz stent is confirmed in other studies, that particular stent would appear to be a more suitable candidate for randomized trials of presently available stents.

Appendix

Participating Centers and Collaborators: Catheterization Laboratory, Thoraxcenter, Rotterdam, The Netherlands: B.H. Strauss, MD, K.J. Beatt, MB BS, M. v.d. Brand, MD, P.J. de Feyter,

MD, H. Suryapranata, MD, I.K. de Scheerder, MD, J.R.T.C. Roelandt, MD, P.W. Serruys, MD; Department of Cardiology, Hopital Cardiologique, Lille, France: M.E. Bertrand; Department of Invasive Cardiology, The Royal Bromptom and National Heart Institute, London, United Kingdom: A.F. Rickards, MD, U Sigwart, MD; Department of Clinical and Experimental Cardiology, CHRU Rangeuil, Toulouse, France: J.P. Bounhoure, MD, A. Courtault, MD, F. Joffre, MD, J. Puel, MD, H. Rousseau, MD; Division of Cardiology, Department of Medicine, CHUV, Lausanne, Switzerland: J.-J. Goy MD, J-C Stauffer, MD, U Kaufmann, MD, L. Kappenberger, MD, P. Urban, MD; Cardiology Center, University Hospital, Geneva, Switzerland: B. Meier, P. Urban.

Acknowledgements

We gratefully acknowledge the assistance of Hanneke Roerade in preparation of the manuscript and Dr. Edward Murphy (Portland, Oregon) for critical comments. We appreciated the technical assistance of Marie-Angèle Morel and Eline Montauban van Swijndregt.

This study was supported in part by grants from the Dutch Ministry of Science and Education, Den Haag, The Netherlands (87159) and the Swiss National Fund (3,835,083).

References

1. Sigwart U, Puel J, Mirkovitch V, Joffre F, Kappenberger L. Intravascular stents to prevent occlusion and restenosis after transluminal angioplasty. N Engl J Med 1987; **316**: 701–6.
2. Serruys PW, Strauss BH, Beatt KJ, et al. Angiographic follow-up after placement of a self-expanding coronary artery stent. N Engl J Med 1991, **324**: 13–7. Comment in: N Engl J Med 1991; **324**: 52–3.
3. Reiber JH, Serruys PW, Kooijman CJ, et al. Assessment of short-, medium-, and long-term variations in arterial dimensions from computer-assisted quantitation of coronary cineangiograms. Circulation 1985; **71**: 280–8.
4. Serruys PW, Luijten HE, Beatt KJ, et al. Incidence of restenosis after successful angioplasty: a time-related phenomenon. A quantitative angiographic study in 342 consecutive patients at 1, 2, 3 and 4 months. Circulation 1988; **77**: 361–71.
5. Leimgruber PP, Roubin GS, Hollman J, et al. Restenosis after successful coronary angioplasty in patients with single-vessel disease. Circulation 1986; **73**: 710–7.
6. Myler RK, Topol EJ, Shaw RE, et al. Multiple vessel coronary angioplasty: classification, results, and patterns of restenosis in 494 consecutive patients. Cathet Cardiovasc Diagn 1987; **13**: 1–15.
7. Vandormael MG, Deligonul U, Kern MJ et al. Multilesion coronary angioplasty:clinical and angiographic follow-up. J Am Coll Cardiol 1987; **10**: 246–52.
8. Mata LA, Bosch X, David PR, Rapold HJ, Corros T, Bourassa MG. Clinical and angiographic assessment 6 months after double vessel percutaneous coronary angioplasty. J Am Coll Cardiol 1985; **6**: 1239–44.
9. Holmes DR Jr., Vlietstra RE, Smith HC, et al. Restenosis after percutaneous transluminal coronary angioplasty (PTCA): a report from the PTCA registry of the National Heart, Lung, and Blood Institute. Am J Cardiol 1984; **53**: 77C–81C.
10. Levine S, Ewels CJ, Rosing DR, Kent KM. Coronary angioplasty: clinical and angiographic follow-up. Am J Cardiol 1985; **55**: 673–6.
11. DiSciascio G, Cowley MJ, Vetrovec GW. Angiographic patterns of restenosis after angioplasty of multiple coronary arteries. Am J Cardiol 1986; **58**: 922–5.

12. Gardner MJ, Altman DG (Eds.), Statistics with confidence: confidence intervals and statistical guidelines. London: British Medical Journal 1989.
13. Kaplan EL, Meier P. Nonparametric estimation from incomplete observations. J Am Stat Assoc 1958; **53**: 457–81.
14. Webb JG, Myler RK, Shaw RE, et al. Coronary angioplasty after coronary bypass surgery: initial results and late outcome in 422 patients. J Am Coll Cardiol 1990; **16**: 812–20.
15. Douglas JS Jr., Gruentzig AR, King SB 3rd, et al. Percutaneous transluminal coronary angioplasty in patients with prior coronary bypass surgery. J Am Coll Cardiol 1983; **2**: 745–54.
16. Block PC, Cowley MJ, Kaltenbach M, Kent KM, Simpson J. Percutaneous angioplasty of stenoses of bypass grafts or of bypass graft anastomosic sites. Am J Cardiol 1984; **53**: 666–8.
17. Bucx JJ, de Scheerder I, Beatt K, et al. The importance of adequate anticoagulation to prevent early thrombosis after stenting of stenosed venous bypass grafts. Am Heart J 1991; **121**; 1389–96.
18. Schatz RA, Baim DS, Leon M, et al. Clinical experience with the Palmaz-Schatz coronary stent. Initial results of a multicenter study. Circulation 1991; **83**: 148–61.
19. Krupski WC, Bass A, Kelly AB, Marzec UM, Hanson SR, Harker LA. Heparin-resistant thrombus formation by endovascular stents in baboons. Interruption by a synthetic antithrombin. Circulation 1990; **82**: 570–7.
20. Serruys PW, Strauss BH, van Beusekom HM, van der Giessen WJ. Stenting of coronary arteries: has a modern Pandora's Box been opened? J Am Coll Cardiol 1991; **17** (6 Suppl B): 143B–154B.
21. Strauss BH, DeScheerder IK, Beatt KJ, Tijssen J, Serruys P.W. Angiographic predictors of restenosis in the coronary Wallstent^R. Circulation 1990; **82** (4 Suppl III): III–540 (Abstract).
22. Austin GE, Ratliff NB, Hollman J, Tabei S, Phillips DF. Intimal proliferation of smooth muscle cells as an explanation for recurrent coronary artery stenosis after percutaneous transluminal coronary angioplasty. J Am Coll Cardiol 1985; **6**: 369–75.
23. Waller BF, Gorfinkel HJ, Rogers FJ, Kent KM, Roberts WC. Early and late morphologic changes in major epicardial coronary arteries after percutaneous transluminal coronary angioplasty. Am J Cardiol 1984; **53**: 42C–47C.
24. Liu MW, Roubin GS, King SB 3rd. Restenosis after coronary angioplasty. Potential biologic determinants and role of intimal hyperplasia. Circulation 1989; **79**: 1374–87.
25. Beatt KJ, Luijten HE, Suryapranata H, de Feyter PJ, Serruys PW. Suboptimal post angioplasty result. The principle risk factor for "restenosis". Circulation 1989; **80** (4 Suppl II): II–257 (Abstract).
26. Liu MW, Roubin GS, King SB 3rd, Gruentzig A. Does an optimal luminal result after PTCA reduce restenosis? Circulation 1989; **80** (4 Suppl II): II–63 (Abstract).
27. Serruys PW, Rutsch W, Heyndrickx G, et al. Effect of long term thromboxane A2 receptor blockade on angiographic restenosis and clinical events after coronary angioplasty. The CARPORT study. J Am Coll Cardiol 1991; **17** (2 Suppl A): 283A (Abstract).
28. Haudenschild CC, Schwartz SM. Endothelial regeneration II. Restitution of endothelial continuity. Lab Invest 1979; **41**: 407–18.
29. Serruys PW, Juilliere Y, Bertrand ME, Puel J, Rickards AF, Sigwart U. Additional improvement of stenosis geometry in human coronary arteries by stenting after balloon dilatation. Am J Cardiol 1988; **61**: 71G–76G.
30. Renkin J, Melin J, Robert A, et al. Detection of restenosis after successful coronary angioplasty: improved clinical decision making with use of a logistic model combining procedural and follow-up variables. J Am Coll Cardiol 1990; **16**: 1333–40.
31. Corbelli J, Franco I, Hollman J, Simpfendorfer C, Galan K. Percutaneous transluminal coronary angioplasty after previous coronary artery bypass surgery. Am J Cardiol 1985; **56**: 398–403.
32. Pinkerton CA, Slack JD, Orr CM, Vantassel JW, Smith ML. Percutaneous transluminal

angioplasty in patients with prior myocardial revascularization surgery. Am J Cardiol 1988; **61**: 15G–22G.

33. Ellis SG, Savage M, Baim D, et al. Intracoronary stenting to prevent restenosis: preliminary results of a multicenter study using the Palmaz-Schatz stent suggest benefit in selected high risk patients. J Am Coll Cardiol 1990; **15** (2 Suppl A): A118 (Abstract).

34. Levine MJ, Leonard BM, Burke JA, et al. Clinical and angiographic results of balloon-expandable intracoronary stents in right coronary artery stenoses. J Am Coll Cardiol 1990; **16**: 332–9.

34. Schatz RA, Goldberg S, Leon MB, Fish RD, Hirshfield JW, Walker CM. Coronary stenting following "suboptimal" coronary angioplasty. Circulation 1990; **82** (4 Suppl III): III–540 (Abstract).

36. Teirstein PS, Cleman MW, Hirshfeld JW, Buchbinder M, Walker C. Influence of prior restenosis on subsequent restenosis after intracoronary stenting. Circulation 1990; **82** (4 Suppl III): III–657 (Abstract).

37. Schwartz RS, Murphy JG, Edwards WD, Camrud AR, Vliestra RE, Holmes DR. Restenosis after balloon angioplasty. A practical proliferative model in porcine coronary arteries. Circulation 1990; **82**: 2190–200.

38. Beatt KJ, Bertrand M, Puel J, Rickards T, Serruys PW, Sigwart U. Additional improvement in vessel lumen in the first 24 hours after stent implantation due to radial dilating force. J Am Coll Cardiol 1989; **13** (2 Suppl A): 224A (Abstract).

39. Van Beusekom HM, Serruys PW, van der Giessen WJ, et al. Histological features 3 to 320 days after stenting of human saphenous vein bypass grafts. J Am Coll Cardiol 1991; **17** (2 Suppl A): 53A (Abstract).

40. Kent KM, Bentivoglio LG, Block PC, et al. Long-term efficacy of percutaneous transluminal coronary angioplasty (PTCA): report from the National Heart, Lung, and Blood Institute PTCA Registry. Am J Cardiol 1984; **53**: 27C–31C.

41. Gruentzig AR, King SB 3rd, Schlumpf M, Siegenthaler W. Long-term follow-up after percutaneous transluminal coronary angioplasty. The early Zürich experience. N Engl J Med 1987; **316**: 1127–32.

42. Detre K, Holubkov R, Kelsey S, et al. One-year follow-up results of the 1985–1986 National Heart, Lung, and Blood Institute's Percutaneous Transluminal Coronary Angioplasty Registry. Circulation 1989; **80**: 421–8.

43. de Feyter PJ, DeScheerder I, van den Brand M, Laarman G, Suryapranata H, Serruys PW. Emergency stenting for refractory acute coronary artery occlusion during coronary angioplasty. Am J Cardiol 1990; **66**: 1147–50.

44. Meester BJ, Samson M, Suryapranata H, et al. Long-term follow-up after attempted angioplasty of saphenous vein grafts: the Thoraxcenter experience 1981–1988. Eur Heart J 1991; **12**: 648–53.

45. Plokker HWT, Meester BH, Serruys PW. The Dutch experience in percutaneous transluminal angioplasty of narrowed saphenous veins used for aortocoronary arterial bypass. Am J Cardiol 1991; **67**: 361–6.

36. Immediate and long-term clinical and angiographic results following Wiktor™ stent implantation in patients with documented restenosis of a native coronary artery lesion following prior balloon angioplasty

PETER DE JAEGERE, PIM J. DE FEYTER and PATRICK W. SERRUYS on behalf of the Wiktor Study Group (MICHEL BERTRAND, VOLKER WIEGAND, GISBERT KOBER, JEAN FRANCOIS MARQUIS, BERNARD VALEIX, RAINER UEBIS and JAN PIESSENS)

Summary

Intracoronary stenting has been introduced as a adjunct to balloon angioplasty, aimed at overcoming its limitations, namely acute vessel closure and late restenosis. This study reports the first experience with the Wiktor stent implanted in the first 50 consecutive patients. All patients had restenosis of a native coronary artery lesion following prior balloon angioplasty. The target coronary artery was the left anterior descending artery in 26 patients, the circumflex artery in 7 patients and the right coronary artery in 17 patients. The implantation success rate was 98% (49/50 patients). There were no procedural deaths. Acute or subacute thrombotic stent occlusion occurred in 5 patients (10%). All 5 patients sustained a nonfatal acute myocardial infarction. Four of these patients were recanalized by means of balloon angioplasty, the remaining patient was referred for bypass surgery. A major bleeding complication occurred in 11 patients (22%): groin bleeding necessitating blood transfusion in 6 patients, gastro-intestinal bleeding in 3 patients and hematuria in 2 patients. Repeat angiography was performed at a mean of 5.6 ± 1.1 months in all implanted patients except one. Restenosis, defined by a reduction of ≥ 0.72 mm in the minimal luminal diameter or a change in diameter stenosis from $<50\%$ to $\geq 50\%$, occurred in 20 patients (45%) and in 13 patients (29%),respectively. In this first experience, the easiness and high technical success rate of Wiktor stent implantation are overshadowed by a high incidence of (sub)acute stent occlusion and bleeding complications. Although direct comparison with balloon angioplasty regarding the incidence of subsequent restenosis rate is not possible, the herein reported incidence compares favorably with data reported in the literature.

J.H.C. Reiber and P.W. Serruys (eds), Advances in Quantitative Coronary Arteriography, 593–607.

Introduction

Percutaneous Transluminal Coronary Angioplasty (PTCA) has established its role as a nonsurgical revascularization procedure in selected patients with obstructive coronary artery disease. Gained operator experience and improved catheter technology has resulted in a high immediate success rate and a low incidence of complications [1]. These favorable initial results are compromized by the unpredictable problem of late restenosis, occurring in 20–40% of the patients following successful balloon angioplasty [2–5]. Furthermore, there is some evidence that the recurrence of subsequent restenosis following repeat balloon angioplasty increases with the number of repeat interventions [6–9]. Intracoronary stents are one of the new technologies that (along with pharmacological interventions, atherectomy and laser techniques) have entered clinical testing to address this problem [10]. Recently, the first experience with the self-expandable Wallstent and the balloon expandable Palmaz-Schatz^R stent have been reported [11, 12]. The stent used in this study is the Medtronic Wiktor^{TM} stent which, in contrast to the Wallstent^R and the Palmaz-Schatz^R stent, is not a mesh made stainless steel device but a coil-like prosthesis made of a single loose interdigitating tantalum wire formed into a sinusoidal wave and configured as a helix. This loose configuration may offer less scaffolding properties compared to the other two stents. Therefore, the purpose of this study is to assess the immediate and the long-term clinical and angiographic results following Wiktor^{TM} stent implantation in the first fifty consecutive patients with restenosis following balloon angioplasty of a native coronary artery lesion.

Methods

Patients. The study population consists of the first 50 consecutive patients in whom a single Wiktor^{TM} stent implantation was attempted (Table 1). All patients had recurrence of angina with objective evidence of ischemia due to restenosis of a native coronary artery lesion following balloon angioplasty. A first restenosis was documented in 33 patients, a second restenosis in 13 patients and a third restenosis in 4 patients. The dilated and stented coronary artery was the left anterior descending artery in 26 patients (52%), the circumflex artery in 7 patients (14%) and the right coronary artery in 17 patients (34%). A written informed consent was required for every patient. The study protocol was approved by the ethics committee of the individual hospitals.

Description of the stent. The endoprosthesis used in this study is a radiopaque balloon-expandable stent (Wiktor^{TM}, Medtronic Inc., Minneapolis, USA) constructed of a single loose interdigitating tantalum wire (0.125 mm in

Table 1. Clinical characteristics

Number of patients	50
age (mean ± s.d. years)	55 ± 9
male	44
Functional class* I	10
II	6
III	14
IV	20
hypertension	7
hypercholesterolemia	7
nicotine	17
diabetes**	6

* According to Canadian Cardiovascular Society.
** All non-insuline dependent.

diameter) formed into a sinusoidal wave and configured as a helix. The prosthesis is crimped onto the deflated polyethylene balloon of a standard angioplasty catheter (Figure 1). The crimped stent profile is approximately 1.5 mm. Upon inflation of the balloon the sinusoidal waves expand to the extent that the stent conforms to the vessel wall. The features of the prosthesis are such that by inflating the balloon the diameter of the stent increases without alteration of its length (14–16 mm). The maximal diameter of the balloon during inflation determines the ultimate size of the prosthesis. The surface of the vascular endothelium covered by a full expanded stent amounts to 6.7, 7.7 and 8.4% for a 4.0, 3.5 and 3.0 mm stent, with an open space of 93.3, 92.3 and 91.6%, respectively. After implantation, the tantalum wire

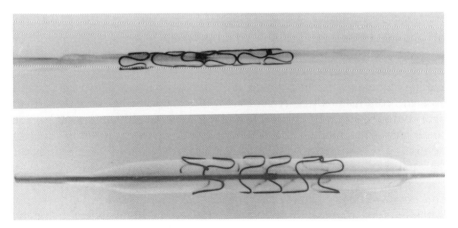

Figure 1. Medtronic Wiktor^{TM} stent mounted on a conventional polyethylene balloon when deflated (upper picture), inflated (lower picture).

undergoes oxidation, resulting in a stable and corrosion resistant oxide (TaO_5).

Stent implantation. One day prior to stent implantation acetylsalicylic acid 300 mg/day was started. Dextran (100cc/hour) was administered 2 hours before the implantation and continued throughout the procedure. A minimum of 500 cc was infused. A total of 20,000 units of heparin was injected intravenously. Full heparinization was maintained until therapeutic levels of coumadin therapy was achieved. Conventional balloon angioplasty was performed prior to stent deployment. After control coronary angiography for subsequent quantitative analysis, the balloon/stent system was advanced over a 0.014 inch steerable guidewire under fluoroscopic control to the treated lesion site. The balloon was inflated until the desired expansion of the stent was achieved. Subsequently the balloon was deflated and the catheter was removed under negative pressure while leaving the stent in place. In case of incomplete expansion of the stent, a repeat balloon dilatation within the stent was performed. The post-procedure drug therapy consisted of coumadin for a minimum of 3 months and acetylsalicylic acid (300 mg/day) for six months.

Quantitative coronary angiography. To assess the immediate and long-term changes in stenosis geometry, all coronary cineangiograms were analyzed at the core laboratory in Rotterdam by means of the computer-assisted Cardiovascular Angiography Analysis System (CAAS), described in detail elsewhere [13]. This system allows an objective and reproducible quantification of a coronary artery stenosis. Briefly, a region of interest (size 6.9×6.9 mm) in a selected cineframe (overall dimensions 18×24 mm) encompassing the desired arterial segment is digitized by a high resolution CCD-camera with resolution of 512×512 pixels and 8 bits of brightness resolution. The coronary segment to be analyzed is determined by selecting a number of centerline points which are connected by linear interpolation. An automated edge detection program determines the arterial contours by assessing the brightness profile along scan lines perpendicular to the centerline. After correction for pincushion distortion and calibration using the guiding catheter as scaling device, a diameter function can be determined from the contour analysis by computing the distances between the left and right contours. From this diameter function, several parameters can be computed such as the minimal luminal diameter, reference diameter and diameter stenosis. The variability, precision and accurracy of the system has been reported previously [14].

End points. Primary clinical end points were death, myocardial infarction, bypass surgery or repeat intervention and bleeding complications. All deaths were considered cardiac, unless an unequivocal non-cardiac cause could be established. The primary angiographic end point was the change in minimal luminal diameter at the dilated and stented segment at 6 months relative to the baseline. If a revascularization procedure involving the stented segment has been performed before 6 months repeat angiography, the last angiogram before this intervention was used to obtain follow-up values, irrespective of the timing of re-PTCA (hours, days or weeks). The secondary angiographic end point was the incidence of restenosis defined according to the following criteria. First, a continuous approach was used in which restenosis was defined by a reduction of $\geqslant 0.72$ mm in the minimal luminal diameter at follow-up. This change in minimal luminal diameter has been found to be a reliable indicator of angiographic progression of vessel narrowing. This value takes into account the limitations of coronary angiographic measurements and represents twice the long-term variability of repeat measurements of a coronary artery obstruction with the Cardiovascular Angiographic Analysis System [14, 15]. Second, a categorical approach was used in which an increase in diameter stenosis of $<50\%$ immediately after stent implantation to $\geqslant 50\%$ at follow-up was used as cutoff point to define restenosis. This criterion was selected since common clinical practice has continued to express lesion severity as a percentage of stenosis.

Statistics. Values obtained by quantitative angiographic analysis are expressed as means $\pm$ s.d. The means for each angiographic variable before PTCA, after PTCA, immediately after stent implantation and at follow-up were compared by analysis of variance. If significant differences were found, two-tailed t-tests were applied to paired data. A statistical probability of less than 0.05 was considered to indicate significance. In the patient with missing follow-up angiogram and no clinical evidence of restenosis, imputation of the minimal luminal diameter at follow-up was performed: the minimal luminal diameter at follow-up of this patient was calculated by adding the mean change of the minimal luminal diameter for the total study population to the minimal luminal diameter immediately post-stent implantation of this particular patient.

Results

Clinical results. The implantation success rate was 98% (49/50 attempted implants). In one patient, the stent could not be delivered at the target site due to inability to cross a tortuous proximal right coronary artery. There were no procedural related deaths. However, (sub)acute thrombotic stent occlusion occurred in 5 patients (10%) while still in the hospital. The occurrence to this trombotic event with respect to the implantation was as follows: day $0 = 1$ patient, day $1 = 1$ patient, day $4 = 1$ patient and day $5 = 2$ patients. Four patients were recanalized by means of conventional balloon angioplasty. In one of these patients adjunctive thrombolytic therapy was

Table 2. Changes in functional class according to the Canadian Cardiovascular Society

	I	II	III	IV
Pre-stent	10	6	14	20
At follow-up*	34	8	4	3

* The patient with unsuccessful stent implantation is not included.

used. The remaining patient was referred for emergency bypass surgery. In this patient, no attempt was made to recanalize the occluded stent either by means of thrombolytic therapy or balloon angioplasty. All five patients sustained a nonfatal acute myocardial infarction (mean ± s.d., creatine phosphokinase 1797 ± 1849 U/l). A major bleeding complication occurred in 11 patients (22%): 6 patients sustained a groin hematoma necessitating blood transfusion, 3 patients had a gastro-intestinal bleeding (2 duodenal ulcers, 1 intestinal polyps) and 2 patients had hematuria. One patient suffered from an infected pharyngeal hematoma caused by acenocoumarol therapy at 3 months post-implant.

During follow-up, 1 patient died 3 months after stent implantation following prostate surgery. Death was considered noncardiac since there was no clinical evidence of restenosis. No patient sustained an acute myocardial infarction. Three patients (6%) underwent bypass surgery (2 patients 3.5 months and 1 patient 6 months after the stent implantation). The changes in functional class are depicted in Table 2.

Angiographic results. The morphologic changes in stenosis geometry immediately after stent implantation and at follow-up along with the associated hemodynamic changes are presented in Tables 3, 4 and 5.

Wiktor^{TM} stent implantation resulted in a further significant increase in minimal luminal diameter from 1.80 ± 0.32 mm immediately following balloon angioplasty to 2.45 ± 0.35 mm immediately after stent implantation. This was associated with a reduction in diameter stenosis from 34 ± 11% to 18 ± 7% (Table 3). There was no change in the reference diameter before and after PTCA (2.81 ± 0.48 mm and 2.80 ± 0.48 mm, respectively, n.s.). However, there was a significant increase following stent implantation (2.98 ± 0.42 mm, $p < 0.00001$), which was confirmed at follow-up (2.91 ± 0.55 mm). Along with the improvement of the minimal luminal diameter, there was an additional increase in minimal luminal cross-sectional area with a concommitant decrease in percentage area. Moreover, there was a significant decrease in plaque area, in- and outflow angle, while the curvature of the lesion was respected (Table 4). These morphologic changes were associated with a decrease in both the calculated turbulent and Poiseuille resistance, as well as the virtual disappearance of the theoretical transstenotic pressure drop for a theoretical flow of 0.5, 1 and 3 ml/s (Table 5).

In most patients the measured diameter of the balloon when fully inflated

Table 3. Immediate and long-term morphologic changes following Wiktor Stent Implantation

	Before PTCA	After PTCA	After stent implantation	At follow-up All patients (N = 49)	At follow-up Pts without (sub) acute occlusion (N = 44)
Minimal luminal diameter (mm)	1.09 ± 0.26	1.80 ± 0.32	2.45 ± 0.35	1.59 ± 0.79	1.78 ± 0.60
Diameter stenosis (%)	61 ± 9	34 ± 11	18 ± 7	45 ± 25	39 ± 18
Minimal luminal Cross Sectional Area	1.00 ± 0.44	2.65 ± 0.91	4.83 ± 1.40	2.49 ± 1.80	2.61 ± 1.72
Area Stenosis	83 ± 8	55 ± 14	31 ± 11	58 ± 19	61 ± 23

$p < 0.00001$ $p < 0.001$ $p < 0.00001$

$p < 0.00001$

All parameters are expressed as mean ± s.d.
Pts: patients.

Table 4. Immediate and long-term morphologic changes following Wiktor stent implantation

	Pre-PTCA	Post-PTCA	Post-Stent	Follow-up	p_1	p_2	p_3
Curvature	23.22 ± 11.87	22.33 ± 9.71	21.39 ± 10.67	24.59 ± 20.71	n.s.	n.s.	n.s.
Plaque area (mm^2)	8.57 ± 4.37	5.20 ± 3.47	3.31 ± 2.32	5.97 ± 4.13	0.0001	0.0002	0.0001
Inflow angle	22.13 ± 6.27	14.68 ± 5.16	6.17 ± 14.54	10.56 ± 7.98	0.0001	0.001	n.s.
Outflow angle	22.05 ± 9.85	15.83 ± 13.91	4.46 ± 14.05	7.41 ± 7.44	0.02	0.0001	n.s.

p_1 p_2 p_3

All parameters are expressed in mean ±s.d.

Table 5. Immediate and long-term hemodynamic changes following Wiktor stent implantation

	Pre-PTCA	Post-PTCA	Post-Stent	Follow-up	p_1	p_2	p_3
Rpois	18.66 ± 39.26	1.24 ± 1.73	0.46 ± 0.25	5.60 ± 12.56	0.003	0.002	0.008
Rturb	11.37 ± 29.47	0.31 ± 0.72	0.02 ± 0.02	1.86 ± 5.26	0.01	0.006	0.02
Pgrad (0.5 ml/s)	30.03 ± 68.36	1.52 ± 2.44	0.48 ± 0.27	7.83 ± 17.93	0.005	0.004	0.008
Pgrad (1 ml/s)	48.68 ± 66.90	3.67 ± 6.30	0.98 ± 0.56	19.41 ± 46.30	0.0001	0.004	0.01
Pgrad (3 ml/s)	92.13 ± 129.07	6.45 ± 11.61	1.49 ± 0.92	34.70 ± 85.17	0.0001	0.004	0.01

———— p_1 ———— p_2 ———— p_3 ————

Rpois: Poiseuille resistance, Rturb: turbulent resistance, Pgrad: pressuredrop. All parameters are expressed in mean ±s.d.

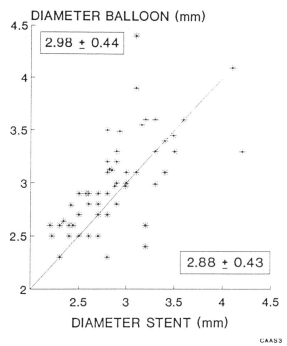

DIAMETER BALLOON (mm)

2.98 ± 0.44

2.88 ± 0.43

CAAS3

DIAMETER STENT (mm)

Figure 2. Difference between the mean diameter of the balloon when fully inflated and stented segment immediately following implantation.

was higher than the measured diameter of the stent (Figure 2). During maximum inflation the mean diameter of the balloon for the total study group was 2.98 ± 0.44 mm. The mean diameter of the stented segment immediately following implantation was 2.88 ± 0.43 mm. This implies a recoil of 0.10 ± 0.36 mm ($p < 0.03$).

Repeat angiography was performed in all patients with successful stent implantation (49 patients), except in 1, who died 3 months after stent implantation following prostate surgery. There was no clinical evidence of restenosis in this patient. The mean time interval between stent implantation and the control study was 5.6 ± 1.1 months. Overall, the minimal luminal diameter was found to have decreased from 2.45 ± 0.35 mm to 1.59 ± 0.79 mm ($p < 0.00001$). The percentage of stenosis had increased from $18 \pm 7\%$ to $45 \pm 25\%$ ($p < 0.0001$, Table 3). When only patients without clinical evidence of (sub)acute vessel closure during hospital stay (44 patients) were included, the minimal luminal diameter and percentage of stenosis were 1.78 ± 0.60 mm and $39 \pm 18\%$, respectively (Table 3). Figure 3 displays the cumulative distribution of the minimal luminal diameter and its changes (immediately after balloon angioplasty and stent implantation and at follow-up). The additional increase in minimal luminal diameter immediately following stent implantation is lost at follow-up.

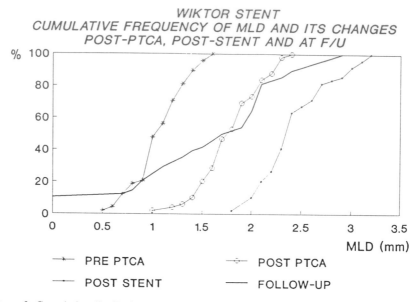

Figure 3. Cumulative distribution of the minimal luminal diameter of the entire study population and its changes immediatley following balloon angioplasty, stent implantation and at follow-up.

The incidence of restenosis depended on the definition used. When a change of ≥0.72 mm in minimal luminal diameter was used as criterion, restenosis was observed within the stent in 19 patients (43%) and in the segment immediately distal to the stent in another patient (2%) out of the 44 patients without clinical evidence of (sub)acute stent occlusion during hospital stay. At follow-up the percentage of stenosis had increased to ≥ 50% within the stent in 12 patients (27%) and in the segment distal to the stent in 1 patient (2%) out of these 44 patients. Therefore, the total restenosis rate was 45% according to the 0.72 mm criterion and 29% according to the 50% diameter stenosis criterion (Figure 4).

Discussion

Clinical results. Intracoronary stents are currently being tested in clinical practice to reduce the incidence of acute vessel occlusion and restenosis following balloon angioplasty. Severall stents are available, each with its own specific design, composition and physico-chemical behaviour once implanted. Implanting foreign body material implies an increased risk for acute thrombosis. Therefore, a stringent anticoagulation protocol is mandatory. Despite such a protocol described above, a thrombotic (sub)acute stent

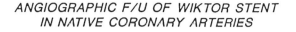

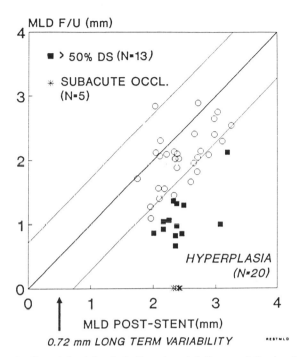

Figure 4. Changes in the minimal luminal diameter at follow-up following Wiktor^{TM} stent implantation. The diameter of each segment immediately after stent implantation is plotted against the diameter at follow-up. The lines on each side of the line of identity (diagonal) represent twice the variability (95% confidence interval) of duplicate measurements (a change $\geqslant 0.72$ mm). Out of the 49 patients, 5 (10%) sustained a (sub)acute stent occlusion (X-axis). In the remaining 44 patients, restenosis was observed in 20 patients (45%) according to the 0.72 mm criterion and in 13 patients (29%) according to the 50% diameter stenosis criterion.

occlusion occurred in 5 patients (10%). Three of these patients did not receive dextran and 1 patient was not properly instituted on acenocoumarol. In the 44 patients without clinical evidence of (sub)acute stent occlusion during hospital stay, only 6 patients (14%) did not receive dextran. Unfortunately, since central assessment of anticoagulation was not performed, the exact role of failure of anticoagulation with respect to (sub)acute thrombotic stent occlusion cannot be elucidated. Although it is tempting to speculate that suboptimal anticoagulation may be the main cause of stent occlusion, other pathophysiological mechanisms may be involved as well. Prior to stent implantation, balloon angioplasty is performed to facilitate stent delivery. The disruptive action of the balloon may cause intimal dissection, which in turn may be the primum movens for an ensuing thrombotic event. Furthermore, patients related factors such as acute ischemic syndromes, procedure related factors such as technical difficult stent implantation and angiography related factors such as small vessel size and/or total occlusion may predispose to trombotic stent occlusion. In this study population, there was no difference in vessel size between the patients with and without (sub)acute stent occlusion (reference diameter 2.8 ± 0.4 and 2.8 ± 0.5 mm, respectively n.s.). The reported (sub)acute stent occlusion rate compares very favorably with the initial Wallstent experience (20% in 105 patients), but is similar to the (sub)acute occlusion rate following the extended Wallstent[R] experience (12% in an additional 160 patients) [11, 16]. However, it contrasts sharply with the incidence of 0.6% following Palmaz-Schatz stent implantation [12]. True comparison is not possible since the studies differ in methods for patient selection, indication for stent implantation and type of vessel stented. Furthermore, the very low incidence of 0.6% reported by Schatz, has not been confirmed by a recent study, using the same device [17]. In this latter study, an incidence of 16% is reported. Probably, the incidence of (sub)acute stent occlusion may be reduced by a more detailed coagulation monitoring. Indeed, recent work indicate that measurement of prothrombin fragment $1 + 2$ and its changes following stent implantation may be predictive for (sub)acute thrombotic stent occlusion [18].

Another matter of concern is the risk of bleeding, inherently associated with aggressive anticoagulation. The incidence of bleeding is negligible following PTCA but is substantial when a combination of intravenous and oral anticoagulant drugs are used [12]. The most dreadful bleeding complication is intracranial hemorrhage which occurred in 1 out of 174 patients following Palmaz-Schatz[R] stent implantation and in 3 out of 265 patients following Wallstent[R] implantation [12, 16]. Another aspect to be considered regarding anticoagulation is the longer period of hospitalization, which in turn increases the overall costs of the procedure [19]. In this study, the hospital stay was (mean ± s.d.) 11.8 ± 7.4 days for the entire study population.

Angiographic results. The smaller mean diameter of the stented segment (2.88 ± 0.43 mm) in comparison with the measured diameter of the fully expanded balloon (2.98 ± 0.44 mm) suggests some recoil of the stented segment. This minimal recoil appears to be a true phenomenon since the accuracy and the precision of the quantitative coronary angiography system used in this study is -30μ and 90μ respectively [14]. Furthermore, recoil has also been observed, although to a larger extent, after Wiktor[TM] stent inplantation in Yorkshire pigs [20]. The more pronounced recoil (10%) observed in the animal model compared to recoil observed in this study (3%) may be explained by the fact that in the former animal study the stent was implanted in normal coronary arteries. All these angiographic data indicate that in contrast to balloon angioplasty, where recoil amounting to 50% has been documented, the Wiktor[TM] stent appropriately scaffolds the vessel [21].

Restenosis and recurrence of restenosis remains the major limitation of (repeat) PTCA. Whether intracoronary stents can address this issue appropriately is still unknown. There are some encouraging data from preliminary reports [22, 23]. However, firm conclusions cannot be drawn, since these data are stemming from nonrandomized studies in which single and multiple stent implantations have been performed in both native coronary arteries and venous bypass grafts in patients with either acute ischemic syndromes or stable angina for a variety of indications (primary stent implantation, restenosis, bail out). Patients undergoing repeat PTCA seems to be at a higher risk for recurrence of restenosis after repeat intervention. The angiographic documented restenosis rate increases from 34% following a second dilatation to 40% following a fourth dilatation [6, 9]. Most likely, this is an underestimation of the actual incidence due to incomplete angiographic follow-up. Repeat angiography is mandatory in all patients, even in patients free of angina at follow-up since approximately 25% of the patients with restenosis are asymptomatic [24]. Taking into account the limitations of these nonrandomized observational studies, as is the herein reported study, the incidence of restenosis of 29% using the 50% diameter stenosis criterion compares favorably with the data from those former studies. It goes without saying that randomized studies are needed to define the exact role of intracoronary stenting in the prevention of (recurrent) restenosis.

Conclusions

Acute and subacute stent occlusion as well as the risk of bleeding following Wiktor^{TM} stent implantation remains a matter of concern. Optimizing the stenosis geometry by stent implantation does not eliminate the late neointimal hyperplasia. However, the further increase in minimal luminal diameter and cross-sectional area after stent implantation compensates to some degree for the restenosis process. To assess the proper role of intracoronary stenting in the prevention of (recurrent) restenosis, further studies with randomized comparisons are needed.

Acknowledgements

We are greatly acknowledged to Marie-Angèle Morel for performing the quantitative analysis, for her assistance in the database management and statistical analysis.

References

1. Detre K, Holubkov R, Kesley S, et al. Percutaneous transluminal coronary angioplasty in

1985–1986 and 1977–1981. The National Heart, Lung and Blood Institute Registry. N Engl J Med 1988; **318**: 265–70.

2. Serruys PW, Luijten HE, Beatt KJ, et al. Incidence of restenosis after successful coronary angioplasty: a time-related phenomenon. A quantitative angiographic study in 342 consecutive patients at 1, 2, 3 and 4 months. Circulation 1988; **77**: 361–71.

3. Leimgruber PP, Roubin GS, Hollman J, et al. Restenosis after successful coronary angioplasty in patients with single-vessel disease. Circulation 1986; **73**: 710–7.

4. Levine S, Ewels CJ, Rosing DR, Kent KM. Coronary angioplasty: clinical and angiographic follow-up. Am J Cardiol 1985; **55**: 673–6.

5. Nobuyoshi M, Kimura T, Nosaka H, et al. Restenosis after successful percutaneous transluminal coronary angioplasty: serial angiographic follow-up of 229 patients. J Am Coll Cardiol 1988; **12**: 616–23.

6. Williams DO, Gruentzig AR, Kent KM, Detre KM, Kelsey SF, To T. Efficacy of repeat percutaneous transluminal coronary angioplasty for coronary restenosis. Am J Cardiol 1984; **53**: 32C–35C.

7. Meier B, King SB III, Gruentzig AR, et al. Repeat coronary angioplasty. J Am Coll Cardiol 1984; **4**: 463–6.

8. Black AJ, Anderson HV, Roubin GS, Powelson SW, Douglas JS Jr, King SB III. Repeat coronary angioplasty: correlates of a second restenosis. J Am Coll Cardiol 1988; **11**: 714–8.

9. Teirstein PS, Hoover CA, Ligon RV, et al. Repeat coronary angioplasty: efficacy of a third angioplasty for a second restenosis. J Am Coll Cardiol 1989; **13**: 291–6.

10. Sigwart U, Puel J, Mirkovitch V, Joffre F, Kappenberger L. Intravascular stents to prevent occlusion and restenosis after transluminal angioplasty. N Engl J Med 1987; **316**: 701–6.

11. Serruys PW, Strauss BH, Beatt KJ, et al. Angiographic follow-up after placement of a self-expanding coronary-artery stent. N Engl J Med 1991; 324: 13–7. Comment in: N Engl J Med 1991; **324**: 52–3.

12. Schatz RA, Baim DS, Leon M, et al. Clinical experience with the Palmaz-Schatz coronary stent. Initial results of a multicenter study. Circulation 1991; **83**: 148–61.

13. Reiber JH, Serruys PW, Slager CJ. Quantitative coronary and left ventricular cineangiography: methodology and clinical applications. Boston: Nijhoff 1986.

14. Reiber JH, Serruys PW, Kooijman CJ, et al. Assessment of short-, medium-, and long-term variations in arterial dimensions from computer-assisted quantitation of coronary cineangiograms. Circulation 1985; **71**: 280–8.

15. Beatt KJ, Serruys PW, Hugenholtz PG. Restenosis after coronary angioplasty: new standards for clinical studies. J Am Coll Cardiol 1990; **15**: 491–8.

16. Strauss BH, Serruys PW, Bertrand M, et al. Quantitative angiographic follow-up of the Coronary Wallstent in native vessels and bypass grafts. European Experience March 1986–March 1990. Am J Cardiol 1992; **69**: 475–81.

17. Haude M, Erbel R, Straub U, Dietz U, Meyer J. Short and long-term results after intracoronary stenting in human coronary arteries: monocenter experience with the balloon-expandable Palmaz-Schatz stent. Br Heart J 1991; **66**: 337–45.

18. Hafner G, Swars H, Erbel R, et al. Monitoring prothrombin fragment + and coagulation factor II to avoid subacute occlusion after coronary stenting. The Lancet, in press.

19. Dick RJ, Popma JJ, Muller DW, Burek KA, Topol EJ. In-hospital costs associated with new percutaneous coronary devices. Am J Cardiol 1991; **68**: 879–85.

20. Van der Giessen WJ, Serruys PW, van Beusekom HMM, et al. Coronary stenting with a new, radiopaque, balloon-expandable endoprosthesis in pigs. Circulation 1991; **83**: 1788–98.

21. Rensing BJ, Hermans WR, Beatt KJ, et al. Quantitative angiographic assessment of elastic recoil after percutaneous transluminal coronary angioplasty. Am J Cardiol 1990; **66**: 1039–44.

22. Shaknovich A, Teirstein PS, Stratienko AA, Walker CM, Cleman MW, Schatz RA. Re-

stenosis in single Palmaz-Schatz coronary stents: effects of prior PTCA and interval to prior PTCA. J Am Coll Cardiol 1991; **17** (2 Suppl A): 269A (Abstract).

23. Marco J, Fajadet J, Cassagncau B, Laurent JP, Robert G. Balloon expandable intracoronary stents: immediate and mean term results in a serie of 122 consecutive patients. Eur Heart J 1990; **11**: (Abstract Suppl): 371 (Abstract).

24. Holmes DR Jr, Schwartz RS, Webster MW. Coronary restenosis: what have we learned from angiography? J Am Coll Cardiol 1991; **17** (6 Suppl B): 14B–22B.

37. Coronary Gianturco-Roubin stents

ADAM D. CANNON and GARY S. ROUBIN

Summary

Coronary revascularization using percutaneous techniques is evolving rapidly as new techniques develop. Despite these recent innovations, acute vessel closure following the procedure, and then restenosis, continue to limit its effectiveness.

The Gianturco-Roubin stent was developed in an attempt to improve the intraluminal results of angioplasty and thereby prevent or control acute vessel closure. Further, by providing an optimal luminal result, the incidence of restenosis my be reduced.

In this chapter, we will briefly describe the early development of this device and then provide detailed technical instruction on the effective deployment of the stent into the coronary artery, based on our experience with over 250 patients. Finally, we will provide some preliminary results from the Cook multicenter database in addition to details of acute success and early follow-up from the experience at the University of Alabama Hospital.

Introduction

The concept of using an intra-arterial prosthetic device to improve the patency of atherosclerotic vessels was first conceived in 1969, by Charles Dotter with the transluminal coil spring tube graft he developed [1]. The device was not widely accepted, and it was not until 1977 when Andreas Gruentzig showed one could safely dilate coronary artery stenoses percutaneously that the impetus for the development of intra-arterial stenting was revived [2].

Following Gruentzig's lead, the technique of balloon angioplasty spread rapidly as a treatment for coronary artery disease. Over the next twelve years, the technique was applied to more and more complex coronary anatomy as operator experience and equipment developed. Currently, the interventional cardiologist has at his disposal, in addition to the balloon, various laser and atherectomy devices for reducing and removing coronary stenoses. Despite

J.H.C. Reiber and P.W. Serruys (eds), Advances in Quantitative Coronary Arteriography, 609–624.
© 1993 Kluwer Academic Publishers. Printed in the Netherlands.

these technological innovations, the effectiveness of coronary angioplasty is limited by two major problems: those of acute closure and restenosis. Acute closure complicates from 2 to 11% of all angioplasties [3–5], accounting for virtually all the major ischemic complications [death, myocardial infarction and coronary artery bypass grafting (CABG) [6, 7]. Restenosis occurs in 30 to 40% of cases [8–10]. Stenting, by controlling the dissection flaps and optimizing the final luminal result with its scaffolding effect, should theoretically reduce both the consequences of acute closure and the incidence of chronic restenosis, for it is well documented that the final angiographic appearance after angioplasty is a significant determinant of both acute and long-term results [11–13] (Figure 1).

The initial work on this balloon-expandable flexible coil stent was done by Cesare Gianturco, a Houston radiologist, beginning in 1981 with the aim of using the stent in peripheral vessels. Difficulties with deployment caused virtual abandonment of the project until further modifications were made by Gianturco and Roubin in 1985, creating an incomplete serpentine, clam shell like coil for application to coronary arteries.

The stent

This balloon-expandable flexible coil stent (Cook Inc., Bloomington, Indiana) is made of mono-filamentous surgical stainless steel suture wire, 0.006" in diameter. The wire is wrapped in a serpentine manner around a compliant polyvinylchloride (PVC) balloon catheter so that every 360° the wire makes a 180° turn (Figure 2). This results in a series of inter-digitating U and inverted U shaped loops, and allows the coil to be expanded in a "clam shell" manner as the balloon inflates. The design also allows expansion without significant shortening of the stent. The coil undergoes some elastic recoil after expansion to the order of 15 to 20% so that the expanding balloon is $\frac{1}{2}$ mm greater in diameter than the nominal stent size. For example, a 3.0 mm diameter stent is deployed using a 3.5 mm diameter balloon, with the compliant balloon material reaching nominal size at 5 atmospheres of pressure. The stent is marked on the balloon by proximal and distal radio-opaque markers positioned approximately 1 mm from either end of the coils. Currently, the stent is manufactured in a 12 and a 20 mm length, mounted on 20 and 30 mm long balloons, respectively.

Company data (Cook Inc.) show that the stent covers from 9 to 17% of the arterial surface area, and from 1 to 4% of the lumen's cross-sectional area allowing adequate free-wall area for branch vessels and adequate luminal area for blood flow.

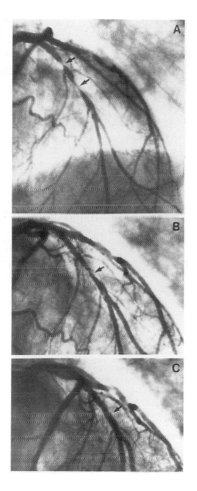

Figure 1. A: RAO angiogram of the LAD showing 2 sequential stenoses in the mid vessel of 80%. B: Post PTCA, showing resolution of the proximal lesion but failure of PTCA to dilate the distal lesion (arrow). There is a residual stenosis of 70%. C: RAO view post stenting showing resolution of the distal stenosis.

Early development

The earliest work concerning the technical utility of this stent prototype was carried out in the coronary arteries of dogs using the femoral artery approach. Results confirmed ease of deployment and long-term patency [14]. Studies using light and scanning electron microscopy were also performed [15]. These revealed that at two to four days the stent wires were embedded into the vessel wall and covered with platelets, red cells and a layer of fibrin. By four days, endothelialization of the wires had begun and was confluent by fourteen

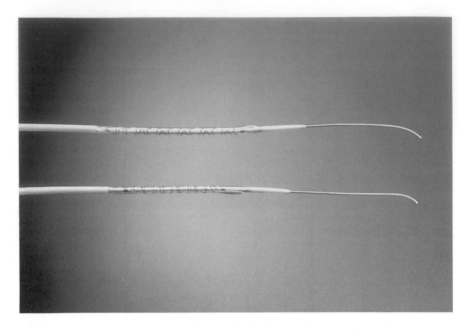

Figure 2. The stent is shown here mounted on the balloon catheter, before inflation. There is an 0.018″ guide wire protruding from the distal tip of the balloon. Note the inter-digitating U and inverse U configuration of the stent wires.

days. At six months, normal-appearing flow-directed endothelium had appeared.

Further studies in atherosclerotic rabbits and swine confirmed the dog findings and also showed that the stent could substantially improve the luminal appearance of dissected vessels [16].

Initial studies in humans were performed in a Phase I study, where the stent was used as a bailout device in the setting of acute closure complicating percutaneous transluminal coronary angioplasty (PTCA) with all patients then going on to CABG. In patients who had a stent placed, none had a Q-wave myocardial infarction, and all left the hospital within eight days [17]. These results led to FDA approval for ongoing studies using the stent to treat acute and threatened closure after PTCA.

Technique of deployment

The Gianturco-Roubin flexible coil stent is deployed into the coronary artery mounted on a standard 0.018″ wire-compatible balloon angioplasty catheter system. While the deployment techniques used are similar to standard over-the-wire PTCA, a number of significant modifications are required. These

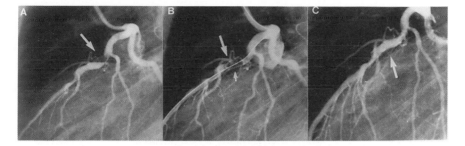

Figure 3. A: LAO cranial view of the LAD showing 2 sequential stenoses (arrows). The severe bend in the 1st stenosis characterizes this as a complex "C" lesion. Note the tapering distal LAD. B: Post PTCA, after repeat inflations, showing a severe dissection between the lesions (arrow) and a narrow perfusion channel (small arrow). There is reduced flow in the 1st septal perforator. C: Final result after placement of a 3.5, 20 mm stent. Due to the tapering of the vessel, the stent was deployed at 5 ATM and then the balloon withdrawn proximally and inflated to higher pressure to further enlarge the proximal stent.

modifications are related to the relative bulk of the stent balloon device compared to current low-profile catheter systems. Although a reasonably trackable device, particularly compared to other stent prototypes, added guide catheter and wire support facilitates deployment.

Consideration of the need for stenting should occur at the initial evaluation of the patient's angiogram before PTCA. The probability of acute or threatened closure can be determined by the appearance of a lesion before PTCA [4, 18] (Figure 3). However, as all experienced angioplasty practitioners know, even a Class A lesion (American Heart Association/American College of Cardiology Classification [19]) can be dilated with an appropriately sized balloon at relatively low pressure and produce a severe dissection; such are the vagaries of angioplasty in atherosclerotic vessels (Figure 4). Our approach is to select a guide catheter, guide wire and balloon system that will allow stenting of a vessel with a minimum of risk should it become necessary.

The standard guide catheter used in our cardiac catheterization laboratory is an 8 French size with a large lumen having an internal diameter of at least .078". This will allow easy tracking of a 2.0, 2.5 and 3.0 mm stent, and provide adequate visualization of the coronary artery. If there is a high-risk lesion in a 3.5 mm or larger vessel, typically a vein graft or large right coronary artery, we will select a large lumen 9 French guide to allow passage of a 3.5 or 4.0 mm stent.

Usually, well-fitting left and right Judkins catheters are used as our standard guides. The left Judkins is frequently the short tipped model, which allows careful deep intubation of the left coronary artery, if necessary for added support. In cases where extra support is necessary, such as in tortuous right and circumflex arteries, then left Amplatz shapes are sometimes used.

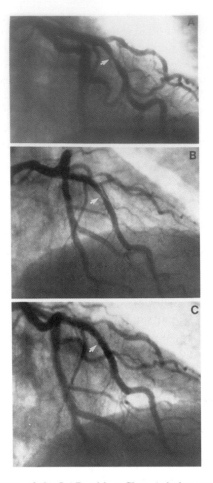

Figure 4. A: RAO angiogram of the LAD with a Class A lesion producing a 70% stenosis (arrow). B: LAD post PTCA with a residual stenosis of 60% and a significant local dissection (arrow). C: LAD after placement of a single 3.0 × 20 mm stent (arrow). There is complete control of the dissection and no residual stenosis.

For angioplasty of vein grafts, a left Amplatz would be used for left-sided conduits, and usually a multi-purpose guide for right coronary artery grafts.

Although it is possible to exchange guide catheters using a guide wire extension system, or even to remove the guide wire and recross the lesion after changing to a more supportive guide catheter, neither is ideal and the risk of not being able to recross a dissected lesion, or worse, to precipitate acute vessel closure, makes appropriate guide catheter choice important at the outset of a PTCA procedure.

Our routine is to use a 0.016″ or 0.018″ flexible tip guide wire for most

PTCA, and certainly in cases where stent deployment could be required. Balloon catheters suitable for use with 0.018" guide wires are routinely used.

It is possible to deploy the stent over standard 0.016" and 0.018" guide wires, and even over a 0.014" wire in a relatively straight segment of artery. However, the use of the 0.018" extra support guide wire (ACS, Santa Barbara, California) docs facilitate deployment. By acting to straighten the vessel, it enhances trackability of the stent. Further, by positioning the wire tip in the vessel as distally as possible, the stiff proximal wire is across the lesion, further easing deployment. These extra support wires are not as steerable as other 0.016" and 0.018" wires, and are therefore not used to initially cross the lesions. When a decision is made to place a stent for acute or threatened closure, the balloon catheter is placed across the lesion so that the tip is well distal to any dissection flap. Then, the current wire is removed and a high support wire substituted. The wire is then extended, and the balloon catheter removed. The stent balloon apparatus is then carefully placed through the Touhy-Borhst adapter ensuring no damage to the stent coils. It is possible to place up to a 3.0 mm stent through a standard adapter; however, our practice is to routinely use large lumen adapters (USCI, Billerica, Massachusetts) to avoid stent damage at this point. The manufacturer also includes a wide bore adapter and introducing sheath in the stent balloon package (Figure 5). Before threading the stent balloon catheter into the guide wire it is also our practice to soften the distal tip of catheter between the thumb and forefinger to aid tracking of the device through the coronary artery (Figure 6). The stent balloon is then advanced to the distal tip of the guiding catheter. Before passing the stent into the vessel, it is important to have pre-dilated any proximal lesions that may impede deployment and tracking of a stent into the desired location. At this point, it is also essential to ensure that the position of the guide catheter in the coronary ostia is optimal and will provide adequate support. It is particularly useful in the right coronary artery to apply clockwise rotation to the guide catheter, thereby coaxially aligning the catheter with the proximal vessel, ensuring sound and stable support. The stent can be advanced into the coronary artery with one operator controlling the guide catheter and advancing the stent balloon catheter, and the assistant maintaining gentle traction on the guide wire. Using this technique, the stent is usually deployed without difficulty, even into a distal and tortuous vessel. We routinely give bolus doses of intracoronary nitroglycerin 200 micrograms (mcgm) before passing the stent into the vessel, and repeat again after deployment, blood pressure permitting. Finally, before balloon inflation, a biplane cine-angiogram is taken to ensure accurate stent placements, as this stainless steel prototype can be difficult to visualize with fluoroscopy alone. This is very important because once balloon inflation has occurred, it is not possible to reposition the stent. Also, local experience has taught us that maximal coverage of any dissection flap is necessary to minimize the incidence of later stent thrombosis. Residual uncovered dissection after stent deployment being a significant risk factor for

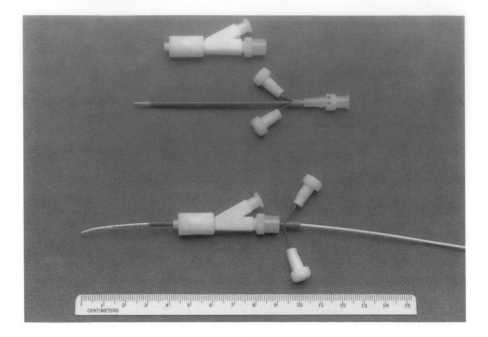

Figure 5. From top to bottom: (a) the large lumen Cook Touhy-Borhst adapter. (b) The peel away stent introducing sheath assembly. (c) A stent balloon inserted into the adapter through the introducing sheath.

this complication [20] (Figure 7). For very long dissections, the first stent deployed should cover the distal dissection, because attempting to deploy a second stent distally through a proximal stent is frequently difficult, and associated with the danger of damaging one or both stents (Figure 8).

The balloon is then inflated to deploy the stent, 5 to 6 atmospheres of pressure being adequate to fully expand the stent to its nominal size. If the stent is in any way undersized compared to the vessel, then taking the balloon to higher pressure will allow up to $\frac{1}{2}$ mm of enlargement at 9 atmospheres of pressure. When inflating the balloon over 5 atmospheres, care must be taken to ensure the vessel distal to the stent is not overdilated, as the stent balloon is $\frac{1}{2}$ mm larger than the stent at this pressure and it protrudes several mm each end of the stent coils. With high pressure this compliant balloon will further enlarge exacerbating distal balloon artery mismatch. This potential problem can be avoided by withdrawing the balloon several mm into the stented arterial segment before inflating to higher pressures. This technique is particularly useful if doing PTCA in a tapering vessel (Figure 3). Early in our experience, this was not fully appreciated and several vessels developed distal dissection. It is recommended that the stent be sized 1:1 with the artery into which it is placed. If the vessel appears a little larger than a nominated

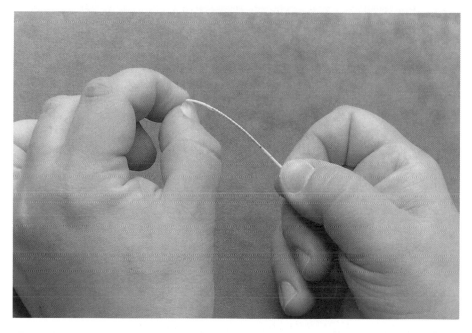

Figure 6. A PTCA operator shows the technique for softening the distal balloon catheter tip. Note the operator's hands are clear of the stent coils.

stent size, for example 3.2 mm, we would suggest using a 3.5 mm stent but deploying the stent at as low a pressure as possible, usually 5 atmospheres. If the post-stent angiogram reveals residual stenosis within the stent, further inflations are recommended to optimize the result. Finally, the balloon catheter is removed after allowing adequate time for full deflation.

On occasions when the stent balloon has been passed into the coronary but satisfactory positioning is not possible, removal is relatively straightforward provided the balloon has not been inflated. Simply, the balloon stent apparatus is withdrawn to the tip of the guide catheter with the proximal end of the stent outside the guide lumen. Then, the guide, stent balloon and wire are withdrawn as one through the femoral sheath. To date, this maneuver has been completely successful without stent displacement. It is important not to attempt to withdraw the stent through the guiding catheter since dislodgement of the stent at the tip of the guiding catheter may occur.

Medical treatment of the stented patient (Table 1)

As the need for stent placement is unpredictable, all of our patients are treated pre-procedure with soluble aspirin 325 mg the night before and the

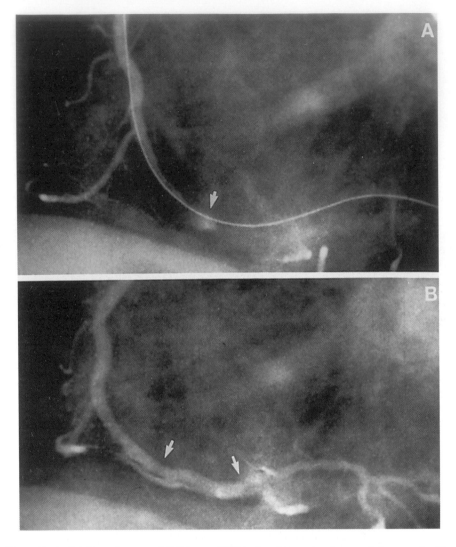

Figure 7. A: LAO angiogram of RCA post-PTCA showing acute closure of the vessel with extra luminal staining of dye (arrow). B: Post-stenting, showing residual dissection (arrows) proximally and distally. This vessel closed distal to the stent at the site of the residual dissection. It could not be opened with PTCA and required CABG.

morning of the procedure, and then daily. In addition, all receive dipyridamole 75 mg three times daily beginning the night before. All patients receive 10,000 units of heparin intra-arterially at the onset of the procedure, and then supplemental bolus doses with the aim of keeping their activated clotting time (ACT) greater than 300 seconds (Hemotech Inc., Colorado. High-range assay). Once a decision to stent is made, they receive a 150 cc bolus of

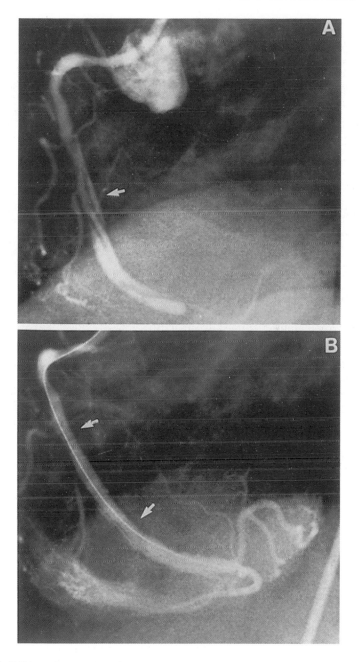

Figure 8. A: RCA angiogram showing a severe spiral dissection extending into the distal vessel with TIMI grade I flow into the posterolateral artery and no flow into the posterior descending artery. B: RCA after placement of 2, 3.0 × 20 mm stents with restoration of flow into the distal branches. The distal stent was placed first. There is some residual dissection marked by the distal arrow. This is well covered by the distal stent and the patient had an uncomplicated post-PTCA course.

Table 1. UAB medical therapy protocol for intracoronary stenting

Pre-Stent/PTCA

ASA 325 mg soluble (>2 doses before PTCA).
Dipyridamole 75 mg tid.
Calcium channel blocker.

During PTCA/Stenting

Heparin 10,000 units IA then supplements to keep ACT > 300 seconds.
Nitroglycerin intracoronary (200 microgram (mcgm) doses).
Dextran 150-200 cc stat then 50 cc/hr.
Methylprednisolone 250 mg IV before Dextran.

Post-Stenting

Heparin IV restarted once sheaths removed (7 units/lb.) No bolus. Aim for PTT of 55–75.
Dextran 40/10%. 50 cc/hr. until heparin recommenced and therapeutic.
Nitroglycerin IV for 12 hours.
Warfarin 10 mg po post procedure then daily. Aim for PT of 17-20 seconds.

intravenous dextran 40, 10% solution with 250 mg of methylprednisolone intravenously. The dextran then continues at an infusion rate of 50 cc's per hour until the sheaths are removed, and the heparin infusion is again therapeutic with a partial thromboplastin time (PTT) of between 55 and 75 seconds. In addition, intravenous nitroglycerin is infused for at least twelve hours post-procedure to counter any tendency to coronary artery spasm in the stented vessels. Heparin is continued for four days and longer if needed, until warfarin therapy is established with a prothrombin time (PT) of 17 to 20 seconds. All patients receive daily calcium channel blockers, aspirin, dipyridamole and warfarin for two months following stenting.

Results

Data from the Cook multi-center registry accumulated from August 1988 to September 1990 show that 95.4% of 306 patients had successful stent deployment. The vessel stenosis was reduced from a mean of 85.9% to 64.2% after angioplasty, and then to 13.9% after placement of a stent. The angiographic assessment was done visually, using hand held digital calipers. Our own data at the University of Alabama Hospital showed 132 of 137 stents (97%) were deployed for acute and threatened closure in a period up to June 1991, producing similar angiographic outcome [21].

The principal reasons for failure of deployment include diffuse proximal atherosclerosis and extreme tortuosity, and in two patients failure occurred when stenting was attempted through an already deployed proximal stent.

Although failure to deploy stent is not common, deployment does not always salvage a badly dissected vessel. In eight patients in our series, stenting

Table 2.

Ischemic Events	UAB Hospital [21]	Multicenter Registry	NHLBI Report [6] 1985–1986
Death (%)	1.7	1.7	5
Total MI (%)	11.2	5.2	40
Total CABG (%) (in hospital)	4.2	6.2	40

failed to produce satisfactory angiographic results, defined as a less than 50% residual stenosis, normal flow and resolution of ischemia. Of these, three had no sequelae, three had non Q-wave myocardial infarction, one patient required coronary artery bypass grafting emergently and there was one death. Thus, while stenting will usually preserve vessel patency, it is not a panacea and other options such as coronary artery bypass grafting must be available.

The incidence of in-hospital major ischemic events (death, Q-wave myocardial infarction and CABG) were low in the registry patients. Emergency CABG was needed in 3.1%, and elective CABG prior to hospital discharge in 3.1%. In this series of patients with acute or threatened closure due to dissection, 6.2% of patients had in-hospital CABG following stenting. The mortality was 1.7%, and 3.1% suffered a Q-wave myocardial infarction with a further 2.1% having non Q-wave infarction. These figures compare favorably with the incidence of in-hospital events in patients with perioprocedural occlusion in the 1985 to 1986 NHLBI registry [6]. In that series, 40% required CABG, mortality was 5% and 40% had a myocardial infarction. Table 2 compares these results and those from our own experience here at the University of Alabama [21].

If we compare six month cumulative events in these two groups, the Cook stent registry patients had a 16% incidence of CABG, a 4% mortality and 6.8% incidence of myocardial infarction compared to 46%, 7% and 42%, respectively, for the NHLBI registry patients.

Metallic stents have two important limitations. These are early stent thrombosis and bleeding complications, usually from the vascular access site. In the Cook registry, only 7.2% of patients had early stent thrombosis in the first month. In our experience, nine patients (7.6%) had this complication in-hospital, and this increased by one to a total of ten (8.5%) in the first month. All but one had their vessel reopened by PTCA. The remaining patient required CABG. Three patients had no sequelae, and six had myocardial infarction (3 Q-wave). Thus, although stent thrombosis was not frequent and was almost always successfully treated with repeat PTCA, it did underlie many of the major ischemic complications of stenting.

Bleeding complications, usually from the femoral vascular access site, were common in the early stages of the registry, occurring in 25% of patients.

However, with modification of the anticoagulation regime and a slower ambulation program post-procedure, the incidence has been reduced to 14%.

Our institutional experience found a significant effect of local learning experience on both these complications. Experience with stent deployment in dissections, the importance of covering distal dissection and familiarity with the anticoagulation regimen and graded ambulation all combined to reduce the incidence of these two complications as our experience grew [20]. The partial thromboplastin time must be critically controlled between 55 and 75 seconds. Excessive anticoagulation is not necessary and predisposes to bleeding problems. Adequate antiplatelet therapy is also critical. Most importantly, patients should undergo 2 to 3 days of bed rest after stenting to avoid femoral bleeding problems.

Currently at the University of Alabama, we have angiographic follow-up available in 81 patients who received Gianturco-Roubin stents in 82 arteries. Overall, restenosis has occurred in 34 of 82 arteries (41%). In 19, the restenosis developed within 3 months of stenting, and in the remainder was detected at the 6 month follow-up angiogram. Analysis of this experience found that restenosis is strongly related to local geometric factors. Stent diameter ≤ 2.5 mm and a stent-to-artery ratio of ≤ 0.9 were both significant predictors of restenosis within the stent with p-values of <0.05. In 37 patients who had a 2.5 mm or less diameter stent deployed restenosis occurred in 19 (51%). This compared to restenosis in 5 of 23 patients (22%) having a 3.0 mm or larger stent. Further, if the stent-to-artery ratio was less than 0.9 mm (28 patients), restenosis occurred in 15 (54%), whereas when this ratio was greater than 0.9, the incidence of restenosis was 24% (7 of 29 patients).

Redilatation within the stenosed segment of artery is relatively straightforward and may be associated with less risk than PTCA in native vessels. In our experience of 37 PTCAs within the stent, the mean stenosis was reduced from 75% to 18%. Only one patient suffered an ischemic complication when an embolus from a saphenous vein graft lesion produced myocardial infarction [22].

Conclusion

The Gianturco-Roubin balloon-expandable stent is a relatively flexible device, and can be deployed into the mid and distal coronary arteries through moderate tortuosity without great difficulty by experienced angioplasty operators. It functions to optimize the geometric result in the arterial lumen by scaffolding the arterial wall against recoil and supporting dissection flaps. It allows control of acute and threatened vessel closure after PTCA in the great majority of patients, and maintains luminal patency and blood flow. Further, it may help reduce the incidence of restenosis by maximizing the reduction in luminal stenosis produced by PTCA. The results appear superior to conventional management of perioprocedural occlusion as reported in the NHLBI registry [6].

The development of a tantalum prototype will enhance visualization, and facilitate deployment. Future developments with polymer coatings and the potential to bond therapeutic agents to target thrombosis and restenosis hold promise for even greater utility of this stent with a lower incidence of complications.

References

1. Dotter CT. Transluminal placed coil spring endarterial tube grafts – long term patency in canine popliteal artery. Invest Radiol 1969; **4**: 329–32.
2. Gruentzig AR, Senning A, Siegenthaler WE. Nonoperative dilatation of coronary artery stenosis: percutaneous transluminal coronary angioplasty. N Engl J Med 1979; **301**: 61–8.
3. Detre K, Holubkov R, Kelsey S, et al. Percutaneous transluminal coronary angioplasty in 1985–1986 and 1977–1981. The National Heart, Lung, and Blood Institute Registry. N Engl J Med 1988; **318**: 265–70.
4. Ellis SG, Vandormael MG, Cowley MJ, et al. Coronary morphologic and clinical determinants of procedural outcome with angioplasty for multivessel coronary disease. Implications for patient selection. Multivessel Angioplasty Prognosis Study Group. Circulation 1990; **82**: 1193–202. Comment in: Circulation 1990; **82**: 1516–8.
5. Simpfendorfer C, Belardi J, Bellamy G, Galan K, Franco I, Hollman J. Frequency, management and follow-up of patients with acute coronary occlusions after percutaneous transluminal coronary angioplasty. Am J Cardiol 1987; **59**: 267–9.
6. Detre KM, Holmes DR Jr, Holubkov R, et al. Incidence and consequences of peri-procedural occlusion: The 1985–1986 National Heart, Blood, and Lung Institute Percutaneous Transluminal Coronary Angioplasty Registry Circulation 1990; **82**: 739 50. Comment in: Circulation 1990; **82**: 1039–43.
7. Bredlau CE, Roubin GS, Leimgruber PP, Douglas JS Jr, King SB 3d, Gruentzig AR. In-hospital morbidity and mortality in patients undergoing elective coronary angioplasty. Circulation 1985; **72**: 1044–52.
8. Leimgruber PP, Roubin GS, Hollman J, et al. Restenosis after successful coronary angioplasty in patients with single vessel disease. Circulation 1986; **73**: 710–7.
9. Roubin GS, King SB 3d, Douglas JS Jr. Restenosis after percutaneous coronary angioplasty – Emory University Hospital experience. Am J Cardiol 1987; **60**: 39B–43B.
10. Gruentzig AR, King SB 3d, Schlumpf M, Siegenthaler W. Long-term follow-up after percutaneous transluminal coronary angioplasty. The early Zurich experience. N Engl J Med 1987; **316**: 1127–32.
11. Black AJR, Namay DL, Niederman AL, Lembo NJ, Roubin GS, Douglas JS Jr, King SB 3d. Tear or dissection after coronary angioplasty. Morphologic correlates of an ischemic complication. Circulation 1989; **79**: 1035–42.
12. Sinclair IN, McCabe CH, Sipperly ME, Baim DS. Abrupt reclosure: predictors, therapeutic options, and long-term outcome. J Am Coll Cardiol 1988; **11** (2 Suppl A): 132A (Abstract).
13. Ellis SG, Roubin GS, King SB 3d, et al. Angiographic and clinical predictors of acute closure after native vessel coronary angioplasty. Circulation 1988; **77**: 372–9.
14. Roubin GS, Robinson KA, King SB 3d, et al. Early and late results of intracoronary arterial stenting after coronary angioplasty in dogs. Circulation 1987; **76**: 891–7.
15. Robinson KA, Roubin GS, Apkarian RP, Black AJ, King SB 3d. Short term effects of intracoronary stenting in the canine: a descriptive scanning electron microscope analysis. Circulation 1987; **76** (4 Suppl IV): IV–26 (Abstract).

16. Robinson KA, Roubin GS, Siegel RJ, Black AJ, Apkarian RP, King SB 3d. Intra-arterial stenting in the atherosclerotic rabbit. Circulation 1988; **78**: 646–53.
17. Roubin GS, Douglas JS Jr, Lembo NJ, Black AJ, King SB 3d. Intracoronary stenting for acute closure following percutaneous transluminal coronary angioplasty (PTCA). Circulation 1988; **78** (Suppl II): II–407 (Abstract).
18. Ischinger T, Gruentzig AR, Meier B, Galan K. Coronary dissection and total coronary occlusion associated with percutaneous transluminal coronary angioplasty: significance of initial angiographic morphology of coronary stenosis. Circulation 1986; **74**: 1371–8.
19. Guidelines for Percutaneous Transluminal Coronary Angioplasty. A report of the American College of Cardiology/American Heart Association Task Force on Assessment of Diagnostic and Therapeutic Cardiovascular Procedures (Subcommittee on Percutaneous Transluminal Coronary Angioplasty). J Am Coll Cardiol 1988; **12**: 529–45.
20. Roubin GS, Agrawal S, Dean LS, et al. What are the predictors of acute complications following coronary artery stenting? Single institutional experience. J Am Coll Cardiol 1991; **17** (2 Suppl A): 281A (Abstract).
21. Roubin GS, Cannon AD, Agrawal SK, et al. Intracoronary stenting for acute and threatened closure complicating percutaneous transluminal coronary angioplasty. Circulation (in press).
22. Macander PJ, Agrawal SK, Cannon AD, et al. Is PTCA within the stenotic coronary stent safer than routine angioplasty? Circulation 1991; **84** (4 Suppl II): II–198 (Abstract).

Index

J.H.C. Reiber and P.W. Serruys (eds), Advances in Quantitative Coronary Arteriography, 625–633.
© 1993 *Kluwer Academic Publishers. Printed in the Netherlands.*

Developments in Cardiovascular Medicine

1. Ch.T. Lancée (ed.): *Echocardiology.* 1979   ISBN 90-247-2209-8
2. J. Baan, A.C. Arntzenius and E.L. Yellin (eds.): *Cardiac Dynamics.* 1980
   ISBN 90-247-2212-8
3. H.J.Th. Thalen and C.C. Meere (eds.): *Fundamentals of Cardiac Pacing.* 1979
   ISBN 90-247-2245-4
4. H.E. Kulbertus and H.J.J. Wellens (eds.): *Sudden Death.* 1980   ISBN 90-247-2290-X
5. L.S. Dreifus and A.N. Brest (eds.): *Clinical Applications of Cardiovascular Drugs.*
   1980   ISBN 90-247-2295-0
6. M.P. Spencer and J.M. Reid: *Cerebrovascular Evaluation with Doppler Ultrasound.*
   With contributions by E.C. Brockenbrough, R.S. Reneman, G.I. Thomas and D.L.
   Davis. 1981   ISBN 90-247-2384-1
7. D.P. Zipes, J.C. Bailey and V. Elharrar (eds.): *The Slow Inward Current and Cardiac
   Arrhythmias.* 1980   ISBN 90-247-2380-9
8. H. Kesteloot and J.V. Joossens (eds.): *Epidemiology of Arterial Blood Pressure.* 1980
   ISBN 90-247-2386-8
9. F.J.Th. Wackers (ed.): *Thallium-201 and Technetium-99m-Pyrophosphate. Myocardial Imaging in the Coronary Care Unit.* 1980   ISBN 90-247-2396-5
10. A. Maseri, C. Marchesi, S. Chierchia and M.G. Trivella (eds.): *Coronary Care Units.*
    Proceedings of a European Seminar (1978). 1981   ISBN 90-247-2456-2
11. J. Morganroth, E.N. Moore, L.S. Dreifus and E.L. Michelson (eds.): *The Evaluation of
    New Antiarrhythmic Drugs.* Proceedings of the First Symposium on New Drugs and
    Devices, held in Philadelphia, Pa., U.S.A. (1980). 1981   ISBN 90-247-2474-0
12. P. Alboni: *Intraventricular Conduction Disturbances.* 1981   ISBN 90-247-2483-X
13. H. Rijsterborgh (ed.): *Echocardiology.* 1981   ISBN 90-247-2491-0
14. G.S. Wagner (ed.): *Myocardial Infarction.* Measurement and Intervention. 1982
    ISBN 90-247-2513-5
15. R.S. Meltzer and J. Roelandt (eds.): *Contrast Echocardiography.* 1982
    ISBN 90-247-2531-3
16. A. Amery, R. Fagard, P. Lijnen and J. Staessen (eds.): *Hypertensive Cardiovascular
    Disease.* Pathophysiology and Treatment. 1982   IBSN 90-247-2534-8
17. L.N. 'Bouman and H.J. Jongsma (eds.): *Cardiac Rate and Rhythm.* Physiological,
    Morphological and Developmental Aspects. 1982   ISBN 90-247-2626-3
18. J. Morganroth and E.N. Moore (eds.): *The Evaluation of Beta Blocker and Calcium
    Antagonist Drugs.* Proceedings of the 2nd Symposium on New Drugs and Devices,
    held in Philadelphia, Pa., U.S.A. (1981). 1982   ISBN 90-247-2642-5
19. M.B. Rosenbaum and M.V. Elizari (eds.): *Frontiers of Cardiac Electrophysiology.*
    1983   ISBN 90-247-2663-8
20. J. Roelandt and P.G. Hugenholtz (eds.): *Long-term Ambulatory Electrocardiography.*
    1982   ISBN 90-247-2664-6
21. A.A.J. Adgey (ed.): *Acute Phase of Ischemic Heart Disease and Myocardial Infarc-
    tion.* 1982   ISBN 90-247-2675-1
22. P. Hanrath, W. Bleifeld and J. Souquet (eds.): *Cardiovascular Diagnosis by Ultra-
    sound.* Transesophageal, Computerized, Contrast, Doppler Echocardiography. 1982
    ISBN 90-247-2692-1
23. J. Roelandt (ed.): *The Practice of M-Mode and Two-dimensional Echocardiography.*
    1983   ISBN 90-247-2745-6
24. J. Meyer, P. Schweizer and R. Erbel (eds.): *Advances in Noninvasive Cardiology.*
    Ultrasound, Computed Tomography, Radioisotopes, Digital Angiography. 1983
    ISBN 0-89838-576-8
25. J. Morganroth and E.N. Moore (eds.): *Sudden Cardiac Death and Congestive Heart
    Failure.* Diagnosis and Treatment. Proceedings of the 3rd Symposium on New Drugs
    and Devices, held in Philadelphia, Pa., U.S.A. (1982). 1983   ISBN 0-89838-580-6
26. H.M. Perry Jr. (ed.): *Lifelong Management of Hypertension.* 1983
    ISBN 0-89838-582-2
27. E.A. Jaffe (ed.): *Biology of Endothelial Cells.* 1984   ISBN 0-89838-587-3

28. B. Surawicz, C.P. Reddy and E.N. Prystowsky (eds.): *Tachycardias*. 1984
ISBN 0-89838-588-1
29. M.P. Spencer (ed.): *Cardiac Doppler Diagnosis*. Proceedings of a Symposium, held in Clearwater, Fla., U.S.A. (1983). 1983
ISBN 0-89838-591-1
30. H. Villarreal and M.P. Sambhi (eds.): *Topics in Pathophysiology of Hypertension*. 1984
ISBN 0-89838-595-4
31. F.H. Messerli (ed.): *Cardiovascular Disease in the Elderly*. 1984
Revised edition, 1988: see below under Volume 76
32. M.L. Simoons and J.H.C. Reiber (eds.): *Nuclear Imaging in Clinical Cardiology*. 1984
ISBN 0-89838-599-7
33. H.E.D.J. ter Keurs and J.J. Schipperheyn (eds.): *Cardiac Left Ventricular Hypertrophy*. 1983
ISBN 0-89838-612-8
34. N. Sperelakis (ed.): *Physiology and Pathology of the Heart*. 1984
Revised edition, 1988: see below under Volume 90
35. F.H. Messerli (ed.): *Kidney in Essential Hypertension*. Proceedings of a Course, held in New Orleans, La., U.S.A. (1983). 1984
ISBN 0-89838-616-0
36. M.P. Sambhi (ed.): *Fundamental Fault in Hypertension*. 1984   ISBN 0-89838-638-1
37. C. Marchesi (ed.): *Ambulatory Monitoring*. Cardiovascular System and Allied Applications. Proceedings of a Workshop, held in Pisa, Italy (1983). 1984
ISBN 0-89838-642-X
38. W. Kupper, R.N. MacAlpin and W. Bleifeld (eds.): *Coronary Tone in Ischemic Heart Disease*. 1984
ISBN 0-89838-646-2
39. N. Sperelakis and J.B. Caulfield (eds.): *Calcium Antagonists*. Mechanism of Action on Cardiac Muscle and Vascular Smooth Muscle. Proceedings of the 5th Annual Meeting of the American Section of the I.S.H.R., held in Hilton Head, S.C., U.S.A. (1983). 1984
ISBN 0-89838-655-1
40. Th. Godfraind, A.G. Herman and D. Wellens (eds.): *Calcium Entry Blockers in Cardiovascular and Cerebral Dysfunctions*. 1984
ISBN 0-89838-658-6
41. J. Morganroth and E.N. Moore (eds.): *Interventions in the Acute Phase of Myocardial Infarction*. Proceedings of the 4th Symposium on New Drugs and Devices, held in Philadelphia, Pa., U.S.A. (1983). 1984
ISBN 0-89838-659-4
42. F.L. Abel and W.H. Newman (eds.): *Functional Aspects of the Normal, Hypertrophied and Failing Heart*. Proceedings of the 5th Annual Meeting of the American Section of the I.S.H.R., held in Hilton Head, S.C., U.S.A. (1983). 1984
ISBN 0-89838-665-9
43. S. Sideman and R. Beyar (eds.): [3-D] *Simulation and Imaging of the Cardiac System*. State of the Heart. Proceedings of the International Henry Goldberg Workshop, held in Haifa, Israel (1984). 1985
ISBN 0-89838-687-X
44. E. van der Wall and K.I. Lie (eds.): *Recent Views on Hypertrophic Cardiomyopathy*. Proceedings of a Symposium, held in Groningen, The Netherlands (1984). 1985
ISBN 0-89838-694-2
45. R.E. Beamish, P.K. Singal and N.S. Dhalla (eds.), *Stress and Heart Disease*. Proceedings of a International Symposium, held in Winnipeg, Canada, 1984 (Vol. 1). 1985
ISBN 0-89838-709-4
46. R.E. Beamish, V. Panagia and N.S. Dhalla (eds.): *Pathogenesis of Stress-induced Heart Disease*. Proceedings of a International Symposium, held in Winnipeg, Canada, 1984 (Vol. 2). 1985
ISBN 0-89838-710-8
47. J. Morganroth and E.N. Moore (eds.): *Cardiac Arrhythmias*. New Therapeutic Drugs and Devices. Proceedings of the 5th Symposium on New Drugs and Devices, held in Philadelphia, Pa., U.S.A. (1984). 1985
ISBN 0-89838-716-7
48. P. Mathes (ed.): *Secondary Prevention in Coronary Artery Disease and Myocardial Infarction*. 1985
ISBN 0-89838-736-1
49. H.L. Stone and W.B. Weglicki (eds.): *Pathobiology of Cardiovascular Injury*. Proceedings of the 6th Annual Meeting of the American Section of the I.S.H.R., held in Oklahoma City, Okla., U.S.A. (1984). 1985
ISBN 0-89838-743-4

Developments in Cardiovascular Medicine

50. J. Meyer, R. Erbel and H.J. Rupprecht (eds.): *Improvement of Myocardial Perfusion.* Thrombolysis, Angioplasty, Bypass Surgery. Proceedings of a Symposium, held in Mainz, F.R.G. (1984). 1985   ISBN 0-89838-748-5
51. J.H.C. Reiber, P.W. Serruys and C.J. Slager (eds.): *Quantitative Coronary and Left Ventricular Cineangiography.* Methodology and Clinical Applications. 1986
                                                                                  ISBN 0-89838-760-4
52. R.H. Fagard and I.E. Bekaert (eds.): *Sports Cardiology.* Exercise in Health and Cardiovascular Disease. Proceedings from an International Conference, held in Knokke, Belgium (1985). 1986   ISBN 0-89838-782-5
53. J.H.C. Reiber and P.W. Serruys (eds.): *State of the Art in Quantitative Cornary Arteriography.* 1986   ISBN 0-89838-804-X
54. J. Roelandt (ed.): *Color Doppler Flow Imaging and Other Advances in Doppler Echocardiography.* 1986   ISBN 0-89838-806-6
55. E.E. van der Wall (ed.): *Noninvasive Imaging of Cardiac Metabolism.* Single Photon Scintigraphy, Position Emission Tomography and Nuclear Magnetic Resonance. 1987
                                                                                  ISBN 0-89838-812-0
56. J. Liebman, R. Plonsey and Y. Rudy (eds.): *Pediatric and Fundamental Electrocardiography.* 1987   ISBN 0-89838-815-5
57. H.H. Hilger, V. Hombach and W.J. Rashkind (eds.), *Invasive Cardiovascular Therapy.* Proceedings of an International Symposium, held in Cologne, F.R.G. (1985). 1987   ISBN 0-89838-818-X
58. P.W. Serruys and G.T. Meester (eds.): *Coronary Angioplasty.* A Controlled Model for Ischemia. 1986   ISBN 0-89838-819-8
59. J.E. Tooke and L.H. Smaje (eds.): *Clinical Investigation of the Microcirculation.* Proceedings of an International Meeting, held in London, U.K. (1985). 1987
                                                                                  ISBN 0-89838-833-3
60. R.Th. van Dam and A. van Oosterom (eds.): *Electrocardiographic Body Surface Mapping.* Proceedings of the 3rd International Symposium on B.S.M., held in Nijmegen, The Netherlands (1985). 1986   ISBN 0-89838-834-1
61. M.P. Spencer (ed.): *Ultrasonic Diagnosis of Cerebrovascular Disease.* Doppler Techniques and Pulse Echo Imaging. 1987   ISBN 0-89838-836-8
62. M.J. Legato (ed.): *The Stressed Heart.* 1987   ISBN 0-89838-849-X
63. M.E. Safar (ed.): *Arterial and Venous Systems in Essential Hypertension.* With Assistance of G.M. London, A.Ch. Simon and Y.A. Weiss. 1987
                                                                                  ISBN 0-89838-857-0
64. J. Roelandt (ed.): *Digital Techniques in Echocardiography.* 1987
                                                                                  ISBN 0-89838-861-9
65. N.S. Dhalla, P.K. Singal and R.E. Beamish (eds.): *Pathology of Heart Disease.* Proceedings of the 8th Annual Meeting of the American Section of the I.S.H.R., held in Winnipeg, Canada, 1986 (Vol. 1). 1987   ISBN 0-89838-864-3
66. N.S. Dhalla, G.N. Pierce and R.E. Beamish (eds.): *Heart Function and Metabolism.* Proceedings of the 8th Annual Meeting of the American Section of the I.S.H.R., held in Winnipeg, Canada, 1986 (Vol. 2). 1987   ISBN 0-89838-865-1
67. N.S. Dhalla, I.R. Innes and R.E. Beamish (eds.): *Myocardial Ischemia.* Proceedings of a Satellite Symposium of the 30th International Physiological Congress, held in Winnipeg, Canada (1986). 1987   ISBN 0-89838-866-X
68. R.E. Beamish, V. Panagia and N.S. Dhalla (eds.): *Pharmacological Aspects of Heart Disease.* Proceedings of an International Symposium, held in Winnipeg, Canada (1986). 1987   ISBN 0-89838-867-8
69. H.E.D.J. ter Keurs and J.V. Tyberg (eds.): *Mechanics of the Circulation.* Proceedings of a Satellite Symposium of the 30th International Physiological Congress, held in Banff, Alberta, Canada (1986). 1987   ISBN 0-89838-870-8
70. S. Sideman and R. Beyar (eds.): *Activation, Metabolism and Perfusion of the Heart.* Simulation and Experimental Models. Proceedings of the 3rd Henry Goldberg Workshop, held in Piscataway, N.J., U.S.A. (1986). 1987   ISBN 0-89838-871-6

Developments in Cardiovascular Medicine

71. E. Aliot and R. Lazzara (eds.): *Ventricular Tachycardias.* From Mechanism to Therapy. 1987   ISBN 0-89838-881-3
72. A. Schneeweiss and G. Schettler: *Cardiovascular Drug Therapoy in the Elderly.* 1988
                                                                    ISBN 0-89838-883-X
73. J.V. Chapman and A. Sgalambro (eds.): *Basic Concepts in Doppler Echocardiography.* Methods of Clinical Applications based on a Multi-modality Doppler Approach. 1987   ISBN 0-89838-888-0
74. S. Chien, J. Dormandy, E. Ernst and A. Matrai (eds.): *Clinical Hemorheology.* Applications in Cardiovascular and Hematological Disease, Diabetes, Surgery and Gynecology. 1987   ISBN 0-89838-807-4
75. J. Morganroth and E.N. Moore (eds.): *Congestive Heart Failure.* Proceedings of the 7th Annual Symposium on New Drugs and Devices, held in Philadelphia, Pa., U.S.A. (1986). 1987   ISBN 0-89838-955-0
76. F.H. Messerli (ed.): *Cardiovascular Disease in the Elderly.* 2nd ed. 1988
                                                                    ISBN 0-89838-962-3
77. P.H. Heintzen and J.H. Bürsch (eds.): *Progress in Digital Angiocardiography.* 1988
                                                                    ISBN 0-89838-965-8
78. M.M. Scheinman (ed.): *Catheter Ablation of Cardiac Arrhythmias.* Basic Bioelectrical Effects and Clinical Indications. 1988   ISBN 0-89838-967-4
79. J.A.E. Spaan, A.V.G. Bruschke and A.C. Gittenberger-De Groot (eds.): *Coronary Circulation.* From Basic Mechanisms to Clinical Implications. 1987
                                                                    ISBN 0-89838-978-X
80. C. Visser, G. Kan and R.S. Meltzer (eds.): *Echocardiography in Coronary Artery Disease.* 1988   ISBN 0-89838-979-8
81. A. Bayés de Luna, A. Betriu and G. Permanyer (eds.): *Therapeutics in Cardiology.* 1988   ISBN 0-89838-981-X
82. D.M. Mirvis (ed.): *Body Surface Electrocardiographic Mapping.* 1988
                                                                    ISBN 0-89838-983-6
83. M.A. Konstam and J.M. Isner (eds.): *The Right Ventricle.* 1988   ISBN 0-89838-987-9
84. C.T. Kappagoda and P.V. Greenwood (eds.): *Long-term Management of Patients after Myocardial Infarction.* 1988   ISBN 0-89838-352-8
85. W.H. Gaasch and H.J. Levine (eds.): *Chronic Aortic Regurgitation.* 1988
                                                                    ISBN 0-89838-364-1
86. P.K. Singal (ed.): *Oxygen Radicals in the Pathophysiology of Heart Disease.* 1988
                                                                    ISBN 0-89838-375-7
87. J.H.C. Reiber and P.W. Serruys (eds.): *New Developments in Quantitative Coronary Arteriography.* 1988   ISBN 0-89838-377-3
88. J. Morganroth and E.N. Moore (eds.): *Silent Myocardial Ischemia.* Proceedings of the 8th Annual Symposium on New Drugs and Devices (1987). 1988
                                                                    ISBN 0-89838-380-3
89. H.E.D.J. ter Keurs and M.I.M. Noble (eds.): *Starling's Law of the Heart Revisted.* 1988   ISBN 0-89838-382-X
90. N. Sperelakis (ed.): *Physiology and Pathophysiology of the Heart.* (Rev. ed.) 1988
                                                                    ISBN 0-89838-388-9
91. J.W. de Jong (ed.): *Myocardial Energy Metabolism.* 1988   ISBN 0-89838-394-3
92. V. Hombach, H.H. Hilger and H.L. Kennedy (eds.): *Electrocardiography and Cardiac Drug Therapy.* Proceedings of an International Symposium, held in Cologne, F.R.G. (1987). 1988   ISBN 0-89838-395-1
93. H. Iwata, J.B. Lombardini and T. Segawa (eds.): *Taurine and the Heart.* 1988
                                                                    ISBN 0-89838-396-X
94. M.R. Rosen and Y. Palti (eds.): *Lethal Arrhythmias Resulting from Myocardial Ischemia and Infarction.* Proceedings of the 2nd Rappaport Symposium, held in Haifa, Israel (1988). 1988   ISBN 0-89838-401-X
95. M. Iwase and I. Sotobata: *Clinical Echocardiography.* With a Foreword by M.P. Spencer. 1989   ISBN 0-7923-0004-1

Developments in Cardiovascular Medicine

96. I. Cikes (ed.): *Echocardiography in Cardiac Interventions.* 1989
                                                    ISBN 0-7923-0088-2
97. E. Rapaport (ed.): *Early Interventions in Acute Myocardial Infarction.* 1989
                                                    ISBN 0-7923-0175-7
98. M.E. Safar and F. Fouad-Tarazi (eds.): *The Heart in Hypertension.* A Tribute to
    Robert C. Tarazi (1925-1986). 1989   ISBN 0-7923-0197-8
99. S. Meerbaum and R. Meltzer (eds.): *Myocardial Contrast Two-dimensional Echocar-
    diography.* 1989   ISBN 0-7923-0205-2
100. J. Morganroth and E.N. Moore (eds.): *Risk/Benefit Analysis for the Use and Approval
    of Thrombolytic, Antiarrhythmic, and Hypolipidemic Agents.* Proceedings of the 9th
    Annual Symposium on New Drugs and Devices (1988). 1989   ISBN 0-7923-0294-X
101. P.W. Serruys, R. Simon and K.J. Beatt (eds.): *PTCA - An Investigational Tool and a
    Non-operative Treatment of Acute Ischemia.* 1990   ISBN 0-7923-0346-6
102. I.S. Anand, P.I. Wahi and N.S. Dhalla (eds.): *Pathophysiology and Pharmacology of
    Heart Disease.* 1989   ISBN 0-7923-0367-9
103. G.S. Abela (ed.): *Lasers in Cardiovascular Medicine and Surgery.* Fundamentals and
    Technique. 1990   ISBN 0-7923-0440-3
104. H.M. Piper (ed.): *Pathophysiology of Severe Ischemic Myocardial Injury.* 1990
                                                    ISBN 0-7923-0459-4
105. S.M. Teague (ed.): *Stress Doppler Echocardiography.* 1990   ISBN 0-7923-0499-3
106. P.R. Saxena, D.I. Wallis, W. Wouters and P. Bevan (eds.): *Cardiovascular Pharmacol-
    ogy of 5-Hydroxytryptamine.* Prospective Therapeutic Applications. 1990 ·
                                                    ISBN 0-7923-0502-7
107. A.P. Shepherd and P.A. Öberg (eds.): *Laser-Doppler Blood Flowmetry.* 1990
                                                    ISBN 0-7923-0508-6
108. J. Soler-Soler, G. Permanyer-Miralda and J. Sagristà-Sauleda (eds.): *Pericardial
    Disease.* New Insights and Old Dilemmas. 1990   ISBN 0-7923-0510-8
109. J.P.M. Hamer: *Practical Echocardiography in the Adult.* With Doppler and Color-
    Doppler Flow Imaging. 1990   ISBN 0-7923-0670-8
110. A. Bayés de Luna, P. Brugada, J. Cosin Aguilar and F. Navarro Lopez (eds.): *Sudden
    Cardiac Death.* 1991   ISBN 0-7923-0716-X
111. E. Andries and R. Stroobandt (eds.): *Hemodynamics in Daily Practice.* 1991
                                                    ISBN 0-7923-0725-9
112. J. Morganroth and E.N. Moore (eds.): *Use and Approval of Antihypertensive Agents
    and Surrogate Endpoints for the Approval of Drugs affecting Antiarrhythmic Heart
    Failure and Hypolipidemia.* Proceedings of the 10th Annual Symposium on New
    Drugs and Devices (1989). 1990   ISBN 0-7923-0756-9
113. S. Iliceto, P. Rizzon and J.R.T.C. Roelandt (eds.): *Ultrasound in Coronary Artery
    Disease.* Present Role and Future Perspectives. 1990   ISBN 0-7923-0784-4
114. J.V. Chapman and G.R. Sutherland (eds.): *The Noninvasive Evaluation of
    Hemodynamics in Congenital Heart Disease.* Doppler Ultrasound Applications in the
    Adult and Pediatric Patient with Congenital Heart Disease. 1990
                                                    ISBN 0-7923-0836-0
115. G.T. Meester and F. Pinciroli (eds.): *Databases for Cardiology.* 1991
                                                    ISBN 0-7923-0886-7
116. B. Korecky and N.S. Dhalla (eds.): *Subcellular Basis of Contractile Failure.* 1990
                                                    ISBN 0-7923-0890-5
117. J.H.C. Reiber and P.W. Serruys (eds.): *Quantitative Coronary Arteriography.* 1991
                                                    ISBN 0-7923-0913-8
118. E. van der Wall and A. de Roos (eds.): *Magnetic Resonance Imaging in Coronary
    Artery Disease.* 1991   ISBN 0-7923-0940-5
119. V. Hombach, M. Kochs and A.J. Camm (eds.): *Interventional Techniques in
    Cardiovascular Medicine.* 1991   ISBN 0-7923-0956-1
120. R. Vos: *Drugs Looking for Diseases.* Innovative Drug Research and the Development
    of the Beta Blockers and the Calcium Antagonists. 1991   ISBN 0-7923-0968-5

Developments in Cardiovascular Medicine

121. S. Sideman, R. Beyar and A.G. Kleber (eds.): *Cardiac Electrophysiology, Circulation, and Transport.* Proceedings of the 7th Henry Goldberg Workshop (Berne, Switzerland, 1990). 1991   ISBN 0-7923-1145-0
122. D.M. Bers: *Excitation-Contraction Coupling and Cardiac Contractile Force.* 1991   ISBN 0-7923-1186-8
123. A.-M. Salmasi and A.N. Nicolaides (eds.): *Occult Atherosclerotic Disease.* Diagnosis, Assessment and Management. 1991   ISBN 0-7923-1188-4
124. J.A.E. Spaan: *Coronary Blood Flow.* Mechanics, Distribution, and Control. 1991   ISBN 0-7923-1210-4
125. R.W. Stout (ed.): *Diabetes and Atherosclerosis.* 1991   ISBN 0-7923-1310-0
126. A.G. Herman (ed.): *Antithrombotics.* Pathophysiological Rationale for Pharmacological Interventions. 1991   ISBN 0-7923-1413-1
127. N.H.J. Pijls: *Maximal Myocardial Perfusion as a Measure of the Functional Significance of Coronary Arteriogram.* From a Pathoanatomic to a Pathophysiologic Interpretation of the Coronary Arteriogram. 1991   ISBN 0-7923-1430-1
128. J.H.C. Reiber and E.E. v.d. Wall (eds.): *Cardiovascular Nuclear Medicine and MRI.* Quantitation and Clinical Applications. 1992   ISBN 0-7923-1467-0
129. E. Andries, P. Brugada and R. Stroobrandt (eds.): *How to Face 'the Faces' of Cardiac Pacing.* 1992   ISBN 0-7923-1528-6
130. M. Nagano, S. Mochizuki and N.S. Dhalla (eds.): *Cardiovascular Disease in Diabetes.* 1992   ISBN 0-7923-1554-5
131. P.W. Serruys, B.H. Strauss and S.B. King III (eds.): *Restenosis after Intervention with New Mechanical Devices.* 1992   ISBN 0-7923-1555-3
132. P.J. Winter (ed.): *Quality of Life after Open Heart Surgery.* 1992   ISBN 0-7923-1580-4
133. E.E. van der Wall, H. Sochor, A. Righetti and M.G. Niemeyer (eds.): *What's new in Cardiac Imaging?* SPECT, PET and MRI. 1992   ISBN 0-7923-1615-0
134. P. Hanrath, R. Uebis and W. Krebs (eds.): *Cardiovascular Imaging by Ultrasound.* 1992   ISBN 0-7923-1755-6
135. F.H. Messerli (ed.): *Cardiovascular Disease in the Elderly.* 3rd ed. 1992   ISBN 0-7923-1859-5
136. J. Hess and G.R. Sutherland (eds.): *Congenital Heart Disease in Adolescents and Adults.* 1992   ISBN 0-7923-1862-5
137. J.H.C. Reiber and P.W. Serruys (eds.): *Advances in Quantitative Coronary Arteriography.* 1993   ISBN 0-7923-1863-3
138. A.-M. Salmasi and A.S. Iskandrian (eds.): *Cardiac Output and Regional Flow in Health and Disease.* 1993 (forthcoming)   ISBN 0-7923-1911-7
139. J.H. Kingma, N.M. van Hemel and K.I. Lie (eds.): *Atrial Fibrillation, a Treatable Disease?* 1992   ISBN 0-7923-2008-5
140. B. Ostadel and N.S. Dhalla (eds.): *Heart Function in Health and Disease.* Proceedings of the Cardiovascular Program (Prague, Czechoslovaki, 1991). 1992   ISBN 0-7923-2052-2

Previous volumes are still available

KLUWER ACADEMIC PUBLISHERS – DORDRECHT / BOSTON / LONDON